Modelling Natural Action Selection

Action selection is a fundamental problem in biology and ecology. It requires determining available alternatives, executing those most appropriate, and resolving conflicts among competing goals and possibilities.

Using advanced computational modelling, this book explores cutting-edge research into action selection in nature from a wide range of disciplines, from neuroscience to behavioural ecology, and even to political science. It delivers new insights into both detailed and systems-level attributes of natural intelligence and demonstrates advances in methodological practice. Contributions from leading researchers cover issues including whether biological action selection is optimal, neural substrates for action selection in the vertebrate brain, perceptual selection in decision making, and interactions between group and individual action selection.

This major integrated review of action selection in nature contains a balance of review and original research material, consolidating current knowledge into a valuable reference for researchers, while illustrating potential paths for future studies.

Anil K. Seth is a Reader in the School of Informatics at the University of Sussex, an EPSRC Leadership Fellow, and Co-Director of the Sackler Centre for Consciousness Science. His research crosses the fields of computational neuroscience, consciousness science, and neurorobotics. In addition to contributing new insights into the mechanisms of action selection, he has developed new ways to link brain activity to conscious experience and he is well known for his research on the statistical analysis of causality.

Tony J. Prescott is Professor of Cognitive Neuroscience at the University of Sheffield where he teaches courses on computational neuroscience and biomimetic robotics. His research lies within the biological and brain sciences, and concerns understanding the evolution, development, and function of natural intelligence. He is particularly well known for his work on modelling the neural substrates for action selection, and building robot models of animal and human behaviour.

Joanna J. Bryson is a Reader in the Department of Computer Science at the University of Bath. She conducts interdisciplinary research on the origins, structure, and construction of human and animal-like intelligence, and is involved in topics ranging from the evolution of altruistic communication to the ethical role of robots in our society. She is recognised for her work in systems AI and the design of action selection. Her most recent work is centred on the application of modelling to understanding the evolution of human social structures and culturally derived behaviour more generally.

Modelling Natural Action Selection

Edited by

ANIL K. SETH
University of Sussex

TONY J. PRESCOTT
University of Sheffield

JOANNA J. BRYSON
University of Bath

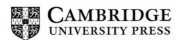

CAMBRIDGE UNIVERSITY PRESS
Cambridge, New York, Melbourne, Madrid, Cape Town,
Singapore, São Paulo, Delhi, Tokyo, Mexico City

Cambridge University Press
The Edinburgh Building, Cambridge CB2 8RU, UK

Published in the United States of America by Cambridge University Press, New York

www.cambridge.org
Information on this title: www.cambridge.org/9781107000490

First published 2012

Printed in the United Kingdom at the University Press, Cambridge

A catalogue record for this publication is available from the British Library

Library of Congress Cataloguing in Publication data
Modelling natural action selection / edited by Anil K. Seth, Tony J. Prescott, Joanna J. Bryson.
   p.   cm.
Includes bibliographical references and index.
ISBN 978-1-107-00049-0
1. Cognitive neuroscience.   2. Neurobiology – Computer simulation.   3. Decision making – Computer
simulation.   I. Seth, Anil K.   II. Prescott, Tony J.   III. Bryson, Joanna J.   IV. Title.
QP360.5.M63   2011
612.8′233 – dc23   2011027497

ISBN 978-1-107-00049-0 Hardback

Contents

Colour plates are to be found between pp. 240 and 241.

Foreword

The sea pen leads a simple life. After floating on the deep-sea currents as a juvenile, it settles down onto a comfortable patch of sand and begins its largely immobile adult life, growing into a feathery shape and swaying in the water while ensnaring whatever edible morsels pass its way. It hardly moves on its own; it just passively filters the world that goes by. No choices need be made, for there are no actions to take. As such, the sea pen will not feature prominently in this book.

For other more active (and more behaviourally interesting) species, life presents a stream of decision points, at which actions must be chosen: stay or move on, ingest or pass by, approach or avoid, wait or strike, court/accept or decline. These are all essentially forms of the exploitation/exploration trade-off that organisms must balance throughout their lives, whenever resources are distributed in space or time and the individual can actively seek them. This is the realm of natural action selection. How do organisms do it?

Action selection mechanisms are decision mechanisms. Like the study of decision mechanisms used for making inferences – a common topic in research on (human) judgement and decision making – the study of action selection mechanisms aims to uncover what the mechanisms are that people and other animals use, how they work, and when and where they work well or do not work – that is, the conditions under which they do or do not produce adaptive (or rational) behaviour. Research on human inference has revealed that there are multiple decision mechanisms that people can use in particular situations – the mind's *adaptive toolbox* – and often several of these can produce similar outcomes. The chapters in this book reveal the range of possible action selection mechanisms that can be used as well. Some of the simple heuristics that have been identified for human inference show that decisions can be made without fully comparing different alternatives on multiple incommensurate dimensions (e.g., by ignoring conflicting dimensions and just deciding on the basis of one factor); some of the models in this book show similar shortcuts or rules of thumb that can work in action selection. One difference between standard decision-making research and that on natural action selection is that, in the former, the possible alternatives that can be selected in an inference task are generally known or specified by the researcher, e.g., which city is larger, Detroit or Milwaukee? The possible actions that an animal might take in nature may not always be explicitly identified and, without knowing precisely the range of possibilities, studying the mechanisms that select among them becomes more difficult.

In the human inference literature, the study of the contents of the adaptive toolbox has led to a further question beyond asking how people choose between alternatives in an inferential task: how do people choose what *mechanism* to use to make their inferences in a particular task? That is, how do people choose which tool to use from the adaptive toolbox? This is an open and challenging question, with different possible answers; sometimes the environment will determine the choice, depending on what types of information are available; other times, individuals may learn through experience or can be taught what decision mechanisms are good to employ in particular settings. If there are multiple competing action selection *mechanisms* in a given situation – not just multiple competing actions themselves – then this kind of meta-selection question will also be important in the study of natural action selection.

Specifying the action selection mechanisms that inhabit the mind's adaptive toolbox means specifying how they work – but how can this be determined? This is also a main theme of this book: exploring the methods that are being employed at the cutting edge of research for understanding the operation of action selection mechanisms. Experiments and field observations are necessary for generating data on action selection in action, but the data must be understood in terms of a theory. Here the theories are instantiated as models, which because they often operate at multiple levels – cognitive, neural, and social – are complex enough that they are best implemented as computer simulations. Ideally, multiple competing models then specify further data to be collected to distinguish between them, and the new data constrain the models (and the theoretical understanding) further, in an ongoing feedback loop. In this book we see multiple stages of that process, and the current state of understanding to which it has led.

This modelling approach can thus be characterised as 'understanding by building'. But once the action selection models have been built and understood, we can also use the models as a way to explore how to change things in important application areas. The applications, like the models, can be at different levels of description. At the neural level, important health implications emerge from understanding clinical conditions such as Parkinson's disease and obsessive–compulsive disorder as disruptions of action selection. And by better knowing how natural action selection works at this level, we can gain better understanding of what is going on when things go wrong – tweaking the models to achieve 'understanding by breaking' – and insights into possible ways of addressing those problems.

At the individual and social level, we may want to help people choose better courses of actions for themselves and others – avoiding the third piece of chocolate cake, or promoting the election of innovative leaders. Again by modelling and understanding the processes of action selection at these levels of description, we can develop, and test, ideas for how to change the action selection process in desired directions, before trying them out in the real world. These methods could involve giving people and groups new ways of selecting their actions – new tools for choosing what and when to eat, or new voting mechanisms, for instance – or could rely on changing the environmental cues that they receive, to 'nudge' people into making different selections. And modelling can help us determine which approach may be more effective, changing environments or changing minds or norms.

Hence, the work in this book is important. And it is incumbent on readers not just to passively filter and accept what is written here, but to actively choose to ingest or pass by, approach or avoid, accept or decline, and above all explore and exploit the ideas presented herein.

Peter M. Todd

Preface

Parts of this book were originally published as an issue of the *Philosophical Transactions of the Royal Society B: Biological Sciences* (Volume 362; Issue 1485) but have been modified and updated. Anil Seth's contribution to the book was supported by EPSRC Leadership Fellowship EP/G007543/1 and by a donation from the Dr Mortimer and Theresa Sackler Foundation. Tony Prescott's contribution was supported by the EU 7th Framework Programme via the projects BIOTACT (ICT-215910) and EFAA (ICT-270490). Joanna Bryson's effort was funded in part by the US Air Force Office of Scientific Research, Air Force Material Command, USAF, under grant number FA8655-10-1-3050.

Contributors

Yasushi Ando
Department of Computer Science, University of Bath, UK

Andrew G. Barto
Department of Computer Science, University of Massachusetts, Amherst, MA, USA

Max Berniker
Bayesian Behavior Lab, Rehabilitation Institute of Chicago, Northwestern University, Chicago, IL, USA

Rafal Bogacz
Department of Computer Science, University of Bristol, UK

Matthew M. Botvinick
Princeton Neuroscience Institute and Department of Psychology, Princeton University, NJ, USA

Joanna J. Bryson
Department of Computer Science, University of Bath, UK

Jonathan M. Chambers
Department of Psychology, University of Sheffield, UK

Paul Cisek
Department of Physiology, University of Montréal, QC, Canada

Guy Cowlishaw
Institute of Zoology, Zoological Society of London, London, UK

Frederick L. Crabbe
Computer Science Department, U.S. Naval Academy, Annapolis, MD, U.S.A.

Eddy J. Davelaar
Department of Psychological Sciences, Birkbeck College, University of London, UK

Anna Dornhaus
Department of Ecology and Evolutionary Biology, University of Arizona, Tucson, AZ, USA

Michael J. Frank
Departments of Psychology and Cognitive and Linguistic Sciences, Brown University, Providence, RI, USA

Nigel R. Franks
School of Biological Sciences, University of Bristol, UK

Kevin N. Gurney
Adaptive Behaviour Research Group, Department of Psychology, University of Sheffield, UK

Thomas E. Hazy
Department of Psychology, University of Colorado Boulder, Boulder, CO, USA

Russell A. Hill
Department of Anthropology, Durham University, UK

James C. Houk
Northwestern University Medical School, Chicago, IL, USA

Alasdair I. Houston
Centre for Behavioural Biology, University of Bristol, UK

Mark D. Humphries
Adaptive Behaviour Research Group, Department of Psychology, University of Sheffield, UK

Konrad Körding
Bayesian Behavior Lab, Rehabilitation Institute of Chicago, Northwestern University, Chicago, IL, USA

Tim Kovacs
Department of Computer Science, University of Bristol, UK

Michael Laver
Department of Politics, New York University, NY, USA

Hagen Lehmann
Department of Computer Science, University of Bath, UK

Brian S. Logan
School of Computer Science, University of Nottingham, UK

James A. R. Marshall
Department of Computer Science, University of Bristol, UK

James L. McClelland
Center for the Neural Bases of Cognition, Carnegie Mellon University, Pittsburgh, PA, USA

John M. McNamara
Centre for Behavioural Biology, University of Bristol, UK

Yael Niv
Princeton Neuroscience Institute and Department of Psychology, Princeton University, NJ, USA

Randall C. O'Reilly
Department of Psychology, University of Colorado Boulder, Boulder, CO, USA

Richard A. Pettifor
Institute of Zoology, Zoological Society of London, London, UK

Robert Planqué
Department of Mathematics, VU University Amsterdam, The Netherlands

Tony J. Prescott
Adaptive Behaviour Research Group, Department of Psychology, University of Sheffield, UK

Sean A. Rands
Centre for Behavioural Biology, University of Bristol, UK

J. Marcus Rowcliffe
Institute of Zoology, Zoological Society of London, London, UK

Anouk Scheres
Department of Psychology, University of Arizona, Tucson, AZ, USA

Michel Schilperoord
Complex and Adaptive Systems Laboratory, University College Dublin, Ireland

William I. Sellers
Faculty of Life Sciences, University of Manchester, UK

Ernest Sergenti
Department of Politics, New York University, NY, USA

Anil K. Seth
Sackler Centre for Consciousness Science, and School of Informatics, University of Sussex, Brighton, UK

Scott J. Sherman
Department of Neurology, University of Arizona, Tucson, AZ, USA

Tom Stafford
Adaptive Behaviour Research Group, Department of Psychology, University of Sheffield, UK

Mark D. Steer
Centre for Behavioural Biology, University of Bristol, UK

Marius Usher
Department of Psychology, Birkbeck College, University of London, UK

Kunlin Wei
Bayesian Behavior Lab, Rehabilitation Institute of Chicago, Northwestern University, Chicago, IL, USA

Julian Zappala
School of Computer Science, University of Nottingham, UK

Jiaxiang Zhang
Department of Computer Science, University of Bristol, UK

1 General introduction

Anil K. Seth, Joanna J. Bryson, and Tony J. Prescott

Action selection is the task of deciding 'what to do next'. As a general problem facing all autonomous entities – animals and artificial agents – it has exercised both the sciences concerned with understanding the biological bases of behaviour (e.g., ethology, neurobiology, psychology) and those concerned with building artefacts (e.g., artificial intelligence, artificial life, and robotics). The problem has two parts: what constitutes an action, and how are actions selected?

This volume is dedicated to advancing our understanding of the behavioural patterns and neural substrates that support action selection in animals, including humans. Its chapters investigate a wide range of issues, including (1) whether biological action selection is optimal, and if so what is optimised; (2) the neural substrates for action selection in the vertebrate brain; (3) the role of perceptual selection in decision making, and (4) the interaction between group and individual decision making. The mechanisms of action selection considered in these contexts include abstract neural circuits (e.g., Bogacz *et al.*, this volume) through specific brain systems (e.g., Stafford and Gurney, this volume) to policy choices exercised by political parties (Laver *et al.*, this volume.) Taken together, this research has broad implications across the natural, social, medical, and computing sciences.

The second aim of the volume is to advance methodological practice, in particular, the practice of computational modelling. Although models cannot generate data about nature, they can generate data about theories. Complex theories can therefore be tested by comparing the outcome of simulation models against other theories in their ability to account for data drawn from nature. Models of 'natural action selection' attempt to account for transitions among different behavioural options, and a wide range of modelling methodologies are currently in use. Formal, mathematical models have been complemented with larger-scale simulations that allow investigation of systems for which analytical solutions are intractable or unknown. These include models of artificial animals (simulated agents or robots) embedded in simulated worlds (individual-based or agent-based models), as well as models of underlying neural control systems (computational neuroscience and connectionist approaches). Over recent years, work in a variety of disciplines has leveraged these and other modelling techniques, as well as analytical

Modelling Natural Action Selection, eds. Anil K. Seth, Tony J. Prescott and Joanna J. Bryson.
Published by Cambridge University Press. © Cambridge University Press 2012.

mathematics, to shed new light on the natural action selection. A comprehensive selection of this work is showcased in the present volume, work which explicitly addresses and integrates both parts of the action selection problem: the 'what' and the 'how'.

Because computational modelling is still a relatively new constituent of the scientific method, it is important to pinpoint exactly what the scientific contributions of computational models can be. For models of natural action selection, several general challenges can be identified: is the model sufficiently constrained by biological data that it captures interesting properties of the target natural system? Do manipulations of the model result in similar outcomes to those seen in nature? Does the model make predictions? Is there a simpler model that could account for the data equally well? Or is the model so abstract that its connection to data seems trivial? A potential pitfall of more detailed models is that they may trade biological fidelity with comprehensibility. The scientist is then left with two systems, one natural and the other artificial, neither of which is well understood. Hence, the best models are generally those that hit upon a good trade-off between accurately mimicking key properties of a target biological system, while at the same time remaining understandable to the extent that new insights into the natural world are generated.

This volume gathers together a remarkable selection of contributions from leading researchers that define the current and future landscape of modelling natural action selection. It has had a substantial gestation period. Back in 2005, we (the editors) convened a two-day meeting entitled 'Modelling Natural Action Selection' which was held at Edinburgh University and supported by the UK Biotechnology and Biological Sciences Research Council (BBSRC). The meeting attracted almost 100 participants, as well as the interest of the Royal Society, who subsequently commissioned a theme issue of their *Philosophical Transactions Series B* dedicated to the same topic, which appeared in 2007 (362:1485). The present volume updates and extends the contents of this theme issue, with the aim of providing a landmark reference in the field. Some of the chapters are revised versions of the corresponding journal papers, incorporating new results and enhanced cross-referencing. Other chapters are entirely new contributions, included in order to better reflect the changing research landscape.

The volume is divided into three sections. The first investigates the question of rational and/or optimal decision making. When an animal does one thing rather than another, it is natural to ask 'why?' A common explanation is that the action is optimal with respect to some goal. Assessing behaviour from a normative perspective has particular value when observations deviate from predictions, because we are forced to consider the origin of the apparently suboptimal behaviour. The seven chapters within this section address a wide variety of action selection problems from the perspective of optimality, and in doing so integrate a number of distinct modelling techniques including analytical optimisation, agent-based modelling combined with numerical optimisation, and Bayesian approaches.

The second section surveys a range of computational neuroscience models examining potential neural mechanisms underlying action selection. An important open question in this area is whether there are specialised neural mechanisms for action selection, or whether selective behaviour 'emerges' from the interactions among brain systems, bodies, and environments. If a dedicated neural mechanism does exist, then arguably it should exhibit the following properties: (1) it should receive inputs that signal internal and external cues relevant to decision making, (2) it should perform some calculation of urgency of salience appropriate to each action, (3) it should possess mechanisms enabling conflict resolution based on salience, and (4) it should generate outputs that allow expression of 'winning' actions while inhibiting losers. A focus of several chapters in this section is the notion that the vertebrate basal ganglia may implement a selection mechanism of this kind. Other chapters discuss alternative possibilities and related issues, including subcortical and brainstem mechanisms, hierarchical architectures, the integration of perception and action via 'affordance competition', feedback in the oculomotor system, and neural disorders of action selection.

The third and final section addresses the important topic of social action selection. In nature, action selection is rarely purely an individual matter; rather, adaptive action selection usually involves a social context. This context supplies a highly dynamic environment, in which the actions of others are generally tightly coupled to the action of the individual. Social action selection is prevalent in many species at many levels of organismal sophistication. Examples include the troop structure of primate species, nest selection by ant colonies, and patterns of voting in democratic societies. Models in this section address each of these topics and others, with a detailed focus on rigorous methodology.

In summary, the study of action selection integrates a broad range of topics including, but not limited to, neuroscience, psychology, ecology, ethology, and even political science. These domains have in common a complexity that benefits from advanced modelling techniques, exemplifying the notion of 'understanding by building'. These techniques can help answer many important questions such as: why animals, including humans, sometimes act irrationally; how damage to neural selection substrates can lead to debilitating neurological disorders; and how action selection by individuals impacts on the organisation of societies. The present volume is dedicated to presenting, integrating, and advancing research at these frontiers.

Acknowledgements

We wish to thank our editors at Cambridge University Press: Martin Griffiths and Lynette Talbot, as well as our authors and our reviewers. We are also very grateful to Dr Gillian Hayes for assistance with indexing and copyediting.

Part I

Rational and optimal decision making

2 Introduction to Part I: rational and optimal decision making

Anil K. Seth, Tony J. Prescott, and Joanna J. Bryson

When an animal does one thing rather than another, it is natural to ask 'why?' A common explanation is that the action is optimal with respect to some goal. For example, when observing the foraging behaviour of a shorebird, one may ask whether the intake of food is being maximised. This 'normative' view, a direct extension of Darwinian principles, has its more recent roots in behavioural ecology (Krebs and Davies, 1997) and optimal foraging theory (Stephens and Krebs, 1986). Adopting a normative perspective on action selection can be very useful in placing constraints on possible underlying mechanisms, for developing and comparing theoretical frameworks relating behaviour to mechanism, and for explaining instances of apparently irrational or suboptimal behaviour. The seven chapters within this section present new insights and modelling results relevant to each of these issues. They also connect with the other parts of this book in important ways. The constraints on underlying mechanisms are thoroughly explored by the computational neuroscience models described in Part II, and patterns of both rational and irrational social behaviour are encountered in a variety of forms in Part III.

2.1 Suboptimality and 'matching'

Assessing animal behaviour from a normative perspective has particular value when observations deviate from predictions, because the scientist is now forced to consider the origin of the apparently suboptimal – or 'irrational' – behaviour. In one important example, many animals behave according to Herrnstein's (1961) 'matching law', in which responses are allocated in proportion to the reward obtained from each response. However, as both Houston *et al.* (this volume) and Seth (this volume) note, matching is not always optimal. One response to this observation is to propose that suboptimal matching arises as a side-effect of some underlying principle of behaviour, such as Thorndike's 'law of effect', which proposes that behaviour shifts towards alternatives that have higher immediate value (Thorndike, 1911). Another is given by the notion of *ecological rationality* – that cognitive mechanisms fit the demands of particular ecological niches and may deliver predictably suboptimal behaviour when operating outside these niches (Gigerenzer *et al.*, 1999). In line with ecological rationality, Seth (this

Modelling Natural Action Selection, eds. Anil K. Seth, Tony J. Prescott and Joanna J. Bryson.
Published by Cambridge University Press. © Cambridge University Press 2012.

volume) shows that simple decision rules that lead to optimal foraging in competitive environments with multiple foragers also lead individual foragers to obey the matching law. The remainder of Seth's chapter describes a novel methodological approach that combines agent-based modelling and optimal/normative approaches via the use of genetic algorithms. The resulting approach, which is given the label 'optimal agent-based modelling', achieves the important task of integrating function and mechanism in explanations of action selection (McNamara and Houston, 2009).

As Houston *et al.* (this volume) discuss, a further possible explanation of apparent irrationality is that we were wrong about what is being optimised. As an example, they consider *violations of transitivity*, showing that such violations can in fact be optimal when decisions are state-dependent and when choice options persist into the future. Another axiom of standard rationality is *independence from irrelevant alternatives*, the notion that the relative preference of one option over another is unaffected by the inclusion of further options into the choice set. However, as Houston *et al.* show, adding a suboptimal option can affect future expectations because, assuming that decision-making errors happen, the suboptimal option is likely to be wrongly chosen in the future. Apparent violations of rationality in human decision making are also discussed by Bogacz *et al.* (this volume), whose contribution we discuss further below.

2.2   Compromise behaviour

A related way we can be mistaken about what is optimised is when behaviour reflects compromises among multiple goals. As Crabbe (this volume) explains, a *compromise action* is defined as an action that, while not necessarily best suited for satisfying any particular goal, may be the best when all (or several) goals are taken into account. For example, a predator stalking two birds might not move directly towards either one of the birds, but in-between the two, hedging its bets in case one of the birds elects to fly away. Crabbe provides a review of approaches to compromise behaviour in relevant literatures finding that, although the intuition that compromise is useful is widespread, data from empirical studies supporting this assertion is rather thin. Crabbe then presents some detailed models directly addressing the question of when compromise behaviour is optimal. The models are restricted to simple situations involving both prescriptive (e.g., food) and proscriptive (e.g., danger areas) goals, but both are spatially explicit and open to analytical characterisation. Perhaps surprisingly, Crabbe finds that compromise behaviour is usually of little benefit in the scenarios analysed. He suggests the interesting proposal that while this may be true for so-called 'low-level' compromise behaviour (e.g., motor actions), it may be less true for 'high-level' compromise, in which the compromise is among competing behaviours (e.g., get food, find shelter) that are less easily 'blended'.

2.3   Optimal perceptual selection

Action selection can be mediated not only by motor control systems but also by perceptual systems. For example, mechanisms of selective attention can guide action selection by linking a specific motor output to one stimulus among a range of stimuli (Posner, 1980). The issue of perceptual selection is raised by a number of chapters in this collection, including Bogacz *et al.* and Stafford and Gurney (see Part II). As an example, take the problem of detecting coherent motion in a cloud of otherwise randomly moving dots. A popular solution to this problem is provided by the *leaky competing accumulator* (LCA) model (Usher and McClelland, 2001), which proposes that during decision making, noisy evidence supporting each of a range of alternatives is accumulated. Importantly, under certain conditions the LCA model can be shown to be optimal (Usher and McClelland, 2001). Bogacz *et al.* (this volume) review various neural implementations of the LCA model from the perspective of optimality, and describe extensions to this work which show that nonlinear neuronal mechanisms can perform better than linear mechanisms in terms of speed of decision making between multiple alternatives. This result raises the interesting hypothesis that nonlinearities in neuronal response functions may have evolved at least in part as a result of selective pressures favouring rapid decision making.

Bogacz *et al.* next extend the LCA framework beyond perceptual selection to account for so-called 'value-based' decisions in which alternatives are compared on the basis of their match to a set of internal motivations as well as to sensory signals. They discuss two examples of apparent irrationality: *risk-aversion*, where humans and other animals prefer the less risky of two alternatives that are equated for expected value, and *preference reversal*, where the preference order between two alternatives can be reversed by the introduction of a third, irrelevant, choice option. They show that the LCA model can account for these phenomena given a nonlinear utility function which is applied to the difference in value between each alternative and a 'referent' which may correspond to the present (or expected) state of the decision maker.

An excellent example of the cross-fertilisation of modelling strategies is evident here. In Part III of this volume, Marshall and colleagues show how the LCA model can be applied to collective decision making by colonies of social insects, via direct competition between evidence accumulating populations. And in Part II, Stafford and Gurney use a similar principle (their 'diffusion' model) to account for behavioural responses in a Stroop paradigm, in which responses are either congruent or incongruent with inducing stimuli.

2.4 Bayesian approaches to action selection

Bayesian theory has become extremely prominent in theoretical biology and especially neuroscience, as a means of combining new sources of information (called 'likelihoods') with expectations or information about the past ('priors'). In the context of action selection, Bayesian decision theory describes how prior beliefs representing action outcomes should be combined with new knowledge (e.g., provided by a visual system) to best approach optimal outcomes as defined by a normative 'utility' function (Körding, 2007). Alternatively, by assuming optimal behaviour, one can use *inverse* Bayesian decision theory to identify the priors and likelihoods used by a decision-making agent. As these observations show, Bayesian decision theory is tightly integrated with normative perspectives on action selection.

In their chapter, Berniker *et al.* provide a comprehensive review of Bayesian approaches to modelling action selection, covering the fundamental issues of combining priors and likelihoods and combining multiple pieces of information. They then address the important problem of Bayesian estimation over time, in which the posterior probabilities from the past are taken to define priors for the future via Kalman filtering, with many applications in motor adaptation (Berniker and Körding, 2008). The problem of estimating environmental structure is then explored, and it is argued that such a process is an essential aspect of any action selection mechanism. Following a discussion of inverse decision theory, the chapter concludes with a discussion of Bayesian inference as a means for expressing optimal control strategies.

2.5   Sequential action selection

The final chapter in this section takes as a starting point the ubiquity of serial ordering in our daily lives. Davelaar notes that action selection mechanisms must convert simultaneously activated representations into a sequence of actions, in order to satisfy constraints of optimality. Instead of focusing on action sequences per se, Davelaar explores sequential memory retrieval, on the grounds that the wealth of modelling material in this domain can be usefully leveraged, and that there are likely to be domain-general mechanisms underlying sequential selection tasks. Davelaar compares two mechanisms: *competitive queuing* and *resampling*, finding that the latter provides a better overall match to empirical data. While both mechanisms create sequences from simultaneously activated representations, they differ in how inter-representation inhibition is applied. The success of the resampling model suggests general constraints on how multiple representations are organised for the expression of adaptive sequences. Moreover, the model is shown to account for deficits in memory selection performance in patients with Alzheimer's and Huntington's diseases.

References

Berniker, M. and K. Körding (2008). Estimating the sources of motor errors for adaptation and generalization. *Nat. Neurosci.* **11**(12): 1454–61.

Gigerenzer, G., P. Todd, and the ABC Research Group (1999). *Simple Heuristics that Make us Smart*. Cambridge: Cambridge University Press.

Herrnstein R. J. (1961). Relative and absolute strength of response as a function of frequency of reinforcement. *J. Exp. Anal. Behav.* **4**: 267–272.

Körding, K. (2007). Decision theory: what 'should' the nervous system do? *Science* **318**(5850): 606–10.

Krebs, J. and N. Davies (1997). *Behavioral Ecology: An Evolutionary Approach*. Oxford: Blackwell Publishers.

McNamara, J. M. and A. I. Houston (2009). Integrating function and mechanism. *Trends Ecol. Evol.* **24**(12): 670–5.

Posner, M. I. (1980). Orienting of attention. *Q. J. Exp. Psychol.* **32**(1): 3–25.

Stephens, D. and J. Krebs (1986). *Foraging Theory*. Princeton, NJ: Princeton University Press.

Thorndike, E. L. (1911). *Animal Intelligence*. New York: Macmillan.

Usher, M. and J. L. McClelland (2001). The time course of perceptual choice: the leaky, competing accumulator model. *Psychol. Rev.* **108**(3): 550–92.

3 Do we expect natural selection to produce rational behaviour?

Alasdair I. Houston, John M. McNamara, and Mark D. Steer

Summary

We expect that natural selection has resulted in behavioural rules that perform well, however, animals (including humans) sometimes make bad decisions. Researchers account for these with a variety of explanations; we concentrate on two of them. One is that the outcome is a side-effect; what matters is how a rule performs (in terms of reproductive success). Several rules may perform well in the environment in which they evolved, but their performance may differ in a 'new' environment (e.g., the lab). Some rules may perform very badly in this environment. We use the debate about whether animals follow the matching law rather than maximising their gains as an illustration. A second possibility is that we were wrong about what is optimal. The general idea here is that the setting in which optimal decisions are investigated is too simple and may not include elements that add extra degrees of freedom to the situation.

3.1 Introduction

The theme of this volume is modelling natural action selection. In this chapter we are concerned with modelling the action of natural selection. Selecting the best action when making a decision can be of great importance to an individual's fitness; we often term making the right choice as being 'rational'. Ultimately, however, decision-making processes are products of an individual's evolutionary history, influenced to a greater or lesser degree by natural selection. Here we are concerned with whether we should expect 'rational' behaviour to be a product of naturally selected systems. In a general sense, rationality involves thinking and behaving reasonably and logically, but the term holds different meanings for researchers in different intellectual fields. The meaning and implications of the term 'rationality' have been discussed at great length. We do not intend to try to review all of these here, but use the categorisations of Kacelnik (2006) as a guide (for further introductions to the debate, see Manktelow and Over, 1993; Moser, 1990; Wilson, 1974). The general area of evolution and rationality is vast and our coverage is highly selective; many issues have not been considered. For other topics

Modelling Natural Action Selection, eds. Anil K. Seth, Tony J. Prescott and Joanna J. Bryson.
Published by Cambridge University Press. © Cambridge University Press 2012.

and perspectives, see Bernardo and Welch (2001), Bogacz *et al.* (this volume), Bateson and Healy (2005), Binmore (1997), Cooper (2001), Dickson (2006, 2008), Kirkpatrick *et al.* (2006), Nozick (1993), Pothos and Busemeyer (2009), Rieskamp *et al.* (2006), Robson (2002; 2003), Shafir and Le Boeuf (2002), Sober (1981), Stein (1996), and Waldman (1994).

Kacelnik (2006) adeptly introduces and summarises three categorisations, representing the different disciplines for which rationality has been of central interest: philosophy and psychology (PP-rationality), economics (E-rationality), and behavioural ecology/evolutionary biology (B-rationality).

Psychologists have traditionally been more interested in the internal mechanisms of behavioural processes, rather than the behavioural outcomes per se. Rational behaviour is distinguished from irrational as a function of the process by which the behaviour became manifest, not by the behaviour itself (cf. Simon's (1978) procedural rationality). An important consequence is that PP-rationality is not understood in terms of observable behaviours, but in terms of internally consistent thoughts and beliefs (Kacelnik, 2006). As a result, it is difficult to carry out experimental analyses of PP-rationality, since it involves examination of the cognitive processes involved in producing behaviour. Human subjects can be questioned about their reasons for choosing particular courses of action, enabling a limited level of investigation into beliefs; such investigation is virtually impossible in the study of non-human behaviour (Kacelnik, 2006).

By contrast with PP-rationality, E-rationality is predominantly a goal-led concept, within certain bounds. The goal is the maximisation of expected utility. E-rationality can therefore be used to predict patterns of observable behaviour (Kacelnik, 2006). For studies of human rationality, utility is most often taken as financial gain, although there are some notable exceptions (e.g., Silberberg *et al.*, 1991); in non-humans utility is most often assumed to be linked to food acquisition, but could involve access to water, mates or conspecifics. However, the plasticity of utility as a term brings its own problems. A forager that seems to be failing to maximise the currency we assume to equal utility may not be behaving irrationally but maximising a different utility. As long as observed choices can be shown to maximise some form of utility, no matter how bizarre, then a decision maker can be classed as acting rationally.

The differences between PP-rationality and E-rationality are relatively straightforward. PP-rationality is a process-based concept dealing with predominantly internal beliefs and not their outcome. On the other hand, E-rationality considers the outcome as being of primary importance, in that utility should be maximised, the process by which this occurs is not taken as being of great interest. B-rationality, springing mainly from the evolutionary literature, has yet another approach.

Natural selection is expected to result in organisms that maximise fitness. This is the basis of B-rationality, also known as ecological rationality (Hutchinson and Gigerenzer, 2005; Stephens *et al.*, 2004; Todd and Gigerenzer, 2000), which can be thought of as a subset of E-rationality in that it replaces the general concept of utility by fitness, which is a more specific concept. An important difference between fitness and utility is that fitness functions can be measured, in terms of reproductive success, independently of the decisions an agent makes, whereas utility functions are derived from the decisions themselves and therefore are not independent of the choice procedure (Houston and Staddon, 1981; Kacelnik, 2006; Luce and Raiffa, 1957). The processes by which an animal reaches a decision are not of primary importance to B-rationality, again similar to E-rationality. However, there is an added caveat: B-rationality assumes that agents are products of naturally selected processes which have shaped the cognitive and emotional machinery of the decision maker to behave in a manner such as to maximise fitness. We cannot expect natural selection, having no foresight, to shape organisms to act rationally in all circumstances, but only in those circumstances which it encounters in its natural setting. Therefore B-rational behaviour (i.e., fitness-maximising behaviour) might not appear when animals are placed in a novel context. As an example take an anecdote concerning the ultimate father of B-rationality, Charles Darwin. Whilst on the Galapagos, Darwin noticed that a frightened marine iguana (*Amblyrhynchus cristatus*) could not be induced to enter the ocean by any means other than picking the animal up and tossing it into the waves (something he did a number of times to one unfortunate individual). He wrote 'perhaps this singular piece of apparent stupidity may be accounted for by the circumstance, that this reptile has no enemy whatever on shore, whereas at sea it must often fall a prey to the numerous sharks. Hence, probably urged by a fixed and hereditary instinct that the shore is its place of safety, whatever the emergency may be, it there takes its refuge.' (Darwin, 1839, Chapter 17). Only when the context of the decision changed with the appearance of a land-based agitator did the iguana's behaviour – heading for land given any danger – appear to be irrational. The general point is that simple rules (heuristics – Todd and Gigerenzer, 2000) can approximate the behaviour of a B-rational agent in natural circumstances, but may seem to be irrational in others (Houston, 2009a; McNamara and Houston, 1980).

To summarise, PP-rationality focuses on how decisions or beliefs are arrived at, but not necessarily on what the decisions or beliefs actually are. Conversely, the focal point of E-rationality is the decision itself, not the process by which it is achieved. E-rationality assumes that an agent will attempt to act in such a way as to maximise utility, utility being an undefined entity. B-rationality, similar to E-rationality, is also most concerned with the end point of a decision-making process, but assumes an animal will maximise fitness when in a relevant context (Kacelnik, 2006). From here on we concentrate on the interplay of E- and B-rationality.

The maximisation of utility means that E-rational preferences should obey a series of conditions including

1. Transitivity: in its simplest form this states that preferences are ordered, so if option *a* is preferred to option *b* and option *b* preferred to option *c* then *a* will be preferred to *c*, and
2. Independence from irrelevant alternatives (IIA; Arrow, 1951; Tversky and Simonson, 1993): the basic idea is that relative preference for one option over another is unaffected by adding or removing options from the choice set (see also Luce, 1959, 1977; Luce and Suppes, 1965).

If either of these conditions is violated, behaviour is classed as irrational. Studies in both biological and psychological literatures have argued that these conditions do not always hold in non-humans e.g., Bateson (2002), Bateson *et al.* (2002, 2003), Hurly and Oseen (1999), Navarick and Fantino (1972, 1974, 1975), Shafir (1994), Shafir *et al.* (2002), Waite (2001a, 2001b). (For work on humans, see Busemeyer and Townsend, 1993, and Shafir and Le Boeuf, 2002.)

A rigorous logician might argue that violations of the axioms of E-rationality can only mean one of two things: either that animals, including humans, cannot be rational or E-rationality cannot be a reasonable description of behaviour. In response it might be argued that E-rationality, on the whole, can provide a good account of behaviour, and the underlying assumptions are only violated in extreme circumstances. It is indeed true that economic concepts of rationality have proved to be effective and useful in predicting behaviour, but the recent boom in experimental economics (see, for example, Hey, 2002; Kahneman, 2003; Smith, 2003), which studies how economic agents actually behave without disregarding deviations from how they ought to behave, illustrates that it has not been totally successful (Hammerstein and Hagen, 2005; Kacelnik, 2006).

As we will show, existing models of choice may predict seemingly irrational behaviours in particular circumstances. Broadly speaking, models of choice are descriptive (they describe observed behaviour), or normative (they specify the behaviour that ought to be observed). Normative models are based on the evaluation of behaviour in terms of some measure (e.g., money or reproductive success). These approaches are linked in that, if rules have been shaped by natural selection, then rules that provide a good description should also make sense in terms of performance. In this chapter, we review examples of behaviour that at first sight does not conform to what we might expect from a rational decision maker. We also present new results on a decision principle known as the delay-reduction hypothesis and bring out general patterns in the behaviour of humans and other animals.

3.2 Descriptive models

The wealth of descriptive models that have been put forward is too great for us to review them all here. Instead, we focus on a few descriptive models from operant psychology that have been influential in the study of choice behaviour.

Matching

The matching law (Herrnstein, 1961, 1970) emerged as a description of how animals in the lab choose between options that provide food. The matching law states that, for two options, the ratio of responses that a decision maker makes on the options equals the ratio of rewards that it has previously received from the options, i.e.,

$$\frac{B_1}{B_2} = \frac{R_1}{R_2} \tag{3.1}$$

where R_i is the number of rewards previously received from option i and B_i is either the number of responses previously made or the amount of time previously spent responding on that option. R_i/B_i is the local rate from option i, so the matching law means that local rates are equal.

Baum (1974) gave the following generalisation of the matching law:

$$\frac{B_1}{B_2} = b \left(\frac{R_1}{R_2} \right)^s$$ (3.2)

where s and b are fitted parameters often referred to as sensitivity and bias, respectively. Houston and colleagues (Houston and McNamara, 1981; Houston and Sumida, 1987) caution that these parameters should be treated simply as fitted parameters since their relationship to actual choice mechanisms is not clear. If both s and $b = 1$ then Herrnstein's original formulation of the matching law ('basic matching') holds. The generalised matching law, however, effectively allows many behavioural patterns which deviate from Equation (3.1) to be explained by fitting the values of s and b to the data.

Since its inception the matching law, especially in its generalised form, has been a successful and popular tool for describing behaviour (e.g., McDowell, 1989; Myerson and Hale, 1984; Pierce and Epling, 1995; Spiga *et al.*, 2005). It has been used to explain behaviours as diverse as wagtail foraging (Houston, 1986a) and shot selection in basketball (Alferink *et al.*, 2009). The relationship between matching and the distribution of animals across habitats is analysed by Houston (2008). Matching and neurophysiology is discussed by, for example, Soltani and Wang (2006) and Sugrue *et al.* (2004). It is important, however, to note that basic matching (Equation (3.1)) may not uniquely specify behaviour; in some settings matching can be produced by a wide range of different behavioural allocations (Houston and McNamara, 1981).

Many studies of matching behaviour have investigated the behaviour of animals (including humans) on concurrent variable interval (VI) schedules. VI schedules are often used in experimental psychology to test choice behaviour. They supply a reward (or stimulus of some sort) following a subject's first response after a given, but variable, time delay has elapsed. For example, a pigeon might be confronted with an illuminated disc (or 'key') that it can peck. During an initial random delay (the variable interval) any pecks that the pigeon makes on the key are unrewarded. Once the delay has elapsed, however, the first peck that the pigeon makes on the key results in a reward being delivered (see Ferster and Skinner, 1957, for further information). If two VI schedules are available to a subject at any one time this is termed a concurrent VI–VI procedure.

Optimal foraging theory is a normative approach that attempts to explain behaviour in terms of the maximisation of fitness (see Stephens and Krebs, 1986 for a review). One simple assumption is that maximising the rate of energetic gain will maximise fitness. Several papers have discussed the relationship between the matching law and rate maximisation. It has been shown that maximising the rate of gain does not necessarily result in matching (e.g., Heyman and Herrnstein, 1986; Heyman and Luce, 1979; Houston, 1983; Houston and McNamara, 1981). Given that matching does not necessarily specify behaviour uniquely, it is not possible to say whether matching behaviour maximises rate of gain. On concurrent VI schedules an infinite number of behavioural allocations can satisfy matching. Some of these allocations will give rates that are close to optimal (Houston and McNamara, 1981). When faced with a VI schedule and a schedule that has a constant probability of giving a reward, matching results in a rate of reward that is well below the optimal rate (Heyman and Herrnstein, 1986; Houston, 1983). Behaviour on such schedules can be described by the generalised matching law (Heyman and Herrnstein, 1986).

VI schedules often use a negative exponential distribution of times between rewards. This means that whether a response is rewarded gives no information about the time until the next reward becomes available. The form of the best strategy when choosing between two such schedules is to repeat a cycle comprising a fixed time t1 on option 1 and a fixed time t2 on option 2 (Houston and McNamara, 1981). In other words, if the animal knows the parameters and is sure that they will not change, it should ignore rewards and get an accurate clock so that it can measure the optimal times t1 and t2. Houston and McNamara (1981) found an exact solution to the problem of maximising rate of gain given a choice between two VI schedules when the mean interval of each schedule is known (see also Belinsky *et al.*, 2004). This approach is not realistic. If we wish to understand the evolution of foraging behaviour we should be looking for rules that perform well under the range of conditions that an animal is likely to experience (cf. Seth, this volume). It should not be assumed that the animal has full knowledge of current conditions. Instead, the animal both learns about and exploits its environment. There are three general features of foraging environments that are relevant here.

1. Rewards may give information about future rewards. This possibility has been thoroughly investigated in the context of how long to stay in a patch that contains a random number of food items (e.g., Iwasa *et al.*, 1981; McNamara, 1982; McNamara and Houston, 1987c).
2. The environment may contain other foragers. A rule that works well for an isolated forager might not work well when that animal has to compete with others. Similarly a forager that utilises a rule that is successful in group situations might perform poorly when in isolation (Seth, 2001, 2006, this volume).
3. The environment may change. If a set of environmental parameters is constant then it is often possible to evolve fixed optimal behaviours. However, these behaviours will become suboptimal given any change in the environment (Dall *et al.*, 1999; McNamara, 1996; McNamara and Houston, 1985; 1987b).

To cope with these aspects of the real world, what is needed is an approach that is based on rules that use information based on rewards obtained to decide between options. A process called melioration uses previous information and results in outcomes that satisfy the matching law. The idea behind melioration is that an animal increases its allocation to the alternative that gives it the highest local rate. At the stable outcome with both options chosen local rates are equal, i.e., matching holds. This is really a framework rather than a detailed model; there are lots of ways in which melioration can be implemented. There are also rules that result in matching without using the principle of melioration (e.g., Harley, 1981; Houston and Sumida, 1987; Seth, 1999). Melioration performs well in many environments but in some environments it results in suboptimal behaviour. This behaviour and the resulting loss in reward rate can be viewed as side-effects of a decision rule that evolved in other circumstances. The results of Heyman and Herrnstein (1986) might be explained by this sort of argument.

3.2.1   The delay reduction hypothesis

Like the matching law, the delay reduction hypothesis (DRH) (Fantino *et al.*, 1993) was developed as a description of choice behaviour in the lab. The DRH can be used to predict choice on what is known as the concurrent chains procedure. In the simplest case, an animal can respond on one of two alternatives, known as initial links. Each alternative has an associated VI schedule, but in contrast to a standard concurrent VI-VI procedure in which the VIs provide rewards, here the VIs provide access to terminal links that result in a reward after a delay has elapsed. This access is indicated by a cue that signals the availability of a reward after a certain delay. During the initial link phase, the animal can choose between the two alternatives, but once a terminal link becomes available, the animal must wait until this link ends in a reward. After this has occurred, the animal can again choose between the initial links. There is some resemblance between the chains procedure and an animal that is searching for two food types at once. From time to time it encounters food items that result in energy after a handling time has elapsed. These items can be thought of as being analogous to the terminal links. Let T be the overall average time to a reward on the concurrent chains procedure. This time depends on both the initial links and the terminal links. To illustrate, assume that each initial link is a VI with the time to its terminal link having an exponential distribution with a mean of 60 s. Then the average time for the first terminal link to become available is 30 s. If one terminal link has a delay of 10 s and the other has a delay of 30 s, then the average time on terminal links is 20 s and so $T = 50$ s. (See Equation (3.10) below for the general equation for T.) The start of the terminal link on option i means that food will be available after a delay D_i. Before this time, the lack of memory associated with an exponential distribution means that the expected time to a reward is T. Thus the start of the terminal link is associated with a reduction in the expected delay to reward of $T - D_i$. Define ρ to be the proportion of responses to option 1, i.e., the number of responses made on the initial link for option 1 divided by the total number of responses made on both initial links. The DRH for two alternatives states that

$$\rho = \frac{T - D_1}{T - D_1 + T - D_2}.$$ (3.3)

This is the equation suggested by Fantino (1969). For modifications in the case of unequal initial links see Fantino and Davison (1983) and Squires and Fantino (1971).

Fantino and Dunn (1983) point out that the DRH predicts the violation of the principle of IIA. Fantino and Dunn (1983) and Mazur (2000) found that adding a third option in a concurrent chains procedure could change the preference of pigeons for the initial pair of options. We now give a formal analysis based on the version of the DRH given in Equation (3.3). Consider a general case with n initial links, each with an exponential VI schedule with mean interval I. Then the mean wait until a terminal link first becomes available is $W_n = I/n$. The DRH states that an animal's preference for an alternative is given by the relative reduction in delay to reward associated with the alternative. If initial link i leads to a terminal link with delay to reward D_i then the overall time to reward is

$$T_n = W_n + \frac{1}{n} \sum_i D_i. \tag{3.4}$$

Denoting the allocation to option i by B_i, we now compare the ratio of allocations to options 1 and 2 with and without option 3 being present. In the case of just two options being available

$$\frac{B_1}{B_2} = \frac{T_2 - D_1}{T_2 - D_2} = \frac{I + D_2 - D_1}{I + D_1 - D_2}. \tag{3.5}$$

When a third option is added the allocation is

$$\frac{B_1}{B_2} = \frac{T_3 - D_1}{T_3 - D_2} = \frac{I + D_2 + D_3 - 2D_1}{I + D_1 + D_3 - 2D_2}. \tag{3.6}$$

It follows from these equations that adding a third alternative can change the allocation of responses to option 1 relative to option 2. In other words we have a violation of IIA. The relative allocation may either increase or decrease; the critical value for a third alternative to produce no change is

$$\hat{D}_3 = \frac{I + D_1 + D_2}{2} = T_2. \tag{3.7}$$

Otherwise adding a third alternative does have an effect.

3.2.1.1 DRH and optimal foraging theory

We now explore the relationship between the DRH (a descriptive account) and optimal foraging theory (a normative account) and present a new result relating the DRH to the costs of deviating from optimality. Consider a foraging animal that searches for food and encounters two types of prey item. The DRH equation for two options (Equation (3.3)) applies to cases in which the animal responds on both initial links. This corresponds to the region of parameter space in which the maximisation of rate of energetic gain predicts that both prey types should be accepted (Fantino and Abarca, 1985; Houston, 1991). This means that the optimal rate of energetic gain, γ, is the rate resulting from taking both types. Assuming equal energy content (which can be set equal to 1 without loss of generality) and denoting the overall time to reward by T,

$$\gamma = \frac{1}{T}. \tag{3.8}$$

Now consider an animal that encounters items that can differ in energy and handling time. An item of type i has energy e_i and handling time D_i. McNamara and Houston (1987a) show that the energetic value of accepting a type i item is

$$H_i = e_i - \gamma D_i. \tag{3.9}$$

As Houston and McNamara (1999) point out, e_i is the energy gained by accepting a type i item and γD_i is the energy that could have been obtained by foraging at rate γ for time D_i rather than spending this time handling the item. Thus H_i is the energetic value of accepting the item. It is optimal to accept all item types for which $H > 0$; i.e., for which $e/D > \gamma$ (Houston and McNamara, 1999). As we have said, the DRH is concerned with parameter values for which both 'types' should be accepted. This means that H_i is positive for both alternatives and is the energy lost if the type is rejected rather than accepted. In other words, H_i is the cost associated with making the error of rejecting type i.

When $e_1 = e_2 = 1$,

$$H_i = 1 - \frac{D_i}{T}. \qquad (3.10)$$

Animals typically make errors in decision making and errors are more likely if the cost is low (Houston, 1987, 1997; McNamara and Houston, 1987a). One possible simple equation that captures this property is

$$\rho = \frac{H_1}{H_1 + H_2} \qquad (3.11)$$

where ρ is the probability of choosing option 1. If we use Equation (3.10) to substitute for H_1 and H_2 in this equation, then we obtain Equation (3.3).

Thus we have shown that the DRH is linked to optimality and the costs of making errors. This might suggest that it is a good rule – even though it was proposed as, and is primarily still, a descriptive model of choice, it has a normative basis.

So far we have discussed the DRH when all rewards have the same magnitude. Data from experiments in which terminal links differ in delay and reward magnitude violate a form of transitivity known as strong stochastic transitivity (Navarick and Fantino, 1972, 1974, 1975). Houston (1991) shows that a generalisation of the DRH to include different reward magnitudes can produce such violations. Houston *et al.* (2005) extend the analysis to include terminal links in which the delay to reward is variable and show that stochastic transitivity can still be violated when reward magnitudes are constant, but the terminal link durations are variable.

3.3   Normative models

We expect rules to be 'good' i.e., natural selection has resulted in rules that perform well. But animals (including humans) sometimes make bad decisions ('humans are not rational' – see Shafir and LeBoeuf, 2002 and Sutherland, 1994 for reviews). Such findings have been explained in a number of ways; we concentrate on two of these explanations.

3.3.1   The outcome is a side-effect

What matters is how a rule performs (in terms of reproductive success). Several rules may perform well in the environment in which they evolved. Their performance may differ in a 'new' environment (e.g., the lab); some rules may perform very badly in this environment. The debate about whether animals follow the matching law rather than maximising their rate of energetic gain can be used as an illustration. It is possible that what has been favoured by natural selection is a rule that performs well in environments that do not resemble experimental procedures and so, when a forager is presented with such procedures, the behavioural outcome is not what we might expect from an E-rational standpoint. It is important to distinguish between rules and outcomes when considering whether a particular behaviour is rational or not. Some behavioural outcomes are non-selected by-products of a decision-making mechanism (rule). Take risk-sensitivity, for example; although there are various normative explanations for the appearance of risk-sensitive responses (e.g., Houston and McNamara, 1999; McNamara and Houston, 1992), it has also been argued that risk-sensitivity can appear as a side-effect of a forager using simple learning rules (e.g., Kacelnik and Bateson, 1996; March, 1996). Arkes and Ayton (1999) suggest that some errors in human reasoning result from overgeneralising a rule that is reasonable in many contexts. For a general discussion of rules and side-effects, see Houston (2009a), Hutchinson and Gigerenzer (2005), McNamara and Houston (1980).

Decision framing is another important factor. There are lots of ways to provide an animal with a particular set of options all of which have the same mathematical characterisation, but which may result in systematic differences in behaviour (Houston, 2009a). The general point is that the details of the experimental procedure can be important (e.g., Heyman and Tanz, 1995; Savastano and Fantino, 1994; Shettleworth, 1989). Shettleworth and Jordan (1986) found that rats preferred receiving sunflower seeds in the husk and removing the husks themselves to simply waiting for a 'handling time' to elapse before being presented with a de-husked seed. Similarly, different time periods within an experimental situation seem to be treated with different degrees of importance by foragers; inter-trial intervals, for example, are often found to be unimportant for guiding choice behaviour, whereas the delay between making a response and receiving food is extremely important (e.g., Kacelnik and Bateson, 1996; Stephens *et al.*, 2004). When seemingly irrational behaviours appear, especially in experimental situations, we need always to ask whether it is the outcome of a well-adapted rule misfiring in a novel environment.

Even if an organism is studied in the environment in which it evolved, natural selection might result in behaviour that is not exactly optimal. As discussed by McNamara and Houston (2009), rules may have to cope with a range of circumstances. Natural selection will tend to favour rules that perform well on average across this range. Such a rule may not act so as to maximise any utility function, so may not even be E-rational.

3.3.2   We were wrong about what is optimal

The idea here is that the context in which optimal decisions are viewed is too simple and may ignore elements that add extra degrees of freedom to the situation. We now present a range of examples.

3.3.2.1   Uncontrolled variation in state

Studies of human irrationality tend to concern one-shot decisions; there can therefore be no differential accumulation of rewards between treatments. This is not always the case for non-humans. Schuck-Paim *et al.* (2004) highlight several cases where analogies have been drawn between similar 'irrational' behaviours in humans and non-humans; they claim, however, that the underlying choice mechanisms are fundamentally different. Their findings hold considerable implications for the comparison of choice behaviour across species. Schuck-Paim *et al.* (2004) show that, at least in some cases, seemingly irrational behaviour in animals can be explained purely as a function of state-dependent preferences. As examples, we discuss work on gray jays (Waite, 2001a) and rufous hummingbirds (Bateson *et al.*, 2002).

Grey jays (*Perisoreus canadensis*) were trained in one of two contexts, both involving choosing between two foraging patches. The patches consisted of a tube in which raisins were placed at different distances from the entrance; increased distance being assumed to correlate with increased perceived predation risk. In context A the jays were offered a series of choices between one and three raisins placed 0.5 m along separate tubes. Birds in context B were offered a series of choices between two identical options: two tubes with a single raisin placed 0.5 m from the entrance. All birds were subsequently offered a choice between three raisins placed 0.7 m along a tube and one raisin just 0.3 m from the entrance of a second tube. Preference for the larger, but riskier, reward was higher among birds that had been trained in context B. The findings were taken as indicating departures from value maximisation as a result of cognitive biases arising as a result of the choice context. The results were seen as mirroring framing effects (Tversky and Kahneman, 1981) in that the same decision was presented to different individuals but in a different scenario, the scenario affecting the final decision. Waite (2001a) compared the results to that of the trade-off contrast hypothesis (Tversky and Simonson, 1993). This predicts that an individual will be more likely to choose a low-quality, cheap item over a high-quality, expensive one if the individual has already experienced a choice between items of similar quality, but with a smaller difference in cost. However, as Schuck-Paim *et al.* (2004) point out, it was not just the previous context in which decisions had been made that differed between the two treatment groups. During the initial phase of the experiment, the jays in context A had gained more than twice as many rewards as those individuals in context B. The problem, therefore, can be thought of in terms of a trade-off between gaining energy and avoiding predation, a trade-off that has been extensively discussed in behavioural ecological systems (e.g., Cuthill *et al.*, 2000; Houston and McNamara, 1999; Houston *et al.*, 1993; McNamara, *et al.*, 2005).

Many species of animal can only increase their rate of energetic gain by also increasing their probability of being killed by a predator (see Lima, 1998 for a review). To predict choice, it is necessary to know the value of energy (gain from foraging) and the value of life (lost if killed) (Houston and McNamara, 1988, 1989, 1999). These will typically depend on the animal's state. In general, animals should accept a risk in order to obtain energy when reserves are low (Clark, 1994; Houston and McNamara, 1988, 1999; McNamara, 1990). The lower energetic state of the individuals in context B means that they should have been more prepared to take the greater risk to achieve the higher payoff than the context A individuals that were more sated. Similarly, seemingly irrational behaviour was reported from rufous hummingbirds (*Selaphorus rufus*; Bateson *et al.*, 2002). The hummingbirds changed their relative preferences for two options in the absence or presence of a decoy option, which provided a lower rate of gain than either of the other two options. Once again, however, the rate of energy gain differed between the two conditions, which could well have led to alterations in choice behaviour consistent with rational theory (Schuck-Paim *et al.*, 2004). Giving weight to their argument Schuck-Paim and her colleagues showed experimentally how seemingly irrational decisions in European starlings (*Sturnus vulgaris*) disappeared when energetic rates were equalised across treatments.

3.3.2.2   Future expectations

The best action to choose at present depends on future expectations (Houston and McNamara, 1999; McNamara and Houston, 1986 and references therein). For example, whether or not an animal should take risks in terms of predation in order to obtain food depends on whether food is likely to be plentiful and easy to obtain in the future. Adding an option to the set of available options changes what is possible in the future, and hence can change future expectations, even if it is not optimal to choose the additional option now. Thus, even if the new option is not chosen when added, its presence can change the current optimal choice. We give two examples of this effect.

Errors

Suppose that there are errors in decision making, with costly errors being rare. Then future gains depend not only on the preferred option, but also on other options that are mistakenly chosen. Adding a suboptimal option now will thus affect future expectations because this option is likely to be wrongly chosen in the future. This means that the value of an option depends on context (i.e., on the other options that are available). As a result violations of transitivity may occur (Houston, 1997). Violations of IIA may also occur.

Possible future states

Schuck-Paim *et al.* (2004) show that uncontrolled variation in state can produce behaviour that appears to be irrational. Houston *et al.* (2007) show how state-dependent effects can produce apparently irrational behaviour even when an animal's choice is measured in the same state. Consider an animal choosing at discrete times between foraging options that differ in terms of expected energetic gain and risk of predation. The animal's state is its level of energy reserves. The animal dies of starvation if its reserves fall to zero. Option A provides little food but has no associated risk of predation. Option B provides slightly better (but still not good) food and involves a risk of predation. Option C provides good food and involves the same risk of predation as Option B. Thus in this model the animal is faced with options that differ in terms of energetic gain and risk of predation. Houston *et al.* considered three environments. In the first environment, options A and B are available. In the second environment, options B and C are available. In the third environment, options A and C are available. In each case McNamara *et al.* used dynamic programming to find the strategy that maximises long-term survival (cf. McNamara and Houston, 1990b). As we would expect, this strategy is state-dependent, i.e., the optimal decision depends on the level of energy reserves. When options A and B are available, it is optimal to choose A when reserves are very high and B otherwise. When options A and C are available, it is optimal to choose A unless reserves are low in which case C is chosen. There is an intuitive explanation for these results. In this example option A is safe, but has a low yield. Thus the option is used when energy reserves are high. When reserves are low the animal should take risks in order to obtain a higher rate of energy gain. When option A is present with option C, because C has a higher yield than B the animal can afford to delay using this risky option until its reserves fall to a lower threshold than had B been present rather than C. Finally, when options B and C are available, option C is always chosen because it yields more food than B and has the same predation risk. From these three results we see that at intermediate levels of reserves, B is preferred to A when these are the two options available, C is preferred to B, and A is preferred to C. In other words, transitivity is violated.

We have given two examples of violations of transitivity, one based on errors (Houston, 1997), the other based on state (Houston *et al.*, 2007). The common principle is that all available options influence choice because they have an effect on future expectations. It is important to emphasise that these examples are based on the assumption that all options currently available will be available in the future. Options are linked to the future either because the animal makes mistakes and hence may choose a suboptimal option or because stochastic changes in state may take it to a state in which an option that is not currently chosen should be used. If this sort of analysis is to be relevant, animals must expect some degree of persistence of options into the future. Whether we might predict animals to have this view will depend on the sort of environment in which they have evolved.

3.3.2.3   **There may be more freedom in behaviour than originally anticipated**

In this section we are concerned with the consequences of changing some aspect of an organism's environment. We show that even if the organism is behaving rationally, the outcome might not correspond to naïve expectations. The reason for the discrepancy is that the expectation is based on too limited a view of the organism and its options. For example, it may seem obvious how a fitness maximising agent should respond to a change in the environment. But, in fact, a different response is optimal because the organism has more degrees of freedom than anticipated.

We start by drawing attention to the contrast between results if behaviour is fixed and results if the animal is free to change its behaviour. The same basic principles can be seen in a range of examples from humans and other animals. Measures such as the introduction of seatbelts or airbags in cars provide an illustration. If behaviour of road-users does not change, then there should be an improvement in safety. The new features may, however, lead to people changing their behaviour, typically by behaving in a more dangerous way. This change may be strong enough to result in an increased level of injury. (For data and discussion see Keeler, 1994; Peltzman, 1975; Peterson and Hoffer, 1994.) Similarly the obvious response to traffic congestion – building more roads – may cause an increase in traffic (e.g., Cervero, 2003; Goodwin and Noland, 2003; Noland and Lem, 2002) to the extent that traffic jams are worse than they were before. Thus when animals are free to change their behaviour the consequences may be an effect on performance that is the opposite of what was expected (and desired). A related physiological example concerns whether a bit of dirt is a good thing. Dirt may have a negative direct effect on disease, but a positive indirect effect through changes in the immune system. The 'hygiene hypothesis' (Strachan, 1989) states that improved hygiene (and reduced family size) have reduced the extent to which children are exposed to infectious agents. The result is a change in the immune system that renders it more likely to give rise to allergic responses such as asthma (see Christen and von Herrath, 2005; Romagnani, 2004; Yazdanbakhsh *et al.*, 2002 for further discussions). Tenner (1996) calls effects like these *revenge effects*. In analysing such examples, two approaches can be adopted. In one, behaviour in response to the change is 'given' (i.e., we adopt a descriptive approach). An alternative is to derive the behavioural response from considerations of optimality (i.e., we adopt a normative approach). This second approach is adopted in models that derive the behaviour of humans from the maximisation of utility. Blomquist (1986) and Janssen and Tenkink (1988) use utility maximisation to derive the dependence of a driver's behaviour on a parameter that corresponds to the level of a safety measure. They show that the effect of an improvement in safety may be substantially reduced by changes in behaviour. We now demonstrate the normative approach in other contexts, starting with examples based on the trade-off between obtaining energy and avoiding predators.

There are two ways of looking at optimal response to a change: (1) change in optimal behaviour (e.g., driving speed in the model of Janssen and Tenkink, 1988) and (2) changes in the resulting levels of some aspect of performance, such as mortality. We show that the relationship between various environmental factors and both the optimal response and the resulting performance may not always be obvious.

1. Changes in optimal behaviour

Consider the following example (see also McNamara and Houston, 1994): a forager has to reach a critical size in order to reproduce. How should it respond to a permanent change in the predation level? The answer depends on how behaviour and predation interact to determine mortality. Assume that the animal has the choice of how hard it works to obtain food. Denote this rate of work by u. The animal's rate of intake of food is proportional to u. Its rate of predation M is given by

$$M(u) = m_0 N(u) + \mu, \tag{3.12}$$

where the function $N(u)$ is increasing and accelerating and determines how predation rate changes with u for a given density of predators (m_0). μ is a background mortality rate. There is thus a trade-off between gaining food and predation risk. We denote the optimal rate of working for food by u^*.

If a change in predation is a result of an increase in m_0, u^* decreases. This is because there will be a marked increase in predation if foraging intensity is high, therefore the best response is to adopt a less dangerous foraging behaviour. In contrast, if μ increases, u^* increases. This is because the same increase in predation rate is imposed on all foraging options. Therefore the best response is to reduce the time exposed to predation by growing faster (i.e., by working harder for food). This shows that the effect of an increase in danger may result in either an increase or a decrease in how hard a B-rational animal works for food.

2. Changes in the performance

When animals can trade off energetic gain against predation risk, the effect of a change in the environment may be counterintuitive (e.g., Abrams, 1993; McNamara and Houston, 1990b). For example, an increase in food availability can lead to a decrease in food intake or an increase in starvation (McNamara and Houston, 1987d, 1990a; see McNamara and Houston, 1994, Figures 2 and 3; also Houston and McNamara, 1999). The effects arise because the animals change their behaviour in adaptive ways (see McNamara and Houston, 1994 for a review). We now give some examples of changes in the performance as a consequence of adaptive behaviour.

McNamara and Buchanan (2005) model a situation in which an animal is exposed to a stressor, such as cold or high predation risk, for a period of time. During this period the animal can choose the level of available resources to direct against the stressor. The more the animal diverts to combating the stressor, the less likely the stressor is to kill the animal. However, diverting resources from essential maintenance reduces the condition of the animal. As condition decreases, the probability of death from disease increases. Thus the animal faces a trade off between dying from the stressor or from the effects of poor condition. McNamara and Buchanan find the allocation to combating the stressor that maximises the probability that the animal will survive. They show that if the likelihood of death from disease at a given level of condition is decreased, the animal allows condition to deteriorate much more. The result is to increase the likelihood that the animal will die from disease. In this model, much of the mortality from disease occurs during recovery of condition after the stressor disappears.

Failure to take account of the fact behaviour is flexible may make it difficult to detect important costs. If we vary a factor, an animal may respond by changing its behaviour or morphology in a way that we have not anticipated. This makes it hard to detect the direct effect of the change. We give an example based on the diving behaviour of animals that hunt for food underwater and return to the surface to breathe (e.g., puffins, otters). A dive cycle starts with the animal at surface. The animal travels to the foraging area at a particular depth, forages there for a time t, and then returns to the surface where it spends a time s gaining oxygen. The amount of oxygen gained is a decelerating function of time at the surface. The total time travelling between the surface and the foraging area is τ. A simple approach assumes that animal should maximise the proportion of time spent in the foraging area, subject to the constraint that the diver balances its oxygen over the cycle (Houston and Carbone, 1992; Kramer, 1988). The rates of oxygen use are m_t and m_τ during foraging and travelling, respectively. If τ is increased with t fixed, then the oxygen constraint means that s is an accelerating function of time underwater. But if the animal is free to adopt the behaviour that maximises the proportion of time spent foraging, then as τ increases, s may be approximately proportional to time underwater (Houston and Carbone, 1992; McNamara et al., 2001). Thus the cost (the effect of a unit increase in τ on s as τ increases) is not apparent when the animal is able to adjust its time budget. Houston et al. (2003) investigate the behaviour of a diving animal that can only catch a single item when hunting underwater. They show that if the diver maximises its rate of energetic gain while hunting for items of two types, then the success of a dive (i.e., the probability of returning to the surface with an item) is not a good indicator of the quality of the environment. For example, as the probability of finding the better type of item increases, the success of the dive may first increase then decrease and then increase again.

It is often assumed that predation risk in birds depends on fat load because heavy birds will be less agile. It is, however, hard to detect the effect of fat on predation because a bird may change both its behaviour and its body composition. As fat loads increase, a bird may adopt safer foraging options. As a result, predation may decrease with mass (Welton and Houston, 2001). Another response to an increased fat load is to increase muscle mass, allowing greater agility and thus preventing an increase in predation.

These examples show that care is needed in choosing the variables that will be measured. If an important variable is not measured, then results may be misleading. For example, in the case of the diver, a better understanding of costs can be obtained if time at the surface is related to time travelling τ and time foraging t rather than to total time underwater $\tau + t$.

3.3.2.4 Fluctuating environments and biased probabilities

It might seem obvious that natural selection should always result in organisms having an accurate view of the world. Models based on evolution in a certain kind of stochastic environment show that this is not the case. Chance acts on many scales in the natural world. At the finest scale, demographic stochasticity describes the good and bad luck that affects individual population members, independently of other population members. At the other extreme, environmental stochasticity concerns fluctuations in the environment as a whole. These fluctuations, which might be due to weather or changes in population size, affect all populations in a similar manner.

Consider first the situation where there is demographic stochasticity, but no environmental stochasticity. Demographic stochasticity will affect the lifetime reproductive success (LRS) of individuals in the population. Let $p(x)$ be the probability that the LRS of a particular individual is x. Then the mean LRS of this individual is

$$r = \sum_x x p(x). \tag{3.13}$$

Here, this mean is an average over demographic stochasticity. The quantity r is the standard fitness measure in this situation, and tends to be maximised by the action of natural selection.

Now suppose that there is also environmental stochasticity. The LRS of an individual will then depend on both demographic good and bad luck and on the state of the environment. Let $p(x|s)$ denote the probability that the LRS of the individual is x when the environmental state is s. The mean LRS given environmental state s is thus

$$r(s) = \sum_x x p(x|s). \tag{3.14}$$

In this situation the standard measure of fitness is the geometric mean, G, of $r(s)$, where the mean is an average over the environmental state s. Equivalently, fitness can be taken to be $g = \log G$, the logarithm of G. This fitness measure can be expressed as

$$g = \sum_s \log(r(s))f(s) \tag{3.15}$$

where $f(s)$ is the probability that the environmental state is s. The quantity g tends to be maximised by the action of natural selection.

Now suppose that the above population is at evolutionary stability, so that population members are maximising the fitness measure g. Let $r^*(s)$ denote the expected LRS of population members when the environmental state is s. Then it can be shown that population members are also maximising

$$\sum_s r(s)f^*(s) \tag{3.16}$$

where f^* is a certain probability distribution on environmental states. Under this distribution the probability, $f^*(s)$, of state s is proportional to $f(s)/r^*(s)$. As this formula shows, the distribution f^* distorts the true probability distribution f, giving extra weight to environmental states for which population members do badly, and reducing the probability of environmental states for which population members do well. Thus population members are maximising their average LRS (averaged over environmental stochasticity), but where the average is based on biased probabilities (McNamara, 1995; cf. Haccou and Iwasa, 1995; Sasaki and Ellner, 1995). For the link between this approach and a general account of optimisation under the action of natural selection, see Grafen (1999).

3.4   Discussion

Given that natural selection maximises fitness, it seems clear that behaviour will satisfy B-rationality. A limitation of this argument is that it is based on choices made by rules that are optimal for particular conditions. We have stressed, however, that problems arise when animals are faced with novel environments (Darwin's iguana, see also McNamara and Houston, 1980; Shettleworth, 1985). Given that animals follow robust rules, side-effects (often referred to as spandrels in this context, e.g., Buss et al., 1998; Gould, 1997; Hampton, 2004; Houston, 2009b) will be ubiquitous. A related point is that we cannot just determine optimal behaviour for the environment of the lab (Houston and McNamara, 1989, 1999). An animal in the lab may be safe from starvation and predation, but it does not 'know' this. It presumably follows rules that evolved to cope with these threats and to deal with competition and changes in the environment. Matching is not optimal in some of the procedures that are used in lab experiments; it may be that matching is a side-effect of decision rules that perform well in a broader context (see also Seth, this volume). We have shown that a version of the DRH can be related to the maximisation of rate of energetic gain given that errors occur but costly errors are rare. Our result suggests that although the DRH may not be strictly optimal, it is likely to be a good principle given that errors occur. The interaction between options that is captured by the DRH can be understood in terms of decisions that are subject to error. On this view, some aspects of the DRH may have appeared to be irrational because we had a limited conception of optimality.

Previous work (e.g., Tversky and Simonson, 1993) has presented models based on plausible psychological principles that can describe irrational behaviour. In this chapter, we have attempted to construct links between descriptive and normative accounts. In addition to showing that the DRH emerges from optimal decision making, subject to errors, we have pointed out that intransitive choice can result from optimal behavioural mechanisms when decisions depend on state and options persist into the future. This result does not rely on uncontrolled variation in state. It emerges because of the effect that options have on future expectations. This general principle deserves further investigation.

We have drawn attention to common themes that arise in the study of humans and other animals, but many analogies have not been explored. For example, the model of driving speed investigated by Janssen and Tenkink (1988) is analogous to models of optimal flight speed (e.g., Norberg, 1981; Houston, 1986b). Whether this resemblance is productive remains to be seen. An area in which a unified account might be useful is optimal defence. In the context of military history, we might be interested in how the builder of a castle should allocate resources to structures that improve the strength of the castle and to features that improve its appearance and hence the prestige of the builder, and consequently the number of descendants that he leaves. Analogous issues arise in several biological contexts, including the interactions between predators and prey (e.g., Abrams, 1986; McNamara et al., 2005), the way in which plants defend themselves against herbivores (e.g., Adler and Karban, 1994; VanDam et al., 1996), the evolution of diseases and the defences against them (e.g., Day and Proulx, 2004; Frank, 1996; Medley, 2002; Shudo and Iwasa, 2001, 2004; van Boven and Weissing, 2004), and the defence of a social insect colony against attack (e.g., Aoki and Kurosu, 2004; Oster and Wilson, 1978). Adler and Karban (1994) make the military analogy explicit, and Jokela et al. (2000) present 'steps towards a unified defence theory', but we suspect that further work on a synthesis of these areas would be instructive.

We also think that the approach to decision making adopted by Fawcett and Johnstone (2003) could be extended. They investigate a model of optimal choice when an animal chooses between objects on the basis of more than one cue. These cues can differ in reliability of the information that they provide and in the cost of assessing them. Fawcett and Johnstone look for the way in which evolution will shape the uses of the cues. This sort of approach may have broad implications for the understanding of apparently irrational behaviour.

Acknowledgements

We thank Alex Kacelnik, Anil Seth and two anonymous referees for comments on previous versions of this manuscript. AIH and JMMcN were supported by Leverhulme Trust Fellowships, MDS by a BBSRC studentship.

References

Abrams, P. A. (1986). Adaptive responses of predators to prey and prey to predators: the failure of the arms race analogy. *Evolution* **40**: 1229–47.

Abrams, P. A. (1993). Why predation rate should not be proportional to predator density. *Ecology* **74**: 726–33.

Adler, F. R. and R. Karban (1994). Defended fortresses or moving targets: another model of inducible defenses inspired by military metaphors. *Am. Nat.* **144**: 813–32.

Alferink L. A, T. S. Critchfield, J. L. Hitt, and W. J. Higgins (2009). Generality of the matching law as a descriptor of basketball shot selection. *J. Appl. Behav. Anal.* **42**: 592–605.

Aoki, S. and U. Kurosu (2004). How many soldiers are optimal for an aphid colony? *J. Theor. Biol.* **230**: 313–17.

Arkes, H. R. and P. Ayton (1999). The sunk cost and Concorde effects: are humans less rational than lower animals? *Psychol. Bull.* **125**: 591–600.

Arrow, K. J. (1951). *Social Choice and Individual Values*. New York: Wiley.

Bateson, M. (2002). Context-dependent foraging choices in risk-sensitive starlings. *Anim. Behav.* **64**: 251–60.

Bateson, M. and S. D. Healy (2005). Comparative evaluation and its implications for mate choice. *Trends Ecol. Evol.* **20**: 659–64.

Bateson, M., S. D. Healy, and T. A. Hurly (2002). Irrational choices in hummingbird foraging behaviour. *Anim. Behav.* **63**: 587–96.

Bateson, M., S. D. Healy, and T. A. Hurly (2003). Context-dependent foraging decisions in rufous hummingbirds. *Proc. R. Soc. Lond. Ser. B. Biol. Sci.* **270**: 1271–6.

Baum, W. M. (1974). On two types of deviation from matching laws: bias and under-matching. *J. Exp. Anal. Behav.* **22**: 231–42.

Belinsky, R., F. Gonzalez, and J. Stahl (2004). Optimal behavior and concurrent variable interval schedules. *J. Math. Psychol.* **48**: 247–62.

Bernardo, A. E. and I. Welch (2001). On the evolution of overconfidence and entrepreneurs. *Journal Econ. Manage. Strat.* **10**: 301–30.

Binmore, K. (1997). Rationality and backward induction. *J. Econ. Met.* **4**: 23–41.

Blomquist, G. (1986). A utility maximization model of driver traffic safety behavior. *Accident Anal. Prev.* **18**: 371–5.

Busemeyer, J. R. and J. T. Townsend (1993). Decision field-theory: a dynamic cognitive approach to decision-making in an uncertain environment. *Psychol. Rev.* **100**: 432–59.

Buss, D. M., M. G. Haselton, T. K. Shackelford, A. L. Bleske, and J. C. Wakefield (1998). Adaptations, exaptations, and spandrels. *Am. Psychol.* **53**: 533–48.

Cervero, R. (2003). Road expansion, urban growth, and induced travel: a path analysis. *J. Amer. Plan. Assoc.* **69**: 145–63.

Christen, U. and M. G. von Herrath (2005). Infections and autoimmunity: good or bad? *J. Immunol.* **174**: 7481–6.

Clark, C. W. (1994). Antipredator behavior and the asset-protection principle. *Behav. Ecol.* **5**: 159–70.

Cooper, W. S. (2001). *The Evolution of Reason*. Cambridge: Cambridge University Press.

Cuthill, I. C., S. A. Maddocks, C. V. Weall, and E. K. M. Jones (2000). Body mass regulation in response to changes in feeding predictability and overnight energy expenditure. *Behav. Ecol.* **11**: 189–95.

Dall, S. R. X., J. M. McNamara, and I. C. Cuthill (1999). Interruptions to foraging and learning in a changing environment. *Anim. Behav.* **57**: 233–41.

Darwin, C. (1839). *Journal of Researches into the Geology and Natural History of the Various Countries Visited by H.M.S. Beagle, Under the Command of Captain Fitzroy, R.N. from 1832 to 1836.* Henry Colburn: London.

Day, T. and S. R. Proulx (2004). A general theory for the evolutionary dynamics of virulence. *Am. Nat.* **163**: E40–E63.

Dickson, E. S. (2006). Rational choice epistemology and belief formation in mass politics. *J. Theor. Polit.* **18**: 454–97.

Dickson, E. S. (2008). Expected utility violations evolve under status-based selection mechanisms. *J. Theor. Biol.* **254**: 650–4.

Fantino, E. (1969). Choice and rate of reinforcement. *J. Exp. Anal. Behav.* **12**: 723.

Fantino, E. and N. Abarca (1985). Choice, optimal foraging, and the delay-reduction hypothesis. *Behav. Brain Sci.* **8**: 315–29.

Fantino, E. and M. Davison (1983). Choice: some quantitative relations. *J. Exp. Anal. Behav.* **40**: 1–13.

Fantino, E. and R. Dunn (1983). The delay-reduction hypothesis: extension to three-alternative choice. *J. Exp. Psychol.-Anim. Behav. Process* 9: 132–46.

Fantino, E., R. A. Preston, and R. Dunn (1993). Delay reduction: current status. *J. Exp. Anal. Behav.* **60**: 159–69.

Fawcett, T. W. and Johnstone R. A. (2003). Optimal assessment of multiple cues. *Proc. R. Soc. Lond. Ser. B. Biol. Sci.* **270**: 1637–43.

Ferster, C. B. and Skinner B. F. (1957). *Schedules of Reinforcement.* Englewood Cliffs, NJ: Prentice Hall.

Frank, S. A. (1996). Models of parasite virulence. *Quart. Rev. Biol.* **71**: 37–78.

Goodwin, P. and R. B. Noland (2003). Building new roads really does create extra traffic: a response to Prakash et al. *Appl. Econ.* **35**: 1451–7.

Gould, S. J. (1997). The exaptive excellence of spandrels as a term and prototype. *Proc. Natl. Acad. Sci. USA* **94**, 10750–5.

Grafen, A. (1999). Formal Darwinism, the individual-as-maximizing-agent analogy and bet-hedging. *Proc. R. Soc. Lond. Ser. B. Biol. Sci.* **266**: 799–803.

Haccou, P. and Y. Iwasa (1995). Optimal mixed strategies in stochastic environments. *Theor. Popul. Biol.* **47**: 212–43.

Hammerstein, P. and E. H. Hagen (2005). The second wave of evolutionary economics in biology. *Trends Ecol. Evol.* **20**: 604–609.

Hampton, S. J. (2004). Domain mismatches, scruffy engineering, exaptations and spandrels. *Theor. Psychol.* **14**: 147–66.

Harley, C. B. (1981). Learning the evolutionarily stable strategy. *J. Theor. Biol.* **89**: 611–33.

Herrnstein, R. J. (1961). Relative and absolute strength of response as a function of frequency of reinforcement. *J. Exp. Anal. Behav.* **4**: 267–272.

Herrnstein, R. J. (1970). On the law of effect. *J. Exp. Anal. Behav.* **13**: 244–66.

Hey, J. D. (2002). Experimental economics and the theory of decision making under risk and uncertainty. *Geneva Pap. Risk Ins.* **27**: 5–21.

Heyman, G. M. and R. J. Herrnstein (1986). More on concurrent interval-ratio schedules: a replication and review. *J. Exp. Anal. Behav.* **46**: 331–51.

Heyman, G. M. and R. D. Luce (1979). Operant matching is not a logical consequence of maximizing reinforcement rate. *Anim. Learn. Behav.* **7**: 133–40.

Heyman, G. M. and L. Tanz (1995). How to teach a pigeon to maximize overall reinforcement rate. *J. Exp. Anal. Behav.* **64**: 277–97.

Houston, A. I. (1983). Optimality theory and matching. *Behav. Anal. Lett.* **3**: 1–15.

Houston, A. I. (1986a). The matching law applies to wagtails' foraging in the wild. *J. Exp. Anal. Behav.* **45**: 15–18.

Houston, A. I. (1986b). The optimal flight velocity for a bird exploiting patches of food. *J. Theor. Biol.* **119**: 345–62.

Houston, A. I. (1987). The control of foraging decisions. In *Quantitative Analysis of Behaviour*, ed. M. L. Commons, A. Kacelnik and S. J. Shettleworth. Hillsdale, NJ: Lawrence Erlbaum, pp. 41–60.

Houston, A. I. (1991). Violations of stochastic transitivity on concurrent chains: Implications for theories and choice. *J. Exp. Anal. Behav.* **55**: 323–335.

Houston, A. I. (1997). Natural selection and context-dependent values. *Proc. R. Soc. Lond. Ser. B. Biol. Sci.* **264**: 1539–41.

Houston, A. I. (2008). Matching and ideal free distributions. *Oikos* **117**: 978–83.

Houston, A. I. (2009a). Flying in the face of nature. *Behav. Proces.* **80**: 295–305.

Houston, A. I. (2009b). San Marco and evolutionary biology. *Biol. Philos.* **24**: 215–230.

Houston, A. I. and C. Carbone (1992). The optimal allocation of time during the diving cycle. *Behav. Ecol.* **3**: 255–65.

Houston, A. I. and J. McNamara (1981). How to maximize reward rate on two variable-interval paradigms. *J. Exp. Anal. Behav.* **35**: 367–96.

Houston, A. I. and J. M. McNamara (1988). A framework for the functional analysis of behavior. *Behav. Brain Sci.* **11**: 117–54.

Houston, A. I. and J. M. McNamara (1989). The value of food: effects of open and closed economies. *Anim. Behav.* **37**: 546–62.

Houston, A. I. and J. M. McNamara (1999). *Models of Adaptive Behaviour: An Approach Based on State.* Cambridge: Cambridge University Press.

Houston, A. I., J. M. McNamara, J. E. Heron, and Z. Barta (2003). The effect of foraging parameters on the probability that a dive is successful. *Proc. R. Soc. Lond. Ser. B. Biol. Sci.* **270**: 2451–5.

Houston, A. I., J. M. McNamara, and J. M. C. Hutchinson (1993). General results concerning the trade-off between gaining energy and avoiding predation. *Philos. Trans. R. Soc. Lond. Ser. B. Biol. Sci.* **341**: 375–97.

Houston, A. I., J. M. McNamara, and M. D. Steer (2007). Violations of transitivity under fitness maximization. *Biol. Letters* **3**: 365–7.

Houston, A. I. and J. E. R. Staddon (1981). Optimality principles and behavior: it's all for the best. *Behav. Brain Sci.* **4**: 395–6.

Houston, A. I., M. D. Steer, P. R. Killeen, and W. A. Thompson (2005). Predicting violations of transitivity when choices involve fixed or variable delays to food. In *Modelling Natural Action Selection: An International Workshop*, ed. J. J. Bryson, T. J. Prescott, and A. K. Seth. Edinburgh: AISB Press, pp. 9–15.

Houston, A. I. and B. H. Sumida (1987). Learning rules, matching and frequency-dependence. *J. Theor. Biol.* **126**: 289–308.

Hurly, T. A. and M. D. Oseen (1999). Context-dependent, risk-sensitive foraging preferences in wild rufous hummingbirds. *Anim. Behav.* **58**: 59–66.

Hutchinson, J. M. C. and G. Gigerenzer (2005). Simple heuristics and rules of thumb: where psychologists and behavioural biologists might meet. *Behav. Processes* **69**: 97–124.

Iwasa, Y., M. Higashi, and N. Yamamura (1981). Prey distribution as a factor determining the choice of optimal foraging strategy. *Am. Nat.* **117**: 710–23.

Janssen, W. H. and E. Tenkink (1988). Considerations on speed selection and risk homeostasis in driving. *Accident Anal. Prev.* **20**: 137–42.

Jokela, J., P. Schmid-Hempel, and M. C. Rigby (2000). Dr Pangloss restrained by the Red Queen: steps towards a unified defence theory. *Oikos* **89**: 267–74.

Kacelnik, A. (2006). Meanings of rationality. In *Rational Animals?* ed. S. Hurley and M. Nudds. Oxford: Oxford University Press, pp. 87–106.

Kacelnik, A. and M. Bateson (1996). Risky theories: the effects of variance on foraging decisions. *Am. Zool.* **36**: 402–34.

Kahneman, D. (2003). Maps of bounded rationality: psychology for behavioral economics. *Am. Econ. Rev.* **93**: 1449–75.

Keeler, T. E. (1994). Highway safety, economic behavior, and driving environment. *Am. Econ. Rev.* **84**: 684–93.

Kramer, D. L. (1988). The behavioral ecology of air breathing by aquatic animals. *Can. J. Zool.* **66**: 89–94.

Kirkpatrick, M., A. S. Rand, and M. J. Ryan (2006). Mate choice rules in animals. *Anim. Behav.* **71**, 1215–25.

Lima, S. L. (1998). Stress and decision making under the risk of predation: recent developments from behavioral, reproductive, and ecological perspectives. In *Advances in the Study of Behavior: Stress and Behavior*, vol. **27**, pp. 215–90.

Luce, R. D. (1959). *Individual Choice Behaviour: A Theoretical Analysis*. New York: John Wiley.

Luce, R. D. (1977). The choice axiom after twenty years. *J. Math. Psychol.* **15**: 215–33.

Luce, R. D. and H. Raiffa (1957). *Games and Decisions*. New York: John Wiley.

Luce R. D. and Suppes P. (1965). Preference, utility, and subjective probability. In *Handbook of Psychology III*, ed. R. D. Luce, R. R. Bush, and E. Galanter. New York: John Wiley, pp. 249–410.

Manktelow, K. I. and D. E. Over (1993). *Rationality: Psychological and Philosophical Perspectives*. London: Routledge.

March, J. G. (1996). Learning to be risk averse. *Psychol. Rev.* **103**: 309–19.

Mazur, J. E. (2000). Two- versus three-alternative concurrent-chain schedules: a test of three models. *J. Exp. Psychol. Anim. Behav. Process.* **26**: 286–93.

McDowell, J. J. (1989). Two modern developments in matching theory. *Behav. Analyst* **12**: 153–66.

McNamara, J. M. (1982). Optimal patch use in a stochastic environment. *Theor. Popul. Biol.* **21**: 269–88.

McNamara, J. M. (1990). The policy which maximizes long-term survival of an animal faced with the risks of starvation and predation. *Adv. Appl. Probab.* **22**: 295–308.

McNamara, J. M. (1995). Implicit frequency-dependence and kin selection in fluctuating environments. *Evol. Ecol.* **9**: 185–203.

McNamara, J. M. (1996). Risk-prone behaviour under rules which have evolved in a changing environment. *Am. Zool.* **36**: 484–95.

McNamara, J. M., Z. Barta, A. I. Houston, and P. Race (2005). A theoretical investigation of the effect of predators on foraging behaviour and energy reserves. *Proc. R. Soc. Lond. Ser. B. Biol. Sci.* **272**: 929–34.

McNamara, J. M. and K. L. Buchanan (2005). Stress, resource allocation, and mortality. *Behav. Ecol. Sociobiol.* **16**: 1008–17.

McNamara, J. M. and A. I. Houston (1980). The application of statistical decision: theory to animal behaviour. *J. Theor. Biol.* **85**: 673–90.

McNamara, J. M. and A. I. Houston (1985). Optimal foraging and learning. *J. Theor. Biol.* **117**: 231–49.

McNamara, J. M. and A. I. Houston (1986). The common currency for behavioral decisions. *Am. Nat.* **127**: 358–78.

McNamara, J. M. and A. I. Houston (1987a). Partial preferences and foraging. *Anim. Behav.* **35**: 1084–99.

McNamara, J. M. and A. I. Houston (1987b). Memory and the efficient use of information. *J. Theor. Biol.* **125**: 385–95.

McNamara, J. M. and A. I. Houston (1987c). Foraging in patches: there's more to life than the marginal value theorem. In *Quantitative Analyses of Behavior*, ed. M. L. Commons, A. Kacelnik, and S. J. Shettleworth. Hillsdale, NJ: Lawrence Erlbaum Associates, pp. 23–39.

McNamara, J. M. and A. I. Houston (1987d). Starvation and predation as factors limiting population size. *Ecology* **68**: 1515–9.

McNamara, J. M. and A. I. Houston (1990a). The value of fat reserves and the trade-off between starvation and predation. *Acta Biotheor.* **38**: 1990.

McNamara, J. M. and A. I. Houston (1990b). Starvation and predation in a patchy environment. In *Living in a Patchy Environment*, ed. I. R. Swingland and B. Shorrocks. Oxford: Oxford University Press, pp. 23–43.

McNamara, J. M. and A. I. Houston (1992). Risk-sensitive foraging: a review of the theory. *Bull. Math. Biol.* **54**: 355–78.

McNamara, J. M. and A. I. Houston (1994). The effect of a change in foraging options on intake rate and predation rate. *Am. Nat.* **144**: 978–1000.

McNamara, J. M. and A. I. Houston (2009). Integrating function and mechanism. *Trends Ecol. Evol.* **24**: 670–5.

McNamara, J. M., A. I. Houston, and E. J. Collins (2001). Optimality models in behavioural biology. *SIAM Rev.* **43**: 413–66.

Medley, G. F. (2002). The epidemiological consequences of optimisation of the individual host immune response. *Parasitology* **125**: S61–S70.

Moser, P. K. (1990). *Rationality in Action: Contemporary Approaches*. Cambridge: Cambridge University Press.

Myerson, J. and S. Hale (1984). Practical implications of the matching law. *J. Appl. Behav. Anal.* **17**: 367–80.

Navarick, D. J. and E. Fantino (1972). Transitivity as a property of choice. *J. Exp. Anal. Behav.* **18**: 389–401.

Navarick, D. J. and E. Fantino (1974). Stochastic transitivity and unidimensional behavior theories. *Psychol. Rev.* **81**: 426–41.

Navarick, D. J. and E. Fantino (1975). Stochastic transitivity and unidimensional control of choice. *Learn. Motiv.* **6**: 179–201.

Noland, R. B. and L. L. Lem (2002). A review of the evidence for induced travel and changes in transportation and environmental policy in the US and the UK. *Transport. Res. D – Tr. E.* **7**: 1–26.

Norberg, R. Å. (1981). Optimal flight speed in birds when feeding young. *J. Anim. Ecol.* **50**: 473–7.

Nozick, R. (1993). *The Nature of Rationality*. Princeton, NJ: Princeton University Press.

Oster, G. F. and E. O. Wilson (1978). *Caste and Ecology in the Social Insects*. Princeton University Press: Princeton, NJ.

Peltzman, S. (1975). Effects of automobile safety regulation. *J. Polit. Econ.* **83**: 677–725.

Peterson, S. P. and G. E. Hoffer (1994). The impact of airbag adoption on relative personal-injury and absolute collision insurance claims. *J. Consum. Res.* **20**: 657–62.

Pierce, W. D. and W. F. Epling (1995). The applied importance of research on the matching law. *J. Appl. Behav. Anal.* **28**: 237–41.

Pothos, E. M. and J. R. Busemeyer (2009). A quantum probability explanation for violations of 'rational' decision theory. *Proc. R. Soc. Lond. Ser. B. Biol. Sci.* **276**: 2171–8.

Rieskamp, J., J. R. Busemeyer, and B. A. Mellers (2006). Extending the bounds of rationality: evidence and theories of preferential choice. *J. Econ. Lit.* **44**: 631–61.

Robson, A. J. (2002). Evolution and human nature. *J. Econ. Perspect.* **16**: 89–106.

Robson, A. J. (2003). The evolution of rationality and the Red Queen. *J. Econ. Theory* **111**: 1–22.

Romagnani, S. (2004). The increased prevalence of allergy and the hygiene hypothesis: missing immune deviation, reduced immune suppression, or both? *Immunology* **112**: 352–63.

Sasaki, A. and S. Ellner (1995). The evolutionarily stable phenotype distribution in a random environment. *Evolution* **49**: 337–50.

Savastano, H. I. and E. Fantino (1994). Human choice in concurrent ratio-interval schedules of reinforcement. *J. Exp. Anal. Behav.* **61**: 453–63.

Schuck-Paim, C., L. Pompilio, and A. Kacelnik (2004). State-dependent decisions cause apparent violations of rationality in animal choice. *PLoS. Biol.* **2**: 2305–15.

Seth, A. K. (1999). Evolving behavioural choice: an investigation into Herrnstein's matching law. In *Advances in Artificial Life: Proceedings of the 5th European Conference (ECAL '99)*, ed. D. Floreano, J.-D. Nicoud, and F. Mondada. Berlin: Springer-Verlag, pp. 225–35.

Seth, A. K. (2001). Modeling group foraging: Individual suboptimality, interference, and a kind of matching. *Adapt. Behav.* **9**: 67–89.

Seth, A. K. (2006). The ecology of action selection: insights from artificial life. *Philos. Trans. R. Soc. Lond. Ser. B. Biol. Sci.* **362**(1485): 670–5.

Shafir, S. (1994). Intransitivity of preferences in honeybees: support for comparative-evaluation of foraging options. *Anim. Behav.* **48**: 55–67.

Shafir, E. and LeBoeuf, R. A. (2002). Rationality. *Annu. Rev. Psychol.* **53**: 491–517.

Shafir S., T. A. Waite, and B. H. Smith (2002). Context-dependent violations of rational choice in honeybees (*Apis mellifera*) and gray jays (*Perisoreus canadensis*). *Behav. Ecol. Sociobiol.* **51**: 180–7.

Shettleworth, S. J. (1985). Foraging, memory, and constraints on learning. *Ann. NY Acad. Sci.* **443**: 216–226.

Shettleworth, S. J. (1989). Animals foraging in the lab: problems and promises. *J. Exp. Psychol. Anim. B.* **15**: 81–7.

Shettleworth, S. J. and V. Jordan (1986). Rats prefer handling food to waiting for it. *Anim. Behav.* **34**: 925–7.

Shudo, E. and Y. Iwasa (2001). Inducible defense against pathogens and parasites: Optimal choice among multiple options. *J. Theor. Biol.* **209**: 233–47.

Shudo, E. and Y. Iwasa (2004). Dynamic optimization of host defense, immune memory, and post-infection pathogen levels in mammals. *J. Theor. Biol.* **228**: 17–29.

Silberberg, A., J. R. Thomas, and N. Berendzen (1991). Human choice on concurrent variable-interval variable-ratio schedules. *J. Exp. Anal. Behav.* **56**: 575–84.

Simon, H. A. (1978). Rationality as process and as product of thought. *Am. Econ. Rev.* **68**: 1–16.

Smith, V. L. (2003). Constructivist and ecological rationality in economics. *Am. Econ. Rev.* **93**: 465–508.

Sober, E. (1981). The evolution of rationality. *Synthese* **46**: 95–120.

Soltani, A. and X. J. Wang (2006). A biophysically based neural model of matching law behavior: Melioration by stochastic synapses. *J. Neurosci.* **26**: 3731–44.

Spiga, R., R. S. Maxwell, R. A. Meisch, and J. Grabowski (2005). Human methadone self-administration and the generalized matching law. *Psychol. Rec.* **55**: 525–38.

Squires, N. and E. Fantino (1971). A model for choice in simple concurrent and concurrent-chains schedules. *J. Exp. Anal. Behav.* **15**: 27–38.

Stein, E. (1996). *Without Good Reason: The Rationality Debate in Philosophy and Cognitive Science*. Oxford: Clarendon Press.

Stephens D. W., B. Kerr, and E. Fernandez-Juricic (2004). Impulsiveness without discounting: the ecological rationality hypothesis. *Proc. R. Soc. Lond. Ser. B. Biol. Sci.* **271**: 2459–65.

Stephens, D. W. and J. R. Krebs (1986). *Foraging Theory*. Princeton, NJ: Princeton University Press.

Strachan, D. P. (1989). Hay-fever, hygiene, and household size. *Brit. Med. J.* **299**: 1259–60.

Sugrue, L. P., G. S. Corrado, and W. T. Newsome (2004). Matching behavior and the representation of value in the parietal cortex. *Science* **304**: 1782–87.

Sutherland, S. (1994). *Irrationality: The Enemy Within*. London: Penguin Books.

Tenner, E. (1996). *Why Things Bite Back: New Technology and the Revenge Effect*. London: Fourth Estate.

Todd, P. M. and G. Gigerenzer (2000). How can we open up the adaptive toolbox? *Behav. Brain Sci.* **23**: 767–80.

Tversky, A. and D. Kahneman (1981). The framing of decisions and the psychology of choice. *Science* **211**, 453–8.

Tversky, A. and I. Simonson (1993). Context-dependent preferences. *Manage. Sci.* **39**: 1179–89.

van Boven, M. and F. J. Weissing (2004). The evolutionary economics of immunity. *Am. Nat.* **163**: 277–94.

VanDam, N. M., T. J. DeJong, Y. Iwasa, and T. Kubo (1996). Optimal distribution of defences: are plants smart investors? *Funct. Ecol.* **10**: 128–36.

Waite, T. A. (2001a). Background context and decision making in hoarding gray jays. *Behav. Ecol.* **12**: 318–24.

Waite, T. A. (2001b). Intransitive preferences in hoarding gray jays (*Perisoreus canadensis*). *Behav. Ecol. Sociobiol.* **50**: 116–21.

Waldman, M. (1994). Systematic errors and the theory of natural selection. *Am. Econ. Rev.* **84**: 482–497.

Welton, N. J. and A. I. Houston (2001). A theoretical investigation into the direct and indirect effects of state on the risk of predation. *J. Theor. Biol.* **123**: 275–97.

Wilson, B. (1974). *Rationality*. Oxford: Basil Blackwell.

Yazdanbakhsh, M., P. G. Kremsner, and R. van Ree (2002). Immunology: allergy, parasites, and the hygiene hypothesis. *Science* **296**: 490–94.

4 Optimised agent-based modelling of action selection

Anil K. Seth

Summary

The problem of action selection has two components: what is selected? How is it selected? To understand *what* is selected, it is necessary to recognise that animals do not choose among behaviours per se; rather, behaviour reflects observed interactions among brains, bodies, and environments (embeddedness). To understand what *guides* selection, it is useful to take a normative, functional perspective that evaluates behaviour in terms of a fitness metric. This perspective can be especially useful for understanding apparently irrational action selection. Bringing together these issues therefore requires integrating function and mechanism in models of action selection. This chapter describes 'optimised agent-based modelling', a methodology that integrates functional and mechanistic perspectives in the context of embedded agent–environment interactions. Using this methodology, I demonstrate that successful action selection can arise from the joint activity of parallel, loosely coupled sensorimotor processes, and I show how an instance of apparently suboptimal decision making (the matching law) can be accounted for by adaptation to competitive foraging environments.

4.1   Introduction

Life is all about action. Bodies and brains have been shaped by natural selection above all for the ability to produce the right action at the right time. This basic fact leads to two observations. First, the neural substrates underpinning action selection must encapsulate mechanisms for perception as well as those supporting motor movements (Friston, 2009), and their operations must be understood in terms of interactions among brains, bodies, and environments. In other words, action selection mechanisms are *embodied* and *embedded*. Second, despite the generality of action selection mechanisms, it is unlikely that they can deliver optimal behaviour in all possible situations. Action selection models therefore need to integrate functional and mechanistic perspectives (McNamara and Houston, 2009), especially when observed behaviour departs from what appears to be optimal or 'rational' (Houston *et al.*, this volume). The goal of this chapter is to describe

Modelling Natural Action Selection, eds. Anil K. Seth, Tony J. Prescott and Joanna J. Bryson.
Published by Cambridge University Press. © Cambridge University Press 2012.

and illustrate a methodology – *optimised agent-based modelling* (oABM; Seth, 2007) – that accommodates both of these observations, and to contrast this methodology with standard techniques in 'optimal foraging theory' (OFT; Stephens and Krebs, 1986). The central idea is that the oABM approach provides a unified framework for modelling natural action selection, 'rational' and otherwise.[1]

4.1.1   Embeddedness and optimal foraging theory

The concept of embeddedness stresses the essential distinction between behaviour and mechanism (Clark, 1997; Hallam and Malcolm, 1994; Hendriks-Jansen, 1996; Seth, 2002a). Very generally, behaviour can be defined as *observed ongoing agent– environment interactivity*, and mechanism as the *agent-side structure subserving this interactivity*. All behaviours (e.g., eating, swimming, building a house) depend on continuous patterns of interaction between agent and environment; there can be no eating without food, no house-building without bricks, no swimming without water. Moreover, external observers impose subjective biases on which segments of agent–environment interactivity warrant which behavioural labels. Different observers may (implicitly or explicitly) select different junctures in observed activity, or they may label the same segments differently. Therefore, critically, the agent-side mechanisms underlying the generation of behaviour should not be assumed to consist of internal correlates, or descriptions, of the behaviours themselves. Models that do not reach down into the details of sensorimotor interactions run the risk of falsely reifying behaviours by proposing mechanisms that incorporate, as components, descriptions of the behaviours they are intended to generate (Hallam and Malcolm, 1994; Seth, 2002a).

The above criticism applies, for instance, to most models within the tradition of OFT, which assumes that behaviour reflects an optimal solution to the problem posed by an environmental niche.[2] Standard OFT models consist of a decision variable, a currency, and a set of constraints (Stephens and Krebs, 1986). Take for example an OFT model of the redshank *Tringa totanus* foraging for worms of different sizes (Goss-Custard, 1977). The decision variable captures the type of choice the animal is assumed to make (e.g., whether a small worm is worth eating), the currency specifies the quantity that the animal is assumed to be maximising (e.g., rate of energy intake), and the constraints govern the relationship between the decision variable and the currency (e.g., the 'handling time' required to eat each worm and their relative prevalence). Given these components, an analytically solvable model can be constructed which predicts how the animal should behave in a particular environment in order to be optimal. Importantly, decision variables – and the foraging strategies that depend on them – are often framed in terms of distinct behaviours (i.e., do behaviour X rather than behaviour Y). This carries the assumption that animals make decisions among entities (behaviours) that are in fact joint products of agents, environments, and observers, and which may not be directly reflected in agent-side mechanisms. A consequence of this assumption is that, since behavioural

---

[1] This chapter is a revised and extended version of Seth (2007).
[2] OFT can be considered as a subset of the more general perspective of behavioural ecology.

complexity is not necessarily reflected in the underlying mechanisms, the complexity of an optimal foraging strategy may be overestimated.[3] Section 4.2 provides a concrete illustration of this reasoning.

4.1.2   Integrating function and mechanism

The importance of integrating function and mechanism is also exposed by OFT. OFT models do not reveal whether or not an animal 'optimises'. Rather, discrepancies between observed and predicted behaviour are taken to imply, either that the assumed currency is wrong, or that relevant constraints have been omitted from the model. In the latter case, one can further distinguish between environmental constraints (e.g., the handling time in the *Tringa totanus* example) and mechanistic constraints, reflecting the possibility that foraging strategies may not be arbitrarily flexible. Although often overlooked in OFT (McNamara and Houston, 2009), alternative perspectives such as ethology have long questioned the assumption of completely flexible behaviour (Tinbergen, 1963). A key challenge for models of action selection is therefore to integrate normative (functional) descriptions with mechanistic constraints. This challenge is exemplified when accounting for apparently suboptimal ('irrational') action selection. For example, many animals behave according to Herrnstein's *matching law*, in which responses are allocated in proportion to the reward obtained from each response (Herrnstein, 1961). Importantly, while matching behaviour is often optimal, it is not always so (see also Houston *et al.*, this volume). A useful framework for conceiving suboptimal behaviour is *ecological rationality*, the idea that cognitive mechanisms which fit the demands of particular ecological niches may deliver predictably suboptimal behaviour when operating outside these niches (Todd and Gigerenzer, 2000). Section 4.5 uses this concept to explore the possibility that matching behaviour may result from foraging in a competitive multi-agent environment.

4.1.3   Organisation

The remainder of this chapter is organised as follows. Section 4.2 describes the methodology of oABM, which aims to integrate function and mechanism in the context of embedded agent–environment interaction (Seth, 2000b; Seth, 2007). Section 4.3 reviews a selection of previous models of action selection and describes a simple oABM which describes a minimal mechanism for action selection that depends on the continuous and concurrent activity of multiple sensorimotor links (Seth, 1998). Section 4.4 describes a second oABM which tests the hypothesis that (potentially suboptimal) matching behaviour may reflect foraging behaviour adapted to a competitive group environment

---

[3] The problem of excessive computational and representational demands of optimal foraging strategies has been discussed extensively. One solution is to consider that animals adopt comparatively simple foraging strategies ('rules of thumb') that approximate optimality (see, for example, Houston and McNamara, 1984; Houston and McNamara, 1999; Iwasa *et al.*, 1981; Marshall *et al.*, this volume; McNamara and Houston, 1980). However, as long as these rules of thumb also utilise decision variables that mediate among distinct behaviours, the possibility of a mismatch between behavioural and mechanistic levels of description remains.

(Seth, 2001a). Section 4.5 models matching behaviour at a higher level of description, connecting more closely with OFT models that describe the equilibrium distribution of foragers over patchy resources (Fretwell, 1972; Seth, 2002b). Finally, Section 4.6 summarises and suggests avenues for future research.

4.2   Optimised agent-based modelling

The oABM methodology derives from the tradition of 'artificial life' and is distinguished by two key features:

1. The use of numerical optimisation algorithms (e.g., genetic algorithms; Mitchell, 1997) to optimise patterns of behaviour within the model with respect to some fitness criterion (e.g., maximisation of resource intake).
2. The modelling of agent–environment and agent–agent interactions at the level of situated perception and action, i.e., via the explicit modelling of sensor input and motor output.

The first of these features serves to *integrate function and mechanism*. More specifically, it provides a natural bridge between OFT models and standard agent-based models (ABMs).[4] OFT models incorporate a functional/normative criterion but generally do not consider aspects of mechanisms beyond arbitrary constructs such as decision variables. ABMs, which have become increasingly popular in ecological modelling (DeAngelis and Gross, 1992; Grimm, 1999; Grimm and Railsback, 2005; Huston *et al.*, 1988) (see also Part III – social action selection – of the present volume), explicitly instantiate individual agents in order to capture the dynamics of their interactions, and they explicitly model the environmental structure that scaffolds these interactions; however, in contrast to OFT standard ABMs generally do not disclose optimal behavioural strategies. The oABM methodology integrates these two modelling strategies. Specifically, ABMs can articulate a very broad range of mechanisms, selected aspects of which can be optimised using numerical techniques in order to ensure near-optimal behavioural solutions.[5]

   The oABM methodology can, in principle, be implemented using any numerical optimisation method. In practice, genetic algorithms (GAs) are suitable due to their flexibility and their extensive history of application to ABMs within artificial life (Mitchell, 1997).[6] A GA is a search algorithm loosely based on natural selection, in which a population of genotypes (e.g., a string of numbers) is decoded into phenotypes (e.g., a neural network controller) which are assessed by a fitness function (e.g., lifespan of the agent, quantity of resources acquired). The fittest individuals are selected to go forward into the

---

[4] I use the term ABM interchangeably with 'individual-based model' (IBM).

[5] This aspect of the oABM approach is similar to the 'evo-mecho' approach recently proposed by McNamara and Houston (2009).

[6] In related approaches such as evolutionary simulation models (Di Paolo *et al.*, 2000; Wheeler and de Bourcier, 1995), GAs are themselves the object of analysis insofar as the models aim to provide insight into evolutionary dynamics phenomena. In oABMs, GAs are used only to specify behaviour and mechanism; evolutionary dynamics per se are not studied.

subsequent generation, and mutation and/or recombination operators are applied to the genotypes of these individuals. Importantly and in contrast to standard OFT, there are few if any restrictions on genotype–phenotype encoding strategies, allowing a high degree of flexibility with regard to the range of potential mechanisms that can be optimised.[7]

The second feature of the oABM approach, modelling at the level of situated perception and action, ensures that oABM models take account of embeddedness and that they accommodate the essential distinction between mechanism and behaviour. From the oABM perspective, the proper mechanistic explanatory targets of action selection are selective mechanisms in both sensory and motor domains that ensure the adaptive coordination of behaviour, which can then be interpreted from a functional point of view by an external observer. An example of a situated architecture would be an artificial neuronal network that translates sensory input, obtained from the perspective of the agent, into motor output; an oABM of just this type is described in the following section. Of course, the first and second features of the oABM approach are closely related; it is because optimisation methods can be applied to arbitrary mechanisms that it becomes possible to implement and explore mechanisms that are properly embodied and embedded.[8]

In short, the oABM approach advocates the construction of computational simulation models which explicitly instantiate internal architectures and environmental constraints, and which generate behaviour via the application of optimisation techniques such as GAs. As I have argued, this approach recognises and operationalises important conceptual distinctions among mechanism, behaviour, and function. It is not, however, without disadvantages. In particular, in common with most simulation modelling and in contrast to standard OFT, oABM models may lack analytical transparency. That is, it may be very difficult or impossible to prove general statements about oABM behaviour. Rather, the models need to be run repeatedly and the data they generate treated in the same way as data garnered from experiments on (non-simulated) biological systems. Nonetheless, it is worth summarising some specific advantages of oABMs over analytic OFT approaches:

- The progressive relaxation of constraints is often easier in a simulation model than in analytically solvable models. For example, representation of non-homogeneous resource distributions can rapidly become intractable for analytic models (see Laver *et al.*, this volume).
- There is no need to assume an explicit decision variable (although such variables can be incorporated if deemed appropriate). Construction of oABMs without explicit decision variables broadens the space of possible internal mechanisms for the implementation

---

[7] GAs cannot guarantee exactly optimal solutions. They may fail to find such solutions for a number of reasons, including insufficient search time, insufficient genetic diversity in the initial population, and overly rugged fitness landscapes in which there exist many local fitness maxima and/or in which genetic operations have widely varying fitness consequences. However, for present purposes it is not necessary that GAs always find exactly optimal solutions. It is sufficient that GAs instantiate a *process* of optimisation so that the resulting behaviour patterns and agent mechanisms can be interpreted from a normative perspective.

[8] The emphasis on embeddedness does not imply that models at higher levels of abstraction are necessarily less valuable. With careful interpretation of the relation between behaviour and mechanism, such models can provide equally useful insights (see Section 4.5).

of foraging strategies, and, in particular, facilitates the generation and evaluation of hypotheses concerning comparatively simple internal mechanisms.

- oABMs are well suited to incorporate *historical* or *stigmergic* constraints that arise from the history of agent–environment interactions, by providing a sufficiently rich medium in which such interactions can create dynamical invariants which constrain, direct, or canalise the future dynamics of the system (Di Paolo *et al.*, 2000). Examples can be found in the construction of termite mounds, or in the formation of ant graveyards.

The above features together offer a distinct strategy for pursuing optimality modelling of behaviour. Standard OFT models are usually incrementally complex. Failures in prediction are attributed to inadequate representation of constraints, prompting a revision of the model. However, only certain aspects of standard OFT models – constraints and currencies – can be incrementally revised. Others, such as the presence of a decision variable, or the absence of situated perception and action, are much harder to manipulate within an analytically tractable framework. oABMs, being simulation-based, can bring into focus aspects of OFT models that are either explicit but potentially unnecessary (e.g., decision variables), or implicit and usually ignored (e.g., embeddedness, historical constraints). Thus, in contrast to an incremental increase in model complexity, oABMs offer the possibility of radically reconfiguring the assumption structure of an optimality model.

4.3   Embedded models of action selection

Recent 'embedded' models of action selection were pioneered by Brooks' subsumption architecture (Brooks, 1986) and by Maes' spreading activation control architecture (Maes, 1990; see Figure 4.1). Brooks decomposed an agent's control structure into a set of task-achieving 'competences' organised into layers, with higher layers subsuming the goals of lower layers and with lower layers interrupting higher layers. For Maes, an organism comprises a 'set of behaviours' with action selection arising via 'parallel local interactions among behaviours and between behaviours and the environment' (Maes, 1990, pp. 238–9). These architectures can be related to ethological principles developed more than 50 years ago by Tinbergen and Lorenz, who considered action selection to depend on a combination of environmental 'sign stimuli' and 'action-specific energy', activating either specific 'behaviour centres' (Tinbergen, 1950) or 'fixed action patterns' (Lorenz, 1937 [1957]). A key issue for these early models was the utility of hierarchical architectures, with some authors viewing hierarchical structure as an essential organising principle (Dawkins, 1976), while others noted that strict hierarchies involve the loss of information at every decision point (Maes, 1990; Rosenblatt and Payton, 1989).

Over the past decade, simulation models of action selection have progressively refined the notion of hierarchical control. In a frequently cited thesis, Tyrrell revised Maes' spreading activation architecture to incorporate *soft-selection* (Rosenblatt and Payton, 1989) in which competing behaviours expressed preferences rather than entering a

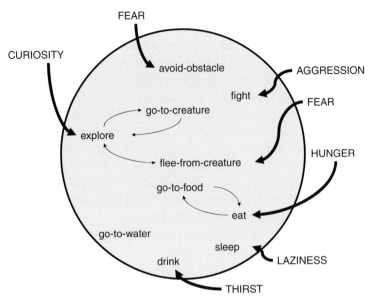

Figure 4.1 Decentralised spreading activation action selection architecture adapted from Maes (1990). Agent behaviour is determined by interactions among internal representations of candidate behaviours, modulated by drives (e.g., curiosity). Notice that the internal mechanism (within the circle) consists of internal correlates of behaviours.

winner-take-all competition (Tyrrell, 1993). At around the same time, Blumberg incorporated inhibition and fatigue into a hierarchical model in order to improve the temporal sequencing of behaviour (Blumberg, 1994). Some years later, Bryson demonstrated that a combination of hierarchical and reactive control outperformed fully parallelised architectures in the action selection task developed by Tyrrell (Bryson, 2000).

Although space limitations preclude a comprehensive review of alternative modelling approaches to action selection, it is worth briefly noting three currently active directions. One is the incorporation of reinforcement learning (Sutton and Barto, 1998), with a recent emphasis on the influences of motivation (Dayan, 2002) and uncertainty (Yu and Dayan, 2005). The second is the incorporation of neuroanatomical constraints, as covered in detail in Part II of the present volume. Notably, Redgrave and colleagues have proposed that the vertebrate basal ganglia implement a winner-take-all competition among inputs with different saliences (Redgrave *et al.*, 1999; see also Hazy *et al.*, this volume). Finally, Friston has recently suggested that effective action selection can take place without any explicit notion of value or salience, but rather as a consequence of a fundamental biological process of minimising informational 'free energy' which corresponds to avoiding surprising exchanges with the world (Friston, 2009; Friston *et al.*, 2009). I return to these issues in Section 4.6.

A feature of many models of action selection (hierarchical or otherwise) is that, on the mechanistic level, they arbitrate among an internal repertoire of behaviours. However, I have already suggested that this assumption is conceptually wrong-headed in that it confuses behavioural and mechanistic levels of description. To illustrate how the oABM approach can successfully avoid such confusion, I now describe a simple oABM designed to show that action selection, at least in a simple situation, need not require internal arbitration among explicitly represented behaviours (Seth, 1998). The architecture of this model was inspired both by Pfeifer's notion of 'parallel, loosely coupled processes' (Pfeifer, 1996) and by Braitenberg's elegant series of thought experiments suggesting that complex behaviour can arise from surprisingly simple internal mechanisms (Braitenberg, 1984). The simulated agent and its environment are shown in Figure 4.2.[9] Briefly, the simulated environment contains three varieties of objects: two types of food (grey and black) as well as 'traps' (open circles, which 'kill' the agent upon contact). The closest instance of each object type can be detected by the agent's sensors. The agent contains two 'batteries' – grey and black – which correspond to the two food types. These batteries diminish at a steady rate and if either becomes empty the agent 'dies'. Encounter with a food item fully replenishes the corresponding battery.

Each sensor is connected directly to the motor output via a set of three *sensorimotor links* (Figure 4.2b). Each link transforms a sensory input signal into a motor output signal via a transfer function, the shape of which can be modulated by the level of one of the two batteries (dashed lines). Left and right wheel speeds are determined by summing motor output signals from all the corresponding links. A GA was used to evolve the shape of each transfer function as well as the parameters governing battery modulation. The fitness function rewarded agents that lived long and that maintained a high average level in both batteries.

Figure 4.2c shows an example of the behaviour of an evolved agent. The agent consumed a series of food items of both types, displayed opportunistic behaviour at point x by consuming a nearby grey item even though it had just consumed such an item, and successfully backtracked to avoid traps at points y and z. Overall agent behaviour was evaluated by a set of behavioural criteria for successful action selection (Table 4.1). Performance on these criteria was evaluated both by analysis of behaviour within the natural environment of the agent (e.g., Figure 4.2c) and by analysis of contrived 'laboratory' situations designed to test specific criteria. For example, the balance between dithering and persistence was tested by placing an evolved agent in between a group of three grey items and a group of three black items. These analyses demonstrated that the evolved agents satisfied all the relevant criteria (Seth, 1998, 2000a).

Examples of evolved transfer functions are shown in Figure 4.2d. Each of these transfer functions showed modulation by a battery level, and each set of three functions was influenced by both batteries (e.g., sensorimotor links sensitive to 'grey' food were modulated by internal levels of *both* grey *and* black batteries). Further analysis of the evolved transfer functions (Seth, 2000a) showed switching between consummatory and appetitive modes (e.g., via a nonlinear response to distance from a food item), and implicit prioritisation (e.g., via disinhibition of forward movement with low battery levels).

It is important to emphasise that this model is intended as a conceptual exercise in what is selected during action selection. Analysis of the model shows that it is possible

---

[9] Full details of the implementation are provided in electronic supplementary material of Seth (2007).

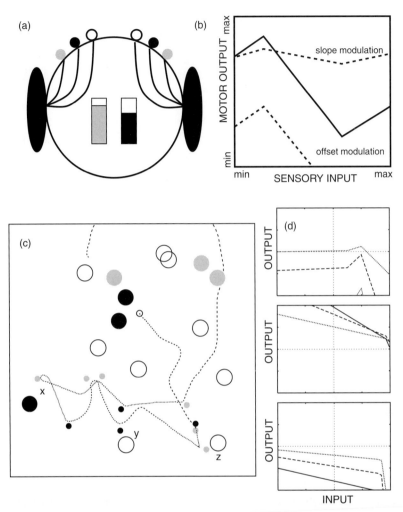

Figure 4.2 A minimal model of action selection. (a) Architecture of the simulated agent. Each wheel is connected to three sensors which respond to distance to the nearest food item (grey and black circles) and 'trap' (large open circles). The agent has two 'batteries' which are replenished by the corresponding food types. (b) The structure of a sensorimotor link (each connection in panel A consists of three of these links). Each link maps a sensory input value into a motor output value via a transfer function (solid line). The 'slope' and the 'offset' of this function can be modulated by the level of one of the two batteries (dashed lines). The transfer function and the parameters governing modulation are encoded as integer values for evolution using a genetic algorithm. (c) Behaviour of an evolved agent (small circles depict consumed resources). The agent displayed opportunistic behaviour at point x by consuming a nearby grey item even though it had just consumed such an item, and showed backtracking to avoid traps at points y and z. (d) Shapes of three example sensorimotor links following evolution [solid line shows the transfer function, dashed and dotted lines show modulation due to low (dashed) and very low (dotted) battery levels].

Table 4.1 Criteria for successful action selection, drawn from Werner (1994).

1 Prioritise behaviour according to current internal requirements.
2 Allow contiguous behavioural sequences to be strung together.
3 Exhibit opportunism; for example, by diverting to a nearby 'grey' food item even if there is a greater immediate need for 'black' food.
4 Balance dithering and persistence; for example, by drinking until full and then eating until full instead of oscillating between eating and drinking.
5 Interrupt current behaviour; for example, by changing course to avoid the sudden appearance of a dangerous object.
6 Privilege *consummatory* actions (i.e., those that are of immediate benefit to the agent, such as eating) over *appetitive* actions (i.e., those that set up conditions in which consummatory actions become more likely).
7 Use all available information.
8 Support real-valued sensors and produce directly usable outputs.

for a simple form of action selection to arise from the concurrent activity of multiple sensorimotor processes with no clear distinctions among sensation, internal processing, or action; without internal behavioural correlates or decision variables, and without any explicit process of internal arbitration. These observations raise the possibility that mechanisms of action selection may not reflect behavioural categories derived by an external observer, and, as a result, may be less complex than supposed on this basis. They also suggest that perceptual selective mechanisms may be as important as motor mechanisms for successful action selection (Cisek, this volume). Having said this, it must be recognised that the particular mechanism implemented in the model is not reflected in biological systems, and may not deliver adaptive behaviour in more complex environments. It is possible that action selection in complex environments will be better served by modular mechanisms that may be more readily scalable in virtue of having fewer interdependencies among functional units. Modularity may also enhance evolvability, the facility with which evolution is able to discover adaptive solutions (Prescott *et al.*, 1999; Wagner and Altenberg, 1996). These issues remain to be decided empirically.

4.4   Probability matching and inter-forager interference

For the remainder of this chapter, the oABM approach is applied to the problem of *suboptimal* action selection, via an exploration of 'matching' behaviour. I first introduce and differentiate two distinct forms of matching: probability matching and the matching law. This section focuses on probability matching, the following section will address the matching law (see also Houston *et al.*, this volume).

In 1961, Richard Herrnstein observed that pigeons match the frequency of their responses to different stimuli in proportion to the rewards *obtained* from each stimulus type (Herrnstein, 1961), a 'matching law' subsequently found to generalise to a wide range of species (Davison and McCarthy, 1988). By contrast, probability matching describes behaviour in which the distribution of responses is matched to the reward probabilities, i.e., the *available* reward (Bitterman, 1965). The difference between these two forms of matching is well illustrated by a simple example. Consider two response alternatives A and B which deliver a fixed reward with probabilities 0.7 and 0.3, respectively. Probability matching would predict that the organism chooses A on 70% of trials and B on 30% of trials. This allocation of responses does *not* satisfy the matching law; the organism would obtain ~85% of its reward from A and ~15% from B. Moreover, probability matching in this example is suboptimal. Clearly, reward maximisation would be achieved by responding exclusively to A. Optimal behaviour does, however, satisfy the matching law, although in a trivial manner: by choosing A in 100% of trials, it is ensured that A is responsible for 100% of the reward obtained. Note, however, that matching does not guarantee optimality: exclusive choice of B would also satisfy the matching law.

Empirical evidence regarding probability matching is mixed. Many studies indicate that both humans and non-human animals show (suboptimal) probability matching in a variety of situations (see Erev and Barron, 2005; Myers, 1976; Vulkan, 2000 for reviews). In human subjects, however, substantial deviations from probability matching have been observed (Friedman and Massaro, 1998; Gluck and Bower, 1988; Silberberg *et al.*, 1991). According to Shanks and colleagues, probability matching in humans can be reduced by increasing reward incentive, providing explicit feedback about correct (i.e., optimal) responses, and allowing extensive training (Shanks *et al.*, 2002). West and Stanovich (2003) found that suboptimal probability matching was rarer in subjects with higher cognitive ability. Although a clear consensus is lacking, it remains likely that probability matching, at least in non-human animals, is a robust phenomenon.

How can this apparently irrational behaviour be accounted for? One possibility is that probability matching may result from reinforcement learning in the context of balancing exploitation and exploration (Niv *et al.*, 2001). Another is that simple behavioural heuristics such as 'win–stay, lose–shift' can generate matching behaviour (Vulkan, 2000). Recently, Gaissmaier and Schooler (2008) proposed that probability matching results from failed attempts to extract patterns from random data, though their conclusions have been contested (Koehler and James, 2009). Here, I explore the different hypothesis that probability matching can arise, in the absence of lifetime learning, as a result of adaptation to a competitive foraging environment (Seth, 1999; Seth, 2001a; see also Houston, 1986; Houston and McNamara, 1988; Houston and Sumida, 1987). The intuition, in the spirit of ecological rationality, is as follows. In an environment containing resources of different values, foragers in the presence of conspecifics may experience different levels of interference with respect to each resource type, where interference refers to the reduction in resource intake as a result of competition among foragers (Seth, 2001b; Sutherland, 1983). Maximisation of overall intake may therefore require distributing responses across resource types, as opposed to responding exclusively to the rich resource type.

To test this hypothesis, I extended the oABM model described in the previous section such that the environment contains two resource types (grey and black) as well as a

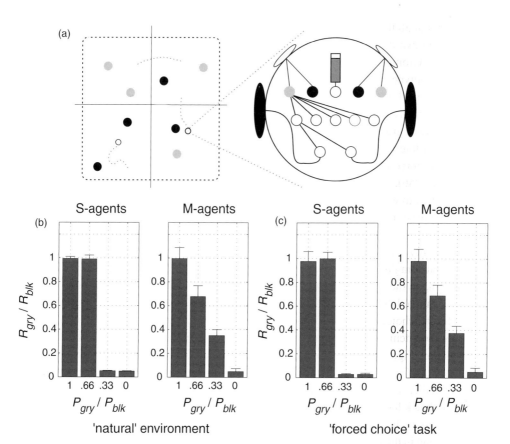

Figure 4.3 Probability matching. (a) Schematic of the simulated environment, containing multiple agents (open circles) and two types of food (grey and black circles). The expansion shows the internal architecture of an agent, which consists of a feedforward neural network (for clarity only a subset of connections are shown). Four of the five input sensors respond to the two food types (grey, black); the fifth sensor input responds to the level of an internal 'battery' (middle). The outputs control left and right wheel speeds. (b) Summary of behaviour when agents were tested in the environment in which they were evolved. Each column represents a set of ten evolutionary runs with the abscissa (x axis) showing the resource distribution, and the ordinate (y axis) showing the proportion of responses to grey food. Agents evolved in isolation (S-agents) showed either indifference or exclusive choice (zero-one behaviour), whereas agents evolved in competitive foraging environments (M-agents) showed probability matching. (c) Summary of behaviour when evolved agents were tested in a forced-choice task (see text), in which probability matching is suboptimal. As in panel B, S-agents showed zero–one behaviour, whereas M-agents showed matching behaviour.

variable number of agents (Figure 4.3a). Each agent has a single internal 'battery', and each resource type is associated with a probability that consumption fully replenishes the battery (P_{gry}, P_{blk}). Each agent is controlled by a simple feedforward neural network (Figure 4.3b) in which four input units respond to the nearest resource of each type (grey and black) and a fifth to the internal battery level, and in which the two outputs control the wheels. A GA was used to evolve parameters of the network controller, including the weights of all the connections and the sensitivity of the sensors to the different resource types, in two different conditions. In the first (condition S), there was only one agent in the environment. In the second (condition M), there were three identical agents (i.e., each genotype in the GA was decoded into three 'clones'). In each condition, agents were evolved in four different environments reflecting different resource distributions. In each environment, black food always replenished the battery ($P_{blk} = 1.0$), whereas the value of grey food (P_{gry}) was chosen from the set $\{1.0, 0.66, 0.33, 0.0\}$.

According to the hypothesis, agents evolved in condition S (S-agents) should treat each resource type in an all-or-none manner (zero–one behaviour; see Stephens and Krebs, 1986), whereas agents evolved in condition M (M-agents) should match their responses to each resource type according to the value of each resource. Results were supportive of the hypothesis. Figure 4.3b shows the proportion of responses to grey food as a function of P_{gry}: whereas S-agents showed zero–one behaviour, M-agents showed probability matching. This suggests that, in the model, zero–one behaviour reflects optimal foraging for an isolated agent, and that probability matching reflects optimal foraging in the competitive foraging environment.

To mimic laboratory tests of probability matching, evolved agents were also tested in a 'forced-choice' task in which they were repeatedly placed equidistant from a single grey food item and a single black food item; both S-agents and M-agents were tested in isolation. Figure 4.3c shows the same pattern of results as in Figure 4.3b, i.e., zero–one behaviour for S-agents and matching behaviour for M-agents. Importantly, in this case probability matching is not optimal for $P_{gry} < 1$ (optimal behaviour would be always to select black food). This result therefore shows that suboptimal probability matching can arise from adaptation to a competitive foraging environment. It is also noteworthy that matching in the model is generated by simple sensorimotor interactions during foraging, as opposed to requiring any dedicated decision-making mechanism.

Further analysis of the model (Seth, 2001a) showed that probability matching arose as an adaptation to patterns of resource instability (upon consumption, a food item disap-peared and reappeared at a different random location). These patterns were generated by sensorimotor interactions among agents and food items during foraging; moreover, they represented historical constraints in the sense that they reflected dynamical invariants that constrained the future dynamics of the system. Both situated agent–environment interactions and rich historical constraints reflect key features of the oABM modelling approach.

4.5   Matching and the ideal free distribution

Recall that Herrnstein's formulation of the matching law predicts that organisms match the frequency of their responses to different stimuli in proportion to the rewards *obtained* from each stimulus type (Herrnstein, 1961). In the model described in the previous section, Herrnstein's law could only be satisfied in the trivial cases of exclusive choice or equal response to both food types. In order to establish a closer correspondence between Herrnstein's matching law and optimal foraging theory, this section describes a model that abstracts away from the details of situated perception and action.

Herrnstein's matching law can be written as:

$$\log \frac{B_A}{B_B} = \log(b) + s \log \frac{R_A}{R_B}, \tag{4.1}$$

where B_A and B_B represent numbers of responses to options A and B, respectively, and R_A and R_B represent resources obtained from options A and B; b and s are bias and sensitivity parameters that can be tuned to account for different data (Baum, 1974). There is robust experimental evidence that in many situations in which matching and reward maximisation are incompatible, humans and other animals will behave according to the matching law (Davison and McCarthy, 1988). Herrnstein's preferred explanation of matching, *melioration*, proposes that the distribution of behaviour shifts towards alternatives that have higher immediate value, regardless of the consequences for overall reinforcement (Herrnstein and Vaughan, 1980). However, melioration, which echoes Thorndike's 'law of effect' (Thorndike, 1911), is a general principle and not a specific mechanistic rule. More recently, a variety of specific mechanisms have been proposed to account for matching. These include a synaptic plasticity rule based on covariance between reward and neural activity (Loewenstein and Seung, 2006), actor–critic learning architectures (Sakai and Fukai, 2008), and, very recently, a suggestion that matching may reflect a Nash equilibrium resulting from mutual defection among multiple 'selves' in an intertemporal prisoner's dilemma (Loewenstein *et al.*, 2009).

Here, I take a different approach, noting that the mathematical form of the matching law is strikingly similar to that of a key concept in OFT: the *ideal free distribution* (IFD). The IFD describes the optimal distribution of foragers (such that no forager can profit by moving elsewhere) in a multi-'patch' environment, where each patch may offer different resource levels (Fretwell, 1972). For a two patch environment, the IFD is written as (Fagen, 1987):

$$\log \frac{N_A}{N_B} = \frac{1}{m} \log \frac{F_A}{F_B}, \tag{4.2}$$

where N_A and N_B represent the number of foragers on patches A and B respectively, F_A and F_B represent the resource densities on patches A and B, and m is an interference constant [0–1]. Field data suggest that many foraging populations fit the IFD (Weber, 1998); an innovative study also found that humans approximated the IFD when foraging in a virtual environment implemented by networked computers in a psychology laboratory (Goldstone and Ashpole, 2004). The concept of the IFD allows the hypothesis of the previous section to be restated with greater clarity: foraging behaviour that leads a population of agents to the IFD may lead individual agents to obey the matching law.

What action selection mechanism could lead both to matching and to the IFD? More than 20 years ago, Harley showed that a *relative payoff sum* (RPS) learning rule, according to which the probability of a response is proportional to its payoff in proportion to the total payoff, leads individual agents to match and leads populations to the IFD (Harley, 1981; Houston and Sumida, 1987). However, it is not surprising that the RPS rule leads to matching since the rule itself directly reflects the matching law; moreover, the RPS rule is computationally costly because it requires all response probabilities to be recalculated at every moment in time. Here, I explore the properties of an alternative foraging strategy, ω-sampling (Seth, 2002b). Unlike the RPS rule, ω-sampling is a moment-to-moment foraging rule (Charnov, 1976; Krebs and Kacelnik, 1991) which does not require response probabilities to be continually recalculated. In the context of the matching law, ω-sampling is related to strategies based on momentary maximisation which specify selection of the best alternative at any given time (Hinson and Staddon, 1983; Shimp, 1966). In a two-patch environment, a ω-sampler initially selects patch A or patch B at random. At each subsequent time step the other patch is sampled with probability p, otherwise the estimate of the current patch is compared with that of the unselected patch, and switching occurs if the former is the lower of the two. The estimate of the current patch (or the sampled patch) is updated at each time step such that more recent rewards are represented more strongly. A formal description of ω-sampling is given in Appendix A.

To test the ability of ω-sampling to lead a population of agents to the IFD, the equilibrium distribution (after 1000 time steps) of 100 ω-samplers was recorded, in a two-patch environment in which each patch provided a reward to each agent, at each time step, as a function of conspecific density, interference (m in Equation (4.2)), and a patch-specific resource density. Figure 4.4a shows equilibrium distributions under various resource density distributions, and with two different levels of interference ($m = 1.0, m = 0.3$). The equilibrium distributions closely match the IFD, indicating that ω-sampling supports optimal foraging in the model.

Figure 4.4b shows the foraging behaviour of individual (isolated) ω-sampling agents under four different reinforcement schedules which reflect those used in experimental studies of matching. In the basic schedule, reward rate is directly proportional to response rate. Empirical data indicate that animals respond exclusively to the most profitable option under this schedule (Davison and McCarthy, 1988), which maximises reward and which also trivially satisfies the matching law. In line with this data, ω-sampling agents also show exclusive choice. In the VR VR (concurrent variable ratio) schedule, each patch must receive a (variable) number of responses before a reward is given. Under this schedule, reward maximisation is again achieved by exclusive choice of the most profitable option. Empirical evidence is more equivocal in this case. As noted in the previous section, although probability matching appears to be a robust phenomenon, many examples of maximisation have been observed (Davison and McCarthy, 1988; Herrnstein, 1997). The behaviour of ω-sampling agents reflects this evidence, showing a preponderance of exclusive choice with occasional deviations. In the VI VI (concurrent variable interval) schedule, which is widely used in matching experiments, a (variable) time delay for each patch must elapse between consecutive rewards. Under this schedule, reward probabilities are non-stationary, reward rate can be largely independent of response rate, and exclusive choice is not optimal. Importantly, matching behaviour can be achieved with a variety of response distributions, including (but not limited to) exclusive choice. The behaviour of ω-samplers is again in line with empirical data in showing matching to obtained reward, in this case without exclusive choice. The final schedule, VI VR, is a mixed schedule in which one patch is rewarded

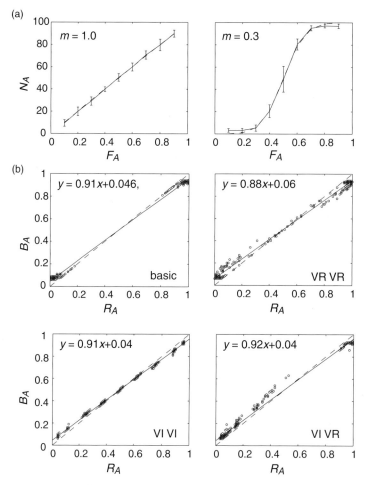

Figure 4.4 (a) Equilibrium population distributions of 100 ω-sampling agents with high interference ($m = 1$) and low interference ($m = 0.3$) in a two-patch environment (patches A and B). F_A shows the proportion of resources in patch A, N_A shows the percentage of the population on patch A. The distribution predicted by the ideal free distribution (IFD) is indicated by the dashed line. (b) Matching performance in four conditions: basic (reward is directly proportional to response), concurrent variable ratio (VR VR), concurrent variable interval (VI VI), and mixed variable interval and variable ratio (VI VR) (see text for details). R_A shows the reward obtained from patch A, B_A shows proportion of time spent on patch A. Matching to obtained resources is shown by the dashed diagonal line. Equations give lines of best fit.

according to a variable interval schedule, and the other according to a variable ratio schedule. Unlike the previous schedules, matching to obtained reward under VI VR is *not* optimal. Nevertheless, both empirical data (Davison and McCarthy, 1988; Herrnstein, 1997) and the behaviour of ω-sampling agents (Figure 4.4b) accord with the matching law.

Together, the above results show that a foraging strategy (ω-sampling) that leads foragers to the optimal (equilibrium) distribution in a competitive foraging environment (the

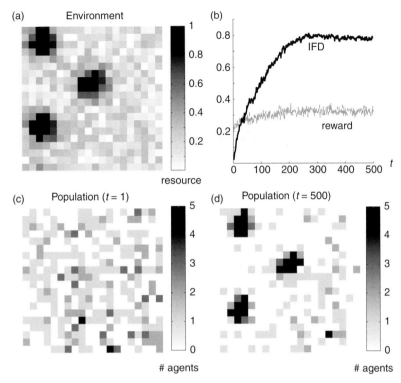

Figure 4.5 Foraging behaviour of 300 ω-sampling agents in an environment with 400 patches (interference $m = 0.5$). (a) Distribution of resources, normalised to maximum across all patches. (b) Match between resource distribution and forager distribution (solid line, IFD) and mean reward (grey dashed line, intake) as a function of time. (c) Initial population distribution. (d) Population distribution after 500 time steps; the population distribution mirrors the resource distribution.

IFD), also leads individual foragers to obey Herrnstein's matching law.[10] Importantly, ω-samplers obey the matching law even when it is suboptimal to do so. Interestingly, VI VI and VI VR schedules involve a non-stationary component (the VI schedule), which may be a common feature of ecological situations in which resources are depleted by foraging and replenished by abstinence.

A final analysis shows that the optimal foraging ability of ω-sampling generalises beyond the two-patch case. Figure 4.5 shows the distribution of 300 ω-sampling agents in an environment consisting of 400 patches in which resources were distributed so as to create three resource density peaks (Figure 4.5a). Agents maintained estimates of the five most recently visited patches, and were able to move, at each time step, to any patch

---

[10] Thuisjman *et al.* (1995) had made similar claims for a related moment-to-moment strategy (ε-sampling), in which foragers retained only a single estimate of environmental quality, as opposed to the multiple estimates required by ω-sampling. However, ε-sampling agents fail to match to obtained reward under the critical VI VI and VI VR schedules (Seth, 2007).

within a radius of three patches. Figure 4.5b–d shows that the distribution of agents, after 500 time steps, closely mirrored the resource distribution, indicating optimal foraging.

4.6   Discussion

If 'all behaviour is choice' (Herrnstein, 1970), then an adequate understanding of action selection will require a broad integration of many disciplines including ecology, psychology, and neuroscience. Ecology provides naturalistic behavioural data as well as a normative perspective, neuroscience and psychology provide controlled experimental conditions as well as insight into internal mechanisms. Successful modelling of action selection will therefore require a computational *lingua franca* to mediate among these disciplines. This chapter has identified steps towards such a lingua franca by describing oABMs which bridge the methods of (normative) OFT and (descriptive) ABMs. oABMs involve explicitly instantiated agents and structured environments (possibly incorporating situated perception and action), as well as a normative component provided by genetic algorithms. I described a series of oABMs showing (1) that successful action selection can arise from the joint activity of parallel, loosely coupled sensorimotor processes, (2) that an instance of apparently suboptimal action selection (matching) can be accounted for by adaptation to a competitive foraging environment.

Ecology has been distinguished by a long tradition of agent-based modelling (DeAngelis and Gross, 1992; Grimm, 1999; Grimm and Railsback, 2005; Huston *et al.*, 1988; Judson, 1994), and recent attention has been given to theoretical analysis and unifying frameworks for such models (Grimm *et al.*, 2005; McNamara and Houston, 2009; Pascual, 2005). Within this context, there are many interesting future challenges in the domain of action selection:

- What features of functional neuroanatomy support optimal action selection? A useful approach would be to incorporate into oABMs more detailed internal mechanisms based, for example, on models of the basal ganglia ((Redgrave *et al.*, 1999; Houk *et al.*, this volume) or on other aspects of the neural mechanisms underlying decision making (Kable and Glimcher, 2009)).
- How do historical/stigmergic constraints affect optimal action selection? Incorporation of situated perception and action into oABMs provides a rich medium for the exploration of historical constraints in a variety of action selection situations.
- How can reinforcement learning be combined with optimality modelling in accounting both for rational, and apparently irrational, action selection? This challenge leads into the territory of behavioural economics (Kahneman and Tversky, 2000) and neuroeconomics (Glimcher and Rustichini, 2004).
- What role do attentional mechanisms play in action selection? oABMs phrased at the level of situated perception and action allow analysis of the influence of perceptual selective mechanisms on behaviour coordination.

Finally, it is heartening to see that there is an increasing recognition of the need to engage in a broader, multi-disciplinary approach to modelling natural action selection. In a recent review, McNamara and Houston (2009) wrote that 'despite the fact that [integration of function and mechanism] has been advocated by many authors for decades, much remains to be done and this integration requires a new impetus'. It is hoped that their article, the present chapter, and an increasing volume of other relevant work, will go some way towards providing that impetus.

Acknowledgements

Drs Jason Fleischer, Alasdair Houston, Emmet Spier, Joanna Bryson, and two anonymous reviewers read a previous version of this manuscript and made a number of useful suggestions. The author is supported by EPSRC Leadership Fellowship EP/G007543/1 and by a donation from the Dr Mortimer and Theresa Sackler foundation.

Appendix A
ω-sampling

Let $\gamma \in [0,1]$ (adaptation rate), and $\varepsilon \in [0,1]$ (sampling rate). Let $M(t) \in \{A, B\}$ represent the patch selected, let $N(t) \in \{A, B\}$ represent the unselected patch, and let $r(t)$ be the reward obtained, at time $t \in \{1,2,3, \ldots, T\}$. Let $E_A(t)$ and $E_B(t)$ represent the estimated values of patches A, B at time t. Define $E_A(1) = E_A(1) = 0$.

For $t \geq 1$, if $M(t) = \mathbf{A}$:

$$E_A(t+1) = \gamma E_A(t) + (1-\gamma)r(t), \; E_B(t+1) = E_B(t), \tag{A.1}$$

otherwise (if $M(t) = \mathbf{B}$):

$$E_A(t+1) = E_A(t), \; E_B(t+1) = \gamma E_B(t) + (1-\gamma)r(t). \tag{A.2}$$

Let $\chi \in [0,1]$ be a random number. Let $A_\varepsilon, B_\varepsilon$ denote the behaviour of choosing patch (**A,B**) with probability (1-ε). The ω-sampling strategy is then defined by playing:

At $t = 1$ use $A_{0.5}$
At $t = 2$ use $M(1)_\varepsilon$
At $t > 2$,

if $\chi < \varepsilon$ or $E_M(t-1) < E_N(t-1)$ choose patch $N(t-1)$,
otherwise choose patch $M(t-1)$.

This strategy has two free parameters: γ and ε. In Seth (2002b), a GA was used to specify values for these parameters for each experimental condition separately. Following evolution, mean parameter values were $\gamma = 0.427$, $\varepsilon = 0.052$.

References

Baum, W. M. (1974). On two types of deviation from the matching law: Bias and undermatching. *J. Exp. Anal. Behav.* **22**: 231–42.
Bitterman, M. E. (1965). Phyletic differences in learning. *Am. Psychol.* **20**: 396–410.

Blumberg, B. (1994). Action selection in Hamsterdam: lessons from ethology. In *From Animals to Animats 3: Proceedings of the Third International Conference on the Simulation of Adaptive Behavior*, ed. D. Cliff, P. Husbands, J. A. Meyer, and S. Wilson. Cambridge, MA: MIT Press, pp. 107–116.

Braitenberg, V. (1984). *Vehicles: Experiments in Synthetic Psychology*. Cambridge, MA: MIT Press.

Brooks, R. A. (1986). A robust layered control system for a mobile robot. *IEEE J. Robotic. Autom.* **2**: 14–23.

Bryson, J. J. (2000). Hierarchy and sequence versus full parallelism in reactive action selection architectures. In *From Animals to Animats 6: Proceedings of the Sixth International Conference on the Simulation of Adaptive Behavior*, ed. J. A. Meyer, A. Berthoz, D. Floreano, H. Roitblat, and S. Wilson. Cambridge, MA: MIT Press, pp. 147–56.

Charnov, E. (1976). Optimal foraging: the marginal value theorem. *Theor. Popul. Biol.* **9**: 129–36.

Clark, A. (1997). *Being There. Putting Brain, Body, and World Together Again*. Cambridge, MA: MIT Press.

Davison, M. and D. McCarthy (1988). *The Matching Law*. Hillsdale, NJ: Erlbaum.

Dawkins, R. (1976). Hierarchical organisation: a candidate principle for ethology. In *Growing Points in Ethology*, ed. P. Bateson and R. Hinde. Cambridge: Cambridge University Press, pp. 7–54.

Dayan, P. (2002). Motivated reinforcement learning. In *Advances in Neural Information Processing Systems*, Vol. 14, ed. T. G. Dietterich, S. Becker, and Z. Ghahramani. Cambridge, MA: MIT Press, pp. 11–18.

DeAngelis, D. L. and L. J. Gross, (eds.) (1992). *Individual-Based Models and Approaches in Ecology: Populations, Communities and Ecosystems*. London: Chapman and Hall.

Di Paolo, E., J. Noble, and S. Bullock (2000). Simulation models as opaque thought experiments. In *Artificial Life VII: The Seventh International Conference on the Simulation and Synthesis of Living Systems*, ed. M. A. Bedau, J. S. McCaskill, N. H. Packard, and S. Rasmussen. Portland, OR: MIT Press, pp. 497–506.

Erev, I. and G. Barron (2005). On adaptation, maximization, and reinforcement learning among cognitive strategies. *Psychol. Rev.* **112**: 912–31.

Fagen, R. (1987). A generalized habitat matching law. *Evol. Ecol.* **1**: 5–10.

Fretwell, S. (1972). *Populations in Seasonal Environments*. Princeton, NJ: Princeton University Press.

Friedman, D. and D. W. Massaro (1998). Understanding variability in binary and continuous choice. *Psycho. B. Rev.* **5**: 370–89.

Friston, K. (2009). The free-energy principle: a rough guide to the brain? *Trends Cogn. Sci.* **13**: 293–301.

Friston, K. J., J. Daunizeau, and S. J. Kiebel (2009). Reinforcement learning or active inference? *PLoS One* **4**: e6421.

Gaissmaier, W. and L. J. Schooler (2008). The smart potential behind probability matching. *Cognition* **109**: 416–22.

Glimcher, P. W. and A. Rustichini (2004). Neuroeconomics: the consilience of brain and decision. *Science* **306**: 447–52.

Gluck, M. A. and G. H. Bower (1988). From conditioning to category learning: an adaptive network model. *J. Exp. Psychol. Gen.* **117**: 227–47.

Goldstone, R. L. and B. C. Ashpole (2004). Human foraging behavior in a virtual environment. *Psychon. B. Rev.* **11**: 508–14.

Goss-Custard, J. (1977). Optimal foraging and size selection of worms by redshank *Tringa totanus* in the field. *Anim. Behav.* **25**: 10–29.

Grimm, V. (1999). Ten years of individual-based modelling in ecology: what have we learnt, and what could we learn in the future? *Ecol. Model.* **115**: 129–48.

Grimm, V. and S. Railsback (2005). *Individual-based Modeling and Ecology.* Princeton, NJ: Princeton University Press.

Grimm, V., E. Revilla, U. Berger, *et al.* (2005). Pattern-oriented modeling of agent-based complex systems: lessons from ecology. *Science* **310**: 987–91.

Hallam, J. and Malcolm, C. (1994). Behaviour: perception, action and intelligence: the view from situated robotics. *Phil. Trans. R. Soc. Lond. A* **349**: 29–42.

Harley, C. B. (1981). Learning the evolutionarily stable strategy. *J. Theor. Biol.* **89**: 611–33.

Hendriks-Jansen, H. (1996). *Catching Ourselves in the Act: Situated Activity, Interactive Emergence, and Human Thought.* Cambridge, MA: MIT Press.

Herrnstein, R. J. (1961). Relative and absolute strength of response as a function of frequency of reinforcement. *J. Exp. Anal. Behav.* **4**: 267–72.

Herrnstein, R. J. (1970). On the law of effect. *J. Exp. Anal. Behav.* **13**: 243–66.

Herrnstein, R. J. (1997). *The Matching Law: Papers in Psychology and Economics.* Cambridge, MA: Harvard University Press.

Herrnstein, R. J. and Vaughan, W. (1980). Melioration and behavioral allocation. In *Limits to Action: The Allocation of Individual Behavior*, ed. J. E. Staddon. New York: Academic Press, pp. 143–76.

Hinson, J. M. and J. E. Staddon (1983). Hill-climbing by pigeons. *J. Exp. Anal. Behav.* **39**: 25–47.

Houston, A. (1986). The matching law applies to wagtails' foraging in the wild. *J. Exp. Anal. Behav.* **45**: 15–18.

Houston, A. and J. McNamara (1984). Imperfectly optimal animals. *Behav. Ecol. Sociobiol.* **15**: 61–4.

Houston, A. and J. McNamara (1988). A framework for the functional analysis of behaviour. *Behav. Brain Sci.* **11**: 117–63.

Houston, A. and J. McNamara (1999). *Models of Adaptive Behavior.* Cambridge: Cambridge University Press.

Houston, A. and B. H. Sumida (1987). Learning rules, matching and frequency dependence. *J. Theor. Biol.* **126**: 289–308.

Huston, M., D. L. DeAngelis, and W. Post (1988). New computer models unify ecological theory. *BioScience* **38**: 682–91.

Iwasa, Y., M. Higashi, and N. Yamamura (1981). Prey distribution as a factor determining the choice of optimal strategy. *Amer. Nat.* **117**: 710–23.

Judson, O. (1994). The rise of the individual-based model in ecology. *Trends Ecol. Evol.* **9**: 9–14.

Kable, J. W. and P. W. Glimcher (2009). The neurobiology of decision: consensus and controversy. *Neuron* **63**: 733–45.

Kahneman, D. and Tversky, A. (eds.) (2000). *Choices, Values, and Frames.* Cambridge: Cambridge University Press.

Koehler, D. J. and G. James (2009). Probability matching in choice under uncertainty: intuition versus deliberation. *Cognition* **113**: 123–7.

Krebs, J. and A. Kacelnik (1991). Decision making. In *Behavioural Ecology: An Evolutionary Approach*, ed. J. Krebs and N. Davies. Oxford: Blackwell Scientific Publishers, pp. 105–37.

Loewenstein, Y., D. Prelec, and H. S. Seung (2009). Operant matching as a Nash equilibrium of an intertemporal game. *Neural Comput.* **21**: 2755–73.

Loewenstein, Y. and H. S. Seung (2006). Operant matching is a generic outcome of synaptic plasticity based on the covariance between reward and neural activity. *Proc. Natl. Acad. Sci. USA* **103**: 15224–9.

Lorenz, K. (1937 [1957]) The nature of instinct: the conception of instinctive behavior. In *Instinctive Behavior: The Development of a Modern Concept*, ed. C. Schiller and K. Lashley. New York: International University Press, pp. 129–75.

Maes, P. (1990). A bottom-up mechanism for behavior selection in an artificial creature. In *From Animals to Animats*, ed. J. Arcady Meyer and S. W. Wilson. Cambridge, MA: MIT Press, pp. 169–75.

McNamara, J. and A. Houston (1980). The application of statistical decision theory to animal behaviour. *J. Theor. Biol.* **85**(4): 673–90.

McNamara, J. M. and A. I. Houston (2009). Integrating function and mechanism. *Trends Ecol. Evol.* **24**: 670–5.

Mitchell, M. (1997). *An Introduction to Genetic Algorithms*. Cambridge, MA: MIT Press.

Myers, J. L. (1976). Probability learning and sequence learning. In *Handbook of Learning and Cognitive Processes: Approaches to Human Learning and Motivation*, ed. W. K. Estes. Hillsdale, NJ: Erlbaum, pp. 171–295.

Niv, Y., D. Joel, I. Meilijson, and E. Ruppin (2001). Evolution of reinforcement learning in uncertain environments: a simple explanation for complex foraging behavior. *Adapt. Behav.* **10**: 5–24.

Pascual, M. (2005). Computational ecology: from the complex to the simple and back. *PLoS Comput Biol.* **1**: 101–5.

Pfeifer, R. (1996). Building 'fungus eaters': design principles of autonomous agents. In *From Animals to Animats 4: Proceedings of the Fourth International Conference on Simulation of Adaptive Behavior*, ed. P. Maes, M. Mataric, J. A. Meyer, J. Pollack, and W. Wilson. Cambridge, MA: MIT Press, pp. 3–12.

Prescott, T. J., P. Redgrave, and K. Gurney (1999). Layered control architectures in robots and vertebrates. *Adapt. Behav.* **7**: 99–127.

Redgrave, P., T. J. Prescott, and K. Gurney (1999). The basal ganglia: a vertebrate solution to the selection problem? *Neuroscience* **89**: 1009–23.

Rosenblatt, K. and D. Payton (1989). A fine-grained alternative to the subsumption architecture for mobile robot control. In *Proceedings of the IEEE/INNS International Joint Conference on Neural Networks*. Washington: IEEE Press, pp. 317–23.

Sakai, Y. and T. Fukai (2008). The actor–critic learning is behind the matching law: matching versus optimal behaviors. *Neural Comput.* **20**: 227–51.

Seth, A. K. (1998). Evolving action selection and selective attention without actions, attention, or selection. In *Proceedings of the Fifth International Conference on the Simulation of Adaptive Behavior*, ed. R. Pfeifer, B. Blumberg, J. A. Meyer, and S. Wilson. Cambridge, MA: MIT Press, pp. 139–47.

Seth, A. K. (1999). Evolving behavioral choice: an investigation of Herrnstein's matching law. In *Proceedings of the Fifth European Conference on Artificial Life*, ed. D. Floreano, J. D. Nicoud, and F. Mondada. Berlin: Springer-Verlag, pp. 225–36.

Seth, A. K. (2000a). On the relations between behaviour, mechanism, and environment: explorations in artificial evolution. D.Phil. thesis, University of Sussex.

Seth, A. K. (2000b). Unorthodox optimal foraging theory. In *From Animals to Animats 6: Proceedings of the Sixth International Conference on the Simulation of Adaptive Behavior*, ed. J. A. Meyer, A. Berthoz, D. Floreano, H. Roitblat, and S. Wilson. Cambridge, MA: MIT Press, pp. 478–81.

Seth, A. K. (2001a), Modeling group foraging: individual suboptimality, interference, and a kind of matching. *Adapt. Behav* **9**: 67–90.

Seth, A. K. (2001b), Spatially explicit models of forager interference. In *Proceedings of the Sixth European Conference on Artificial Life*, ed. J. Kelemen and P. Sosik. Berlin: Springer-Verlag, pp. 151–62.

Seth, A. K. (2002a), Agent-based modelling and the environmental complexity thesis. In *From Animals to Animats 7: Proceedings of the Seventh International Conference on the Simulation of Adaptive Behavior*, ed. B. Hallam, D. Floreano, J. Hallam, G. Heyes, and J. A. Meyer. Cambridge, MA: MIT Press, pp. 13–24.

Seth, A. K. (2002b), Competitive foraging, decision making, and the ecological rationality of the matching law. In *From Animals to Animats 7: Proceedings of the Seventh International Conference on the Simulation of Adaptive Behavior*, ed. B. Hallam, D. Floreano, J. Hallam, G. Heyes, and J. A. Meyer. Cambridge, MA: MIT Press, pp. 359–68.

Seth, A. K. (2007). The ecology of action selection: insights from artificial life. *Phil. Trans. R. Soc. Lond. B Biol. Sci.* **362**: 1545–58.

Shanks, D. R., R. J. Tunney, and J. D. McCarthy (2002). A re-examination of probability matching and rational choice. *J. Behav. Decis. Making* **15**: 233–50.

Shimp, C. P. (1966). Probabalistically reinforced choice behavior in pigeons. *J. Exp. Anal. Behav.* **9**: 443–55.

Silberberg, A., J. R. Thomas, and N. Berendzen (1991). Human choice on concurrent variable-interval variable-ratio schedules. *J. Exp. Anal. Behav.* **56**: 575–84.

Stephens, D. and Krebs, J. (1986). *Foraging Theory*. Monographs in Behavior and Ecology. Princeton, NJ: Princeton University Press.

Sutherland, W. (1983). Aggregation and the 'ideal free' distribution. *J. Anim. Ecol.* **52**: 821–28.

Sutton, R. and A. Barto (1998). *Reinforcement Learning*. Cambridge, MA: MIT Press.

Thorndike, E. L. (1911). *Animal Intelligence*. New York: Macmillan.

Thuisjman, F., B. Peleg, M. Amitai, and A. Shmida (1995). Automata, matching, and foraging behavior of bees. *J. Theor. Biol.* **175**: 305–16.

Tinbergen, N. (1950). The hierarchical organisation of nervous mechanisms underlying instinctive behavior. *Sym. Soc. Exp. Biol.* **4**: 305–12.

Tinbergen, N. (1963). On the aims and methods of ethology. *Zeitschr. Tierpsychol.* **20**: 410–33.

Todd, P. M. and G. Gigerenzer (2000). Precis of simple heuristics that make us smart. *Behav. Brain Sci.* **23**: 727–41; Discussion, 742–80.

Tyrrell, T. (1993). The use of hierarchies for action selection. *Adapt. Behav.* **1**: 387–420.

Vulkan, N. (2000). An economist's perspective on probability matching. *J. Econ Surv.* **14**: 101–18.

Wagner, G. P. and L. A. Altenberg (1996). Complex adaptations and the evolution of evolvability. *Evolution* **50**: 967–76.

Weber, T. (1998). News from the realm of the ideal free distribution. *Trends Ecol. Evol.* **13**: 89–90.

Werner, G. (1994). Using second-order neural connections for motivation of behavioral choice. In *From Animals to Animats 3: Proceedings of the Third International Conference on the Simulation of Adaptive Behavior*, ed. D. Cliff, P. Husbands, J. A. Meyer, and S. Wilson. Cambridge, MA: MIT Press, pp. 154–64.

West, R. and K. Stanovich (2003). Is probability matching smart? Associations between probabilistic choices and cognitive ability. *Mem. Cognition* **31**: 243–51.

Wheeler, M. and P. de Bourcier (1995). How not to murder your neighbor: using synthetic behavioral ecology to study aggressive signalling. *Adapt. Behav.* **3**: 235–71.

Yu, A. J. and P. Dayan (2005). Uncertainty, neuromodulation, and attention. *Neuron* **46**: 681–92.

5   Compromise strategies for action selection

Frederick L. Crabbe

Summary

Among many properties suggested for action selection mechanisms, a prominent one is the ability to select compromise actions, i.e., actions that are not the best to satisfy any active goal in isolation, but rather compromise between the multiple goals. This chapter briefly reviews the history of compromise behaviour and performs experimental analyses of it in an attempt to determine how much compromise behaviour aids an agent. It concludes that optimal compromise behaviour has a surprisingly small benefit over non-compromise behaviour in the experiments performed, it presents some reasons why this may be true, and hypothesises cases where compromise behaviour is truly useful. In particular, it hypothesises that a crucial factor is the level at which an action is taken (low level actions are specific, such as 'move left leg'; high level actions are vague, such as 'forage for food'). The chapter hypothesises that compromise behaviour is more beneficial for high-level actions than low-level actions.

5.1   Introduction

Agents act. An agent, be it a robot, animal, or piece of software, must repeatedly select actions from a set of candidates. A *controller* is the mechanism within an agent that selects the action. The question of how to design controllers for such agents is the *action selection problem*. Researchers who consider the action selection problem have identified potential properties of these controllers. One such property is the ability to exhibit *compromise behaviour*. A controller exhibits compromise behaviour when the agent has multiple conflicting goals, yet the action selected is not the optimal action for achieving any single one of those goals, but is good for achieving several of those goals in conjunction. For example, a predator stalking two prey might not move directly toward one of the prey, but in between the two, in case one flees (Hutchinson, 1999). The action would not be optimal for individual goals to catch either prey, instead being a compromise between them.

Modelling Natural Action Selection, eds. Anil K. Seth, Tony J. Prescott and Joanna J. Bryson.
Published by Cambridge University Press. © Cambridge University Press 2012.

The ability to select a compromise action conveys a benefit to an agent: the optimal action changes in light of other of the agent's goals. There has been disagreement on the beneficiality of compromise behaviour in both animals and artificial agents. This chapter investigates the history of compromise behaviour, its various definitions, and the degree to which (under the most common definitions) it confers a behavioural advantage, concluding that the disagreement about the utility of compromise behaviour arises from a fundamentally imprecise notion of what it is. Finally, this chapter proposes a new hypothesis for when compromise behaviour is truly beneficial: when the agent selects actions at a high level rather than a low one.

5.2   Background

In order to understand compromise behaviour, it is instructive to examine its history in terms of ethology, comparative psychology, behavioural ecology, artificial intelligence (AI), planning, and robotics. After describing some basic background, this section will describe each of these disciplines in turn, with an emphasis on their relation to the question of compromise behaviour.

5.2.1   Definitions of compromise

In many approaches to animal behaviour, the full ramifications of an action are weighed in light of the current situation (see Section 5.2.4). Because this can be computationally expensive (see Section 5.2.5), a computational simplification is to divide the action selection problem into subgoals, solve those optimally, and combine the solutions (see Section 5.2.2). It is with respect to this latter strategy that compromise behaviour (acting such that no single subgoal is optimally satisfied) is most often considered (Tyrrell, 1993).

Definitions of compromise behaviour can be categorised on two major dimensions, the level of the action and whether the goals are prescriptive or proscriptive. Each of these dimensions is defined in detail below.

One of the primary characteristics of the different versions of compromise depends upon the abstraction level of the actions selected by the agent. For instance, a low-level action might be for an agent to contract left quadriceps 3 cm. A higher level action might be to transfer itself to a particular location. At the highest levels, an action might be to forage for food or mates. The distinction is based on the level of specificity given by the action; the first is as specific as possible, while the third leaves flexibility as to how it is to be accomplished. The nature of a particular action selection situation varies based on the level of the actions involved. As will be seen, different authors consider compromise behaviour at different levels.

The other dimension of distinction is the prescriptive or proscriptive nature of the agent's goals. Prescriptive goals are those that are satisfied by the execution of an act, such as the consumption of a resource. Proscriptive goals encourage an agent to not perform certain actions in certain situations. These goals are not satisfied by a particular action, but can be said to have been satisfied over a period of time if offending actions are not performed. These goals include avoidance goals, such as remaining at a safe distance from a predator. This chapter will not explicitly consider evolutionary goals that are always active for the life of the agent, such as maximising the chance of survival or maximising the chance of reproductive success.

The remainder of this section will review the history of the concept of compromise behaviour from the point of view of the above mentioned fields, demonstrating how the perspectives of compromise behaviour developed.

5.2.2   Ethology

Ethology (the study of animal behaviour) and the study of artificial agents are both concerned with the nature of behaviour and the selection of action. The former considers animal behaviour descriptively and analytically (Tinbergen, 1950), while the latter considers it synthetically via the construction of agents (Pfeifer and Scheier, 1999; Todd, 1992).

Traditionally, the ethologist studies animals in their natural environment, focusing on how they behave in the presence of multiple simultaneous drives. One of the main results of ethology is the identification of fixed action patterns (FAPs) (Brigant, 2005; Dewsbury, 1978; Lorenz, 1981), where an animal exhibits fixed behaviour when it receives a particular type of stimulus. One common example is of the greylag goose (*Anser anser*), which will exhibit a behaviour of rolling an egg back into its nest using a fixed motion pattern, completing the motion pattern even if the egg is removed (Lorenz, 1981). Careful observation of this and similar behaviours led researchers to hypothesise that these individual action patterns are controlled by separate innate modules that compete for expression in the animal's behaviour (Burkhardt, 2004).

The idea that the modules might compete for expression in behaviour led to investigations into how these conflicts might be resolved. Hinde (1966) lists nine different resolution mechanisms observed in animals. These mechanisms include exhibiting just one behaviour, alternating between multiple behaviours, and compromise behaviour.

Natural compromise behaviour takes multiple forms. First, it is either unimodal or bimodal in input. In unimodal input, signals from different sensors of the same type (each ear, for example) cause the animal to consider each a separate goal (Lund *et al.*, 1997). Bimodal input combines signals from two different types of sensors (eyes and ears, for example) for compromise. In both cases, compromise is typically considered a result of competition for effector mechanisms at a low level (Hinde, 1966). Thus, if one FAP controls only leg motion while another only head movement, their simultaneous expression would not be considered compromise behaviour but rather superposition.

Low-level, prescriptive, unimodal compromise has been observed in the crustacean *Armadillium* when performing tropotaxis toward two light sources (Müller, 1925), and katydids when performing phonotaxis (Bailey *et al.*, 1990; Latimer and Sippel, 1987; Morris *et al.*, 1978). The fish *Crenilabris* displays low-level prescriptive, bimodal compromise in its orientation behaviour between its reaction to light and its reaction to the direction of gravity (von Holst, 1935).

Evidence for high-level compromise behaviour in nature is less clear, though it may be argued that it can be seen in blue herons, which select suboptimal feeding patches to avoid predation by hawks in years when hawk attacks are frequent (Caldwell, 1986). Similar behaviour has been shown in minnows (Fraser and Cerri, 1982), sparrows (Grubb and Greenwald, 1982), pike, and sticklebacks (Milinksi, 1986). Indeed, a great many studies suggest that animals balance the risk of predation against foraging or other benefits (Brown and Kotler, 2004; Lima, 1998). Mesterton-Gibbons (1989) reinterpreted the data of Krebs *et al.* (1977) to show that great tits *Parus major* appear to compromise between time and energy consumption in foraging, though it is not clear whether this compromise fits into our definition as 'time saving' is not an explicit FAP that an agent can select.

5.2.3   Comparative psychology

Concurrent with the developments in ethology was a competing branch of study, comparative psychology, that examined many of the same issues (Dewsbury, 1978). This approach differed from ethology in that individual phenomena were studied in isolation, and there was much greater emphasis placed on learning over that of innate mechanisms (Thorpe, 1979). In their experiments, researchers went to great lengths to ensure that only one drive was active in the test animal (Dewsbury, 1992). This enabled the experimenter to delve deeply into questions about that particular behaviour without interference from others, but it limited investigation into interaction of behaviours. In recent years, the branches of ethology and comparative psychology have been synthesised (Dewsbury, 1992), but early theoretical work had important influences in AI (see Section 5.2.5).

5.2.4   Optimal biological approaches

Modern trends in biology have employed formal models and optimisation techniques borrowed from decision theory and operations research (Clemen, 1996; Hillier and Lieberman, 2002); and recently, statistical physics (Bartumeus and Catalan, 2009) in order to determine optimal behaviour. Behavioural ecology is the study of the interaction between an organism's environment and its behaviour, as shaped via natural selection (Krebs and Davies, 1997). Under the assumption that selection optimises behaviour to maximise reproductive success, to understand animal behaviour it is important to analyse it with techniques that optimise objective functions that describe reproductive success. For example, in the field of foraging theory (Stephens and Krebs, 1986), techniques such as linear programming (Hillier and Lieberman, 2002) or dynamic programming (Bertsekas, 2005) are used to find optimal foraging behaviour in terms of such features as maximising energy intake and minimising exposure to predators (Brown and Kotler, 2004; Houston *et al.*, 2007; Lima, 1998; McNamara and Houston, 1994; Seth, 2007). In these studies, optimisation is used as a basis of comparison and as an explanation for natural selection; it is not posited as the decision-making process the animal itself uses. Optimisation is computationally expensive, such that the time to compute solutions grows exponentially with the complexity. Complicated problems cannot be solved in short periods of time (Bertsekas, 2005).

When examining behavioural choice with these optimal techniques, compromise behaviour is not an explicit issue because the techniques combine the subgoals into a single objective function to be optimised. As such, optimal solutions to the individual subgoals are not considered, only the solution to the overall objective function.

5.2.5   Artificial intelligence and planning

The field of planning within AI was delayed in development until the advent of robotic hardware sufficiently sophisticated to exhibit agent-like behaviour (Fikes and Nilsson, 1971). The approaches used came from the operations research and computer science communities (with influence from comparative psychology; Newell and Simon, 1976), where the agent attempted to formulate a mathematical proof of the correct action to take in the agent's current situation.

A typical planning problem is represented as a conjunction of logical relatively high-level predicates. For example, a hypothetical hospital robot might have a planning goal: Have(robot,medicine003)ˆIn(robot,room342), indicating that the robot should both be in possession of the medicine and be in the correct hospital room.

From the planning perspective, this is a single goal that is achieved by achieving each of its component parts such that there comes a time when both are simultaneously true. The individual predicates, also known as subgoals, can conflict with each other. For example the robot can take actions so as to make the In(robot,room342) true while Have(robot,*medicine003*) is false. The robot must then take actions to make *Have(robot,medicine003)* that may in turn make *In(robot,room342)* false. This conflict is different from the conflict between FAPs in that it arises from the order actions are performed, not in which subgoal will be achieved. If multiple subgoals are inherently in conflict such that they cannot both be simultaneously true, then the overall goal is unattainable. Further, because subgoals cannot be partially satisfied (they are simply true or false) it is impossible for the agent to trade in some quality in the satisfaction of one subgoal in order to improve the quality of others. A survey of the state of the art in planning can be found in Ghallab *et al.* (2004).

Other features of the planning problem also resemble features of the compromise behaviour question. For instance, often a single action can move the agent closer to the satisfaction of more than one of the goal literals. This 'positive interference' (Russell and Norvig, 2010) is unlike compromise behaviour, however, in that there is nothing lost in the selection of this action. Negated literals in a goal (e.g., *In(robot,room342)*) are unlike proscriptive goals in that they must only be not true at some point for the goal to be satisfied, as opposed to never becoming true. Recently, there has been interest in *multi-criteria* planning (Gerevini *et al.*, 2008; Hoffmann, 2003; Refanidis and Vlahavas, 2003). A multi-criteria problem is different from a multiple goal problem in that the former, as with standard planning, has a single goal to achieve. The multiple criteria are used to measure solution quality. Proscriptive goals can be similar to quality criteria when the criteria measure such properties as agent safety, which encourage the agent to not take certain actions.

For the reasons described above, the notion of compromise behaviour was unfamiliar to AI researchers until the 1980s (Brooks, 1986), and optimality under compromise was unexamined.

A major drawback of the AI approaches is that attempts to prove correct actions can be prohibitively expensive in moderately complex environments. If an agent is limited to just ten actions at any time, then each step into the future increases the number of possible outcomes to consider by a factor of ten. If the solution to the current problem is twenty steps long, then the program must examine on the order of 10^{20} possible sequences (Russell and Norvig, 2010). For comparison, there have been (estimated) 10^{18} seconds since the beginning of the universe (Bridle *et al.*, 2003). This high computation cost prevents using these techniques for planning behaviour with low-level actions, where solutions to problems might be many hundreds of steps long.

5.2.6   Behaviour-based robotics

Eventually, the inability of robotic systems to solve certain problems of the real world (such as those with multiple simultaneous goals) forced roboticists to re-evaluate their approach. In the real world, agents have conflicting goals that must be selected from, and they must be able to adjust quickly to unforeseen events. For instance, the agent may find a previously unknown obstacle or discover that an action did not have the desired effect.

The result of the re-evaluation, *behaviour-based robotics*, borrows from ethology the idea that there are multiple innate behaviours that are triggered by sensory input. In the extreme formulation, advocates maintain that all intelligent behaviour can be constructed out of suites of these competing mechanisms (Arkin, 1998; Brooks, 1986, 1997). Some have attempted to explain human-level cognition using similar modular approaches (Carruthers, 2004). One advantage to the behaviour-based approach is that the innate reactive systems do not need to plan with low-level actions, and thus are practical to implement. Another advantage is that conflicting goals can be represented.

Because the approach borrows heavily from the ethological tradition, it has the same concerns. These concerns include how conflicts between innate behaviours can be resolved, and whether compromise behaviour itself is an important property for controllers. In 1993, Tyrrell introduced a list of 14 requirements for action selection mechanisms drawn from ethology. Of these, number 12 was 'Compromise Candidates: the need to be able to choose actions that, while not the best choice for any one sub-problem alone, are best when all sub-problems are considered simultaneously' (Tyrrell, 1993, p. 174). In justifying this rule, Tyrrell used a 'council-of-ministers' analogy. In this perspective, there are a collection of 'ministers' or experts on achieving each of the agent's goals. Each minister casts votes for courses of action that it predicts will solve the goal with which that minister is associated. For example, it might cast five votes for its highest ranked action, four for the next highest ranked, and so on. The agent then selects the action that receives the most votes. Note that this characterisation of compromise is of high-level compromise. Tyrrell's list has had significant impact on the action selection field (Bryson, 2000; Decugis and Ferber, 1998; Girard *et al.*, 2002; Humphrys, 1996), and a number of researchers have developed systems to meet the criteria he set out (Antonelli *et al.*, 2008; Avila-Garcia and Canamero, 2004; Blumberg, 1994; Blumberg *et al.*, 1996; Crabbe and Dyer, 1999; Hurdus and Hong, 2009; Maes, 1990; Montes-Gonzales *et al.*, 2000; Werner, 1994). Recently fuzzy logic controllers have become popular, in part, because they include compromise naturally (Jaafar and McKenzie, 2008; Luo and Jennings, 2007).

5.2.7   Current status

Although some researchers in behaviour-based robotics considered it 'obviously preferable to combine [the] demand [to avoid a hazard] with a preference to head toward food, if the two don't clash, rather than to head diametrically away from the hazard because the only system being considered is that of avoid hazard' (Tyrrell, 1993), more recent modelling work generated results that seem to contradict the claim (Bryson, 2000; Crabbe, 2004; Jones *et al.*, 1999), in that artificial agents without the ability to select compromise actions often perform as well on tasks as those that can select compromise actions. If valid, these results suggest that the appropriation of this idea from ethology was not necessary for high-performing artificial agents. A central thesis of this chapter is that this error occurred in the case of compromise behaviour because it had been poorly defined, in particular, that no distinction was drawn between high-level compromise and low-level compromise. Although low-level compromise is what is seen in much of the action selection literature, its existence was justified by arguments concerning high-level compromise. This equivocation has caused confusion on these topics.

Some artificial agent researchers who use ethological ideas directly are those that design systems not to perform better in the sense of scoring higher on a metric, but to appear more natural to observers. These systems appear in the areas of computer graphics and video gaming, where a naturalistic appearance to a human viewer is necessary to maintain the desired illusion (Iglesias and Luengo, 2005; de Sevin *et al.*, 2001; Thorisson, 1996; Tu, 1996).

Although work mentioned above (Bryson, 2000; Crabbe, 2004; Jones *et al.*, 1999) implies that compromise behaviour is less useful than originally thought, this work is not conclusive. The next section will attempt to analyse the nature of low-level compromise behaviour more thoroughly.

5.3   Experiments

In order to understand the properties of compromise behaviour, it is helpful to examine the optimal behaviour in potential compromise situations. As discussed above, there are multiple formulations of the action selection problem. The experiments here will closely examine those most often described in the ethological and behaviour-based robotics literature, *low-level prescriptive* and *low-level proscriptive*. As the compromise formulations investigated here are low-level, the domain is defined to be that of navigation of a mobile agent, similar to several authors' simulated domains (Maes, 1990; Tyrrell, 1993) or to navigating mobile robots (Choset *et al.*, 2005). In the simulations, space is continuous, but time is discrete, such that the action at each time step is defined as a movement of one distance unit at any angle. Slightly different models are required for each of the proscriptive or prescriptive situations.

5.3.1   Prescriptive experiments

The initial experiments test a scenario where an agent has a goal to be co-located with one of two target locations in the environment. These could be locations of food, water, potential mates, or shelter, etc. At any moment either or both of the targets can disappear from the environment, simulating the intrusion of environmental factors. The agent must select an action that maximises its chances of co-locating with a target before it is removed from the environment.

This scenario is approximated by placing an agent at the origin on a plane. Two targets are placed on the plane, one in the first and one in the second quadrant in the y-range of $(0; 100)$, and x-ranges of $(-100; 0)$ for one target and $(100; 0)$ for the other. Targets will be referred to as t_a and t_b. The agent can sense the location of each target. Sensor information takes the form of complete knowledge of the locations of both targets' (x, y) coordinates. Because the quality of the individual targets may vary, or the types of the targets may be different, the agent has two independent goals to be co-located with them. The strength of the goals are in the range $(0; 100)$. Each goal will be referred to as G_a and G_b. The dynamism in the environment is represented with a probability p. This is the probability that any object in the environment will still exist after each time step. That is, any object will spontaneously disappear from the environment at each time step with probability $1 - p$. Time is divided into discrete, equal sized time steps. The agent moves at a constant speed, and therefore a constant distance per time step. All distances are measured in the number of time steps it takes the agent to travel that distance. Notationally, $\overline{ij}$ is the distance from some location i to some location j. An agent's action selection problem is to select an angle θ in which direction to move for the next time step. θ is continuous, so the environment is also continuous and the size of the set of actions being selected from is infinite.

Once the agent has executed its action, it is again faced with the same action selection problem. If one of the targets has disappeared, the best action is to move directly to the other target. Compromise behaviour in this task is the selection of any direction to move that is not directly toward either target. Any action selected that is in the direction of one of the targets cannot be a compromise action because it is also the action that is optimal for achieving one of the subgoals. As the agent repeatedly selects an action, the path it follows resembles a piece-wise linear approximation of a curved path to one of the targets.

5.3.1.1 Formal model

An analysis of compromise candidates is performed using Utility Theory (Howard, 1977). Utility Theory assigns a set of numerical values (utilities) to states of the world. These utilities represent the usefulness of that state to an agent. Expected utility (*EU*) is a prediction of the eventual total utility an agent will receive if it takes a particular action in a particular state. The *EU* of taking an action A_i in a state S_j is the sum of the product of the probability of each outcome that could occur and the utility of that outcome:

$$EU(A_i|S_j) = \sum_{S_o \in O} P(S_o|A_i, S_j)U_h(S_o) \tag{5.1}$$

where O is the set of possible outcome states, $P(S_o|A_i, S_j)$ is the probability of outcome S_o occurring given that the agent takes action A_i in state S_j, and $U_h(S_o)$ is the historical utility of outcome S_o (defined below).

Let $U(t)$ be the utility to the agent of consuming t. Assuming the agent is rational, the set of goals to consume objects will be order isomorphic to the set of the agent's utilities of having consumed the objects. That is, every possible utility corresponds to a matching goal value, such that the order of the utilities from least to greatest is the same as the order of the corresponding goals. Therefore, *EU* calculated with utilities is order isomorphic with *EU* calculated with goals instead. For the purposes here, it will be assumed that the goals and utilities are equivalent ($U(t) = G_t$).

A rational agent is expected to select the action with the largest *EU*. The historical utility of a state is defined as the utility of the state plus future utility, or the maximum of the expected utility of the actions possible in each state:

$$U_h(S) = U(S) + \max_{A_i \in A} EU(A_i|S_J) \tag{5.2}$$

where A is the set of possible actions. The maximum is found because of the assumption that a rational agent will always act to maximise its expected utility. An agent can calculate *EU* using multiple actions in the future by recursively applying Equations (5.1) and (5.2).

Low-level prescriptive compromise behaviour is analysed by comparing an approximation of optimal behaviour with several non-optimal but easy to generate behaviours. The optimal behaviour is approximated based on the dynamic programming technique used by Hutchinson (1999). The technique overlays a grid of points on top of the problem space and calculates the maximal expected utility of each location given optimal future actions. This is done recursively starting at the target locations and moving outward until stable values have been generated for all grid points. As with similar dynamic programming techniques, the time to convergence increases as the number and variety of targets increases.

The value calculated is the expected utility of optimal action at an environmental location when the two targets still remain: $EU(A_\theta|t_a, t_b, \lambda)$. λ is the agent's location in the environment, θ is the angle of the optimal move for the agent and λ' is 1 unit away from λ in direction θ. By Equations (5.1) and (5.2) the expected utility of being at λ is:

$$EU(A_\theta|t_a, t_b, \lambda) = p^2 EU(A_\theta|t_a, t_b, \lambda') + p(1 - p)EU(A_\theta|t_a, \lambda')$$
$$+ p(1 - p)EU(A_\theta|t_b, \lambda'), \tag{5.3}$$
$$EU(A_\theta|t_a, \lambda') = G_a p^{\overline{\lambda' t_a}}, \quad \text{and} \tag{5.4}$$
$$EU(A_\theta|t_b, \lambda') = G_b p^{\overline{\lambda' t_b}}. \tag{5.5}$$

The total expected utility (Equation 5.3) is the expectation over four possible situations after an action: both targets there, both targets gone, t_a there but t_b gone, and vice versa (the EU of both targets gone is zero). When one of the targets disappears from the environment, the optimal action for the agent to take is to move directly to the other target, as shown in Equations (5.4) and (5.5). A formal specification of the algorithm is given in the supplementary material in Crabbe (2007).

It is typically computationally prohibitive for an agent to calculate the optimal action using a technique similar to the one described here (the program used for these experiments takes between 5 and 20 minutes to converge in these two target scenarios). Instead, many researchers propose easy to compute action selection mechanisms that are intended to approximate the optimal action. (Cannings and Cruz Orive, 1975; Fraenkel and Gunn, 1961; Houston *et al.*, 2007; Hutchinson and Gigerenzer, 2005; McNamara and Houston, 1980; Römer, 1993; Seth, 2007; Stephens and Krebs, 1986). The mechanisms can be divided into two categories: those that select a single target and move directly toward it, and those that exhibit some sort of compromise behaviour. In the former category, considered here are:

- Closest (C): select the closest target.
- Maximum utility (MU): select the target with the higher utility.
- Maximum expected utility (MEU): select the target with the higher expected utility if it were the only target in the environment (MEU is a non-compromise strategy because it can only select a direction to move that is directly toward one of the targets, and is therefore optimal for one of the agent's subgoals in isolation).

Of the action selection mechanisms that exhibit compromise behaviour, examined here are:

- Forces (F): the agent behaves as if it has two forces acting on it, where the strength of the force is proportional to the utility of the target divided by the square of the distance between the agent and the target location. Let AngleTo() be a function of two locations that returns the angle from the first location to the second. If V_a is the force vector from T_a, the direction of V_a is AngleTo(λ, T_a) and the magnitude of V_a is $G_a/\overline{\lambda T}_a^2$. The direction the agent moves (θ) is:

$$\theta = \text{AngleTo}(\lambda, V_a + V_b) \tag{5.6}$$

- Signal gradient (SG): the agent behaves as if it is following a signal gradient. The targets emit a simulated 'odour' that falls with the square of the distance from the target. The initial strength of the odour is proportional to the utility of the target. The agent moves to the neighbouring location that has the strongest odour calculated as the sum of the odour emanating from each of the two targets. That is,

$$\theta = \text{AngleTo}(\lambda, \text{argmax}_{\lambda'}(G_a/\lambda' T_a^2 + G_b/\lambda' T_b^2)) \tag{5.7}$$

- Exponentially weakening forces (EWF): this strategy is identical to the forces strategy, except the pulling effects of the targets fall exponentially with distance, rather than quadratically. The magnitudes of the two vectors are $G_a p^{\overline{\lambda T_a}}$ and $G_b p^{\overline{\lambda T_b}}$. It is predicted that since expected utility falls exponentially with distance, this strategy may perform better than forces.

The expected utility of each of these non-optimal mechanisms can be calculated for any particular scenario by using Equations (5.3), (5.4) and (5.5), where the action θ is the one recommended by the strategy, not the optimal action.

5.3.1.2   Prescriptive results

The results reported here are based on 50 000 scenarios. Each scenario was a set of parameters (G_a, G_b, t_a, t_b) selected randomly from a uniform distribution. The simulations were written in Lisp, compiled in Franz Allegro Common Lisp, version 7.0, and run on a cluster of 25 Sun Blade 1500s, for 347 computer-days. Detailed discussion of the implementation can be found in the electronic supplementary materials in Crabbe (2007). For each scenario, the expected utility of each of the action selection mechanisms described in the previous section were computed: closest (C), maximum utility (MU), maximum expected utility (MEU), forces (F), signal gradient (SG), and exponentially weakening forces (EWF). The expected utilities of optimal behaviour using the dynamic programming technique were computed (an example of the optimal behaviour is shown in Figure 5.1). Table 5.1 compares the three non-compromise mechanisms (C, MU, and MEU), using the worst performer (MU) as a baseline. The table reports the average percentage improvement of the strategy over MU (e.g., the closest strategy performs on average 9% better than the maximum utility strategy). It also reports the percentage of cases where the strategy selected the correct action of the two possible. MEU is the best of the three as it selects the better target in most cases and its overall expected utility is 15% better than MU. MEU selects the worse target only 0.68% of the time. The table also shows that C is a better strategy than MU. This may be so because the expected utility of a target falls exponentially with distance, so that closer targets have higher expected utility than targets with higher raw utilities.

Table 5.2 compares the compromise-based mechanisms with the best non-compromise strategy, MEU. It shows both the average percentage improvement over MEU and the percentage improvement over MEU in the single best scenario. There are three important aspects of this table. The first is that the optimal strategy is only 1.1% better than the non-compromise based MEU. This contradicts the intuition (discussed above) that optimal

Table 5.1 Comparison of non-compromise strategies. Each strategy is listed in the columns. The first row reports the percentage of times that strategy makes the correct selection. The second row reports the strategy's performance improvement over maximum utility (MU). Numbers in parentheses are the standard deviation. The numbers are generated from the 50 000 trials. Percentage improvement is calculated as (Score of Strategy A − Score of MU)/Score of MU. All differences were significant in a Mann–Whitney U-test to a confidence level of 0:999.

	MaxUtility	Closest	MaxExpectedUtility
% correct	70.29	79.99	99.32
% over MU	0.0	9.35 (3.97)	15.31 (3.44)

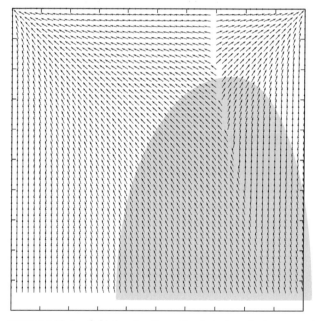

Figure 5.1 Vector field showing the optimal strategy for two prescriptive goal scenarios. t_a is located in the upper left corner, and t_b is located in the upper right. G_a is 100, G_b is 50. The arrows' lengths are uniform and have no significance. Each arrow direction represents the optimal direction of movement for the agent at that location. A greater proportion of the arrows point toward the upper left, reflecting the larger value of G_a. While the arrows near the targets point directly at the respective targets (indicating non-compromise behaviour is optimal), many of the arrows, especially those in the shaded region in the lower right, do not point directly at either target, indicating that in those regions, compromise actions are indeed optimal.

behaviour would be significantly better than a non-compromise approach. The result is consistent, however, with the non-continuous space experiments of Crabbe (2002) and the study in Hutchinson (1999).

The second important aspect is that all of the non-optimal compromise-based strategies performed *worse* than the MEU strategy. These results may help explain why some researchers have found that compromise behaviour is unhelpful (Bryson, 2000; Crabbe,

Table 5.2 Comparison of compromise strategies to the non-compromise maximum expected utility (MEU). For each strategy, the average expected utility improvement over MEU is given in the first line. The best expected utility improvement over MEU in a single scenario is provided in the second line. The optimal strategy performs the best, but is less beneficial than expected. The non-optimal strategies (F, SG, and EWF) are all worse than the non-compromise MEU, though EWF is the best of that set. Differences in the averages were significant in a Mann–Whitney U-test to a confidence level of 0.99.

	F	SG	EWF	Optimal
% Over MaxExpectedUtility	−4.07	−2.79	−2.47	1.12
% Over MaxExpectedUtility (best case)	4.84	4.82	20.56	22.73

2004; Jones *et al.*, 1999): the commonly used *tractable* compromise strategies perform worse than a non-compromise strategy.

The final aspect of Table 5.2 to note is that EWF is the best performing of the easy to compute compromise strategies tested. While it is not conclusive, this may imply that the approach of decreasing the influence of farther targets exponentially is a good one for developing action selection strategies. Examining the score for the *best* scenario for EWF shows that it is nearly as high as the best scenario for optimal.

5.3.1.3   Prescriptive discussion

With respect to animals and natural action selection, the results presented here imply that animals that exhibit low-level prescriptive compromise behaviour are either: behaving non-optimally; using an as yet unproposed compromise-based action selection strategy; or behaving in that manner for reasons other than purely to compromise between two targets. Hutchinson (1999) suggests three possible reasons for what appears to be low-level prescriptive compromise behaviour: (1) a desire not to tip off potential prey that it is being stalked, (2) it is a part of a strategy to gather more sense data before committing to a target, or (3) that computational issues yield simple mechanisms that exhibit compromise-style behaviour. Hutchinson's reasons are particularly interesting in light of MEU being the best non-compromise strategy. This strategy requires not only detailed knowledge of the targets' locations and worths, but also that the agent knows p. It may be that apparent low-level compromise is an attempt to gather more information about the targets, or that, lacking knowledge of p, animals are unable to use the MEU strategy, in which case the compromise signal gradient or EWF strategies might be the best (although results from foraging theory suggest that animals are able to estimate p accurately; Stephens and Krebs, 1986)). Regarding Hutchinson's third suggestion, Houston *et al.* (2007) suggest that behavioural characteristics can be 'side-effects' of rules that evolved in environments that differ from where they are being used, or that the objective function and criteria being maximised are more complex than the scenarios in which they are being tested.

Ghez *et al.* (1997) showed that when humans performed a reaching task, a narrow angle between targets led to low-level compromise behaviour, while a wide angle did not. They hypothesised that for widely separated targets, the brain treated each as a separate concept or category, but that for narrowly separated targets, the brain is unable to tease them apart, thus reacting to their superposition. By analysing reaction time, Favilla (2002) showed that humans do appear to be switching mental strategies when changing between compromise and non-compromise behaviour, even when the tasks remain the same. These results may indicate that low-level compromise is a side-effect of other computational mechanisms. This switching may be solely an artefact of other mechanisms, or it may be an attempt to display compromise behaviour only in situations where it is likely to occur. Section 5.3.1.4 will look further at conditions where compromise strategies appear to be most beneficial.

With respect to higher-level actions, the behavioural ecology evidence is much less clear that natural compromise is occurring. For instance in the cases of an animal using suboptimal feeding patches to avoid heightened predator activity, this behaviour could be explained by the animal downgrading the quality of a feeding patch (the G_x) because of the presence of the predators. The animal then compares the utilities of the two patches directly rather than considering compromise behaviour (Stephens and Krebs, 1986). Alternatively, the animal could be abstracting the problem so that it might be solved optimally.

5.3.1.4   Prescriptive analysis

While on average low-level compromise appears to have little benefit, there may be scenarios where the optimal or EWF strategies are significantly better than the MEU. This might explain the exhibition of compromise in animals in some situations and not others, as well as provide strategies for the construction of artificial agents. This section uses the idea of information gain from information theory to attempt to determine when compromise strategies might be a benefit.

Information gain is the technique used in the decision tree algorithms ID3 and C4.5 (Mitchell, 1997; Quinlan, 1983, 1993). The technique begins with a data set and a classification of the data elements. The data here are the situations generated in the prescriptive experiments, and the classification is whether or not the scenario has a compromise strategy (either EWF or optimal) with an EU better than MEU. The technique then considers a set of n-ary attributes which partition the data set. The attributes are properties of the starting scenario that might indicate whether compromise is beneficial, such as the distance between the two targets, or the value of p. For each attribute, the technique considers the information gain of applying that attribute to partition the data set. Information gain is the decrease in entropy of the data set, where entropy is:

$$E(S) = \sum_{i \in C} -p_i \log_2 p_i \qquad (5.8)$$

S is a data set, i is a category of the classification, and p_i is the proportion of S categorised as i. Entropy measures the inverse of the purity of a data set with respect to the classification. A set is most pure when all the data have the same classification, and least pure when the data is classified evenly across all categories.

The information gain of dividing set S based on attribute A is defined as:

$$Gain(S, A) = E(S) - \sum_{v \in V(A)} \frac{|S_v|}{|S|} E(S_v), \qquad (5.9)$$

where v is a value of an attribute, $|S|$ is a size of set S, S_v is the subset of S for which attribute A takes value v, and $V(A)$ is the set of values the attribute might take (e.g., the attribute *colour* might take the values red, green, or blue). The attribute with the largest information gain is the attribute which best partitions the data set, and in our case is the property of a situation which most determines if there is a good compromise candidate.

The data describing any situation is continuous information, but attributes are n-ary classifiers. To cope with this, the attributes partition the values into ranges, such as every 0.05. The attributes used are listed below:

- $\overline{\lambda t_a}, \overline{\lambda t_b}, \overline{t_a t_b}$. These three attributes are the distances between the key locations in the scenario. The distances can be anywhere from 0 to 224, and the attributes break them up into ranges of 5 units.
- G_a, G_b. The goal values from 0 to 100, broken into ranges of 5 units.
- p. The value of p from 0 to 1, broken into ranges of 0.005.
- $R(\overline{\lambda t_a}, \overline{\lambda t_b})$. This encodes the relationship between $\overline{\lambda t_a}$ and $\overline{\lambda t_b}$, while keeping the values between 0 and 1 using the formula $\frac{\overline{\lambda t_a}}{\overline{\lambda t_a} + \overline{\lambda t_b}}$. It is broken into ranges of 0.05.
- $R(\overline{\lambda t_a}, \overline{t_a t_b})$. This encodes the relationship between $\overline{\lambda t_a}$ and $\overline{t_a t_b}$, while keeping the values between 0 and 1 using the formula $\frac{\overline{\lambda t_a}}{\overline{\lambda t_a} + \overline{t_a t_b}}$. It is broken into ranges of 0.05.
- $R(\overline{\lambda t_b}, \overline{t_a t_b})$. This encodes the relationship between $\overline{\lambda t_b}$ and $\overline{t_a t_b}$, while keeping the values between 0 and 1 using the formula $\frac{\overline{\lambda t_b}}{\overline{\lambda t_b} + \overline{t_a t_b}}$. It is broken into ranges of 0.05.
- $R(G_a, G_b)$. This encodes the relationship between G_a and G_b, while keeping the values between 0 and 1 using the formula $\frac{G_a}{G_a + G_b}$. It is broken into ranges of 0.05.
- $R_l(G_a, \overline{\lambda t_a}, G_b, \overline{\lambda t_b})$. This encodes a *linear* relationship between $G_a, \overline{\lambda t_a}, G_b$, and $\overline{\lambda t_b}$, while keeping the values between 0 and 1 using the formula $\frac{G_a \overline{\lambda t_a}}{G_a \overline{\lambda t_a} + G_b \overline{\lambda t_b}}$. It is broken into ranges of 0.05.
- $R_e(G_a, \overline{\lambda t_a}, G_b, \overline{\lambda t_b})$. This encodes an *exponential* relationship between $G_a, \overline{\lambda t_a}, G_b$, and $\overline{\lambda t_b}$, while keeping the values between 0 and 1 using the formula $\frac{G_a p^{\overline{\lambda t_a}}}{G_a p^{\overline{\lambda t_a}} + G_b p^{\overline{\lambda t_b}}}$. It is broken into ranges of 0.05.

5.3.1.5   Analysis experiments

The data is first classified based on whether the performance of the optimal behaviour is a 1% or greater improvement over the performance of MEU for that scenario. Using Equation (5.9), it can be seen that the attribute with the largest information gain is $R_e(G_a, \overline{\lambda t_a}, G_b, \overline{\lambda t_b})$ with a gain of 0.07243. Figure 5.2 shows a breakdown of the data as partitioned by the attribute. The x-axis is the range of values of the attribute, and the y-axis is the percentage of the data that falls in that range and is positively classified (the performance of the optimal behaviour is a 1% or greater improvement over the performance of MEU). The figure shows that the greatest likelihood of good

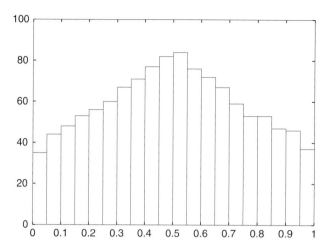

Figure 5.2 Breakdown of attribute $R_e(G_a, \overline{\lambda t_a}, G_b, \overline{\lambda t_b})$ when comparing optimal to MEU. Each bar represents the fraction of scenarios with the attribute in that value range where the optimal strategy is at least 1% better than MEU. For example, when R_a is between 0.45 and 0.55, over 80% of the time the optimal strategy is more than 1% better than MEU.

compromise behaviour is when the attribute is close to 0.5. This means that if $G_a p^{\overline{\lambda t_a}}$ is close to $G_b p^{\overline{\lambda t_b}}$ (when the expected utilities of the two targets are roughly equal), it is more likely that optimal behaviour will confer a large advantage.

The second largest information gain is $R(\overline{\lambda t_a}, \overline{\lambda t_b})$ with a gain of 0.06917. The next two attributes with high gain are $R(\overline{\lambda t_a}, \overline{t_a t_b})$ and $R(\overline{\lambda t_b}, \overline{t_a t_b})$, both with a gain of 0.027.

Although on average EWF performs worse than MEU, it is interesting to analyse the situations in which it performs better. If these situations could be recognised, then EWF could be applied only when they occur. Furthermore, it may lead to insight on why EWF outperformed the other non-optimal strategies. The data is analysed as done for the case of optimal vs. MEU, and classified based on whether or not EWF out performs MEU. The top two attributes in terms of information gain are $R(\overline{\lambda t_a}, \overline{t_a t_b})$ and $R(\overline{\lambda t_b}, \overline{t_a t_b})$, with gains of 0.1620 and 0.1569 respectively. Figure 5.3 shows a breakdown of the data as classified by $R(\overline{\lambda t_a}, \overline{t_a t_b})$.

These results strongly suggest that good compromises using EWF occur when the targets are relatively far away from the origin and close to each other.

5.3.1.6   Prescriptive analysis discussion

The analysis shows that there are good compromises when the expected utility is roughly equal. This is not too surprising, as expected utility incorporates both the goal value and the likelihood of obtaining the target, such that when one target has a value much greater than the other, the strategy of MEU should be close to the optimal. The high gain associated with $R(\overline{\lambda t_a}, \overline{\lambda t_b})$ is probably an extension of this property, as the distances are a major component of the expected utility.

Interestingly, for both the optimal strategy, as well as for EWF, the ratio of the distance to one target to the distance between the targets plays an important role. When

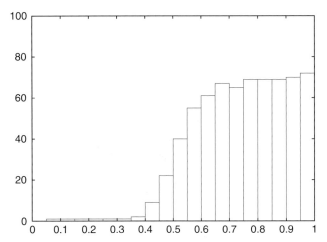

Figure 5.3 Breakdown of attribute $R(\overline{\lambda t_a}, \overline{t_a t_b})$ when comparing EWF to MEU. Each bar represents the fraction of scenarios with the attribute in that value range where the optimal strategy is at least 1% more than MEU. For example, when R is between 0.5 and 0.55, approximately 40% of the time the optimal strategy is more than 1% better than MEU.

the targets are close together and far from the agent, then there are better options for compromise behaviour. This is consistent with the results of Ghez, *et al.* discussed in Section 5.3.1.3. This may explain why humans exhibit compromise when targets are close together. If so, it does not indicate which phenomenon preceded the other: did low-level compromise exist in all reaching behaviours and was then evolved out in all but the most beneficial cases, or was compromise behaviour an addition in some cases because it was so beneficial?

5.3.2   Proscriptive experiments

Although in the low-level prescriptive experiments compromise behaviour had less benefit than predicted, it could be argued that the prescriptive case is not best suited for eliciting positive results. It may be that compromise is more useful in cases where there is one prescriptive goal and one proscriptive goal:

proscriptive sub-problems such as avoiding hazards should place a demand on the animal's actions that it does not approach the hazard, rather than positively prescribing any particular action. It is obviously preferable to combine this demand with a preference to head toward food, if the two don't clash, rather than to head diametrically away from the hazard because the only system being considered is that of avoid hazard (Tyrrell, 1993, p. 170).

This section tests this claim by performing experiments similar to the prescriptive case, but with one proscriptive goal. In these experiments, the environment contains a target and a danger in fixed locations. The danger can 'strike' the agent from a limited distance. The agent has a prescriptive goal to be co-located with the target, and a proscriptive goal to avoid being struck by the danger.

5.3.2.1   Formal model

The model described in Section 5.3.1 requires modification to match this new scenario. The two environmental objects, the target (t) and the danger (d) are treated separately with individual probabilities of remaining in the environment (p_t and p_d, respectively). At each time step, there is a probability $p_n(\lambda)$ that the predator will *not* strike or pounce on the agent. This probability is a function of the distance between the agent and the danger, calculated from the agent's position λ. The experiments use four different versions of the $p_n(\lambda)$ function. The agent also has a goal level associated with the target and the danger, (G_t and G_d) that can vary with the quality of the resource and the damage due to the predator. Other notation remains the same.

The application of Equations (5.1) and (5.2) calculate the expected utility of being at λ:

$$EU(A_\theta|t, d, \lambda) = p_t p_d p_n(\lambda) EU(A_\theta|t, d, \lambda') + p_t(1 - p_d) EU(A_\theta|t, \lambda')$$
$$+ p_d(1 - p_n(\lambda)) G_d + (1 - p_t) p_d p_n(\lambda) EU(A_\theta|d, \lambda') \quad (5.10)$$

$$EU(A_\theta|t, \lambda) = G_t p^{\overline{\lambda t}}, \quad \text{and} \quad (5.11)$$

$$EU(A_\theta|d, \lambda) = p_n(\lambda') p_d EU(A_\theta|d, \lambda') + (1 - p_n(\lambda')) G_d. \quad (5.12)$$

The total expected utility (Equation 5.10) is the expectation over four possible situations: both target and danger are still there, but the danger does not strike; the target remains, but the danger disappears (no possibility of a strike now); the danger remains and strikes the agent (status of the target is not relevant); and the target disappears, the danger remains but the danger does not strike. When only the target remains, the optimal strategy is to go straight to the target, as in Equation (5.11). When the target disappears but the danger remains, the agent must flee to a safe distance from the danger, as in Equation (5.12). A safe distance is a variable parameter called the danger radius. Once the agent is outside the danger radius, it presumes that it is safe from the danger. The area inside the danger radius is the danger zone.

In addition to the optimal strategy described above, three other action selection strategies are examined:

- MEU: the agent moves in accordance with the maximum expected utility strategy, as described in Section 5.3.1. Movement is directly to the target, ignoring the danger, because the target has the higher utility. This is a non-compromise strategy that could be expected to do poorly.
- Active goal: this strategy considers only one goal at a time: the danger when in the danger zone and the target otherwise. Using this, the agent moves directly to the target unless within the danger zone. Within the danger zone, the agent moves directly away from the danger until it leaves the zone. This strategy zig-zags along the edge of the danger zone as the agent moves toward the target. Active goal is also a non-compromise strategy that only acts upon one goal at a time.
- Skirt: this strategy moves directly toward the target unless such a move would enter the danger zone. In such a position, the agent moves along the tangent edge of the danger zone until it can resume heading directly to the target. Skirt is primarily a

non-compromise strategy. Outside the danger radius, the agent moves straight to the target. Inside the danger radius the agent moves straight away from the danger.

The expected utility of each of these non-optimal mechanisms can be calculated for any particular scenario by using Equations (5.10), (5.11), and (5.12), as in the previous experiments.

For these experiments, four $p_n(\lambda)$ functions are used, all with a danger radius of 20:

- Linear A: $p_n(\lambda) = 0.04 \times \overline{d\lambda} + 0.2$ when $\overline{d\lambda} \leq 20$, 1 otherwise.
- Linear B: $p_n(\lambda) = 0.005 \times \overline{d\lambda} + .9$ when $\overline{d\lambda} \leq 20$, 1 otherwise.
- Quadratic: $p_n(\lambda) = (\overline{d\lambda})^2/400$ when, $\overline{d\lambda} \leq 20$, 1 otherwise.
- Sigmoid: $p_n(\lambda) = 1/(1 + 1.8^{10-\overline{d\lambda}})$ everywhere.

Linear A is a baseline strategy where the probability of a strike is high near the danger, but low at the edge of the danger zone. Linear B makes the chance of a strike low overall, thus increasing the tendency of the agent to remain in the danger zone. This may generate more compromise behaviour. Quadratic has a high probability of a strike for much of the danger zone, but drops off sharply at the edge. This may encourage compromise behaviour near the edge of the danger radius but not at the centre. Sigmoid should resemble quadratic, but the area with low strike probability is larger, and there is the possibility of some strike for every location in the environment, not just inside the danger radius.

5.3.2.2   Proscriptive results

A total of 1000 scenarios were generated with a target at (50, 90) with a $G_t = 100$ and a danger at (60, 50) with $G_d = -100$. p_t was varied systematically in range (0.95; 1) and p_d was varied systematically in the range (0.5; 1). These ranges were selected because they contain the most interesting behaviour. For instance, when p_t is too low, the probability that an agent will reach the target quickly approaches zero. Related studies (Crabbe, 2002) indicated that compromise behaviour was greater when $p_t > 0.95$). Once the scenario was generated, the expected utility for each of the three non-optimal strategies and the optimal strategy was calculated for 200 points in the environment, for 200 000 data points calculated over 312 computer-days.

Figure 5.4 shows the results of the optimal strategy when $p_t = 0.995$, $p_d = 0.99$, and $p_n(\lambda)$, is Linear A. Within the danger zone, there is little display of compromise action; the agent flees directly away from the danger at all locations, ignoring the target. There is compromise action displayed outside the danger zone, to the lower right. The vectors point not at the target, but along the tangent of the danger zone. This phenomenon occurs because the agent moves along the shortest path around the danger zone to maximise the likelihood that the target will remain in the environment until the agent arrives. The compromise in the lower right does not match the common implementations of compromise action. In most architectures, the goal to avoid the danger would not be active when the agent is in that area of the environment (since the agent is

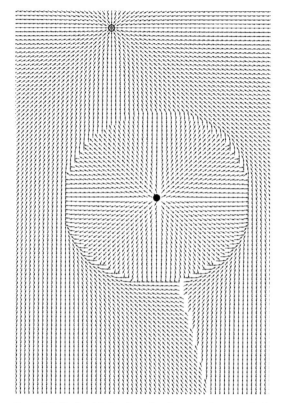

Figure 5.4 Optimal behaviour for the agent in proscriptive scenarios. The target is located along the top of the plot, indicated by an open circle. The danger is located near the centre of the plot, indicated by a filled circle. The large circle on the plots is formed by the vectors pointing away from the danger in areas inside the danger zone. Outside the danger zone, the vectors point toward the target. The probability of the target remaining is high ($p_t = 0.995$), the probability of the danger remaining is high ($p_d = 0.99$) and p_n (λ) is linear A. In most locations, the optimal strategy is to move directly toward the target. Inside the danger zone, the optimal strategy is to move directly away from the danger. On the side of the danger zone opposite the target, the optimal strategy is to move to the target along the shortest path while not entering the danger zone.

too far away from the danger; Arkin, 1998; Brooks, 1986). Thus one would expect it to have no effect of the action selected.

When p_d is reduced to 0.5 the compromise action in the lower right is less pronounced (Figure 5.5). The optimal strategy is to act as if the danger will disappear before the agent enters the danger zone. This property is seen in all the other experiments, i.e., when p_d is high, optimal behaviour avoids the danger zone and exhibits compromise behaviour in the lower right region, but when p_d is low, the agent moves straight to the target in that region.

When lowering p_t to 0.95 (with $p_d = 0.99$, and $p_n(\lambda)$ as Linear A), the results are qualitatively identical to Figure 5.4. (This and other additional plots can be found in the electronic supplementary materials in Crabbe (2007). When $p_t = 0.95$,

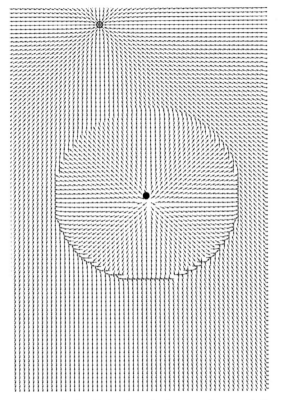

Figure 5.5 Optimal behaviour for the agent in proscriptive scenarios, similar to Figure 5.4. The parameters are the same as in Figure 5.4, but the probability of the danger remaining is low ($p_d =$ 0.5). The optimal behaviour is qualitatively the same as for Figure 5.4 except in the area on the side of the danger zone opposite the target, where optimal behaviour is to move directly toward the target (see text).

$p_d = 0.5$, and $p_n(\lambda)$, is Linear A, (i.e., low p_t and low p_d) predicted compromise behaviour emerges (Figure 5.6). The combination of both the urgency to get to the target with the likelihood that the danger will disappear leads to more target-focused behaviour in the danger zone.

Examining the nonlinear $p_n(\lambda)$ functions, compromise action is seen clearly in all cases. Figure 5.7 shows $p_t = 0.995$, $p_d = 0.99$, and $p_n(\lambda)$ is sigmoid. The compromise behaviour is evident both near the centre of the danger zone and again near the edges as the probability of a strike drops gradually from the danger. This also occurs when the $p_n(\lambda)$ is quadratic, though the transition at the edge of the danger zone has the same discontinuity seen with the linear functions.

Comparison between the optimal strategy and the other strategies described above is shown in Table 5.3. The table uses active goal as a baseline and compares skirt and the optimal strategy to it. The MEU strategy was poor (less than half as good as the other strategies across all trials, and one-sixth as good inside the danger zone), so was omitted from the table. The percentages are of the average expected utility for each strategy

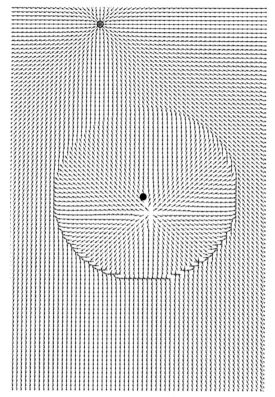

Figure 5.6 Optimal behaviour in situations where more compromise behaviour is shown. The figure should be interpreted in the same manner as Figure 5.4. Both the probability of the target and the danger remaining are low ($p_t = 0.95$, $p_d = 0.5$) and $p_n(\lambda)$ is Linear A. Compromise behaviour is evident inside the danger zone because the optimal direction of movement is no longer directly away from the danger.

across all the starting positions and scenarios (200 000 data points). Across all samples, the optimal behaviour performs 29.6% better than active goal, but skirt is nearly as good, performing 29.1% better than active goal. When considering just those locations on the other side of the danger zone from the target, the benefit is greater for optimal over active goal, but still only slightly so over skirt. This trend continues for locations inside the danger zone, and samples from each of the $p_n(\lambda)$ functions.

5.3.2.3   Proscriptive discussion

An examination of the data reveals properties of the optimal strategy that were not initially predicted (see Section 5.3.2). In stable environments (Figures 5.4 and 5.5), the priority is to flee the danger. Even in cases where the target is likely to disappear and the danger unlikely to remain more than a few time steps, with a moderate chance of a strike, the optimal action is to flee the danger first (Figure 5.5).

Compromise behaviour can be induced by reducing the p_t and p_d, and using the functions that reduce the chance of a strike, making the danger zone safer, and the target

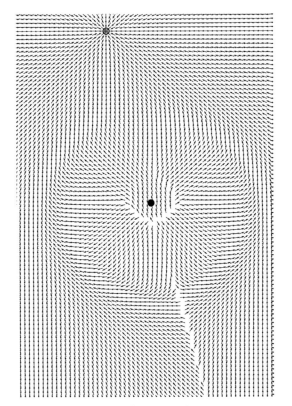

Figure 5.7 Optimal behavior in situations where more compromise behavior is shown, similar to Figure 5.6. The probability of the target remaining is high ($p_t = 0.995$), the probability of the danger remaining is high ($p_d = 0.99$), but p_n (λ) is Sigmoid. Within the centre of the danger zone, the optimal behaviour is to ignore the danger and move directly toward the target. In areas closer to the edge of the danger zone, the optimal strategy shifts to moving away from the danger. At the extremity of the danger radius, the optimal strategy gradually shifts back to moving toward the target.

more urgent. The nonlinear functions had the most unusual qualitative result, the area in the centre of the danger zone where the danger is ignored. It is thought that this is because the probability of the strike is so high that the agent would certainly fall victim, and the only differentiating property between possible moves is the target p_t.

While low-level compromise is shown to be beneficial in the proscriptive experiments, the experiments also show that it is not beneficial in the manner expected, namely that instead of inside the danger zone, low-level compromise is most beneficial outside the danger zone. Indeed, the comparison between the optimal and the skirt strategies shows that the majority of the benefit comes not from finding a compromise between two goals, but from preventing the oscillation between acting on each goal, thus generating longer than necessary paths along the edge of the danger zone. In the cases where the transition at the edge of the danger zone was less behaviourly severe (i.e., the $p_n(\lambda)$ was unlikely to generate a strike, so that optimal behaviour just inside and just outside the zone were

Table 5.3 Results comparing optimal and skirt strategies to the active goal. The values reflect the average per cent expected utility improvement of the samples. The rows are subsets of the data set. 'All' is across all scenarios and starting positions; 'opposite' is just the starting positions that are opposite from the target (the lower right region); 'Danger Zone' is across the starting positions inside the danger radius; 'Linear A', 'Linear B', 'Quadratic', and 'Sigmoid' are all positions when the $p_n(\lambda)$ is each of the named functions. The data consistently shows that the skirt strategy is nearly as good as the optimal one in all cases. All differences over active goal were significant in a Mann–Whitney U-test to a confidence level of 0.999.

Scenarios	Optimal over active goal	Skirt over active goal
All	29.6%	29.1%
Opposite	64.9%	63.3%
Danger Zone	26.2%	26.1%
Linear A	40.9%	40.8%
Linear B	13.5%	13.1%
Quadratic	48.6%	48.5%
Sigmoid	16.7%	15.2%

similar when $p_n(\lambda)$ is Linear B or Sigmoid) then the benefit of the optimal strategy is only 13–18% greater than the active goal strategy that zig-zags in and out of the danger zone.

5.4   Final discussion

This chapter has presented two sets of experiments analysing low-level compromise behaviour. The experimental setup was based on situations predicted to be amenable toward good compromise actions (Tyrrell, 1993), and used environments that are commonly seen in the artificial agent community (Blumberg *et al.*, 1996). The results show that compromise was not as beneficial as predicted in the prescriptive cases, and while it was beneficial in the proscriptive cases, it: (1) took forms different from what was expected, and (2) the vast majority of benefit came from low-level compromise that served primarily to shorten the overall path of the agent. This section will discuss the implications of these findings.

5.4.1   High versus low-level actions

Mounting experimental evidence (in this chapter and in other papers; Bryson, 2000; Crabbe, 2004; Jones *et al.*, 1999) appears to show that compromise behaviour is less helpful than predicted, and yet the intuition that compromise must have greater impact can still be strong. A simple thought experiment makes it appear even more so. Imagine an agent at a location l_0 that needs some of resource a and some of resource b. There is a quality source of a at l_1, a location far from a quality source of b at l_2. There is a single low-quality source of both a and b at l_3. Let the utility of a at location l_n be a_n. If there is some cost of movement c (a chance of the resource moving away or a direct cost such as energy consumed) then the agent should move to l_3 whenever $a_3 + b_3 - c(\overline{l_o l_3}) > a_1 + b_2 - c \times \min(\overline{l_o l_1} + \overline{l_1 l_2}, \overline{l_o l_2} + \overline{l_1 l_2})$. Using the council-of-ministers analogy, the a minister would cast some votes for l_1, but also some for l_3. Similarly, the b minister would cast votes for both l_2 and l_3. The agent might then select moving l_3 as its compromise choice when it is beneficial.

The key difference between the scenario just described and the experiments described in earlier sections is the nature of the actions selected. The experiments closely resembled the sort of compromise shown often in the ethological literature, where the actions selected appear as a continuous blend of the non-compromise actions, whereas the justification for compromise was posed as a discrete voting system. With voting, the compromise action selected can be radically different from the non-compromise actions, whereas blends tend to resemble the actions they are a blend of.

This difference arises due to the level at which the action is defined. Blending compromises take place at the lower levels, where the outputs are the motor commands for the agent. Thus changes allow for little variation in the output. Voting compromises take place at a higher level, where each choice can result in many varied low-level actions. Although this distinction is highlighted here, it is not common in literature. Tyrrell for example used the two definitions interchangeably (it may be that this distinction was not made by the early researchers in action selection in part because their experimental environments were entirely discrete and grid-based, thus affording few action options to the agent). As discussed in Section 5.2, selection of optimal actions at the low level is much more computationally difficult than selecting actions at a high level.

It should be noted that the 'three-layer architectures' in robotics do explicitly make this action level distinction, where higher layers select between multiple possible high-level behaviours, and then at lower layers, active behaviours select low-level actions. (Bonasso et al., 1997; Evans et al., 2008; Gat, 1991). In existing systems, when and where compromise behaviour is included varies from instance to instance in an ad hoc manner. Many modern hierarchical action selection mechanisms that explicitly use voting-base compromise tend to do so at the behaviour level only (Bryson, 2000; Pirjanian, 2000; Pirjanian et al., 1998).

5.4.2   Compromise behaviour hypothesis

The experiments and insights discussed above, lead us to propose the following Compromise Behaviour Hypothesis:

Compromise at low levels confers less overall benefit to an agent than does compromise at high levels. Compromise behaviour is progressively more useful as one moves upward in the level of abstraction at which the decision is made, for the following reasons: (1) In simple environments (e.g., two prescriptive goals), optimal compromise actions are similar to the possible non-optimal compromise actions as well as the possible non-compromise actions. As such, they offer limited benefit. In these environments there is no possibility of compromise at the higher levels. (2) In complex environments (e.g., where multiple resources are to be consumed in succession) good compromise behaviour can be very different from the active non-compromise behaviours, endowing it with the potential to be greatly superior to the non-compromise. (3) In complex environments, optimal or even very good non-optimal low-level actions are prohibitively difficult to calculate, whereas good higher level actions are not. Furthermore, easy to compute heuristics are unlikely to generate the radically different actions required for good compromise.

This hypothesis predicts that compromise behaviour will be beneficial in more complex environments, where the computational cost of selecting an action at a low level is prohibitive. In these environments, action selection at a high level, with compromise, may be the best strategy.

5.5   Conclusion

The notion of compromise behaviour has been influential in the action selection community despite disagreements about what precisely it might be. By examining the most common forms of compromise behaviour described by ethologists or implemented by computer scientists (low-level prescriptive and proscriptive), this chapter adds credence the idea that while it may exist in nature, low-level compromise behaviour affords little benefit. The chapter proposes that compromise is not especially useful at the low levels, but *is* useful at higher levels. Future work will revolve around testing, validation or refutation of this Compromise Behaviour Hypothesis.

Acknowledgements

We would like to thank Chris Brown and Rebecca Hwa for wonderful discussions. We would also like to thank the editors and anonymous reviewers for many helpful comments. This work was sponsored in part by a grant from the Office of Naval Research, number N0001404WR20377.

References

Antonelli, G., F. Arrichiello, and S. Chiaverini (2008). The null-space-based behavioral control for autonomous robotic systems. *Intell. Serv. Rob.* **1**(1): 27–39.

Arkin, R. (1998). *Behavior-based Robotics*. Cambridge, MA: MIT Press.

Avila-Garcia, O. and L. Canamero (2004). Using hormonal feedback to modulate action selection in a competitive scenario. In *From Animals to Animats 8: Proceedings of the Eighth International Conference on Simulation of Adaptive Behavior*, ed. S. Schaal, A. J. Ijspeert, A. Billard, *et al.* Cambridge, MA: MIT Press, pp. 243–54.

Bailey, W. J., R. J. Cunningham, and L. Lebel (1990). Song power, spectral distribution and female phonotaxis in the bushcricket *Requena verticalis* (Tettigoniiddae: Orthoptera): active female choice or passive attraction. *Anim. Behav.* **40**: 33–42.

Bartumeus, F. and J. Catalan (2009). Optimal search behavior and classic foraging theory. *J. Phys. A-Math. Theor.* **42**: 434002.

Bertsekas, D. P. (2005). *Dynamic Programming and Optimal Control.* Vol. 1. Belmont, MA: Athena Scientific.

Blumberg, B. M. (1994). Action-selection in Hamsterdam: lessons from ethology. In *From Animals to Animats 3: Proceedings of the Third International Conference on the Simulation of Adaptive Behavior*, ed. D. Cliff, P. Husbands, J. A. Meyer, and S. Wilson. Cambridge, MA: MIT Press, pp. 108–117.

Blumberg, B. M., P. M. Todd, and P. Maes (1996). No bad dogs: ethological lessons for learning in Hamsterdam. In *From Animals to Animats 4: Proceedings of the Fourth International Conference on Simulation of Adaptive Behavior*, ed. P. Maes, M. Mataric, J. A. Meyer, J. Pollack, and W. Wilson. Cambridge, MA: MIT Press, pp. 295–304.

Bonasso, R. P., R. J. Firby, E. Gat, D. Kortenkamp, and D. Miller (1997). Experiences with an architecture for intelligent, reactive agents. *J. Exp. Theor. Artif. In.* **9**(2): 237–56.

Bridle, S. L., O. Lahav, J. P. Ostriker, and P. J. Steinhardt (2003). Precision cosmology? Not just yet. *Science* **299**: 1532.

Brigant, I. (2005). The instinct concept of the early Konrad Lorenz. *J. Hist. Biol.* **38**(3): 571–608.

Brooks, R. (1986). A robust layered control system for a mobile robot. *IEEE J. Robotic. Autom.* **RA-2**: 14–23.

Brooks, R. (1997). From earwigs to humans. *Robot. Auton. Syst.* **20**(2–4): 291–304.

Brown, J. S. and B. Kotler (2004). Hazardous duty pay and the foraging cost of predation. *Ecol. Lett.* **7**: 999–1014.

Bryson, J. (2000). Hierarchy and sequence vs. full parallelism in action selection. In *From Animals to Animats 6: Proceedings of the Sixth International Conference on the Simulation of Adaptive Behavior*, ed. J. A. Meyer, A. Berthoz, D. Floreano, H. Roitblat, and S. Wilson. Cambridge, MA: MIT Press, pp. 147–56.

Burkhardt, R. W. (2004). *Patterns of Behavior: Konrad Lorenz, Niko Tinbergen, and the Founding of Ethology.* Chicago: Chicago University Press.

Caldwell, G. (1986). Predation as a selective force on foraging herons: effects of plumage color and flocking. *Auk* **103**: 494–505.

Cannings, C. and L. M. Cruz Orive (1975). On the adjustment of the sex ratio and the gregarious behavior of animal populations. *J. Theor. Biol.* **55**: 115–36.

Carruthers, P. (2004). Practical reasoning in a modular mind. *Mind Lang.* **19**(3): 259–78.

Choset, H., K. M. Lynch, S. Hutchinson, *et al.* (2005). *Principles of Robot Motion: Theory, Algorithms, and Implementations.* Cambridge, MA: MIT Press.

Clemen, R. (1996). *Making Hard Decisions: An Introduction to Decision Analysis.* Belmont, CA: Duxbury Press.

Crabbe, F. L. (2002). Compromise Candidates in Positive Goal Scenarios. In *From Animals to Animats 7: Proceedings of the Seventh International Conference on the Simulation of Adaptive Behavior*, ed. B. Hallam, D. Floreano, J. Hallam, G. Heyes, and J. A. Meyer. Cambridge, MA: MIT Press, pp. 105–106.

Crabbe, F. L. (2004). Optimal and non-optimal compromise strategies in action selection. In *From Animals to Animats 8: Proceedings of the Eighth International Conference on Simulation of Adaptive Behavior*, ed. S. Schaal, A. J. Ijspeert, A. Billard, *et al.* Cambridge, MA: MIT Press, pp. 233–42.

Crabbe, F. L. (2007). Compromise strategies for action selection. *Phil. Trans. R. Soc. Lond. B Biol. Sci.* **362**(1485): 1559–71.

Crabbe, F. L. and M. G. Dyer (1999). Second-order networks for wall-building agents. In *Proceedings of the International Joint Conference on Neural Networks*, ed. D. Brown. Washington, DC, USA: IEEE.

de Sevin, E., M. Kallmann, and D. Thalmann (2001). Towards real time virtual human life simulations. In *Computer Graphics International*. Hong Kong: IEEE Computer Society Press, pp. 31–4.

Decugis, V. and J. Ferber (1998). An extension of Maes' action selection mechanism for animats. In *From Animals to Animats 5: Proceedings of the Fifth International Conference on Simulation of Adaptive Behavior*, ed. R. Pfeifer, B. Blumberg, J-A. Meyer, and S. W. Wilson. Cambridge, MA: MIT Press, pp. 153–8.

Dewsbury, D. A. (1978). What is (was?) the 'fixed action pattern?' *Anim. Behav.* **26**: 310–11.

Dewsbury, D. A. (1992). Comparative psychology and ethology: a reassessment. *Am. Psychol.* **47**: 208–15.

Evans, J., P. Patron, B. Smith, and . M. Lane (2008). Design and evaluation of a reactive and deliberative collision avoidance and escape architecture for autonomous robots. *Auton. Rob.* **24**(3): 247–66.

Favilla, M. (2002). Reaching movements: mode of motor programming influences programming by time itself. *Exp Brain Res.* **144**: 414–18.

Fikes, R. E. and N. J. Nilsson (1971). STRIPS: a new approach to the application of theorem proving to problem solving. *Artif. Intell.* **2**(3–4): 189–208.

Fraenkel, G. S., and D. L. Gunn (1961). *The Orientation of Animals*. New York: Dover.

Fraser, D. F., and R. D. Cerri (1982). Experimental evaluation of predator–prey relationships in a patchy environment: consequences for habitat use patterns in minnows. *Ecology*, **63**(2): 307–13.

Gat, E. (1991). *Reliable goal-directed reactive control for real-world autonomous mobile robots*. Ph.D. thesis, Virginia Polytechnic Institute and State University, Blacksburg, VA.

Gerevini, A. E., A. Saetti, and I. Serina (2008). An approach to efficient planning with numerical fluents and multi-criteria plan quality. *Artif. Intell.* **172**(8–9): 899–944.

Ghallab, M., D. Nau, and P. Traverso (2004). *Automated Planning: Theory and Practice*. San Francisco, CA: Morgan Kaufmann Publishers Inc.

Ghez, C., M. Favilla, M. F. Ghilardi, *et al.* (1997). Discrete and continuous planning of hand movements and isometric force trajectories. *Exp. Brain Res.* **115**: 217–33.

Girard, B., V. Cuzin, A. Guillot, K. N. Gurney, and T. J. Prescott (2002). Comparing a brain-inspired robot action selection mechanism with 'winner-takes-all'. In *From Animals to Animats 7: Proceedings of the Seventh International Conference on the Simulation of Adaptive Behavior*, ed. B. Hallam, D. Floreano, J. Hallam, G. Heyes, and J. A. Meyer. Cambridge, MA: MIT Press, pp. 75–84.

Grubb, T. C. and L. Greenwald (1982). Sparrows and a brushpile: foraging responses to different combinations of predation risk and energy cost. *Anim. Behav.* **30**: 637–40.

Hillier, F. S. and G. J. Lieberman (2002). *Introduction to Operations Research*. New York: McGraw-Hill.

Hinde, R. A. (1966). *Animal Behaviour*. New York: McGraw-Hill.

Hoffmann, J. (2003). The Metric-FF planning system: translating ignoring delete lists to numeric state variables. *J. Artif. Intell. Res.* **20**(20): 291–341.

Houston, A. I., J. M. McNamara, and S. Steer (2007). Do we expect natural selection to produce rational behavior. *Phil. Trans. Roy. Soc. B* **362**(1485): 1531–43.

Howard, R. A. (1977). Risk preference. In *Readings in Decision Analysis*. Menlo Park, CA: SRI International.

Humphrys, M. (1996). *Action Selection Methods Using Reinforcement Learning*. Ph.D. thesis, University of Cambridge, Cambridge, UK.

Hurdus, J. G. and D. W. Hong (2009). Behavioral programming with hierarchy and parallelism in the DARPA Urban Challenge and RoboCup. In *Multisensor Fusion and Integration for Intelligent Systems*. ed. H. Hahn, H. Ko, and S. Lee. Berlin: Springer, pp. 255–69.

Hutchinson, J. M. C. (1999). Bet-hedging when targets may disappear: optimal mate-seeking or prey-catching trajectories and the stability of leks and herds. *J. Theor. Biol.* **196**: 33–49.

Hutchinson, J. M. C. and G. Gigerenzer (2005). Simple heuristics and rules of thumb: where psychologists and behavioural biologists might meet. *Behav. Process.* **69**: 97–124.

Iglesias, A. and F. Luengo (2005). New goal selection scheme for behavioral animation of intelligent virtual agents. *IEICE Trans. Inf. and Syst.* **E88-D**(5): 865–71.

Jaafar, J. and E. McKenzie (2008). A fuzzy action selection method for virtual agent navigation in unknown virtual environments. *J. Uncertain Syst.* **2**(2): 144–54.

Jones, R. M., J. E. Laird, P. E. Nielsen, *et al.* (1999). Automated intelligent pilots for combat flight simulation. *AI Magazine*, **20**(1): 27–42.

Krebs, J. R. and N. Davies, eds (1997). *Behavioural Ecology: An Evolutionary Approach*. Oxford: Blackwell Publishers.

Krebs, J. R., J. T. Erichsen, M. I. Webber, and E. L. Charnov (1977). Optimal prey selection in the great tit (*Parus major*). *Anim. Behav.* **25**: 30–8.

Latimer, W. and M. Sippel (1987). Acoustic cues for female choice and male competition in *Tettigonia cantans*. *Anim. Behav.* **35**: 887–900.

Lima, S. L. (1998). Stress and decision making under the risk of predation: recent developments from behavioral, reproductive, and ecological perspectives. *Adv. Stud. Behav.* **27**: 215–90.

Lorenz, K. Z. (1981). *The Foundations of Ethology*. New York: Springer-Verlag.

Lund, H. H., B. Webb, and J. Hallam (1997). A robot attracted to the cricket species *Gryllus bimaculatus*. In *Fourth European Conference on Artificial Life*, ed. P. Husbands and I. Harvey. Brighton, UK: MIT Press/Bradford Books, pp. 246–55.

Luo, X. and N. R. Jennings (2007). A spectrum of compromise aggregation operators for multi-attribute decision making. *Artif. Intell.* **171**(2–3): 161–184.

Maes, P. (1990). How to do the right thing. *Connect. Sci., Special Issue on Hybrid Systems* **1**: 291–323.

McNamara, J. M. and A. I. Houston (1980). The application of statistical decision theory to animal behaviour. *J. Theor. Biol.* **85**: 673–90.

McNamara, J. M. and A. I. Houston (1994). The effect of a change in foraging options on intake rate and predation rate. *Am. Nat.* **144**: 978–1000.

Mesterton-Gibbons, M. (1989). On compromise in foraging and an experiment by Krebs *et al.* (1977). *J. Math. Biol.* **27**: 273–96.

Milinksi, M. (1986). Constraints places by predators on feeding behavior. In *The behavior of teleost fishes*, ed. T. J. Pitcher. London: Croom Helm, pp. 236–56.

Mitchell, T. M. (1997). *Machine Learning*. Boston: McGraw-Hill.

Montes-Gonzales, F., T. J. Prescott, K. Gurney, M. Humphrys, and P. Redgrave (2000). An embodied model of action selection mechanisms in the vertebrate brain. In *From Animals to Animats 6: Proceedings of the Sixth International Conference on the Simulation of Adaptive*

Behavior, ed. J. A. Meyer, A. Berthoz, D. Floreano, H. Roitblat, and S. Wilson. Cambridge, MA: MIT Press, pp. 157–66.

Morris, G. K., G. E. Kerr, and J. H. Fullard (1978). Phonotactic preferences of female meadow katydids. *Can. J. Zool.* **56**: 1479–87.

Müller, A. (1925). Über Lichtreaktionen von Landasseln. *Z. vergl. Physiol.* **3**: 113–44.

Newell, A. and H. A. Simon (1976). Computer science as empirical inquiry: symbols and search. *Comm. ACM* **19**(3): 113–26.

Pfeifer, R. and C. Scheier (1999). *Understanding Intelligence*. Cambridge, MA: MIT Press.

Pirjanian, P. (2000). Multiple objective behavior-based control. *J. Robot. Auton. Syst.* **31**(1–2): 53–60.

Pirjanian, P, H. I. Christensen, and J. A. Fayman (1998). Application of voting to fusion of purposive modules: an experimental investigation. *J. Robot. Auton. Syst.* **23**(4): 253–66.

Quinlan, J. R. (1983). Learning efficient classification procedures and their application to chess and games. In *Machine Learning: an artificial intelligence approach*, ed. R. S. Michalski, J. G. Carbonell, and T. M. Mitchell. San Mateo, CA: Morgan Kaufmann, pp. 463–82.

Quinlan, J. R. (1993). *C4.5: Programs for Machine Learning*. San Mateo, CA: Morgan Kaufmann.

Refanidis, I. and I. Vlahavas (2003). Multiobjective heuristic state-space planning. *Artif. Intell.* **145**(1–2): 1–32.

Römer, H. (1993). Environmental and biological constraints for the evolution of long-range signalling and hearing in acoustic insects. *Phil. Trans. Roy. Soc. B*. **340**: 179–85.

Russell, S. and P. Norvig (2010). *Artificial Intelligence. A Modern Approach*. 3rd edn. Cambridge, MA: MIT Press.

Seth, A. K. (2007). The ecology of action selection. *Phil. Trans. Roy. Soc. B*. **362**(1485): 1545–58.

Stephens, W. and J. R. Krebs (1986). *Foraging Theory*. Princeton, NJ: Princeton University Press.

Thorisson, K. R. (1996). Communicative humanoids: a computational model of psychosocial dialogue skills. Ph.D. thesis, Massachusetts Institute of Technology, Cambridge, MA.

Thorpe, W. H. (1979). *The Origins and Rise of Ethology*. New York: Preager.

Tinbergen, N. (1950). The hierarchical organisation of nervous mechanisms underlying instinctive behavior. *Sympos. Soc. Exper. Biol.* **4**: 305–12.

Todd, P. M. (1992). Machine intelligence – the animat path to intelligent adaptive behaviour. *IEEE Computer* **25**(11): 78–81.

Tu, X. (1996). Artificial animals for computer animation: biomechanics, locomotion, perception, and behavior. Ph.D. thesis, University of Toronto, Department of Computer Science.

Tyrrell, T. (1993). Computational mechanism for action selection. Ph.D. thesis, University of Edinburgh.

von Holst, E. (1935). Über den Lichtruchenreflex bei Fischen. *Publ. Staz. Zool.* **15**: 143–58.

Werner, G. M. (1994). Using second order neural connection for motivation of behavioral choices. In *Proceedings of the Third International Conference on Simulation of Adaptive Behavior*, ed. D. Cliff, P. Husbands, J-A. Meyer, and S. W. Wilson. Brighton, UK: MIT Press, pp. 154–61.

6 Extending a biologically inspired model of choice: multi-alternatives, nonlinearity, and value-based multidimensional choice

Rafal Bogacz, Marius Usher, Jiaxiang Zhang, and James L. McClelland

Summary

The Leaky Competing Accumulator (LCA) is a biologically inspired model of choice. It describes the processes of leaky accumulation and competition observed in neuronal populations during choice tasks and it accounts for reaction time distributions observed in psychophysical experiments. This chapter discusses recent analyses and extensions of the LCA model. First, it reviews the dynamics and it examines the conditions that make the model achieve optimal performance. Second, it shows that nonlinearities of the type present in biological neurons improve performance when the number of choice-alternatives increases. Third, the model is extended to value-based choice, where it is shown that nonlinearities in the value function, explain risk-aversion in risky-choice and preference reversals in choice between alternatives characterised across multiple dimensions.

6.1 Introduction

Making choices on the basis of visual perceptions is an ubiquitous and central element of human and animal life, which has been studied extensively in experimental psychology. Within the last half century, mathematical models of choice reaction times have been proposed which assume that, during the choice process, noisy evidence supporting the alternatives is accumulated (Laming, 1968; Ratcliff, 1978; Stone, 1960; Vickers, 1970). Within the last decade, data from neurobiological experiments have shed further light on the neural bases of such choice. For example, it has been reported that while a monkey decides which of two stimuli is presented, certain neuronal populations gradually increase their firing rate, thereby accumulating evidence supporting the alternatives (Gold and Shadlen, 2002; Schall, 2001; Shadlen and Newsome, 2001). Recently, a series of neurocomputational models have offered an explanation of the neural mechanism

Modelling Natural Action Selection, eds. Anil K. Seth, Tony J. Prescott and Joanna J. Bryson.
Published by Cambridge University Press. © Cambridge University Press 2012.

underlying both, psychological measures like reaction times and neurophysiological data of choice. One such model, is the Leaky Competing Accumulator (LCA; Usher and McClelland, 2001), which is sufficiently simple to allow a detailed mathematical analysis. Furthermore, as we will discuss, this model can, for certain values of its parameters, approximate the same computations carried out by a series of mathematical models of choice (Busemeyer and Townsend, 1993; Ratcliff, 1978; Shadlen and Newsome, 2001; Vickers, 1970; Wang, 2002).

Since its original publication, the LCA model (Usher and McClelland, 2001) has been analysed mathematically and extended in a number of directions (Bogacz *et al.*, 2006; Brown *et al.*, 2005; Brown and Holmes, 2001; McMillen and Holmes, 2006). In particular, which values of parameters achieve an optimal performance have been investigated. This matter is important, because if 'we expect natural selection to produce rational behaviour', as discussed by Houston *et al.* (2006), then the values of parameters revealed by these analyses should be found in the neural networks mediating choice processes. In this chapter, we will use the word 'optimal' to describe the theoretically best possible performance. In some cases, decision networks cannot achieve the optimal performance, e.g., due to some biological constraints, however, it is still of interest to investigate which parameters give best possible performance within the constraints considered – we use the word 'optimised' to refer to such performance.

It has been shown that for choices between two alternatives, the LCA model achieves optimal performance for particular values of parameters when its processing is linear (Bogacz *et al.*, 2006) or remains in a linear range (Brown *et al.*, 2005) (the precise meaning of these conditions will be reviewed later). However, it is known that information processing in biological neurons is nonlinear and two questions remain open: (1) is linear processing also optimal for choice between multiple alternatives, and (2) what are the parameters of the nonlinear LCA model that optimise its performance?

This chapter has two aims. First, it reviews the biological mechanisms assumed in the LCA model, and reviews an analysis of the dynamics and performance of the linear and nonlinear LCA models (Section 6.2). Second, it presents new developed extensions connected with the introduction of nonlinearities. In Section 6.3 we show that nonlinearities (of the type present in biological neurons) may improve performance in choice between multiple alternatives. In Section 6.4 we discuss how to optimise the performance of the nonlinear LCA model for two alternatives. Finally, in Section 6.5 we show how nonlinearities in the LCA model also explain counterintuitive results from choice experiments involving multiple goals or stimulus dimensions.

6.2   Review of the LCA model

In this section we briefly review the experimental data on neurophysiology of choice and models proposed to describe them, focusing on the LCA model. We examine the linear version and nonlinear versions of this model and we analyse its dynamics and performance.

6.2.1   Neurophysiology of choice

The neurophysiology of choice processes has been the subject of a number of recent reviews (Schall, 2001; Sugrue *et al.*, 2005). We start by describing a typical task used to study perceptual choice, which makes use of three important processes: representation of noisy evidence, integration of evidence, and meeting a decision criterion.

In a typical experiment used to study neural bases of perceptual choice, animals are presented with a cloud of moving dots on a computer screen (Britten *et al.*, 1993). In each trial, a proportion of the dots are moving coherently in one direction, while the remaining dots are moving randomly. The animal has to indicate the direction of prevalent dot movement by making a saccade in the corresponding direction. There are two versions of this task. The first one is the *free-response* paradigm, in which participants are allowed to respond at any moment of time. The second paradigm is the *interrogation* (or response–signal) paradigm, in which participants are required to continuously observe the stimulus until a particular signal (whose delay is controlled) is provided and which prompts an immediate response.

During the choice process, sensory areas (e.g., motion area MT) provide noisy evidence supporting the alternatives, which is represented in the firing rates of motion-sensitive neurons tuned to specific directions (Britten *et al.*, 1993; Schall, 2001). Let us denote the mean activity of the population providing evidence supporting alternative i by I_i. The perceptual choice problem may be formulated simply as finding which I_i is the highest. However, this question is not trivial, as the activity levels of these input neurons are noisy (Britten *et al.*, 1993), and hence answering this question requires sampling the inputs for a certain period.

It has been observed that in this task neurons in certain cortical regions including the lateral intraparietal area (LIP) and the frontal eye field (FEF) gradually increase their firing rates (Schall, 2001; Shadlen and Newsome, 2001). Furthermore, because the easier the task, the faster is the rate of this increase (Shadlen and Newsome, 2001), it has been suggested that these neurons integrate the evidence from sensory neurons over time (Schall, 2001; Shadlen and Newsome, 2001). This integration averages out the noise present in sensory neurons allowing the accuracy of the choice to increase with time. Moreover, because (in the free-response paradigm) the firing rate, just before the saccade, does not differ between difficulty levels of the task (Roitman and Shadlen, 2002), it is believed that the choice is made when the activity of the neuronal population representing one of the alternatives reaches a decision threshold.

6.2.2   Biologically inspired models of perceptual choice

A number of computational models have been proposed to describe the choice process described above, and their architectures are shown in Figure 6.1 for the case of two alternatives (Mazurek *et al.*, 2003; Usher and McClelland, 2001; Wang, 2002). All of these models include two units (bottom circles in Figure 6.1) corresponding to neuronal populations providing noisy evidence, and two accumulator units (denoted by y_1 and y_2

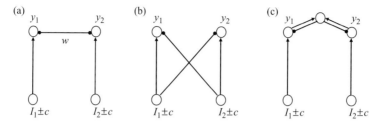

Figure 6.1 Architectures of the models of choice. Arrows denote excitatory connections, lines with filled circles denote inhibitory connections. (a) LCA model (Usher and McClelland, 2001) (b) Mazurek *et al.* (2003) model, (c) Wang (2002) model.

in Figure 6.1) integrating the evidence. The models differ in the way inhibition affects the integration process: in the LCA model (Figure 6.1a) the accumulators inhibit each other, in the Mazurek *et al.* (2003) model (Figure 6.1b) the accumulators receive inhibition from the other inputs, and in the Wang (2002) model (Figure 6.1c) the accumulators inhibit each other via a population of inhibitory inter-neurons. It has been shown that for certain values of their parameters, these models become computationally equivalent, as they all implement the same optimal algorithm for decision between two alternatives (Bogacz *et al.*, 2006). In this chapter, we thus focus on the LCA model, and we review its optimality (analogous analysis for the other two models is described in Bogacz *et al.*, 2006).

6.2.3   Linear LCA model

Figure 6.1a shows the architecture of the LCA model for the two alternative choice tasks (Usher and McClelland, 2001). The accumulator units are modelled as leaky integrators with activity levels denoted by y_1 and y_2. Each accumulator unit integrates evidence from an input unit with mean activity I_i and independent white noise fluctuations dW_i of amplitude c_i (dW_i denote independent Wiener processes). These units also inhibit each other by way of a connection of weight w. Hence, during the choice process, information is accumulated according to (Usher and McClelland, 2001):

$$\begin{cases} dy_1 = (-ky_1 - wy_2 + I_1)\,dt + c_1 dW_1 \\ dy_2 = (-ky_2 - wy_1 + I_2)\,dt + c_2 dW_2 \end{cases}, \quad y_1(0) = y_2(0) = 0. \qquad (6.1)$$

In the equations above, the term k denotes the decay rate of the accumulators' activity (i.e., the leak) and $-wy_i$ denotes the mutual inhibition. For simplicity, it is assumed that integration starts from $y_1(0) = y_2(0) = 0$ (cf. Bogacz *et al.*, 2006).

The LCA model can be used to describe the two paradigms described in Subsection 6.2.1. In the free-response paradigm, the model is assumed to make a response as soon as either accumulator exceeds a preassigned threshold, Z. The interrogation paradigm is modelled by assuming that at the interrogation time the choice is made in favour of the alternative with higher y_i at the moment when the choice is requested.

Because the goal of the choice process is to select the alternative with highest mean input I_i, in the following analyses and simulations we always set $I_1 > I_2$. Hence a simulated choice is considered to be correct if the first alternative is chosen; this will happen in the majority of simulated trials. However, in some trials, due to noise, another alternative may be chosen; such trials correspond to incorrect responses. By simulating the model multiple times expected error rate (ER) may be estimated. In addition, in the free-response paradigm, the average decision time (DT) from choice onset to reaching the threshold can be computed.

The LCA model can be naturally extended to N alternatives. In this case, the dynamics of each accumulator i is described by the following equation (Usher and McClelland, 2001):

$$dy_i = \left(-ky_i - w \sum_{\substack{j=1 \\ j \neq i}}^{N} y_j + I_i \right) dt + c_i dW_i, \quad y_i(0) = 0. \tag{6.2}$$

When the decay and inhibition parameters are equal to zero, the terms in Equations (6.1) and (6.2) describing leak and competition disappear, and the linear LCA model reduces to another model known in psychological literature as the *race* model (Vickers, 1970; 1979), in which accumulators integrate noisy evidence independent of one another.

6.2.4 Dynamics of the model

The review of dynamics of the linear LCA model in this subsection is based on Bogacz *et al.* (2006). In the case of two alternatives, the state of the model at a given moment in time is described by the values of y_1 and y_2, and may therefore be represented as a point on a plane whose horizontal and vertical axes correspond to y_1 and y_2; the evolution of activities of the accumulator units during the choice process may be visualised as a path in this plane. Representative paths for three different parameter ranges in this plane are shown in Figure 6.2. In each case the choice process starts from $y_1 = 0$ and $y_2 = 0$, i.e., from the bottom left corner of each panel. Initially the activities of both accumulators increase due to stimulus onset, which is represented by a path going in an upper-right direction. But as the accumulators become more active, mutual inhibition causes the activity of the 'weaker' accumulator to decrease and the path moves toward the threshold for the more strongly activated accumulator (i.e., the correct choice).

To better understand the dynamics of the model, Figure 6.2 shows its *vector fields*. Each arrow shows the average direction in which the state moves from the point indicated by the arrow's tail, and its length corresponds to the speed of movement (i.e., rate of change) in the absence of noise. Note that in all three panels of Figure 6.2 there is a line, indicated by a thick grey line, to which all states are attracted: the arrows point towards this line from both sides. The location along this line represents an important variable: the difference in activity between the two accumulators. As most of the choice-determining dynamics occur along this line, it is helpful to make use of new coordinates rotated clockwise by 45° with respect to the y_1 and y_2 coordinates. These new coordinates are shown in Figure 6.2b: x_1 is parallel to the attracting line and describes the difference

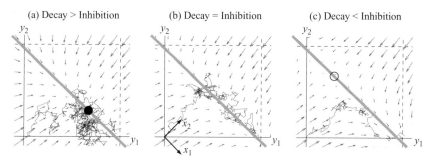

Figure 6.2 Examples of the evolution of the LCA model, showing paths in the state space of the model. The horizontal axes denote the activation of the first accumulator; the vertical axes denote the activation of the second accumulator. The paths show the choice process from stimulus onset (where $y_1 = y_2 = 0$) to reaching a threshold (thresholds are shown by dashed lines). The model was simulated for the following parameters: $I_1 = 4.41$, $I_2 = 3$, $c = 0.33$, $Z = 0.4$. The sum of inhibition (w) and decay (k) is kept constant in all panels, by setting $k + w = 20$, but the parameters themselves have different values in different panels: (a) $w = 7$, $k = 13$; (b) $w = 10$, $k = 10$; (c) $w = 13$, $k = 7$. The simulations were performed using the Euler method with timestep $\Delta t = 0.01$. To simulate the Wiener processes, at every step of integration, each of the variables y_1 and y_2 was increased by a random number from the normal distribution with mean 0 and variance $c^2 \Delta t$. The arrows show the average direction of movement of LCA model in the state space. The thick grey lines symbolise the attracting lines. The filled circle in panel (a) indicates the attractor. The open circle in panel (c) indicates the unstable fixed point.

between activities of the two accumulators; while x_2 describes the sum of their activities. The transformation from y to x coordinates is given by (cf. Seung, 2003):

$$
\begin{cases}
x_1 = \dfrac{y_1 - y_2}{\sqrt{2}}, \\[2mm]
x_2 = \dfrac{y_1 + y_2}{\sqrt{2}}.
\end{cases}
\tag{6.3}
$$

In these new coordinates Equations (6.1) become (Bogacz *et al.*, 2006):

$$
dx_1 = \left((w - k)x_1 + \frac{I_1 - I_2}{\sqrt{2}} \right) dt + \frac{c_1}{\sqrt{2}} dW_1 - \frac{c_2}{\sqrt{2}} dW_2,
\tag{6.4}
$$

$$
dx_2 = \left((-k - w)x_2 + \frac{I_1 + I_2}{\sqrt{2}} \right) dt + \frac{c_1}{\sqrt{2}} dW_1 + \frac{c_2}{\sqrt{2}} dW_2.
\tag{6.5}
$$

Equations (6.4) and (6.5) are *uncoupled*; that is, the rate of change of each x_i depends only on x_i itself (this was not the case for y_1 and y_2 in Equations (6.1)). Hence, the evolution of x_1 and x_2 may be analysed separately.

We first consider the dynamics in the x_2 direction, corresponding to the summed activity of the two accumulators, which has the faster dynamics. As noted above, on all panels of Figure 6.2 there is a line to whose proximity the state is attracted, implying that x_2 initially increases and then fluctuates around the value corresponding to the position of the attracting line. The magnitude of these fluctuations depends on the inhibition and decay parameters; the larger the sum of inhibition and decay, the smaller the fluctuation (i.e., the closer the system stays to the attracting line).

Figure 6.2 also shows that the dynamics of the system in the direction of coordinate x_1. These dynamics are slower than the x_2 dynamics and correspond to a motion along the line. Their characteristics depend on the relative values of inhibitory weight w and decay k. When decay is larger than inhibition, there are also attractor dynamics for the x_1 dynamics, as shown in Figure 6.2a. The system is attracted towards this point and fluctuates in its vicinity. In Figure 6.2a the threshold is reached when noise pushes the system away from the attractor. When inhibition is larger than decay, x_1-dynamics are characterised by repulsion from the fixed point, as shown in Figure 6.2c.

When inhibition equals decay, the term $(w - k) x_1$ in Equation (6.4) disappears, and Equation (6.4) describing the evolution along the attracting line can be written as:

$$dx_1 = \left(\frac{I_1}{\sqrt{2}} dt + \frac{c_1}{\sqrt{2}} dW_1 \right) - \left(\frac{I_2}{\sqrt{2}} dt + \frac{c_2}{\sqrt{2}} dW_2 \right). \qquad (6.6)$$

In the remainder of this chapter we refer to the linear LCA model with inhibition equal to decay as *balanced*. The vector field for this case is shown in Figure 6.2b. In this case, according to Equation (6.6) the value of x_1 changes according to the difference in evidence in support of two alternatives, hence the value of x_1 is equal to the *accumulated* difference in evidence in support of two alternatives.

The three cases illustrated in Figure 6.2 make different predictions about the impact of temporal information on choice in the interrogation paradigm. If inhibition is larger than decay (Figure 6.2c), and the repulsion is high, the state is likely to remain on the same side of the fixed point. This causes a *primacy effect* (Busemeyer and Townsend, 1993; Usher and McClelland, 2001): the inputs at the beginning of the trial determine to which side of the fixed point the state of the network moves, and then due to repulsion, late inputs before the interrogation time have little effect on choice made. Analogously, decay larger than inhibition produces a *recency effect*: the inputs later in the trial have more influence on the choice than inputs at the beginning, whose impact has decayed (Busemeyer and Townsend, 1993; Usher and McClelland, 2001). If the decay is equal to inhibition, inputs during the whole trial (from the stimulus onset to the interrogation signal) influence the choice equally, resulting in a balanced choice (with maximal detection accuracy; see below). Usher and McClelland (2001) tested whether the effects described above are present in human decision makers by manipulating the time flow of input favouring two alternatives, and reported significant individual differences: some participants showed primacy, others showed recency and some were balanced and optimal in their choice.

6.2.5   Performance of linear LCA model

In this subsection we review parameters of the model (w, k) that result in an optimal performance of the linear LCA model in the free-response paradigm for given parameters of the inputs (I_i, c_i). We start with the two alternatives in the free-response paradigm (Bogacz *et al.*, 2006), then we discuss multiple alternatives (see also McMillen and Holmes, 2006), and the interrogation paradigm.

When inhibition and decay are both fairly strong (as in Figure 6.2b), the state evolves very closely to the attracting line (see above) reaching the decision threshold very close to the intersection of the decision threshold and attracting line (see Figure 6.2b). Thus in this case, the LCA model exceeds one of the decision thresholds approximately when the variable x_1 exceeds a positive value (corresponding to y_1 exceeding Z) or decreases below a certain negative value (corresponding to y_2 exceeding Z).

The above analysis shows that when the LCA model is balanced and both inhibition and decay are high, a choice is made approximately when x_1 representing the accumulated difference between the evidence supporting the two alternatives exceeds a positive or negative threshold. This is the characteristic of a mathematical choice model known as the diffusion model (Laming, 1968; Ratcliff, 1978; Stone, 1960), which implements the optimal statistical test for choice in the free-response paradigm: the Sequential Probability Ratio Test (SPRT) (Barnard, 1946; Wald, 1947). The SPRT is optimal in the following sense: among all possible procedures for solving this choice problem given a certain ER, it minimises the average DT.

In summary, when the linear LCA model of choice between two alternatives is balanced and both inhibition and decay are high, the model approximates the optimal SPRT and makes the fastest decisions for fixed ERs (Bogacz *et al.*, 2006).

In the case of multiple alternatives the performance of the linear LCA model is also optimised when inhibition is equal to decay and both have high values (McMillen and Holmes, 2006). However, in contrast to the case of two alternatives, the LCA model with the above parameters does not achieve as good performance as the statistically (asymptotically) optimal tests: the Multiple SPRT (MSPRT) (Dragalin *et al.*, 1999). The MSPRT tests require much more complex neuronal implementation than the LCA model (McMillen and Holmes, 2006). For example, one of the MSPRT tests may be implemented by the 'max vs. next' procedure (McMillen and Holmes, 2006), in which the following quantities are calculated for each alternative at each moment of time: $L_i = y_i\text{-max}_{j \neq i} y_j$, where y_i is the evidence supporting alternative i accumulated according to the race model. The choice is made whenever any of the L_i exceeds a threshold.

Although the linear and balanced LCA with high inhibition and decay achieves shorter DT for fixed ER than the linear LCA model with other values of parameters (e.g., inhibition different from decay, or both equal to zero), it is slower than MSPRT (McMillen and Holmes, 2006). Furthermore, as the number of alternatives for N increases, the best achievable DT for a fixed ER of the linear balanced LCA model approaches that of the race model (McMillen and Holmes, 2006).

In the interrogation paradigm, the LCA model achieves optimal performance when it is balanced both for two alternatives (it then implements the Neyman–Pearson test (Bogacz *et al.*, 2006; Neyman and Pearson, 1933)) and for multiple alternatives (McMillen and Holmes, 2006). However, by contrast to the free-response paradigm, in the interrogation paradigm, the high value of decay and inhibition is not necessary for optimal performance and the balanced LCA model (even with high inhibition and decay) achieves the same performance as the race model.

Table 6.1 summarises conditions necessary for the linear LCA model to implement the optimal algorithm for a given type of choice problem. Note that the linear LCA model can implement the algorithms achieving best possible performance for all cases except of choice between multiple alternatives in the free-response paradigm. Hence this is the only case in which there exists room for improvement of the LCA model – this case is addressed in Section 6.3.

Table 6.1 Summary of conditions the linear LCA model must satisfy to implement the optimal choice algorithms.

	# of alternatives	
Paradigm	$N = 2$	$N > 2$
Free response	Inhibition = Decay and both high	*Optimality not attainable*
Interrogation	Inhibition = Decay	Inhibition = Decay
(response-signal)		

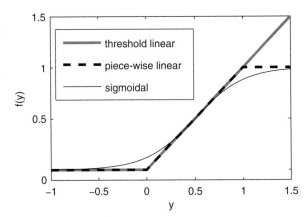

Figure 6.3 Nonlinear input–output functions used in the LCA model. Threshold linear: $f(y) = y$ for $y \geq 0$ and $f(y) = 0$ for $y < 0$ (Usher and McClelland, 2001). Piece-wise linear: $f(y) = 0$ for $y < 0$, $f(y) = 1$ for $y > 1$, and $f(y) = y$ otherwise (Brown *et al.*, 2005). Sigmoidal: $f(y) = 1 / (1 + e^{-4(y-0.5)})$ (Brown *et al.*, 2005; Brown and Holmes, 2001).

6.2.6   Nonlinear LCA model

In the linear version of the LCA model described so far, during the course of the choice process, the activity levels of accumulators can achieve arbitrarily large or small (including negative) values. However, the firing rate of biological neurons cannot be negative and cannot exceed a certain level (due to the refractory period of biological neurons). A number of ways of capturing these limits in the LCA model has been proposed, starting with the original version (Usher and McClelland, 2001), where the values of y_1 and y_2 are transformed through a nonlinear activation function $f(y)$ before they influence (inhibit) each other:

$$dy_i = \left(-ky_i - w \sum_{\substack{j=1 \\ j \neq i}}^{N} f\left(y_j\right) + I_i \right) dt + c_i dW_i, \quad y_i(0) = 0. \tag{6.7}$$

Figure 6.3 shows three functions $f(y)$ proposed in the literature: threshold linear (Usher and McClelland, 2001), piece-wise linear (Brown *et al.*, 2005), and sigmoidal (Brown *et al.*, 2005; Brown and Holmes, 2001). The threshold linear function corresponds to the

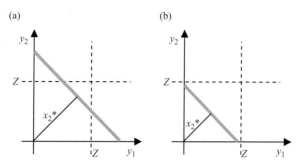

Figure 6.4 State plane analysis of the LCA model. Thick grey lines symbolise attracting lines in the y_1y_2 plane. The position of the attracting line is shown for parameters used in simulations in Figure 6.5a and b, respectively. Thus the distance x_2^* of the attracting line from the origin is equal to 0.26 and 0.12, respectively (from Equation (6.8)). The dashed lines indicate the thresholds. The values of the threshold are shown that produce ER $= 10\%$ in simulations of the unbounded (linear) LCA model for $N = 2$ alternatives in Figure 6.5a and b respectively, i.e., 0.25 and 0.17.

constraint that actual neural activity is bounded (by zero) at its low end. The piece-wise linear and sigmoidal functions bound the activity levels of accumulators at both ends (the maximum level of activity being equal to 1). In the free-response paradigm, the threshold of the model with piece-wise linear activation function (Brown *et al.*, 2005) must be lower than 1 (as otherwise a choice would never be made). Hence, in the free-response paradigm the nonlinear model with piece-wise linear activation function is equivalent to the model with the threshold linear function (Usher and McClelland, 2001) (the upper boundary cannot be reached); these models only differ in the interrogation paradigm.

One way to simplify the analysis is to use linear Equation (6.2) (rather than (6.7)) and add reflecting boundaries on y_j at 0, preventing any of y_j from being negative (Usher and McClelland, 2001), and we refer to such model as *bounded*. In every step of the simulation of the bounded LCA model, the activity level of an accumulator y_j is being reset to 0 if a negative value is obtained. The bounded model behaves very similarly to the nonlinear models with threshold linear, piece-wise linear and even sigmoidal activation functions and provides a good approximation for them (see Appendix A of Usher and McClelland, 2001, for detailed comparison between the bounded and nonlinear LCA models).

6.2.7   Performance of bounded LCA model

For two alternatives, the bounded model implements the optimal choice algorithm, as long as decay is equal to inhibition and both are large (see Subsection 6.2.5) and the model remains in the linear range (i.e., the levels of accumulators never decrease to zero; cf. Brown *et al.*, 2005). Since during the choice process the state of the model moves rapidly towards the attracting line, the levels of y_j are likely to remain positive, if the attracting line crosses the decision thresholds before the axes as shown in Figure 6.4a

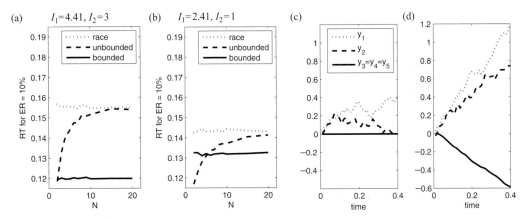

Figure 6.5 Performance and dynamics of choice models with only two accumulators receiving inputs. All models were simulated using the Euler method with $\Delta t = 0.01$s. (a), (b) Decision time for a threshold resulting in an error rate (ER) of 10% of different choice models as a function of the number of alternatives N (shown on x-axis). Three models are shown: the race model, the unbounded (i.e., linear) LCA model, and the bounded LCA model (see key). The parameters of the LCA model are equal to $w = k = 10$. The parameters of the first two inputs were chosen such that $c_1 = c_2 = 0.33$, $I_1 - I_2 = 1.41$ (values estimated from data of a sample participant of Experiment 1 in the study of Bogacz et al., 2006), while the other inputs were equal to 0, $I_3 = \ldots = I_N = 0$, $c_3 = \ldots = c_N = 0$. The panels differ in the total mean input to the first two accumulators: in panel (a) $I_2 = 3$, while in panel (b) $I_2 = 1$. For each set of parameters, a threshold was found numerically that resulted in ER of $10 \pm 0.2\%$ (s.e.); this search for the threshold was repeated 20 times. For each of these 20 thresholds, the decision time was then found by simulation and their average used to construct the data points. Standard error of the mean was lower than 2 ms for all data points hence the error bars are not shown. (c), (d) Examples of the evolution of the bounded (c) and the unbounded (d) LCA model, showing y_i as functions of time. The models were simulated for the same parameters as in panel (a), and for $N = 5$ alternatives. Panels (c) and (d) were simulated for the same initial seed of the random number generator hence in both cases the networks received exactly the same inputs.

(but not in Figure 6.4b). The distance of the attracting line from the origin of the plane is equal to (Bogacz et al., 2006):

$$x_2^* = \frac{I_1 + I_2}{\sqrt{2}\,(k + w)}. \tag{6.8}$$

According to Equation (6.8), the larger the sum of mean inputs $I_1 + I_2$, the further the attracting line is from the origin. Figure 6.5 compares the performance of the bounded LCA model and the linear LCA model without boundaries, which we refer to as *unbounded*. Figure 6.4a shows the position of the attracting line relative to thresholds for the parameters used in the simulations of the unbounded LCA model for $N = 2$ alternatives in Figure 6.5. For $N = 2$, adding the reflecting boundaries at $y_i = 0$ does not affect the performance of the model (the left end of the solid line coincides with the left end of the dashed line). This can be expected since for the parameters used in simulations, the attracting line crosses the threshold before the axes, as shown in Figure 6.4a.

(a)   (b)

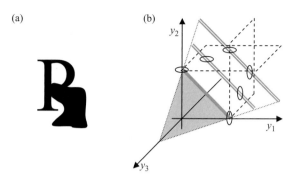

Figure 6.6 (a) Example of a stimulus providing strong evidence in favour of two letters (P and R) and very weak evidence in favour of any other letter. (b) State space analysis of the LCA model for three alternatives. The grey triangle indicates the attracting plane, and dotted lines indicate the intersection of the attracting plane with the y_1y_3 plane and the y_2y_3 plane. Thick grey line symbolises the attracting line in the y_1y_2 plane. The double grey lines show sample positions of the attracting line in the y_1y_2 plane for two negative values of y_3. The two planes surrounded by dashed lines indicate positions of the decision thresholds for alternatives 1 and 2. The ellipses indicate the intersections of the attracting lines in the y_1y_2 plane with the decision thresholds.

Figure 6.4b shows the position of the attracting line for the parameters used in simulations of the unbounded LCA model for $N = 2$ alternatives in Figure 6.5b. For $N = 2$, adding the reflecting boundaries at $y_i = 0$ degrades the performance of the model (the left end of the solid line lies above the left end of the dashed line). This happens because the attracting line reaches the axes before crossing the threshold, as shown in Figure 6.4b and hence the state is likely to hit the boundaries before reaching the threshold.

McMillen and Holmes (2006) tested the performance of the bounded LCA model for multiple alternatives, for the following parameters: $I_1 = 2, I_2 = \ldots = I_N = 0, c_1 = \ldots = c_N = 1$ (all accumulators received noise of equal standard deviation), $w = k = 1$, and N varying from 2 to 16. They found that the DT of bounded LCA for ER = 10% was slower than that of the unbounded LCA model. However, it will be shown here that this is not the case for more biologically realistic types of inputs.

6.3   The advantage of nonlinearity in multiple choice

Most real-life decisions involve the need to select between multiple alternatives, on the basis of partial evidence that supports a small subset of them. One ubiquitous example could correspond to a letter (or word) classification task, based on occluded (or partial) information. This is illustrated in Figure 6.6a for a visual stimulus that provides strong evidence in favour of P/R and very weak evidence in favour of any other letter (a simple analogue for the case of word-classification would consist of a word-stem consistent with few word completions). Note the need to select among multiple alternatives, based on input that supports only a few of them.

We compare the performance of the bounded and unbounded LCA models in the tasks of type described above within the free-response paradigm: we will discuss two cases (with regards to the type of evidence and noise parameters), which may arise in such situations. We start with a simplified case, which is helpful for the purpose of mathematical analysis, followed by a more realistic situation.

6.3.1   Case 1: only two accumulators receive input and noise

Consider a model of N accumulators y_i (corresponding to N alternatives), two of which receive input (supporting evidence; with means I_1, I_2 and standard deviation c), while other accumulators do not, so that $I_3 = \ldots = I_N = c_3 = \ldots = c_N = 0$. Let us examine first the dynamics of the bounded LCA model (with $y_1, y_2 \geq 0$). In this case, the other accumulators $y_3, \ldots, y_N$ do not receive any input but only inhibition from y_1, y_2 and hence they remain equal to 0 (i.e., $y_i = 0$ for all $i > 2$; see Figure 6.5c). Therefore, the choice process simplifies to a model of two alternatives, as described by Equation (6.1). Hence, when the boundaries are present, the performance of the model does not depend on the total number of alternatives N. This is illustrated in Figure 6.5a and b for sample parameters of the model. Note that DTs for fixed ER in each panel (shown by solid lines) do not differ significantly between different values of N.

Figure 6.5c and d compare the evolution of bounded and unbounded LCA models for $N = 5$ alternatives. Figure 6.5c shows the evolution of the bounded LCA model in which accumulators y_1, y_2 evolve in the way typical for the LCA model for two alternatives (compare with Figure 6.2b): the competition between accumulators y_1, y_2 is resolved and as y_1 increases, y_2 decreases towards 0. Figure 6.5d shows that during the evolution of the unbounded model, the accumulators $y_3, \ldots, y_N$ become more and more negative. Hence the inhibition received by y_1, y_2 from $y_3, \ldots, y_N$ is actually positive, and increases the value of *both* y_1, y_2. Therefore, in Figure 6.5d (by contrast to Figure 6.5c) the activation of the 'losing' accumulator, y_2, also increases.

To better illustrate the difference between the bounded and unbounded choice behaviour, consider the dynamics of the unbounded model (Equation (6.1)) for $N = 3$ alternatives. In such a case, the state is attracted to a plane (indicated in Figure 6.6b; McMillen and Holmes, 2006). However, since only alternatives 1 and 2 can be chosen, it is still useful to examine the dynamics in the $y_1 y_2$ plane. In the $y_1 y_2$ plane the state of the model is attracted to a line, and the position of this line is determined by the value of y_3. For example, if $y_3 = 0$, then the attracting line in the $y_1 y_2$ plane is the intersection of the attracting plane and the $y_1 y_2$ plane, i.e., the thick grey line in Figure 6.6b. For other values of y_3, the attracting line in the $y_1 y_2$ plane is the intersection of the attracting plane and the plane parallel to the $y_1 y_2$ plane intersecting y_3 axis in the current value of y_3. For example, the double grey lines in Figure 6.6b show the attracting lines in the $y_1 y_2$ plane for two negative values of y_3.

During the choice process of unbounded LCA of Equation (6.1), accumulator y_3 becomes more and more negative (as it receives more and more inhibition from y_1 and y_2), as illustrated in Figure 6.5d. Hence the attracting line in the $y_1 y_2$ plane moves further and further away from the origin of the $y_1 y_2$ plane. For example, the thick grey line in

Figure 6.6b shows the position of the attracting line in the $y_1 y_2$ plane at the beginning of the choice process and the double grey lines show the positions at two later time points. Therefore, the choice involves two processes: evolution along the attracting line (the optimal process) and evolution of this line's position (which depends on the total input integrated so far). Due to the presence of the second process the performance of the unbounded LCA model for $N = 3$ departs from that for $N = 2$, which is visible in Figure 6.5a and b. Also note in Figure 6.6b that as y_3 becomes more and more negative, the relative positions of the decision thresholds and the attracting line change, and the part of the attracting line between the thresholds becomes shorter and shorter. Hence relative to the attractive line, the thresholds move during the choice process. This situation is in contrast to the case of the bounded LCA model, in which y_3 is constant (as stated above), and hence the position of the attracting line in the $y_1 y_2$ plane (and thus its relation to the thresholds) does not change.

In summary, in the case of choice between multiple alternatives with only two alternatives receiving supporting evidence, the boundaries allow the LCA model to achieve the performance of the LCA model for two alternatives (close to the optimal performance). The performance of the unbounded LCA model is lower – approaching that of the race model as the number of alternatives increases.

6.3.2   Case 2: biologically realistic input parameters for choice with continuous variables

We assumed above that only two integrators receive input while the others received none: $I_3 = \ldots = I_N = 0$. However, in many situations, it might be expected that there is a more graded similarity among the different inputs, with the strength of the input falling off as a continuous function of similarity. This would be the case, for example, in tasks where the stimuli were arranged along a continuum, as they might be in a wavelength or length discrimination task. Here we consider the case of stimuli arranged at N equally spaced positions around a ring, an organisation that is relevant to many tasks used in psychophysical and physiological experiments, where the ring may be defined in terms of positions, orientations, or directions of motion. We use the motion case since it is well studied in the perceptual decision-making literature but the analysis applies equally to other such cases as well, and may be instructive for the larger class of cases in which stimuli are positioned at various points in a space.

Considering the motion discrimination case, motion-sensitive neurons in area MT are thought to provide evidence of the direction of stimulus motion. Neurons providing evidence for alternative i respond with a mean firing rate that is a function of the angular distance d_i between the direction of coherent motion in the stimulus and their preferred direction. This function is called a tuning curve, and can be well approximated by a Gaussian (Snowden *et al.*, 1992):

$$I_i = r_{\min} + (r_{\max} - r_{\min}) \exp \left(-\frac{d_i^2}{2\sigma^2} \right) \qquad (6.9)$$

(a)

(b)

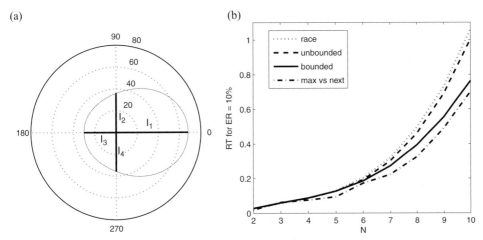

Figure 6.7 Simulation of the motion discrimination task. (a) Tuning curve describing the simulated firing rate of MT neurons (network inputs) as a function of angular difference d_i between the direction of coherent motion in the stimulus and neurons' preferred direction. We used the following parameters of the tuning curve $\sigma = 46.5°$ (the average value over tuning curves fitted to 30 MT neurons by Snowden *et al.*, 1992), $r_{min} = 30$ Hz, $r_{max} = 68$ Hz (values from a neuron analysed in Britten *et al.*, 1993). Thick lines show sample values of I_i in case of $N = 4$, which were computed in the following way. Since we assume that the first alternative is correct and alternatives are equally distributed around 360°, we computed $d_i = 360°(i-1)/N$, then if $d_i > 180°$, we made $d_i = d_i - 360°$, and then we computed I_i from Equation (6.9). (b) Decision time with a threshold resulting in error rate of 10% of different models as a function of the number of alternatives N (shown on *x*-axis). Four models are shown: the race model, the unbounded LCA model, the bounded LCA model, and max vs. next (see key). Methods of simulations as in Figure 6.5. The parameters of LCA model are equal to $w = k = 4$; this value was chosen as it optimised performance of the bonded LCA model for the inputs described in panel (a).

where r_{min} and r_{max} denote the minimum and the maximum firing rate of the neuron, and σ describes the width of the tuning curve. In our simulation we use the parameter values that generate the tuning curve function shown in Figure 6.7a.

Furthermore, we simulated the input to the accumulators as spikes (rather than values chosen from a Gaussian distribution). In particular, we assumed that the input to accumulator i comes from the Poisson process with mean I_i, because the Poisson process captures many aspects of firing of cortical neurons (Shadlen and Newsome, 1998). Thus the input to accumulator i within a very short interval dt is chosen stochastically such that it is equal to 1 with probability $I_i dt$ (that corresponds to a spike being produced by sensory population i), and 0 with probability $1 - I_i dt$.

Figure 6.7b shows the DTs under the assumptions described above. The DT grows rapidly as N increases, because as N grows, the difference between the largest input (I_1) and the next two largest inputs (I_2 and I_N) decreases. Importantly, in the simulation, introduction of boundaries to the LCA model reduce DT (for a fixed ER of 10%) very significantly, as N increases. For example, for $N = 10$ the boundaries reduce the DT by about 25%. Figure 6.7b also shows that the performance of bounded LCA model is close to that of the max vs. next procedure (that implements asymptotically optimal test; see Subsection 6.2.5).

In summary, this simulation shows that the introduction of the biologically realistic assumption that the firing rate of accumulator neurons cannot be negative, may not only improve the performance of choice networks for biologically realistic parameters of inputs, but it also allows the LCA model to approximate the optimal performance.

6.4   Optimisation of performance of bounded LCA model in the interrogation paradigm

It is typically assumed that in the interrogation paradigm the decision threshold is no longer used to render a choice. Instead, the alternative with the highest activity level is chosen when the interrogation signal appears (Usher and McClelland, 2001). However, a more complex assumption regarding the process that terminates decisions in the interrogation paradigm is also possible. As suggested by Roger Ratcliff (1988), a response criterion is still in place (as in the free-response paradigm) and participants use a response criterion (like in free-response paradigm) and when the activation reaches this criterion, they make a preliminary decision (and stop integrating input). Accordingly there are two type of trials: (1) those that reach criterion (as above), and (2) those that do not reach criterion until the interrogation signal is received and where the choice is determined by the unit with highest activation. This is mathematically equivalent to the introduction of an absorbing upper boundary on the accumulator trajectories; once an accumulator hits the upper boundary, it terminates the decision process, so that the state of the model does not change from that moment until the interrogation time (Mazurek *et al.*, 2003; Ratcliff, 1988). Mazurek *et al.* (2003) point out that the dynamics of the model with absorbing upper boundaries is consistent with the observation that in the motion discrimination task under interrogation paradigm, the time courses of average responses from population of LIP neurons cease increasing after a certain period following the stimulus onset, and are maintained until the interrogation time (Roitman and Shadlen, 2002).

In Subsection 6.2.5, we showed that the unbounded LCA model achieves optimal performance when the decay is equal to inhibition. Then the following question arises: does the balance of decay and inhibition still optimise the performance of the bounded LCA model in the interrogation paradigm, when an absorbing upper boundary is assumed (to account for pre-interrogation decisions)? Figure 6.8 illustrates the ER of bounded LCA model for $N = 2$ alternatives. To make the position of the attracting line stable (cf. Equation (6.8)), we fixed parameters $w + k$ but varied $w - k$. The results illustrate that by increasing inhibition relative to decay the bounded model can achieve lower ER in the interrogation paradigm. This happens because in this case, there is an attracting point to which state of the model is attracted, as shown in Figure 6.2a, and this attraction prevents the model from hitting the absorbing boundary prematurely due to noise; thus the biasing effect of early input leading to premature choice is minimised. In summary,

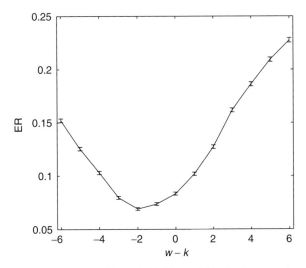

Figure 6.8 The ER of bounded LCA model in the interrogation paradigm. The models were simulated with parameters: $I_1 = 5.414$, $I_2 = 4$, $c_1 = c_2 = 0.8$, $B = 1.4$, $T = 2.5$. The sum of decay and inhibition was fixed $w + k = 6$, while their difference changed from -6 to 6. Data is averaged from 10 000 trials.

in contrast to the unbounded model, a balance of decay and inhibition did not optimise ER in the interrogation paradigm for the bounded model. Instead, optimal performance within the tested range was achieved when inhibition was smaller than decay.

6.5   Value-based decisions

The LCA model and its extensions discussed so far are targeting an important, but special type of choice; the type deployed in perceptual classification judgements. A different type of choice, of no less importance to humans and animals, is deciding between alternatives on the basis of their match to a set of internal motivations. Typically, this comes under the label of decision making. While human decision making is a mature field, where much data and theories have been accumulated (Kahneman and Tversky, 2000), more recently neurophysiological studies of value-based decisions have also been conducted on behaving animals (Platt and Glimcher, 1999; Sugrue *et al.*, 2004).

Although both the perceptual and the value/motivational decisions involve a common selection mechanism, the basis on which this selection operates differs. The aim of this section is to discuss the underlying principles of value-based decisions and to suggest ways in which a simple LCA type of mechanism can be used to explain the underlying cognitive processes. We start with a brief review of these principles and of some puzzling challenges they raise for an optimal theory of choice, before we explore a computational model that addresses the underlying processes.

6.5.1   Value and motivation-based choice

Unlike in perceptual choice, the decisions we consider here cannot be settled on the basis of perceptual information alone. Rather, each alternative (typically an action, such as purchasing a laptop from a set of alternatives) needs to be evaluated in relation to its potential consequences and its match to internal motivations. Often, this is a complex process, where the preferences for the various alternatives are being constructed as part of the decision process itself (Slovic, 1995). In some situations, where the consequences are obvious or explicitly described, the process can be simplified. Consider, for example, a choice between three laptops, which vary in their properties as described by a number of dimensions (screen size, price, etc.) or a choice between lotteries described in terms of their potential win and corresponding risks. The immediate challenge facing a choice in such situations is the need to convert between the different currencies, associated with the various dimensions. The concept of *value* is central to decision making, as a way to provide such a universal internal currency.

Assuming the existence of a value function, associated with each dimension, a simple normative rule of decision making, the *expected-additive-value*, seems to result. Accordingly, one should add the values that an alternative has on each dimension and compute expectation values when the consequences of the alternatives are probabilistic. Such a rule is then bound to generate a fixed and stable preference order for the various alternatives. Behavioural research in decision making indicates, however, that humans and animals violate expected-value prescriptions and change their preferences between a set of options depending on the way the options are described and on a set of contextual factors.

6.5.2   Violations of expected-value and preference reversals

First, consider the pattern of *risk-aversion* for gains. Humans and animals prefer the less risky of two options that are equated for expected value (Kahneman and Tversky, 2000). For example most people prefer a *sure* gain of £100 to a lottery with a probability 0.5 of winning £200 and nothing otherwise. An opposite pattern, *risk-seeking* is apparent for losses: most people prefer to play lottery with a chance 0.5 of losing £200 (and nothing otherwise) to a *sure* loss of £100.

Second, the preference between alternatives depends on a reference, which corresponds either to the present state of the decision maker, or even to an *expected* state, which is subject to manipulation. Consider, for example the following situation (Figure 6.9a). When offered a choice between two job alternatives A and B, described on two dimensions (e.g., distance from home and salary) to replace an hypothetical job that is being terminated – the *reference* (R_A or R_B, which is manipulated between groups) – participants prefer the option that is more similar to the reference (Tversky and Kahneman, 1991).

Third, it has been shown that the preference order between two options can be modified by the introduction of a third option, even when this option is not being chosen. Three such situations have been widely discussed in the decision-making literature, resulting

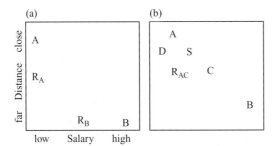

Figure 6.9 Configurations of alternatives in the attribute space. In each panel the two axes denote two attributes of the alternatives (sample attributes' labels are given in panel (a). The capital letters denote the positions of the alternative choices in the attribute space, while letters R_i denote the reference points. (a) Reference effect in multi-attribute decision making (after Tversky and Kahneman, 1991). (b) Contextual preference reversal: similarity, attraction and the compromise effects. Alternatives A, B, C, S lie on the indifference line.

in the *similarity*, the *attraction* and the *compromise* effects. To illustrate these effects consider a set of options, A, B, C, and S, which are characterised by two attributes (or dimensions) and which are located on a decision-maker indifference curve: the person is of equal preference on a choice between any two of these options (Figure 6.9b). The similarity effect is the finding that the preference between A and B can be modified in the favour of B by the introduction of a new option, S, similar to A in the choice-set. The attraction effect corresponds to the finding that, when a new option similar to A, D, and dominated by it (D is worse than A on both dimensions) is introduced into the choice set, the choice preference is modified in favour of A (the similar option; note that while the similarity effects favours the dissimilar option, the attraction effect favours the similar one). Finally, the compromise effect corresponds to the finding that, when a new option such as B is introduced into the choice set of two options A and C, the choice is now biased in favour of the intermediate one, C, the compromise.

The traditional way in which the decision-making literature addresses such deviations from the normative (additive-expected-value) theory is via the introduction of a set of disparate heuristics, each addressing some other aspect of these deviations (LeBoef and Shafir, 2005). One notable exception is work by Tversky and colleagues (Tversky, 1972; Tversky and Simonson, 1993), who developed a mathematical, context-dependent-advantage model that accounts for reference effects and preference reversal in multidimensional choice. However, as observed by Roe *et al.* (2001), the context-dependent-advantage model cannot explain the preference reversals in similarity effect situations (interestingly, a much earlier model by Tversky (1972), the elimination by aspects, accounts for the similarity effect but not for the attraction, the compromise or other reference effect). In turn, Roe *et al.* (2001), have proposed a neurocomputational account of preference reversal in multidimensional choice, termed the Decision Field Theory (DFT; see also Busemeyer and Townsend, 1993). More recently, Usher and McClelland (2004) have proposed a neurocomputational account of the same findings, using the LCA framework extended to include some assumptions regarding nonlinearities in value functions and reference effects introduced by Tversky and colleagues.

The DFT and the LCA models share many principles but also differ on some. While DFT is a linear model (where excitation by negated inhibition, of the type described in Section 6.2, is allowed) and where the degree of lateral inhibition depends on the similarity between the alternatives, in the LCA account the lateral inhibition is constant (not similarity dependent) but we impose two types of nonlinearity. The first type corresponds to a zero-activation threshold (discussed in Section 6.3), while the second one involves a convex utility-value function (Kahneman and Tversky, 2000).

It is beyond the scope of this chapter to compare detailed predictions of the two models (but see Usher and McClelland, 2004, and reply by Busemeyer *et al.*, 2005). We believe, however, that there is enough independent motivation for nonlinearity and reference dependency of the value functions. In the next subsection we discuss some principles underlying value evaluation and then we show how a simple LCA type model, taking these principles on board, can address value-based decisions.

6.5.3   Nonlinear utility functions and the Weber law

The need for a nonlinear relation between internal utility and objective value was noticed by Daniel Bernoulli (1738 [1954]), almost two centuries ago. Bernoulli proposed a logarithmic type of nonlinearity in the value function in response to the so-called St. Petersburg Paradox. (The paradox was first noticed by the casino operators of St. Petersburg. See for example Martin, 2004, and Glimcher, 2004, pp. 188–92 for good descriptions of the paradox and of Bernoulli's solution). Due to its simple logic and intuitive appeal, we reiterate it here.

Consider the option of entering a game, where you are allowed to repeatedly toss a fair coin until 'head' comes. If the 'head' comes in the first toss you receive £2. If the 'head' comes in the second toss, you receive £4, if in the third toss, £8, and so on (with each new toss needed to obtain a 'head' the value is doubled). The question is what is the price that a person should be willing to pay for playing this game. The puzzle is that although the expected value of the game is infinite ($E = \Sigma_{i=1,\ldots,\infty} \frac{1}{2}^i 2^i = \Sigma_{i=1,\ldots,\infty} 1 = \infty$), as the casino operators in St. Petersburg discovered, most people are not willing to pay more than £4 for playing the game and very few more than £25 (Hacking, 1980). Most people show *risk-aversion*. (In this game, most often one wins small amounts (75% to win less than £5), but in few cases one can win a lot. Paying a large amount to play the game results in a high probability of making a loss and a small probability of a high win. Hence the low value that people are willing to pay reflects risk-aversion.)

Bernoulli's assumption, that internal utility is nonlinearly (with diminishing returns) related to objective value, offers a solution to this paradox (the utility of a twice larger value is less than twice the utility of the original value) and has been included in the dominant theory of risky choice, the prospect theory (Tversky and Kahneman, 1979). A logarithmic value function $u(x) = \log_{10}(x)$, used as the expected utility, gives a value of about £4 for the St. Petersburg game.

Note that the need to trade between the utility associated with different objective values arises, not only in risky choice between options associated with monetary values but also in cases of multidimensional choice (as illustrated in Figure 6.9) where the

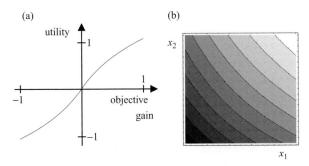

Figure 6.10 (a) Utility function, $u(x) = \log(1 + kx)$ for $x > 0$, and $-\gamma \log(1 - kx)$, for $x < 0$. ($k = 2$, $\gamma = 1$). (b) Combined 2D-utility function for gains ($x_1 > 0$, $x_2 > 0$).

options are characterised by their value on two or more dimensions. Moreover, as such values are examples of analogue magnitude representations, one attractive idea is to assume that their evaluation obeys a psychophysical principle that applies to magnitude judgements, in general: the Weber law. The Weber law states that to be able to discriminate between two magnitudes (e.g., weights), x and $x + dx$, the just-noticeable-difference, dx, is proportional to x itself.

One simple way to satisfy the Weber law is to assume that there are neural representations that transform their input (which corresponds to objective value) under a logarithmic type of nonlinearity and that the output is subject to additional independent noise of constant variance. This explanation for the Weber law is consistent with neurophysiological data from a task in which monkeys discriminated between stimuli differing in the number of dots, that suggest that prefrontal neurons represent the logarithms of numbers (Dehaene, 2003).

As proposed by Bernoulli (1738 [1954]) a logarithmic nonlinearity also accounts for risk aversion. Here we assume a logarithmic nonlinearity of the type, $u(x) = \log(1 + kx)$ for $x > 0$, and $u(x) = -\gamma \log(1 - kx)$, for $x < 0$ ($x > 0$ corresponds to gains and $x < 0$ to losses); the constant of 1 in the logarithm corresponds to a baseline of present value before any gains or losses are received). [In prospect theory (Kahneman and Tversky, 2000; Tversky and Simonson, 1993) one chooses, $\gamma > 1$, indicating a higher slope for losses than for gains. This is also assumed in Usher and McClelland (2004). Here we use $\gamma = 1$ in order to explore the simplest set of assumptions that can result in these reversal effects; increasing γ strengthens the effects.] As shown in Figure 6.10a, function $u(x)$ starts linearly and then is subject to diminishing returns, which is a good approximation to the neuronal input–output response function of neurons at low to intermediate firing rates (Usher and Niebur, 1996).

There is a third rationale for a logarithmic utility function, which relates to the need to combine utilities across dimensions. When summing such a utility function across multiple dimensions, one obtains (for two dimensions), $U(x_1,x_2) = u(x_1) + u(x_2) = \log[1 + k(x_1 + x_2) + k^2 x_1 x_2]$. Note that to maximise this utility function one has to maximise a combination of linear and multiplicative terms. The inclusion of a multiplicative term in the utility optimisation is supported by a survival rationale: to survive animals needs to ensure the joined (rather than separate) possession of essential resources (like food and water). Figure 6.10b illustrates a contour plot of this 2D utility function. One can observe that equal preference curves are now curved in the x_1–x_2 continuum: the compromise (0.5,0.5) has a much better utility than the (1,0) option.

Another component of the utility evaluation is its reference dependence. Moreover, as discussed in Subsection 6.5.2, the reference depends on the subjective expectations and on the information accessible to the decision maker (Kahneman, 2003). As we show below, the combination of nonlinear utility and reference dependence explains the presence of contextual preference reversals. Finally, when choice alternatives are characterised over multiple dimensions, we assume (following Tversky's elimination by aspects, Tversky, 1972, and the various DFT applications, Busemeyer and Townsend, 1993; Roe *et al.*, 2001) that decision makers switch their attention, stochastically, from dimension to dimension. Thus at every time step the evaluation is performed with regard to one of the dimensions and the preference is integrated by the leaky competing accumulators. In the following subsection, these components of utility evaluations are introduced into an LCA model and applied to the value-based decision patterns described above.

6.5.4   Modelling value-based choice in the LCA framework

To allow for the switching between the alternative dimensions, the LCA simulations are done using a discretised version of the LCA model of Equation (6.2) (single step of Euler method; note a threshold nonlinearity at zero is imposed: only $y_i > 0$ are allowed)

$$y_i\,(t + \Delta t) = y_i\,(t) + \Delta t\left(-ky_i - w\sum_{\substack{j=1\\j\neq i}}^{N} y_j + I_i + I_0 + noise\right) \qquad (6.10)$$

where I_i were evaluated according to the utility function described above and I_0 is a constant input added to all choice units, which is forcing a choice (in all simulations reported here this value is chosen as 0.6). To account for the stochastic nature of human choice each integrator received the noise that was Gaussian distributed (with standard deviation (SD) of 0.5). During all simulations the following parameters were chosen, $\Delta t = 0.05$, $k = w = 1$ (balanced network). When a reference location is explicitly provided (as in the situation depicted in Figure 6.9) the utility is computed relative to that reference. When no explicit reference is given, a number of possibilities for implicit reference are considered.

In all the simulations we present, the decision is monitored (as in Roe *et al.*, 2001, and in Usher and McClelland, 2004) via an interrogation-like procedure. The response units are allowed to accumulate their preference-evaluation for T-time steps. A total of 500 trials of this type are simulated and the probability of choosing an option as a function of time, $P_i(t)$ is computed by counting the fraction of trials in which the corresponding unit has the highest activation (relative to all other units) at time-t. We start with a simple

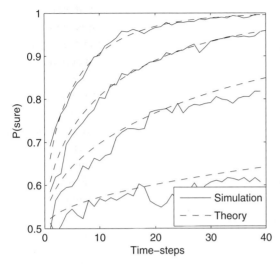

Figure 6.11 Probability of choosing the sure option as a function of deliberation time for five values of risk (indicated in the plot). Solid lines were obtained from simulations of the LCA model for the following parameters $W = 1$, $I_0 = 0.6$, SD $= .5$, and the utility function from Figure 6.10. Dashed lines show corresponding probabilities derived in Bogacz *et al.* (2007).

demonstration of risk-aversion in probabilistic monetary choice and then we turn to preference reversals in multidimensional choice.

6.5.4.1 Risk-aversion in probabilistic choice

We simulate here a choice between two options. The first one corresponds to a 'sure' win, W, while the second one to a probabilistic win of W/p, with probability p (note that the two have equal expected objective value, W, and that p provides a measure of risk: lower p is more risky). The model assumes that decision makers undergo a 'mental simulation' process, in which the utility of the gain drives the value accumulator, thus the sure unit receives a constant input $I_0 + u(W)$, while the probabilistic unit receives probabilistic input, chosen to be $I_0 + u(W/p)$ with probability p, and I_0 otherwise. In addition, a constant noise input (SD $= 0.5$) is applied to both units at all time steps. Note that due to the shape of utility function u, the average input to the sure unit $(I_0 + u(W))$ is larger than to the probabilistic unit $(I_0 + u(W/p)p)$. In Figure 6.11 we show the probability of choosing the sure option as a function of deliberation time for five risk levels, p (small p corresponds to large risk and p close to 1 to low risk). Thus the higher the risk the more likely is the bias of choosing the sure option (this bias starts at value approximately proportional to $1 - p$ and increases due to time integration to asymptotic value). This is consistent with experimental data, except for low p, where as explained by the Prospect Theory (Tversky and Kahneman, 1979), decision makers show an overestimative discrepancy between subjective and objective probability, which we do not address here (but see Hertwig *et al.*, 2004). Risk seeking for losses can be simulated analogously.

6.5.4.2   Multidimensional choice: reference effects and preference reversal

Three simulations are reported. In all of them, at each time step, one dimension is probabilistically chosen (with $p = 0.5$) for evaluation. The preferences are then accumulated across time and the choices for the various options are reported as a function of deliberation time.

First, we examine how the choice between two options, corresponding to A and B in Figure 6.9a is affected by a change of the reference, R_A versus R_B. The options are defined on two dimensions as follows: $A = (0.2, 0.8)$, $B = (0.8, 0.2)$, $R_A = (0.2, 0.6)$ and $R_B = (0.6, 0.2)$. Thus, for example, in simulations with reference R_A, when the first dimension is considered, the inputs I_A and I_B are $I_0 + u(0)$ and $I_0 + u(0.6)$ while when the second dimension is considered the inputs are $I_0 + u(0.2)$ and $I_0 + u(-0.4)$ (this follows from the fact that $A - R_A = (0,0.2)$ and $B - R_A = (0.6, -0.4)$). We observe (Figure 6.12a) that the R_A reference increases the probability of choosing the similar A-option (top curve) and that the choice preference reverses with the R_B reference (the middle curve corresponds to a neutral $(0,0)$ reference point). This happens because with reference R_A the average input to A is larger than to B (as $u(0) + u(0.2) = u(0.2) > u(0.6) - u(0.4) = u(0.6) + u(-0.4)$) and vice versa. [If $I_0 = 0$, the net advantage in utility for the nearby option is partially cancelled by an advantage for the distant option due to the zero-activation boundary (negative inputs are reflected by the boundary). The value of I_0 does not affect the other results (compromise or similarity)].

Second, we examine the compromise effect. The options correspond to a choice situation with three alternatives A, B, and C differing on two dimensions as shown in Figure 6.9b. A and B are defined as before and C is defined as $(0.5, 0.5)$. We assume that when all three choices are available the reference is neutral $(0, 0)$. We observe (Figure 6.12b) that the compromise alternative is preferred among the three. This is a direct result of 2D utility function (Figure 6.10b). For binary choice between A and C we assume that the reference point is moved to a point of neutrality between A and C, such as $R_{AC} = (0.2, 0.5)$, which corresponds to a new baseline relative to which the options A and C can be easily evaluated as having only gains and no losses (alternatively, one can assume that each option serves as a reference for the evaluation of the other ones; Usher and McClelland, 2004). This maintains an equal preference between C and the extremes in binary choice. Note also the dynamics of the compromise effect. This takes time to develop; at short times the preference is larger for the extremes, depending on the dimension evaluated first. Experimental data indicates that, indeed, the magnitude of the compromise effect increases with the deliberation time (Dhar *et al.*, 2000).

Third, we examine the similarity effect. In this situation, the option $S = (0.2, 0.7)$ (similar to A) is added to the choice set of A and B. The reference is again neutral $(0, 0)$. We observe that the dissimilar option, B (Figure 6.12c, solid curve), is preferred. This effect is due to the correlation in the activation of the similar alternatives (A and S), which is caused by their co-activation by the same dimensional evaluation. When the supporting dimension is evaluated both of the similar options rise in activation and they split their choices, while the dissimilar option peaks at different times and has a relative advantage. Note also a small compromise effect in this situation. Among the similar options, S (which is a compromise) has a higher choice probability. The attraction effect

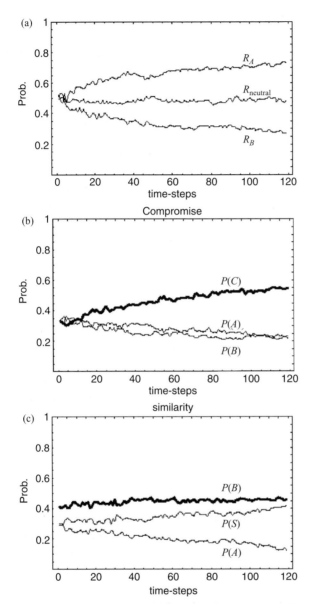

Figure 6.12 Contextual preference reversal. (a) Reference effects in binary choice. (b) Compromise effect. (c) Similarity effect.

is similar to the reference effect. One simple way to explain it is to assume that the reference moves towards the dominated option. (Alternatively, each option may serve as a reference for every other option; Tversky and Simonson, 1993; Usher and McClelland, 2004).

To summarise, we have shown that when the input to LCA choice units is evaluated according to a nonlinear utility function of the type proposed by Bernoulli, which is applied to differences in value between options and a referent, the model can account for a number of choice patterns that 'appear' to violate normativity. For example, the model provides a plausible neural implementation and extension of the Prospect Theory (Tversky and Kahneman, 1979), displaying risk aversion (it prefers the sure option on a risky one of equal expected value) and a series of preference reversals that are due to the effect of context on the choice-reference.

6.6   Discussion

In this chapter we have reviewed the conditions under which various versions of the LCA model (linear and nonlinear) achieve optimal performance for different experimental conditions (free-response and interrogation). We have also shown how the LCA model can be extended to value-based decisions to account for risk aversion and contextual preference reversals.

We have shown that the linear LCA model can implement the optimal choice algorithm for all tasks except the choice between multiple alternatives receiving similar amounts of supporting evidence in the free-response paradigm. Moreover, we have shown that for the choice involving multiple alternatives in the free-response paradigm, the nonlinearities of type present in a biological decision network can improve the performance, and in fact may allow the networks to approximate the optimal choice algorithm. This raises an intriguing possibility, that these nonlinearities are not a result of constraints of biological neurons, but may rather be a result of evolutionary pressure for speed of decisions.

We have also identified a condition (see Section 6.4) in which performance can be optimised by an elevation/decrease in the level of lateral inhibition relative to the leak (this may be achieved via neuromodulation, e.g., Usher and Davelaar, 2002). It will be interesting to test whether the behavioural manifestations of unbalance of decay and inhibition (Usher and McClelland, 2001) can be experimentally observed under these conditions.

One interesting comment relates to Hick's law, according to which the DT is proportional to the logarithm of the number of alternatives (Teichner and Krebs, 1974). In the simulations of bounded LCA model in Figure 6.5a and b, the DT does not depend on the number of potentially available alternatives. Note, however, this simulation was designed to model the task described at the beginning of Section 6.3 (Figure 6.6a) in which the choice is mainly between two alternatives, which match the ambiguous input (in this simulation only two accumulators receive any input or noise). If all accumulators received equal levels of noise and the bounded LCA model remained in the linear range, it would satisfy Hick's law, because when the bounded LCA model is in linear range, it is equivalent to the linear model, and the linear model satisfies Hick's law when accumulators receive equal level of noise (McMillen and Holmes, 2006). However, it has been recently reported that in tasks where one of the alternatives receives much more support than all the others, Hick's law is indeed violated and the DT does not depend on the number of alternatives (Kveraga *et al.*, 2002). Thus it would be interesting to investigate the prediction of our theory that a similar independence may occur when two alternatives receive much larger input than the others.

It has been recently proposed that if the balanced LCA model projects to a complex network with architecture resembling that of the basal ganglia, the system as a whole may implement the MSPRT (Bogacz and Gurney, 2007) – the optimal algorithm for this condition. The system involving the basal ganglia may thus optimally make choices between motor actions. However, many other choices (e.g., perceptual or motivational) are likely to be implemented in the cortex. The complexity of MSPRT prevents any obvious cortical implementations, hence it is still of great interest to investigate the parameters optimising the LCA model which can be viewed as an abstraction of cortical processing.

The extension to value based decisions brings the model in closer contact with the topic of action selection. Actions need to be selected according to the value of their consequences, and this requires an estimation of utility and its integration across dimensions. The LCA model is also related to many models of choice on the basis of noisy data presented in this book. In particular, it is very similar to the model of action selection in the cerebral cortex by Cisek (2006), which also includes accumulation of evidence and competition between neuronal populations corresponding to different alternatives.

Acknowledgements

This work was supported by EPSRC grant EP/C514416/1. We thank Andrew Lulham for reading the manuscript and for his very useful comments. Matlab codes for simulation and finding decision time of LCA model can be downloaded from: http://www.cs.bris.ac.uk/home/rafal/optimal/.

References

Barnard, G. (1946). Sequential tests in industrial statistics. *J. Roy. Stat. Soc. Suppl.* **8**: 1–26.

Bernoulli, D. (1738 [1954]). Exposition of a new theory on the measurement of risk. *Ekonometrica* **22**: 23–36.

Bogacz, R., E. Brown, J. Moehlis, P. Holmes, and J. D. Cohen (2006). The physics of optimal decision making: a formal analysis of models of performance in two-alternative forced choice tasks. *Psychol. Rev.* **113**: 700–65.

Bogacz, R. and K. Gurney (2007). The basal ganglia and cortex implement optimal decision making between alternative actions. *Neural Comput.* **19**: 442–77.

Bogacz, R., M. Usher, J. Zhang, and J. L. McClelland (2007). Extending a biologically inspired model of choice: multi-alternatives, nonlinearity and value-based multidimensional choice. *Phil. Trans. Roy. Soc. B.* **362**: 1655–70.

Britten, K. H., M. N. Shadlen, W. T. Newsome, and J. A. Movshon (1993). Responses of neurons in macaque MT to stochastic motion signals. *Vis. Neurosci.* **10**(6): 1157–69.

Brown, E., J. Gao, P. Holmes, *et al.* (2005). Simple networks that optimize decisions. *Int. J. Bifurcat. Chaos* **15**: 803–26.

Brown, E. and P. Holmes (2001). Modeling a simple choice task: stochastic dynamics of mutually inhibitory neural groups. *Stoch. Dynam.* **1**: 159–91.

Busemeyer, J. R. and J. T. Townsend (1993). Decision field theory: a dynamic-cognitive approach to decision making in uncertain environment. *Psychol. Rev.* **100**: 432–59.

Busemeyer, J. R., J. T. Townsend, A. Diederich, and R. Barkan (2005). Contrast effects or loss aversion? Comment on Usher and McClelland (2004). *Psychol. Rev.* **111**: 757–69.

Cisek, P. (2006). Cortical mechanisms of action selection: the affordance competition hypothesis. *Phil. Trans. Roy. Soc. B.* **362**: 1585–600.

Dehaene, S. (2003). The neural basis of the Weber–Fechner law: a logarithmic mental number line. *Trends Cog. Sci.* **7**: 145–7.

Dhar, R., S. M. Nowlis, and S. J. Sherman (2000). Trying hard or hardly trying: an analysis of context effects in choice. *J. Con. Psych.* **9**: 189–200.

Dragalin, V. P., A. G. Tertakovsky, and V. V. Veeravalli (1999). Multihypothesis sequential probability ratio tests – part I: asymptotic optimality. *IEEE Trans. I.T.* **45**: 2448–61.

Glimcher, P. W. (2004). *Decisions, Uncertainty, and the Brain: The Science of Neuroeconomics.* Cambridge, MA: MIT Press.

Gold, J. I. and M. N. Shadlen (2002). Banburismus and the brain: decoding the relationship between sensory stimuli, decisions, and reward. *Neuron* **36**(2): 299–308.

Hacking, I. (1980). Strange expectations. *Phil. Sci.* **47**: 562–7.

Hertwig, R., G. Barron, E. U. Weber, and I. Erev (2004). Decisions from experience and the effect of rare events in risky choice. *Psych. Sci.* **15**: 534–9.

Houston, A. I., J. McNamara, and M. Steer (2006). Do we expect natural selection to produce rational behaviour? *Phil. Trans. Roy. Soc. B* **362**: 1531–44.

Kahneman, D. (2003). Maps of bounded rationality: psychology for behavioral economics. *Am. Econ. Rev.* **93**: 1449–75.

Kahneman, D. and A. Tversky, eds. (2000). *Choices, Values and Frames.* Cambridge: Cambridge University Press.

Kveraga, K., L. Boucher, and H. C. Hughes (2002). Saccades operate in violation of Hick's law. *Exp. Brain Res.* **146**(3): 307–14.

Laming, D. R. J. (1968). *Information Theory of Choice Reaction Time.* New York: Wiley.

LeBoef, R. and E. B. Shafir (2005). Decision-making. In *Cambridge Handbook of Thinking and Reasoning*, ed. K. J. Holyoak and R. G. Morisson. Cambridge: Cambridge University Press, pp. 243–66.

Martin, R. (2004). The St. Petersburg Paradox. In *The Stanford Encyclopedia of Philosophy*, ed. E. Zalta. Stanford, CA: The Metaphysics Research Lab. Available at http://plato.stanford.edu/archives/fall2008/entries/paradox-stpetersburg/.

Mazurek, M. E., J. D. Roitman, J. Ditterich, and M. N. Shadlen (2003). A role for neural integrators in perceptual decision making. *Cereb. Cortex* **13**(11): 1257–69.

McMillen, T. and P. Holmes, (2006). The dynamics of choice among multiple alternatives. *J. Math. Psych.* **50**: 30–57.

Neyman, J. and E. S. Pearson (1933). On the problem of the most efficient tests of statistical hypotheses. *Phil. Trans. Roy. Soc. A* **231**: 289–337.

Platt, M. L. and P. W. Glimcher (1999). Neural correlates of decision variables in parietal cortex. *Nature* **400**(6741): 233–8.

Ratcliff, R. (1978). A theory of memory retrieval. *Psychol. Rev.* **83**: 59–108.

Ratcliff, R. (1988). Continuous versus discrete information processing: modeling accumulation of partial information. *Psychol. Rev.* **95**: 238–55.

Roe, R. M., J. R. Busemeyer, and J. T. Townsend (2001). Multialternative decision field theory: a dynamic connectionist model of decision making. *Psychol. Rev.* **108**: 370–92.

Roitman, J. D. and M. N. Shadlen (2002). Response of neurons in the lateral intraparietal area during a combined visual discrimination reaction time task. *J. Neurosci.* **22**(21): 9475–89.

Schall, J. D. (2001). Neural basis of deciding, choosing and acting. *Nat. Rev. Neurosci.* **2**(1): 33–42.

Seung, H. S. (2003). Amplification, attenuation, and integration. In *The Handbook of Brain Theory and Neural Networks*, 2nd edn, ed. M. A. Adbib. Cambridge, MA: MIT Press, pp. 94–7.

Shadlen, M. N. and W. T. Newsome (1998). The variable discharge of cortical neurons: implications for connectivity, computation, and information coding. *J. Neurosci.* **18**(10): 3870–96.

Shadlen, M. N. and W. T. Newsome (2001). Neural basis of a perceptual decision in the parietal cortex (area LIP) of the rhesus monkey. *J. Neurophysiol.* **86**(4): 1916–36.

Slovic, P. (1995). The construction of preference. *Am. Psychol.* **50**: 364–71.

Snowden, R. J., S. Treue, and R. A. Andersen (1992). The response of neurons in areas V1 and MT of the alert rhesus monkey to moving random dot patterns. *Exp. Brain Res.* **88**(2): 389–400.

Stone, M. (1960). Models for choice reaction time. *Psychometrika* **25**: 251–60.

Sugrue, L. P., G. S. Corrado, and W. T. Newsome (2004). Matching behavior and the representation of value in the parietal cortex. *Science* **304**(5678): 1782–7.

Sugrue, L. P., G. S. Corrado, and W. T. Newsome, (2005). Choosing the greater of two goods: neural currencies for valuation and decision making. *Nat. Rev. Neurosci.* **6**(5): 363–75.

Teichner, W. H. and M. J. Krebs (1974). Laws of visual choice reaction time. *Psychol. Rev.* **81**: 75–98.

Tversky, A. (1972). Elimination by aspects: a theory of choice. *Psychol. Rev.* **79**: 281–99.

Tversky, A. and D. Kahneman (1979). Prospect theory: an analysis of decision under risk. *Econometrica* **47**: 263–92.

Tversky, A. and D. Kahneman (1991). Loss aversion in riskless choice: a reference-dependent model. *Q. J. Economet.* **106**: 1039–61.

Tversky, A. and I. Simonson (1993). Context-dependent preferences. *Manage. Sci.* **39**: 1179–89.

Usher, M. and E. J. Davelaar (2002). Neuromodulation of decision and response selection. *Neural Networks* **15**: 635–45.

Usher, M. and J. L. McClelland (2001). The time course of perceptual choice: the leaky, competing accumulator model. *Psychol. Rev.* **108**(3): 550–92.

Usher, M. and J. L. McClelland (2004). Loss aversion and inhibition in dynamical models of multialternative choice. *Psychol. Rev.* **111**: 759–69.

Usher, M. and N. Niebur (1996). Modeling the Temporal Dynamics of IT Neurons in Visual Search: A Mechanism for Top-Down Selective Attention. *J. Cog. Neurosci.* **8**: 311–27.

Vickers, D. (1970). Evidence for an accumulator model of psychophysical discrimination. *Ergonomics* **13**: 37–58.

Vickers, D. (1979). *Decision Processes in Perception*. New York: Academic Press.

Wald, A. (1947). *Sequential Analysis*. New York: Wiley.

Wang, X. J. (2002). Probabilistic decision making by slow reverberation in cortical circuits. *Neuron* **36**(5): 955–968.

7 Bayesian approaches to modelling action selection

Max Berniker, Kunlin Wei, and Konrad Körding

Summary

We live in an uncertain world, and each decision may have many possible outcomes; choosing the best decision is thus complicated. This chapter describes recent research in Bayesian decision theory, which formalises the problem of decision making in the presence of uncertainty and often provides compact models that predict observed behaviour. With its elegant formalisation of the problems faced by the nervous system, it promises to become a major inspiration for studies in neuroscience.

7.1 Introduction

Choosing the right action relies on our having the right information. The more information we have, the more capable we become at making intelligent decisions. Ideally, we want to know what the current state of the world is, what possible actions we can take in response to it, and what the outcomes of these actions will be. When we choose actions that will most clearly bring about our desired results, we are said to be behaving rationally (see Chapter 2). Equivalently, we could say that rational behaviour is optimal, in that this behaviour executes the best actions for achieving our desired results (see Chapters 3 and 4). Thus behaving rationally is equivalent to solving an optimality problem: what actions should we select to best achieve our goals?

The mathematics that formalise these types of optimality problems are well developed under the study of *decision theory* and *optimal control*. Using these approaches, all possible actions can be assessed in terms of their ability to achieve our goals. Thus the optimal action can be identified and executed. To quantify the relative merit of one action over another, we must define a cost function (sometimes referred to as a loss function). In its most general form, the cost function assigns a value to a choice of action and the resulting outcome, within the context of our goals. In essence, it mathematically quantifies our goals and our strategy for achieving them. Therefore, by selecting actions that minimise this cost, we can best achieve our goals. To illustrate, consider a simplified game of darts. Assume the actions we can choose amongst uniquely specify where the

Modelling Natural Action Selection, eds. Anil K. Seth, Tony J. Prescott and Joanna J. Bryson.
Published by Cambridge University Press. © Cambridge University Press 2012.

dart lands on the board, the outcome of our action. Assuming our goal is to get the highest score possible, our 'cost' function is inversely proportional to our score; that is, we achieve the lowest cost by getting the highest score. The optimal choice of action is the one (or any of the many actions, see Chapter 5) that result in the dart landing on the triple 20 (60 points, better than a bull's eye). Mathematically, we would express this optimal action as,

$$a^o = \arg\max_a \{\text{cost}(\text{outcome}(a), a)\}. \tag{7.1}$$

Here a is shorthand for the possible actions, and a^o is the optimal action. The above example, while valuable in portraying the general approach to selecting optimal actions, requires more elaboration before we can analyse human motor behaviours. Certainly a more realistic description of the example would include temporal dynamics of our limb and the dart, and perhaps nonlinearities associated with them (we'll address both below), but first and foremost, we shall argue that we must take into account uncertainty. That is, we've assumed we deterministically choose a command and can be sure of its outcome. Yet, most action selection problems are stochastic in nature, and action outcomes are affected by uncertainty. Under more realistic conditions we cannot simply choose the action that lands the dart on the triple 20, since we cannot be certain of this outcome. Instead, we must account for the statistics of the task. To continue the example, if we aim at the centre of the dartboard we are not certain to hit the bull's eye with the dart (even if we are a seasoned champion). Indeed, if we aim at the centre and throw many times we will end up with a distribution of dart positions. This distribution characterises the likelihood of each outcome, the dart landing at a certain position on the board, given that we aimed at the centre. This distribution helps to define a new optimisation problem: what action minimises the likely cost?

Taking the uncertainty of our aims into account, our new optimal action minimises the so-called expected cost: the average cost when weighted by the probability of the various outcomes.

In the darts example, the best aiming point is a point where we will receive high scores even if we make large mistakes. In fact, both amateur and world-class players are known to adopt a strategy that is well predicted by this approach. Mathematically, we would express this best action as,

$$a^o = \arg\max_a \left\{ \sum_{\text{outcomes}} \text{cost}(\text{outcome}(a), a) p(\text{outcome}|a) \right\}. \tag{7.2}$$

Here $p(\text{outcome}|a)$ is the probability of an outcome conditioned on the choice of action, a.

While playing darts, our uncertainty in the dart's location arises largely from motor noise (Figure 7.1a). However, there are many sensory sources of uncertainty as well. For example, our visual system is noisy and our sense of the location of the dartboard relative to our body is uncertain (Figure 7.1a). Moreover, our proprioceptive system is noisy as well; the orientation of our hand and arm as we release the dart are uncertain (Figure 7.1a). These and many other sources of uncertainty combine to produce variability in the motor outcome given our actions.

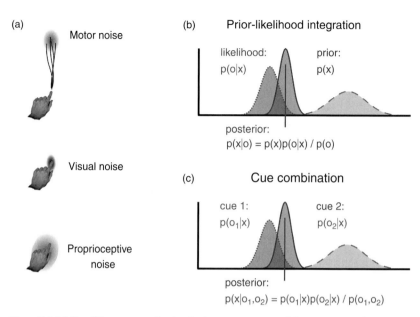

Figure 7.1 (a) Possible sources of noise in the motor system. Motor commands possess noise and result in uncertain movements. Visual and proprioceptive senses too, contain inherent uncertainties. (b) Bayesian integration of a prior and likelihood. The prior, denoted with the dashed curve, represents the probability of a state, x. The likelihood, denoted with the dotted curve, represents the probability of observing the data, o, given x. The posterior is the probability that x is the state, given our observation, o. (c) Bayes' rule applied to cue combinations is mathematically equivalent, only instead of using a prior and likelihood, we integrate two likelihoods.

Pressing our example further, we can examine more sophisticated and realistic action selection problems. For instance, a more sensible description of dart throwing recognises that the task is dynamic. The dart's final position on the board depends on the ballistic trajectory it takes once it has been released from our hand. The motion of the dart up until the moment we release it is dictated by the inertial mechanics of our limb and the force generating properties of our muscles. Clearly, our description of the dart-throwing problem can take on greater and greater levels of detail and physical accuracy. Nevertheless, our problem is still to select the best possible action, albeit an action that varies in time due to the dynamic nature of the problem. The minimisation to be performed at each instant is a sum over both the statistics of the possible outcomes at the current time, and the statistics of future possible outcomes that unfold as a result of the current choice of action.

For a dynamic task such as this, we need to know the state of the system to compute the optimal action. For our dart-throwing example, depending on how we modelled the problem, the state might be the orientation and velocity of our hand. To measure this state we would use sensory feedback. Yet this information is subject to noise and its own statistics. Each of our sensory modalities offers only a limited level of precision, which can vary depending on the situation. Vision is limited under dim light or extra-foveal conditions, hearing becomes unreliable for weak sounds, and proprioception drifts without calibration from vision (Deneve, 2008; Hoyer and Hyvärinen, 2003; Pouget *et al.*, 2003; Zemel *et al.*, 1998). Therefore, in addition to the uncertainty concerning the outcome of our motor actions, we must cope with the further uncertainty of the state.

Despite the varying complexity of the above examples, we can still formulate the action selection problem as one of an optimisation. We must solve a statistical problem concerning likely motor outcomes conditioned on the actions we choose. The difficulty with this problem, and action selection in general, is that computing the probability of an outcome given an action can be onerous. Doing so demands the specification of many variables that are uncertain and subject to their own statistics. This includes information about our body, the world and how they interact. Integrating all this uncertain information requires a statistical approach. Bayesian integration is the mathematical framework that calculates how uncertain information from multiple sources can be optimally combined. It results in a coherent and maximally accurate estimate of a set of observations, crucial for ultimately selecting the best action.

As explained above, before we can rationally, or optimally, select an action, we must be well informed, i.e., we must know the state of the world, the actions we can take, and their outcomes. In this chapter we focus on the process of constructing a state estimate. A number of recent psychophysics and computational studies have analysed how people and animals integrate uncertain information to make sensorimotor decisions. Below we will discuss some of these findings in the context of action selection. In particular, we discuss how Bayesian integration allows us to combine multiple pieces of information into a single distribution, how we can update this distribution over time as we continue to gain new information about it, and finally, how we can use our observations to update our beliefs about the structure of the world, that is, what processes are responsible for shaping our observations.

7.2   Bayesian estimation

7.2.1   Combining prior knowledge with new evidence

Combining uncertain information to produce a coherent and accurate estimate of our body and the world is integral to action selection. Sometimes the source of this uncertain information is our senses, and we must compare it against what we would expect before it can be of benefit. As an example, consider the task of descending a staircase. Based on our familiarity with walking down stairs, we have strong assumptions for things like the distance between steps, their height and their general shape. These assumptions form a prior over stairs, a belief in their typical properties. Often these priors are strong enough that we feel comfortable taking stairs without even observing them, as when we descend stairs without looking at our feet, or in the dark. Normally though, we'll first observe how far we'll need to step. Vision does not provide perfect measurements however. The visual system provides us with an estimate, or likelihood of the step's height. This likelihood is the probability of having a particular sensory observation for a given stair height. Bayes' rule defines how to combine the prior and the likelihood to make an optimal estimate of the step's height.

Bayes' rule states that the probability of the step's height being value x, given our observation, o, is the product of the prior probability of the stair height and the likelihood, normalised by the probability of the observation. Mathematically, this is expressed as,

$$p(x|o) = p(x)p(o|x)/p(o). \tag{7.3}$$

The distribution produced by Equation (7.3) is known as the posterior probability (this is shown graphically in Figure 7.1b). We can also interpret Bayes' rule as the 'optimal' means of combining a prior and a likelihood, as it produces an estimate with minimal uncertainty.

Several studies, using many sensory modalities, have shown that when subjects combine preceding knowledge with new information their behaviour reflects the integration of a prior and likelihood in a manner prescribed by Bayes' rule (Körding, 2007). In a typical study (Körding and Wolpert, 2004a), subjects will indicate their estimate of a target's location through a motor task. On each trial, the target's location is drawn from a normal distribution, the prior. Noisy feedback of the target's location is then provided, the likelihood. The distribution used for the prior or the likelihood can be fixed, or vary across subjects as an experimental condition. Bayesian statistics predicts how subjects should combine the likelihood and the prior. These predictions are then compared against human performance, often revealing a high degree of similarity.

These paradigms have been applied to a wide range of topics spanning sensorimotor integration, force estimation, timing estimations, speed estimations, stance regulation, the interpretation of visual scenes, and even cognitive estimates (Chater *et al.*, 2006; Knill and Richards, 1996; Körding and Wolpert, 2006; Körding *et al.*, 2004; Miyazaki *et al.*, 2005, 2006; Peterka and Loughlin, 2004; Tassinari *et al.*, 2006; Weiss *et al.*, 2002). Together these studies demonstrate that people are adept at combining prior knowledge with new evidence in a manner predicted by Bayesian statistics; a necessary first step in action selection.

7.2.2 Combining multiple pieces of information

In many cases it is not new information that is combined with prior knowledge, but rather two or more different pieces of information available to the nervous system, that are combined. For example, we may see and feel an object at the same time (Ernst and Banks, 2002). We can then use our sense of vision and touch to estimate a common property of the object, for instance, its size or its texture. This type of task is what is commonly referred to as *cue combination*; two or more sensory cues are combined to form a common, or joint, estimate. Just as before, Bayesian statistics prescribes how we should combine the likelihoods to compute an optimal estimate from the posterior distribution (Figure 7.1c). Again, only by accurately combining these sensory cues can we optimally select the appropriate action.

Recent studies have found that when combining information from multiple senses, people are also similar to optimal. As an example study, we consider how people combine visual and auditory information to estimate the position of a target. First the precision of visual and auditory perceptions are separately measured for each subject (Alais and Burr, 2004). This is done to characterise the subject's likelihood for the two sensory modalities. Then the precision and accuracy of perception is measured when subjects use both senses. Their performance in these cue combination trials can be predicted using the rules of Bayesian integration, further evidencing people's ability to cope with uncertain information in a statistically optimal manner.

In addition to auditory and visual cues, combinations of other sensory modalities have been analysed in a good number of studies (Ernst and Banks, 2002; Ernst and Bulthoff, 2004; Geisler and Kersten, 2002; Kersten and Yuille, 2003; Knill, 2007; Knill and Richards, 1996; Körding, 2007; Rosas et al., 2005; van Ee et al., 2003). In all reported cases, cues are combined by the subjects in a fashion that is close to the optimum prescribed by Bayesian statistics.

7.2.3   Credit assignment

The rules of Bayesian statistics reviewed above prescribe how we bring new information to bear upon our beliefs. As just illustrated, at times we are only concerned with estimating a single property. However, sometimes we are concerned with estimating many properties at once. For instance, suppose we hold two blocks in our hand, one sitting atop the other, and we want to estimate their individual weights. Our observation of their combined weight upon our hand is indicative of their individual weights, namely the magnitude of their sum. However, this information is not sufficient to accurately establish their individual weights. To estimate them, we need to solve a credit assignment problem; that is, how does each property (individual weight) contribute to our observation (overall weight). Bayesian statistics also prescribes an optimal solution to this problem.

Our observation of their combined weight forms a likelihood, a probability of having a particular sensory observation of their combined weight, for each value of their individual weights. By combining this with a prior over the object's weight, perhaps based on their size (Flanagan et al., 2008), we can compute a posterior distribution of their individual weights. Again, this distribution will provide an optimal estimate of their individual weights, simultaneously solving the credit assignment problem: how much does each block contribute to the total weight I feel? Recent research (Berniker and Körding, 2008) addresses this type of problem by integrating information over time.

7.3   Bayesian estimation across time

In our discussions above we were concerned with estimating what we assumed were static properties, such as the weight of a block or the location of an auditory cue. However, the world is dynamic, and as such its properties and our perception of them are continually changing. Thus we constantly need to integrate newly obtained information with our

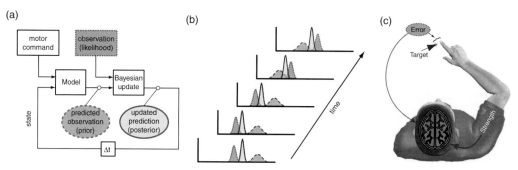

Figure 7.2 (a) Typical procedure for optimally estimating the world's state in modern control theory. A model of the world, combined with a motor command is used to estimate a predicted state (the prior). Observations of the world dictate the likelihood of a particular observation given the current world state. A Kalman filter is used to make a Bayesian update of our belief in the world's current state. (b) This process of Bayesian inference repeats itself at each time step, using the posterior from one time step, as the prior for the following time step. (c) Motor adaptation can be framed as an analogous update procedure. Our prior belief in muscle properties (e.g., muscle strength, labelled in green) is integrated with our observed motor errors to update estimates in our muscle properties.

current beliefs to inform new estimates of the world if we are to behave rationally. This implies that Bayesian integration should take place in an ongoing, or continuous manner.

This ongoing integration of information is an approach taken extensively in modern applications of control theory through the use of a Kalman filter. Kalman filtering is a procedure for using a model and our observations to continuously update our beliefs (Figure 7.2a). At each update the Kalman filter combines a model's estimate of the world's state (the prior) with a measured observation (the likelihood) to update a prediction of the world's current state, represented by a posterior (Figure 7.2b). At any point of time, the posterior from the past defines the prior for the future. This formalism is well developed and used in a wide range of applications from aeronautics to humanoid robotics (Stengel, 1994; Todorov, 2006). Indeed, even the motor control problems of two applications as disparate as controlling a jet and controlling our bodies, share many computational analogies. In both cases, continuously incoming information needs to be assessed to move precisely (albeit on different timescales). Only recently has the methodology of Kalman filtering been applied to make quantitative predictions of human movement behaviour.

As an example of this approach we consider a recent study of motor adaptation (Berniker and Körding, 2008). Since the properties of our bodies change continuously throughout our lives, it is imperative that we monitor these changes if we are to control our motor behaviours accurately and precisely. For example, errors in the perceived strength of our muscles will translate to movement errors. However, we can use these errors to obtain a likelihood characterising how strong our muscles are. According to Bayesian statistics we should combine this newly obtained information, our motor errors, with our prior beliefs. Accordingly we infer new and improved estimates of our muscles (Figure 7.2c).

It has been found that motor adaptation across time can be understood using the predictions of Kalman filtering. For instance, evidence suggests how people estimate the position of their hand (Wolpert *et al.*, 1995), adapt to robot-rendered force fields (Berniker and Körding, 2008), and even balance a pole upon their hand (Mehta and Schaal, 2002) can all be explained using this strategy. Taken together, these studies highlight the hypothesis that when people integrate information over time, they seem to do so in a fashion that is consistent with the optimal Bayesian solution. These findings have important consequences for optimal action selection, where finding the best action relies on accurate estimates of the world's state.

7.4   Bayesian estimation of structure

In our discussion above, cue-combination studies have provided evidence that the nervous system combines multiple pieces of information for estimating states in an optimal fashion. However, the brain receives a very large number of sensory cues, and not all cues should be combined; many cues may simply be irrelevant. To make sense of the world then, the nervous system should only combine those sensory cues that are likely to provide information about the same characters of the world.

Consider the example of a ventriloquist: he or she synchronises his or her voice with the movement of the puppet's mouth. Due to visuo-auditory cue combination, the audience experiences the illusion of a talking puppet, or more precisely, that a voice is being emitted from the puppet's mouth. If the ventriloquist's voice is out of sync with the puppet's movements, this illusion will immediately break down. In this example, the temporal proximity of cues is an overriding factor in inducing the merging of cues. Similarly, spatial proximity or disparity can also influence whether we combine different cues into a single percept: if a thundering sound is emitted close to a flash of light, these two cues are readily interpreted as an explosion; in contrast, if the sound is far away from the flash, these two stimuli may be perceived as independent events. The nervous system combines cues that appear to originate from the same source. In other words, it seems that the nervous system estimates the *structure* of the world, i.e., what causes the perceived cues.

Traditional Bayesian analyses of cue combination examine tasks where the experimental cues are close to coincident, and implicitly assume that the cues are caused by the same event, or source. New studies have tested subject performance in situations where two cues are dissimilar from one another. In the simplest case, a visual cue and an auditory cue are simultaneously presented for estimating the location of an object. These two cues can either have the same cause or have different causes. In the same-cause case, these two cues should be combined to form a single estimate; in the different-cause case, these two cues should be processed separately (Figure 7.3a). The optimal estimate should weigh each cause with respect to its likelihood. This likelihood is a function expressing the probability of observing the cues when they arise from the same cause, or not. Not surprisingly, this likelihood depends on spatial and temporal disparity between cues, with increasing disparity between the cues subjects' belief in a common cause decreases

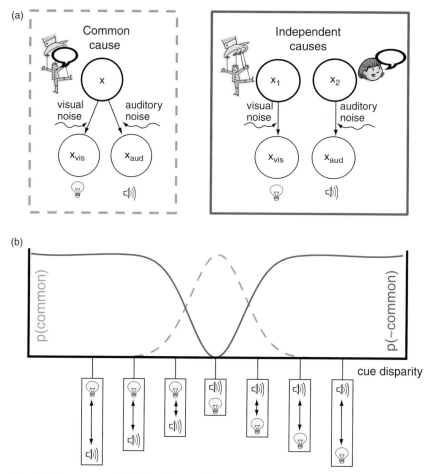

Figure 7.3 Two structural beliefs of the world. (a) If two cues are adequately coincident, subjects perceive them as having a common cause (the dashed box), a phenomenon typified through ventriloquism. In this case, the two cues should be integrated according to Bayes' rule. If the cues are disparate in time or space, subjects perceive them as having independent causes (the solid box). (b) Subject's belief of a common cause. As the spatial disparity of two cues, a voice and a puppet's motions, or a light flash and a tone, is experimentally controlled the belief in a common cause can be manipulated.

(Figure 7.3b). Recent studies have provided support for the predictions of Bayesian models of causal inference for cross-modality cue combination (Körding *et al.*, 2006; Shams *et al.*, 2005), depth perception (Knill, 2007), and estimation of stimuli numbers (Wozny *et al.*, 2008). These studies highlight that the nervous system estimates state with consideration of causal structures among sensory cues in a way that is close to statistical optimum.

One central feature of the human movement system is that it adapts continuously to changes in the environment and in the body. It has been suggested that this adaptation is largely driven by movement errors. However, errors are subject to unknown causal structures. For example, if an error is caused by changes in the motor apparatus, such as strength changes due to muscle fatigue, the nervous system should adapt its estimates of the body. On the other hand, if an error is caused by random external perturbations, the nervous system should not adapt its estimates of the body, as this error is irrelevant. Given the inherent ambiguity in errors, the best choice of adaptive action should be a function of the probability of error being relevant. Bayesian models can predict the optimal adaptation to errors with unknown causal relationship. These predictions have been confirmed in a recent study on motor adaptation in a visuomotor task (Wei and Körding, 2008). It appears that in these sensorimotor tasks the nervous system not only estimates the state but also estimates the causal structure of perceptual information.

The statistical problem that subjects solve in cue combination implicitly involves an inference about the causal structure of the stimuli, e.g., did the flash of light cause the auditory tone, did the tone cause the flash, was there an unknown cause for them both, or were they simply coincidental? The problem faced by the nervous system is thus similar to those studied extensively in psychology and cognitive science that occur in the context of causal induction (Gopnik *et al.*, 2004; Griffiths and Tenenbaum, 2005; Michotte, 1963; Sperber and Premack, 1995; Tenenbaum *et al.*, 2006). Many experiments demonstrate that people interpret events in terms of cause and effect. The results presented here show that sensorimotor integration exhibits some of the same factors found in human cognition. Incorporating the causal relationships among state variables, it appears the nervous system estimates a structural view of the world. Once again, this process is necessary to optimally select actions, whether they be for motor, or any other behaviours.

7.5   Bayesian decision theory and inverse decision theory

We have surveyed a great amount of evidence on how people judge, gauge, and generally make sense of their perceptions of the world. We have shown that they estimate the structure of the world, using models to predict how its property values evolve over time, and combine multiple sensory cues or their prior experience, to form a best estimate. Conceptually, however, this is only the first step in action selection. Once we have estimated the state of the world, we need to assess the relative value of all available actions in terms of the statistics of their outcomes. Only then can we choose the action that will best achieve our goals. Mathematically this is expressed as minimising our expected costs (Equation (7.2)). This formalism of choosing optimal actions by combining the statistics of outcomes and the resulting costs falls under the study of *decision theory* and *optimal control*. In all but the simplest cases, computing these optimal commands is very difficult.

Consider one such simple case, that of pea shooting. Those that pursue this hobby blow dried peas through a small hollow tube, or pea shooter. Once the pea leaves the shooter, its fate is dictated by wind, aerodynamics, etc. Assuming you have total control over the position and orientation of your pea tube (and in the World Pea Shooting Championship, it is not unheard of for contestants to use laser targeting for this express purpose), where your aim will dictate a distribution of possible locations the pea will land within the target. Referring again to equation (7.2), choosing the best aiming location requires considering the likely score a distribution of pea locations will yield for any given aim point. However, if you are unsure where exactly you are aiming (or your laser is faulty), then you must also integrate your uncertainty in your aiming point into your final decision.

Often, when we are examining the behaviours of a human subject or animal, we want to compare them against what is optimal (see Chapter 3). Assuming we can overcome the difficulties outlined above, we can move forward with our analysis, and compare experimental evidence against our theoretical predictions. Yet, there is a fundamental hurdle in this comparison. For this type of analysis to be constructive, we must know beforehand what it is the experimental subject is trying to achieve; that is, what their cost function is. With this in mind, researchers have designed experiments where the cost of the task is relatively explicit, such as in the dartboard example. In a set of reaching studies not unlike throwing a dart, it was observed that people are remarkably close to the optimal choices prescribed by decision theory (Maloney *et al.*, 2006; Trommershäuser *et al.*, 2003, 2005). Similar experiments have studied visual tasks (Najemnik and Geisler, 2005, 2008, 2009) and force-producing tasks (Körding and Wolpert, 2004b; Körding *et al.*, 2004; see also, Part II). This further demonstrates people's abilities to integrate statistical information in a Bayes-optimal manner, not just for estimation, but also for action selection.

In general though, even when subjects are given explicit rewards and penalties, the cost function they actually use is unknown to us. For instance, one may value a 2 point reward more than twice that of a 1 point reward. Fortunately, the mechanisms of decision theory may be inverted and computational techniques can be used to infer not only the costs subjects use, but also their priors and likelihoods to make their decisions. This pursuit is referred to as inverse decision theory. Though this technique has long been employed in economics (Kagel and Roth, 1995), and agent-based modelling (see Part III) only recently has this approach been used in neuroscience and motor control.

Using inverse decision theory, recent studies have examined both implicit cost functions that subjects use when performing motor tasks (Körding *et al.*, 2004) and when penalising target errors (Körding and Wolpert, 2004b, see Figure 7.4). These inferred cost functions have highly nonlinear and nontrivial forms (Todorov, 2004). These findings highlight a crucial problem in decision theory; good fits to behaviour may be obtained with incorrect cost functions. Inverse decision theory can thus be used as a means of searching for violations in the assumptions we make using the Bayesian approach to decision making.

As mentioned, inverse decision theory also allows for the analysis of subject priors and likelihoods. For example, studies have found that subjects sometimes use a non-Gaussian prior, and underestimate the speed of visual motion (Stocker and Simoncelli, 2006; Weiss *et al.*, 2002). While this approach is enticing for future studies, it also has its weaknesses. Inverse decision theory will always yield a cost function, or likelihood, or prior, for which the observed behaviour is optimal. Like other models built to explain data, over-fitting is also a problem for these decision theoretic models. Researchers must

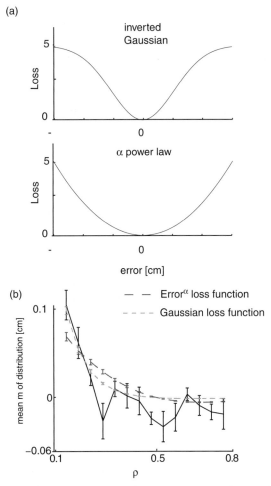

Figure 7.4 Inverse decision theory. (a) Cost functions are proposed for penalising motor errors. In this example, the upper cost function penalises errors with an inverted Gaussian, and the lower cost function with a power law. (b) In a motor task the free parameter, the skewness of targets, ρ, is varied to examine the subject's performance. The best fits for the two cost functions are overlaid on human data (taken from Körding and Wolpert, 2004b).

take steps to ensure this character does not bias their results, or experiments can be designed to independently test these results.

7.6   Bayesian decision theory in dynamical systems: optimal control

7.6.1   The optimal control problem

Up to this point, the actions we've been considering are relatively simple choices, discrete actions that instantly effect outcomes, e.g., where we aim the pea shooter or dart. However, as we pointed out in the introduction, many, if not most of the choices we take under more realistic conditions are dynamical in nature. Again, a more realistic description of dart throwing considers the forces and motions of the dart, the inertial mechanics of our limb and the force generating properties of our muscles (all of which we can only infer through noisy information). As the state of the dart evolves in time, so too must our actions. Under these more realistic conditions our possible actions move from a range of aiming points, to a list of possible muscles to excite, and the time-history of how these muscles should be excited. Clearly, the relationship between our actions under this scenario and the dart's trajectory and eventual landing place on the board are complicated to say the least.

Under these dynamic conditions, our costs too, are no longer immediately evident, and instead may evolve over time, or may not even be apparent until some delayed period of time after we've taken them. For instance, how hard we throw the dart will influence its path once it leaves our hands and eventually hits its target. Moreover, how hard we throw will influence how quickly we tire, influencing our later throws. How we perform during the dart game may influence our physical and emotional wellbeing for the remainder of the afternoon as well. Taking these considerations into account, one can see how choosing our optimal actions can quickly become a daunting task. Mathematically, we still express our optimal actions in essentially the same form as Equation (7.2), however, now the actions are functions of time and state, and the costs too must be integrated across time. This time- and state-dependent series of actions is often referred to as a policy: a plan of action to control decisions and achieve our desired outcome.

The best possible policy dictates the action we should take at this instant, knowing how it will influence both future states and the actions we can take at that future time. In a sense, to be optimal we need to know the future; we need to be aware of the possible future states and actions that will result from the decision we make now. Under very simple scenarios these future states and actions could be learned through trial and error. However, more generally the future is inferred through models of the world. These models, referred to as forward models, require hypothesis about the nature of the world (Bayesian estimation of structure) and how it evolves (Bayesian estimation across time). Regardless of how the future states are estimated, we need to know how choosing an action based on our current state will affect future states and the costs associated with them. Mathematically, this is compactly represented by what is referred to as the value function. The value function quantifies the cost of being in any state, and acting according to a given policy for all future times. Not surprisingly, computing this value function is very difficult, as it is akin to seeing into the future. However, once we know this value function, we can relatively easily asses the value of being in any given state, and choose the action that moves us to a state with the best value.

7.6.2   Solution strategies in optimal control

Because this value function is such an integral component to solving for optimal actions, a whole field of numerical techniques has been spawned to achieve this goal (e.g., see Bryson and Ho, 1975; Stuart and Peter, 2003). Difficult to compute analytically, many techniques have been developed to approximate the value function and the accompanying optimal policy. As the problem descriptions get more complicated (e.g., as when we move from choosing where to aim a dart to choosing muscle activation patterns), the likelihood that these techniques will provide an accurate solution diminishes. As such, approximating the optimal actions is often the best one can hope for. Regardless of the difficulty in solving these problems, the same basic principles hold; we represent the necessary statistics of actions and how they impact the statistics of outcomes.

When our observations of the state of the world are relatively certain, we can attempt to approximate the value function directly. There are two widely used approaches. Value iteration is a boot-strapping algorithm, initialised with a naïve value function and repeatedly updated until the estimate is acceptably accurate. Using the current estimate of the value function, the algorithm sweeps across all world states, updating the value of being in that state given that state's cost and the value of the best possible future state. The policy is never explicitly computed, instead actions are chosen by evaluating the value function's estimate. In a similar approach, policy iteration uses a current estimate of the value function to compute a policy. This policy is then used to converge on an estimate of the value function. These steps are repeated until both the policy and value function converge. Value and policy iteration techniques are particularly applicable to problems with a finite and discrete number of world states and actions. When our certainty of the world and how our actions will influence it is less certain we must rely on other methods. In reinforcement learning algorithms, rather than using accurate distributions of states and costs, empirical observations are used (Sutton and Barto, 1998). By observing world states and actions taken, an intermediate function is computed that can be used to estimate the optimal policy.

While the above algorithms are very successful for a large class of problems, a more general approach to solving optimal control problems is found through the Hamilton–Jacobi–Bellman equation (or simply the Bellman equation when dealing with discrete time). These equations define the necessary and sufficient conditions for optimality in terms of the value function. Under limited conditions, these equations can be used to find analytical solutions to the optimal policy. For example, the widely popular method of dynamic programming can be used to solve for an optimal policy when the states and actions are discrete and finite. What's more, for linear problems with Gaussian noise, these equations can be used to derive the value function and the optimal policy, the so-called linear quadratic Gaussian regulator (LQG) problem. Under more general conditions, these equations can be used to approximate, perhaps iteratively, the value function and an optimal policy (Stengel, 1994). A wide range of numerical techniques is available to solve problems of optimal control and these techniques generally incorporate Bayesian updating.

7.6.3   Optimal control as Bayesian inference

Interestingly, recent advanced statistical techniques suggest that these traditional methods for computing optimal actions may be supplemented, or even altogether abandoned for what promises to be a truly Bayesian inference formalism. To motivate this new approach, we first point out that in the simplest of cases, it is well known that there is a correspondence between how to choose optimal actions, and how to make optimal inferences. In the linear setting, the optimal estimation problem is the mathematical dual to the optimal control problem (e.g., Stengel, 1994). The defining equations for the solutions to these two problems are identical. Practically speaking, this means the same numerical techniques can be employed to solve either problem. Theoretically, the implication is that choosing an optimal action is a similar problem to optimally estimating the world's state.

Recent work has extended this duality to a larger class of problems. Making some broad assumptions concerning system dynamics and probability distributions of the optimal solutions, this duality has been extended to a large class of nonlinear problems (Todorov, 2008, 2009). There is a correspondence between the distribution of states under optimal conditions, and the solution to the value function. This work further emphasises the implicit connection between optimal actions and optimal inference.

Taking another approach, recent work has neglected a cost function altogether and reformulated the problem of optimal action selection as a problem of optimal Bayesian inference (Friston, 2009; Friston *et al.*, 2009; Toussaint, 2009, 2010). This new work replaces the traditional cost function with a desired distribution over states. Actions are selected to reduce uncertainty in our expectations of the world. These new methods, which are purely inference processes, subsume the problem of optimal action selection and optimal inference into a more general Bayesian inference procedure.

7.7   Experimental investigation of learnt statistics

We began this chapter discussing how noise and uncertainty must be considered when choosing our actions. As such, we introduced the Bayesian formalism for making the optimal estimates necessary for choosing our actions. In particular, we reviewed how new evidence should be combined with prior knowledge, and experimental results that demonstrate human subjects appear to do this rationally. We then discussed how these estimates could be updated as evidence is accumulated across time. These estimates could then be used to choose actions according to Bayesian decision theory and optimal control. Having reviewed the necessary theory and background we now present some recent experimental work that examines an important aspect of action selection: representing prior beliefs.

Based on a growing body of evidence, many animals, and humans in particular, appear to make estimates, and choose actions, consistent with the predictions of Bayesian statistics. Implicit in these choices is our prior knowledge; the knowledge we have accumulated throughout life, as well as the knowledge we accumulate during the course of an experimental manipulation, represented as a statistical distribution. While these studies have shown that human subjects can efficiently use prior information, little is known about the way such priors are learned. It is clear priors can change as we accumulate knowledge, however, it is unclear *how* these priors change over time, if they converge to the veridical distribution, and over what timescales they change.

We recently set out to examine just these questions. We designed two simple 'coin catching' experiments to examine if subjects could not only accurately estimate a prior, but also the timescale over which it was learned. As many Bayesian experiments rely on a subject's use of an appropriate prior, these results would have an important impact on future studies.

In these experiments we investigated how subjects adapted their expectation of coin locations (a prior) in response to changes in the underlying distribution. Subjects had to estimate the location of a virtual target coin, randomly drawn from a normal distribution. On every trial, subjects were given noisy information of the coin's current location, in the form of a single 'cue coin' and were then asked to guess the location of the 'target coin'. To successfully estimate the target coin's location, subjects needed to integrate the coin's likelihood (obtained from the cue coin) with its prior (the distribution of previous target coin locations). By collecting data on where the subjects estimated the target coin to be, we could then estimate the prior used by the subject and analyse its temporal evolution.

In the first experiment, the target coins were drawn from a normally distributed prior. One of two priors was used for each subject; one prior had a relatively narrow distribution, and the other a relatively wide distribution. This first experiment determined whether or not subjects could accurately learn the prior, and if so, the timescale over which it was learned. In the second experiment naïve subjects were recruited to participate in a modified task. Halfway through the experiment, the variance of the prior would switch. The same two variances used in experiment 1 were used. One of these two values was randomly chosen at the start of the experiment and assigned to the prior. After half of the trials the prior's variance would switch to the other value. This allowed us to further probe how subjects learned a prior, and to observe if the learning rate remained constant.

To infer each subject's estimate of the prior's variance, we measured the relative weighting subject's placed on the cue coin relative to the prior's mean, when estimating the target coin's location. This gain, r, is a measure of the subject's estimate of the prior (see Section 7.2.1). If subjects believed the prior had a wide distribution, r would be close to 1.0, indicating the cue coin was the best proxy for the target coin's location. Similarly, if the subjects believed the prior had a narrow distribution, the gain r, would be close to 0, indicating the prior's mean was the best proxy for the target coin. In both experiments r was either 0.8 or 0.2. We computed this gain over bins of 10 consecutive trials.

Across all subjects, r took on relatively large values in the first trials, indicating the subjects' belief in a 'flat' prior; e.g., the subjects displayed little preference for initially believing the coins would appear in any particular location. However, as the experiment progressed r converged to the correct value. For subjects in the narrow variance group of experiment 1, the data averaged across subjects indicated that approximately 200 trials (20 bins) were required to correctly estimate the variance of the prior (see Figure 7.5c), and on average converged to the correct value. The subjects in wide variance group of experiment 1 essentially began the experiment with the correct gain (see Figure 7.5a). In addition to this analysis, we also inferred the subjects' estimate of the mean of the prior. This too was found to be accurately estimated, albeit on a much faster timescale (data not shown). Using the values inferred for the mean and variance, we were able to

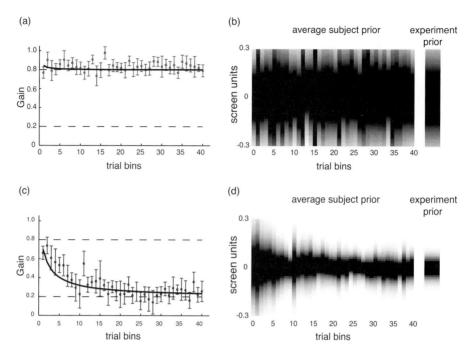

Figure 7.5 Learning a fixed prior. (a) Across-subject averages for the gain, *r*, in the wide variance group (mean ± standard error). The bold black line indicates the Bayesian inference model fits to the experimental data. (b) The inferred average prior as it evolved over the experiment. (c) and (d) Across-subject averages for the gain, *r*, in the narrow variance group and the inferred prior as it evolved (taken from Berniker *et al.*, 2010).

reconstruct the subjects' estimated prior during the course of learning (Figure 7.5b and c). This analysis shows that human subjects converge to the correct variance of the prior with a timescale on the order of a hundred trials.

To interpret the subjects' results in a Bayesian framework, we postulated an optimal inference model assigned to the same task, and questioned how it would perform. By observing the cue and target coin locations, the model accurately applied the rules of Bayesian statistics to update a joint distribution of the prior's estimated mean and variance. For this inference, we used an often-assumed normal-scaled inverse gamma distribution. This uses a normal distribution to represent a belief in the mean, and an inverse gamma distribution to represent a belief in the variance. The model contains four free parameters that needed to be specified before we could compare its results with those of the subjects. Therefore, we used the data from the first half of the experiment to fit the model's parameters and then proceeded to compute the model's results for the second half of the experiment. With more knowledge about the task than the subjects, the model represents the upper limit in accuracy on what could be observed experimentally.

Just as with the data shown above, during the first 250 trials of experiment 2, the subjects quickly acquired the mean of the prior and the correct variance over a slower timescale (statistically indistinguishable from the first 250 trials of experiment 1).

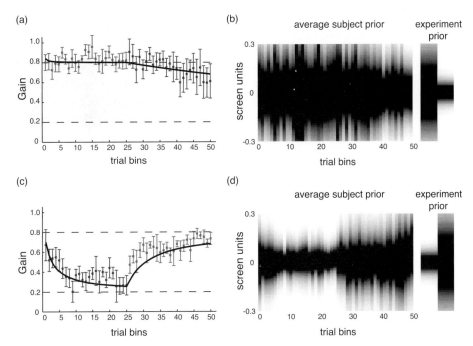

Figure 7.6 Learning a switching prior. (a) Across-subject averages for the gain, *r*, in the wide variance first group (mean ± standard error). The bold black line indicates the Bayesian inference model's predicted result based on the fit from experiment 1. (b) The inferred average prior as it evolved over the experiment. (c) and (d) Across-subject averages for the gain, *r*, in the narrow variance first group and the inferred prior as it evolved (taken from Berniker *et al.*, 2010).

However, the second 250 trials were distinct, and there were clear differences in the apparent rate at which subjects learned the prior's variance. The learning rate during the second half of experiment 2 was smaller than the apparent learning rate of the first half (or equivalently, the first half of experiment 1). For example, with the wide variance first group, after 500 trials the average behaviour did not yet reflect an accurate estimate for the variance as it did in the first half of the experiment (Figure 7.6a). Inferring the average subject prior using the measured gains and means we could track the prior as it changed over the course of learning (Figure 7.6b). It appeared as if learning the first prior somehow acted to impede subjects' ability to adapt to the second prior. This is especially evident when transitioning from a large variance to a small variance; the change in the subjects' prior was gradual (Figure 7.6a and b).

A good fit to experiment 1 was obtained with the Bayesian inference model by minimising the log-likelihood of the subject data (see Figure 7.5a and c). This model was then used to predict the results of experiment 2. The model's behaviour was qualitatively similar to the subjects' (see Figure 7.6a and c, black lines). In particular, note that the inference model correctly predicts a slower learning rate for the second half of the experiment; just as with the subject's data, the model is slow to infer the last half of experiment 2 relative to the first half of experiment 2. Initially, the model is relatively uncertain of the prior and predisposed to estimating large changes in the variance based on the observed distribution of coins. As the experiment progresses, the model's estimate of the variance becomes more certain. By the 250th trial, the model's certainty in the prior's variance makes it insensitive to the new observations of the coin's distribution, now indicating a different variance. As a result, the model is now slow to estimate the new variance, qualitatively similar to the subjects' behaviour.

Overall, we find that subjects can learn an accurate prior, and appear to do so in a rational way. They relatively quickly learn the mean of a distribution (as sample statistics would suggest, the certainty in the mean is higher than the certainty in the variance) and the variance is learned accurately, and in a manner consistent with a Bayesian interpretation. Together this suggests humans can accurately and efficiently learn a prior for making optimal action selections.

7.8   Discussion

Here we have reviewed the results from a wide range of studies that probe cue combination, sensorimotor integration, and motor control using experiments with human volunteers. These studies have found that information such as trial-by-trial error is not sufficient to describe their error. Instead, what has been found is that the statistics of movements play an important role and that quantitative predictions of behaviour can be obtained from the Bayesian formalism.

Estimating the relevant variables needed for motor behaviours happens on many timescales. Traditionally, depending on the timescales involved, different terms are used to refer to this process. Estimations performed on a very fast timescale are usually referred to as information integration; e.g., cue combination or state estimation. Phenomena that require estimations over medium durations are often called motor adaptation; e.g., adapting to a visuomotor disturbance. Estimations over relatively long timescales are usually called motor learning; e.g., learning the structure of a disturbance. These three terms are used widely in different areas of the motor control literature. In this article we have discussed all three phenomena in the same context, highlighting the fact that the same Bayesian ideas can be used to explore many distinct classes of motor behaviour.

Related issues are the phenomena of consolidation and interference. Under some conditions, subjects can acquire a new motor behaviour, and recall the behaviour for later use, even after significant periods of time and with other movements happening in between. The phenomena of preserving a motor behaviour has been termed consolidation (e.g., Brashers-Krug *et al.*, 1996). However, it is often found that the act of adapting to one motor behaviour can have adverse effects on our ability to retain a previously adapted motor behaviour; thus one motor behaviour interferes with the consolidation of another. A Bayesian analysis of motor adaptation has already demonstrated how adaptation can lead to new estimates of multiple parameters if they have similar likelihoods (Berniker and Körding, 2008). Thus it could be that adapting to one motor behaviour inadvertently influences the parameters of another. Further, it is not difficult to speculate how prolonged practice with a new motor behaviour increases the certainty in its properties. A Bayesian model would translate this certainty into strong priors, making the behaviour relatively unsusceptible to re-adaptation, a form of consolidation.

As we have shown, the general problem of choosing actions can be modelled as an optimal control problem. This approach has been successfully applied in a number of fields. It is worth noting that different fields sometimes use different formulations to refer to the same problem. As a result, many researchers examine choice selection under the banner of Markov decision processes, while others use the wording of stochastic optimal control. However, the same mathematics, requiring Bayesian statistics, govern both approaches. Moreover, this same formalism is not limited to action selection and motor control, but is also widely used to model cognitive processes and the more general problem of intelligence or even social intelligence (see Part III).

Most Bayesian models discussed above assume that noise sources are Gaussian and that the interactions between the subject and the world have linear dynamics. A set of recent approaches in Bayesian statistics allows a powerful framework well beyond these simple assumptions to be applied. For instance, the structure inference problem is a simple case of non-Gaussian probability distributions. Methods that may be applied to such problems range from linearisation techniques such as extended Kalman filters over variational techniques, to particle filtering methods (Bishop 2006; MacKay, 2003). Clearly more realistic models of the motor system will benefit from further advances in machine learning.

The evidence reviewed for Bayesian integration in the nervous system has been based on psychophysical experiments where human behaviour is measured and the underlying neural processes are unobserved. The Bayesian models proposed are often interpreted as archetypes for the neural computations responsible for the motor behaviours. Recent studies though are looking for evidence of these computations at the neuronal level. Purely computational studies now show how neurons might easily solve some of the needed computations (Ma et al., 2006). Other studies are looking for neural correlates of uncertainty (Cisek and Kalaska, 2005; Gold and Shadlen, 2001, 2003; Kiani and Shadlen, 2009) and electrophysiological evidence of multimodal cue combination in the context of uncertainty (Angelaki et al., 2004). Future studies might focus on imaging or electrophysiological studies to find more evidence for the neural substrates of these computations (see also, Part II).

The human nervous system clearly has limitations and it would be very surprising if our behaviour were optimal for all tasks. Indeed, many past experiments have found deviations from optimality. For example, in situations requiring economic decisions, human subjects systematically overestimate small probabilities and exhibit so-called framing effects (Kahneman and Tversky, 1979). As a result of these biases it is known that we are not optimal at speculating on, for example, the stock market. The phenomena that we reviewed here where near optimal Bayesian behaviour is observed are all rather low-level phenomena – simple perceptual and sensorimotor tasks. The optimality observed for these phenomena does not appear to carry over to the range of high-level decision-making tasks that have been characterised in behavioural economics. However, we have yet to find the limits of the Bayesian approach for modelling action selection.

7.9   Conclusions

Recognising the inherent uncertainty in motor tasks, many motor control problems have been successfully described by applying the rules of Bayesian statistics to analyse their solutions.

This same method holds promise for many of the outstanding problems in cue combination, motor control, cognitive science, and neuroscience, in general. Bayesian statistics and normative modelling are complementary to descriptive studies of the nervous system. As such, combining the two approaches will provide models that not only predict, but explain how the nervous system solves the problems it is confronted with. This insight into the purpose, and detail of structure, will provide a deeper understanding of the nervous system.

References

Alais, D. and D. Burr (2004). The ventriloquist effect results from near-optimal bimodal integration. *Curr. Biol.* **14**(3): 257–62.

Angelaki, D. E., A. G. Shaikh, A. M. Green, *et al.* (2004). Neurons compute internal models of the physical laws of motion. *Nature* **430**(6999): 560–4.

Berniker, M. and K. Körding (2008). Estimating the sources of motor errors for adaptation and generalization. *Nat. Neurosci.* **11**(12): 1454–61.

Berniker, M., M. Voss, and K. Körding (2010). Learning priors for Bayesian computations in the nervous system. *PLoS One* **5**(9): e12686.

Bishop, C. (2006). *Pattern Recognition and Machine Learning*. Berlin: Springer.

Brashers-Krug, T., R. Shadmehr, and E. Bizzi (1996). Consolidation in human motor memory. *Nature* **382**(6588): 252–5.

Bryson, A. E. and Y. C. Ho (1975). *Applied Optimal Control: Optimization, Estimation, and Control*. London: Taylor and Francis Group.

Chater, N., J. B. Tenenbaum, and A. Yuille (2006). Probabilistic models of cognition: where next? *Trends Cogn. Sci.* **10**(7): 292–3.

Cisek, P. and J. F. Kalaska (2005). Neural correlates of reaching decisions in dorsal premotor cortex: specification of multiple direction choices and final selection of action. *Neuron* **45**(5): 801–14.

Deneve, S. (2008). Bayesian spiking neurons I: inference. *Neural Comput.* **20**(1): 91–117.

Ernst, M. O. and M. S. Banks (2002). Humans integrate visual and haptic information in a statistically optimal fashion. *Nature* **415**(6870): 429–33.

Ernst, M. O. and H. H. Bulthoff (2004). Merging the senses into a robust percept. *Trends Cogn. Sci.* **8**(4): 162–9.

Flanagan, J. R., J. P. Bittner, and R. S. Johansson (2008). Experience can change distinct size-weight priors engaged in lifting objects and judging their weights. *Curr. Biol.* **18**: 1742–7.

Friston, K. (2009). The free-energy principle: a rough guide to the brain? *Trends Cogn. Sci.* **13**(7): 293–301.

Friston, K. J., J. Daunizeau, and S. J. Kiebel (2009). Reinforcement learning or active inference? *PLoS One* **4**(7).

Geisler, W. S. and D. Kersten (2002). Illusions, perception and Bayes. *Nat. Neurosci.* **5**(6): 508–10.

Gold, J. I. and M. N. Shadlen (2001). Neural computations that underlie decisions about sensory stimuli. *Trends Cogn. Sci.* **5**(1): 10–16.

Gold, J. I. and M. N. Shadlen (2003). The influence of behavioral context on the representation of a perceptual decision in developing oculomotor commands. *J. Neurosci.* **23**(2): 632.

Gopnik, A., C. Glymour, D. Sobel, *et al.* (2004). A theory of causal learning in children: causal maps and Bayes nets. *Psychol. Rev.* **111**(1): 3–32.

Griffiths, T. L. and J. B. Tenenbaum (2005). Structure and strength in causal induction. *Cognit. Psychol.* **51**(4): 334–84.

Hoyer, P. O. and A. Hyvärinen (2003). Interpreting neural response variability as Monte Carlo sampling of the posterior. In *Neural Information Processing Systems*, Vol. 15. Cambridge, MA: MIT Press.

Kagel, J. H. and A. E. Roth, eds. (1995). *The Handbook of Experimental Economics*. Princeton, NJ: Princeton University Press.

Kahneman, D. and A. Tversky (1979). Prospect theory: an analysis of decision under risk. *Econometrica* **XLVII**: 263–291.

Kersten, D. and A. Yuille (2003). Bayesian models of object perception. *Curr. Opin. Neurobiol.* **13**(2): 150–8.

Kiani, R. and M. N. Shadlen (2009). Representation of confidence associated with a decision by neurons in the parietal cortex. *Science* **324**(5928): 759.

Knill, D. C. (2007). Robust cue integration: a Bayesian model and evidence from cue-conflict studies with stereoscopic and figure cues to slant. *J. Vis.* **7**(7): 5 1–24.

Knill, D. and W. Richards, eds. (1996). *Perception as Bayesian Inference*, Cambridge: Cambridge University Press.

Körding, K. (2007). Decision theory: what 'should' the nervous system do? *Science* **318**(5850): 606–10.

Körding, K., J. Tenenbaum, *et al.* (2006). A generative model based approach to motor adaptation. In *Neural Information Processing Systems*, Vol. 15. Cambridge, MA: MIT Press.

Körding, K. P., I. Fukunaga, I. Howard, *et al.* (2004). A neuroeconomics approach to inferring utility functions in sensorimotor control. *PLoS Biol.* **2**(10): e330.

Körding, K. P., S. P. Ku, and D. M. Wolpert (2004). Bayesian integration in force estimation. *J. Neurophys.* **92**(5): 3161–5.

Körding, K. P. and D. M. Wolpert (2004a). Bayesian integration in sensorimotor learning. *Nature* **427**(6971): 244–7.

Körding, K. P. and D. M. Wolpert (2004b). The loss function of sensorimotor learning. *Proc. Natl. Acad. Sci. USA* **101**(26): 9839–42.

Körding, K. P. and D. M. Wolpert (2006). Bayesian decision theory in sensorimotor control. *Trends Cogn Sci.* **10**(7): 319–26.

Ma, W. J., J. M. Beck, P. E. Latham, and A. Pouget (2006). Bayesian inference with probabilistic population codes. *Nat. Neurosci.* **9**(11): 1432–8.

MacKay, D. J. C. (2003). *Information Theory, Inference, and Learning Algorithms*. Cambridge: Cambridge University Press.

Maloney, L. T., J. Trommershäuser, *et al.* (2006). Questions without words: A comparison between decision making under risk and movement planning under risk. In *Integrated Models of Cognitive Systems*, ed. W. Gray. New York, NY: Oxford University Press, pp. 297–314.

Mehta, B. and S. Schaal (2002). Forward models in visuomotor control. *J. Neurophysiol.* **88**(2): 942–53.

Michotte, A. (1963). *The Perception of Causality*. London: Methuen.

Miyazaki, M., D. Nozaki, and Y. Nakajima (2005). Testing Bayesian models of human coincidence timing. *J. Neurophysiol.* **94**(1): 395–9.

Miyazaki, M., S. Yamamoto, S. Uchida, and S. Kitazawa (2006). Bayesian calibration of simultaneity in tactile temporal order judgment. *Nat. Neurosci.* **9**(7): 875–7.

Najemnik, J. and W. S. Geisler (2005). Optimal eye movement strategies in visual search. *Nature* **434**(7031): 387–91.

Najemnik, J. and W. S. Geisler (2008). Eye movement statistics in humans are consistent with an optimal search strategy. *J. Vis.* **8**(3): 1–14.

Najemnik, J. and W. S. Geisler (2009). Simple summation rule for optimal fixation selection in visual search. *Vision Res.* **49**: 1286–94.

Peterka, R. J. and P. J. Loughlin (2004). Dynamic regulation of sensorimotor integration in human postural control. *J. Neurophysiol.* **91**(1): 410–23.

Pouget, A., P. Dayan, and R. S. Zemel (2003). Inference and computation with population codes. *An. Rev. Neurosci.* **26**: 381–410.

Rosas, P., J. Wagemans, M. O. Ernst, and F. A. Wichmann (2005). Texture and haptic cues in slant discrimination: reliability-based cue weighting without statistically optimal cue combination. *J. Opt. Soc. Am. A* **22**(5): 801–809.

Shams, L., W. J. Ma, S. Tanaka, *et al.* (2005). Sound-induced flash illusion as an optimal percept. *Neuroreport* **16**(17): 1923–7.

Sperber, D. and D. Premack (1995). *Causal Cognition: A Multidisciplinary Debate*. Oxford: Oxford University Press.

Stengel, R. F. (1994). *Optimal Control and Estimation*. New York: Dover Publications.

Stocker, A. A. and E. P. Simoncelli (2006). Noise characteristics and prior expectations in human visual speed perception. *Nat. Neurosci.* **9**(4): 578–85.

Stuart, J. R. and N. Peter (2003). *Artificial Intelligence: A Modern Approach*. Harlow, UK: Pearson Education.

Sutton, R. S. and A. G. Barto (1998). *Reinforcement Learning*. Cambridge, MA: MIT Press.

Tassinari, H., T. E. Hudson, and M. S. Landy (2006). Combining priors and noisy visual cues in a rapid pointing task. *J. Neurosci.* **26**(40): 10154–63.

Tenenbaum, J. B., T. L. Griffiths, and C. Kemp (2006). Theory-based Bayesian models of inductive learning and reasoning. *Trends Cogn. Sci.* **10**(7): 309–18.

Todorov, E. (2004). Optimality principles in sensorimotor control. *Nat. Neurosci.* **7**(9): 907–15.

Todorov, E. (2006). Optimal Control Theory. In *Bayesian Brain*, ed. K. Doya. Cambridge, MA, MIT Press, pp. 269–98.

Todorov, E. (2008). General duality between optimal control and estimation. Proceedings of the 47th IEEE Conference on Decision and Control, Cancun, Mexico, pp. 4286–92.

Todorov, E. (2009). Efficient computation of optimal actions. *Proc. Natl. Acad. Sci. USA* **106**(28): 11478–83.

Toussaint, M. (2009). Robot trajectory optimization using approximate inference. 26th International Conference on Machine Learning (ICML 2009), ACM New York, NY, USA, pp. 449–56.

Toussaint, M. (2010). *A Bayesian View on Motor Control and Planning*. Berlin: Springer.

Trommershäuser, J., S. Gepshtein, L. T. Maloney, M. S. Landy, and M. S. Banks (2005). Optimal compensation for changes in task-relevant movement variability. *J. Neurosci.* **25**(31): 7169–78.

Trommershäuser, J., L. T. Maloney, and M. S. Landy (2003). Statistical decision theory and the selection of rapid, goal-directed movements. *J. Opt. Soc. Am. A* **20**: 1419–33.

van Ee, R., W. J. Adams, and P. Mamassian (2003). Bayesian modeling of cue interaction: bistability in stereoscopic slant perception. *J. Opt. Soc. Am. A* **20**(7): 1398–406.

Wei, K. and K. P. Körding (2008). Relevance of error: what drives motor adaptation? *J. Neurophys.* **90545**: 2008.

Weiss, Y., E. P. Simoncelli, and E. H. Adelson (2002). Motion illusions as optimal percepts. *Nat. Neurosci.* **5**(6): 598–604.

Wolpert, D. M., Z. Ghahramani, and M. I. Jordan (1995). An internal model for sensorimotor integration. *Science* **269**(5232): 1880–2.

Wozny, D. R., U. R. Beierholm, and L. Shams (2008). Human trimodal perception follows optimal statistical inference. *J. Vis.* **8**(3): 1–11.

Zemel, R. S., P. Dayan, and A. Pouget (1998). Probabilistic interpretation of population codes. *Neural Comput.* **10**(2): 403–30.

8 Post-retrieval inhibition in sequential memory search[1]

Eddy J. Davelaar

Summary

Sequential behaviour is observed in various domains of cognitive psychology, including free recall paradigms. In this chapter, within a neurocomputational framework resampling (RS) mechanisms are compared with competitive queuing (CQ) mechanisms. While both types of implementations select the most active representation, the subsequent inhibition is at the level of selection for RS models and at the level of (re)activation for CQ models. It is shown that despite the overwhelming success of CQ models in serial recall (with regard to types of sequencing error), RS models outperform CQ models with regard to interresponse times in a free recall task. Additional analyses show that decay of response suppression reduces the difference between the models. The RS model is sensitive to the size of the search set and accounts for memory selection performance in patients with Alzheimer's dementia or Huntington's disease.

8.1 Introduction

In many complex systems that exhibit sequential ordering of actions, a selection mechanism converts simultaneously activated representations into a sequence of actions. The simplest form this selection mechanism can take is one by which one action is selected and then executed, after which another action is activated (from zero), selected, and executed, and so on. However, research within psychology has demonstrated that this type of selection mechanism is inconsistent with detailed error analyses in serial recall (Henson *et al.*, 1996) and typing (see Salthouse, 1986), as it would, for example, be unable to account for the smooth transitions between successive actions. Instead, evidence points towards a two-stage mechanism, by which in the first stage all task-appropriate representations are activated in parallel (instead of sequentially), and in the second stage representations are selected one at a time to produce its corresponding

---

[1] This chapter is a revised version of an original article. The final, definitive version of this paper has been published in *Adaptive Behavior*, **15**(1), 51–71, March 2007 doi: 10.1177/1059712306076250 by SAGE Publications Ltd. All rights reserved.

Modelling Natural Action Selection, eds. Anil K. Seth, Tony J. Prescott and Joanna J. Bryson.
Published by Cambridge University Press. © Cambridge University Press 2012.

action. Although most of the initial knowledge was gathered from motor behaviour, with typing as one familiar example (see the review by Salthouse, 1986, and references therein), researchers have suggested that this two-stage mechanism may also be central to other forms of sequential behaviour, from walking through a room or grasping a mug to producing speech, preparing coffee, or even memorising words. Given the ubiquity of serial ordering in our daily lives, it may come as no surprise that models exist in which simultaneously activated representations produce serially ordered actions. Two of these models are highlighted in this chapter and relate to sequential retrieval from memory.

The reason for focusing on memory retrieval is twofold. First, a long tradition of mathematical sampling models has led to a wide range of memory models that are used to account for memory phenomena. During the 1990s, a new generation of models emerged that were embedded in a connectionist framework and used a particular mechanism called 'competitive queuing', which is able to transform an activation gradient over to-be-reported memoranda into a sequential order of reports. As is shown here, the two mechanisms make different predictions with regard to the timing of actions. This difference may be important beyond the memory literature in other areas in which sequential selection of parallel-activated actions is a common implementational choice. A modeller would need to know which mechanism to use to account for a particular type of data and empirical researchers (psychologists, biologists) would need to know what the behavioural signatures of these mechanisms are. For example, it is useful to know that if a certain mechanism underlies higher-order behaviour (e.g., parallel activation and sequential selection), specific implementational details may lead to different behaviour at a more finely grained level (in this chapter, the profile of the timing between successive actions). Second, in recent years, evidence has been found that favours some components and disfavours other components of competitive queuing. Given the wide applicability of a two-stage activation-selection mechanism, it could be beneficial to re-examine the components. This chapter aims at directly comparing two well-known mechanisms that were never before compared in this way. The memory literature contains much of the data needed for this comparison, and is used here.

Throughout, the term 'action selection' is used loosely and relates to the selection of representations that when executed has a behavioural consequence. Thus, retrieving a word from memory will eventually lead to the spoken or typed version of that word. Similarly, retrieving a plan of actions (e.g., making coffee) will eventually lead to the selection of a series of goal-directed movements. This chapter therefore deals only with situations in which a higher-order action plan (retrieving memoranda) activates lower-order plans (producing a word) that eventually lead to a behavioural response that can be measured in real-time. The chapter does not deal with situations that require unpacking of a motor sequence, such as walking or throwing a ball.

Section 8.2 outlines the competitive queuing and sampling mechanisms, which is then followed by a brief introduction of the retrieval latencies that differentiate these mechanisms. A generic computational model is presented in which both mechanisms are implemented. This model is then used to demonstrate the impact of the different mechanisms on retrieval latencies, and is used to show its ability to qualitatively account for psychological data. The chapter closes with implications of the computational evaluation for models of memory, action selection, and other domains.

8.2   Competitive queuing versus resampling

This section presents the two mechanisms that will be compared in a generic model. The focus here is on free recall or sequential selection in any order for three reasons. First, neurocomputational models of free recall are developed (Davelaar *et al.*, 2005, 2006), but still rely on the non-dynamic retrieval process, as used in current mathematical models. This work is then extended by incorporating the dynamical mechanisms of sequential selection from the literature on serial recall. Second, detailed analyses of retrieval latencies exist for free recall (see Section 8.3), which form a benchmark for model evaluation. Although data for serial recall exist (Farrell and Lewandowsky, 2004; Kahana and Jacobs, 2000), similar rigorous analyses have not yet been conducted. Third, as free recall is by definition free from any constraints on output order, the task is highly suitable to investigate mechanisms of sequential selection. Just as the properties of inherent circadian rhythm in agents (humans, animals, plants) can be investigated by taking away external cues of time, so can the sequential selection mechanism of agents be investigated by taking away external constraints of sequencing (i.e., the requirement to produce actions or report words in a pre-specified order). Given that sequential selection is central to behaviour in general, the analyses in the following support the view that measuring latencies between successive behaviours can provide insight into the type of underlying selection mechanism that led to the sequence of behaviours.

8.2.1   Competitive queuing

Grossberg (1978a, b) developed a model in which sequential output can be obtained from parallel activation in a dynamical model with excitatory feedforward and inhibitory feedback connections. The basic architecture is shown in Figure 8.1. The profile of activations in the activation layer is fed into the selection layer. This profile may originate from an activation-based short-term buffer, or from long-term memory with or without a static signal. There are three critical components. First, the activation profile shows the degree of activations for all yet-to-be executed plans, with the desired sequential order being from most active to least active. Second, the activations compete, that is, the representations in the activation layer all inhibit each other. A non-specific arousal signal arrives at the selection layer, which brings the activations above a response threshold. Third, as soon as a plan is selected (e.g., for moving the fingers to the desired key for typing, or flexing the muscles for articulation of a word), the representation in the selection layer inhibits the representation from which it received input. This prevents perseverative behaviour and allows the next strongest representation to become selected for output.

This two-layer output module produces all actions corresponding to the activated representations in the correct serial order with smooth transitions from one selected

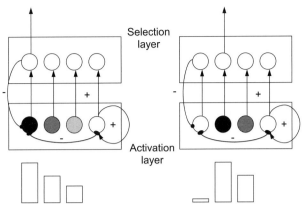

Figure 8.1 Architecture of the model used in Grossberg (1978a, b). Each unit in the activation layer has self-recurrent excitatory connection and inhibits all other units in the same layer. The feedforward one-to-one connections from the activation layer to the selection layer are excitatory, whereas the feedback one-to-one connections are inhibitory. At the lower end is a snapshot of the activation gradient in the activation layer. On the left, the left-most unit is the most active and leads to a response. After that, the feedback inhibition causes that unit to be lowered in activation. Due to decrease in the amount of inhibition in the activation layer, the unit with the next-highest activation level can increase in activation and will lead to the next response. This cycle continues until all units who received activation have produced an output.

action to the next. By adding noise to any of the three critical components, the model can account for sequencing errors seen in human behaviour, from typing (e.g., Salthouse, 1986) to memory for serial order.

In the 1990s, starting with Houghton (1990), this architecture received much attention in the memory literature (Brown *et al.*, 2000; Burgess and Hitch, 1999; Henson, 1998; Page and Norris, 1998; for a review, see Page and Henson, 2001) and related areas – planning (Cooper and Shallice, 2000), spelling (Glasspool and Houghton, 2005), and speech production (Hartley and Houghton, 1996) – leading to a range of models employing the select-then-inhibit dynamics (for review, see Glasspool, 2005). The models are collectively referred to as competitive-queuing (CQ) models, as the activations are placed in a competitive queue before being selected.[2]

It should be noted, however, that these models of serial ordered recall differ from the original model of Grossberg (1978b) in at least two critical aspects. First, in the Grossberg model, the inhibition of the representation in the activation layer is complete (i.e., total response suppression), whereas the CQ models were aimed at capturing errors,

---

[2] The literature seems to be inconsistent in its definition of which post-Houghton (1990) models can be called CQ models. Here, the following definition is used: a CQ model is a model in which given the same context, the layer immediately preceding the selection (or sampling) layer, (1) drives the selection, (2) has multiple representations active, and (3) has its activation profile altered as a consequence of the selection layer. This captures the notion of a queue that is altered with subsequent selection. Within this definition, models like the Primacy model (Page and Norris, 1998) and the Start-End model (Henson, 1998), and also the Grossberg (1978b) model are CQ models. Models of free recall, such as SAM (Raaijmakers and Shiffrin, 1980, 1981) do not alter the activation profile given the same context, and thus are not considered CQ models, but instead are here referred to as RS models.

such as repetitions, and thus assume a need for a gradually decaying inhibition (for a non-decaying inhibition account, see Farrell and Lewandowsky, 2002). If the set of activated representations in the activation layer is called the search set, then the Grossberg model could be referred to as a sampling-without-replacement model and the CQ models could be referred to as sampling-with-delayed-replacement models. Secondly, whereas the Grossberg model focuses on producing sequential behaviour given a single activation gradient, the aforementioned CQ models (except the primacy model by Page and Norris, 1998, which follows Grossberg in this regard) have addressed various forms of changing the source of activation during the course of retrieval. A contextual representation is incorporated in those models that changes along a certain dimension (e.g., temporal, absolute, or relative position in the list) and becomes linked with the representations of the to-be-remembered items. During retrieval, this context signal is replayed leading to serial recall. Not surprisingly, this context signal contributes greatly to variations in the timing of actions. However, these models have yet to be extended to account for retrieval latencies.

Neurophysiological studies support the dynamics assumed in these types of models. For example, Averbeck *et al.* (2002) trained macaque monkeys to draw geometric figures (triangle, square, trapezoid, inverted triangle). After training, the recorded neural firing patterns of neurons in the prefrontal cortex during drawing suggested that representations of all segments of a figure were coactivated before the initiation of the first action. During drawing, the firing rate of neurons corresponding to the upcoming action increased and then decreased before and after the action, respectively, in the same manner as predicted by the Grossberg model and CQ models that use a single context representation. However, the results did not show that the activation of the selected-and-then-inhibited representations gradually increased, as is critical for CQ models to account for repetition errors. Although it is certainly possible that the motor task of drawing figures by monkeys is not comparable to human memory performance, recent research on human memory has questioned the existence of a gradual decaying inhibition and employed other forms of response suppression (Duncan and Lewandowsky, 2005; Farrell and Lewandowsky, 2002, 2004). Nevertheless, the first simulation study will consider both the sampling-without-replacement (CQ^0) and the sampling-with-gradual-replacement (CQ^Δ) versions.

8.2.2   Resampling models

Although the CQ models gained much success, a different approach to producing sequential retrieval has been employed in global memory models, such as Search of Associative Memory (SAM; Raaijmakers and Shiffrin, 1980, 1981), MINERVA 2 (Hintzman, 1984), and Theory Of Distributed Memory (TODAM; Murdock, 1982). Here, SAM is used to exemplify the retrieval process, which is broken down into three critical components. First, a search set is defined based on available retrieval cues, which in most models is the list context, but could also be categories (e.g., Gronlund and Shiffrin, 1986) or chunks (e.g., Anderson and Matessa, 1997; Anderson *et al.*, 1998). Second, a single trace is selected (sampled) from the search set and used to recover the full memory representation. This could correspond to recovering the phonemic representation in order to utter the word or to the execution of the motor plan for typing the word. Third, after successful recovery, the trace is allowed to compete for resampling (RS) if the same cue is used to probe the memory system, but will not produce an output. Because of the possibility of RS (but not re-recovery) of an item, SAM could be seen as a RS or selection-with-replacement model. In order to compare the CQ model with the RS model, it is assumed that the first two components of both models are equivalent, and that the critical difference lies in the post-response suppression mechanism. The assumption in SAM that a resampled representation never leads to an output can be relaxed and the assumption of gradual decay of inhibition can be used instead. Such a model has never been used in the SAM framework, but will be used in the simulation study for completeness.

Functional imaging data support the view that the brain has separate components for activation and selection (Badre *et al.*, 2005). For example, in a study by Badre *et al.* (2005), participants performed a number of tasks that have previously been used in investigations on memory retrieval and have been argued to rely to different degrees on the ability to select the correct response among distractors. The authors were interested in whether selection and activation mechanisms are subserved by the same or by different neural substrates. Factor analysis on the behavioural results produced two factors that were labelled as selection and non-selection components. These behaviourally defined factors were associated with variance in different brain regions, with the anterior ventrolateral pre-frontal cortex (aVLPFC) and the inferior-temporal cortex (IT) related to activation of information and the mid-ventrolateral pre-frontal cortex (mVLPFC) related to selection of task-appropriate representations. This two-stage model of retrieval supports the global memory models, but does not necessarily falsify the CQ mechanism. Nevertheless, the retrieval dynamics are different for the two mechanisms, as discussed in Section 8.3.

8.3   Retrieval dynamics

This section summarises the data patterns that are used to compare and validate the above two models. Recall latencies provide information on the underlying memory processes and distinguish different patient populations.

8.3.1   Recall latencies

In a series of analytical studies, Rohrer and Wixted (Rohrer, 1996, 2002; Rohrer and Wixted, 1994; Wixted and Rohrer, 1993) investigated the temporal dynamics in free recall of words. This work, which extends the limited number of previous empirical investigations (e.g., Murdock and Okada, 1970; Patterson, Meltzer and Mandler, 1971; for a review, see Wixted and Rohrer, 1994), provided critical insight regarding the sampling and recovery of items. In a typical experiment, a participant memorises a number of words and after a distractor task reports as many words as possible in any order. During the retrieval phase, the time taken to retrieve an item is measured as the main dependent variable. The basic findings are as follows. The time needed to retrieve an item increases with the number of items that were memorised (set size effect). The interresponse time (IRT), the elapsed time between two consecutive responses, increases during the retrieval phase and is a function of the number of words yet to be recalled. These findings have been interpreted to support the RS mechanism of selection, where the recall latency reflects the size of the search set. The larger the search set, the longer it takes to select an item from the set.

8.3.2   Utility of retrieval latencies

The analysis of recall latencies has provided an empirical tool for measuring the size of the memory search set, dissociating the effect of episodic and semantic cues (Rohrer, 2002), and measuring the loss of semantic memory in patients with Alzheimer's dementia (AD). After analysing the recall latencies (minus the first recall latency), Rohrer *et al.* (1995) argued that patients with AD have a structural memory deficit. The loss of neural tissue in AD leads to a smaller size of the memory set, which in turn is observed as shorter recall latencies for patients with AD compared to controls. This contrasts the longer recall latencies observed in patients with Huntington's disease (HD; Rohrer *et al.*, 1999). Whereas patients with AD and HD have lower total recall compared to controls, the retrieval latencies revealed marked differences.

8.3.3   Model predictions

As mentioned above, CQ and RS models have a stage in which all target representations are activated by a cue. It takes time for the first item to be selected and produce an output. Given that no differences exist between these two models at this initial stage, both models will produce the same first retrieval latency. However, after the first item is retrieved, in CQ models the representation of this item is inhibited (i.e., deleted from the queue). As every output is followed by inhibition of the retrieved item representation, there is an ever-decreasing competition during the retrieval phase. This model therefore predicts that the time needed for selecting a new item decreases: IRTs become shorter. In RS models, the item representation is still activated by the cue and can therefore be sampled, even though it will not be output. The more items have been output, the lower the probability (and therefore the longer it will take) that a new not-yet retrieved item will be sampled. This model predicts that the time needed to report the next item depends on the activation gradient, and therefore reflects the size of the memory set. This model therefore predicts that the time needed for selecting a new item increases: IRTs become longer.

8.4   Generic model

In order to evaluate the mechanisms, a generic model is presented in which RS and CQ mechanisms can be explored. The main dependent measures are the IRTs and the

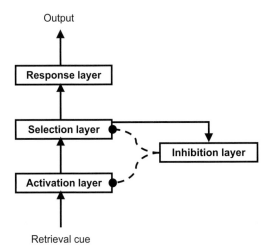

Figure 8.2 Model architecture. The model consists of four interconnected layers. The arrows ending in pointed heads and circled heads are excitatory and inhibitory connections, respectively. A number of representations are activated at the activation layer which feeds activation to the selection layer. When a unit in the selection layer reaches a selection threshold, the inputs to the inhibition and response layers receive a sharp pulse. Depending on the employed mechanism, the output of the inhibition layer inhibits the selection (in the RS model) or the activation (in the CQ model) layer.

distributions of recall latencies. As Study 1 makes clear that the CQ mechanism does not capture the IRTs, Study 2 only addresses the applicability of the RS model.

8.4.1   Model architecture

The model consists of four layers (see Figure 8.2). Each layer contains 20 localistic representations that are connected to corresponding representations in other layers. Each unit corresponds to a large number of neurons that together participate in the neural code for that particular representation. For every unit in each layer, its current activation depends on the activation value on the previous time step, the self-recurrent excitation, the inhibition felt from every other unit in the same layer, the external input and some random noise. The activations of all units in the model are updated at each time step according the following differential equation (see also Davelaar *et al.*, 2005, 2006; Usher and McClelland, 2001):

$$x_i(t+1) = \lambda x_i(t) + (1-\lambda)\{\alpha F[x_i(t)] + I_i(t) - \beta \Sigma_j F[x_j(t)] + \xi\}. \qquad (8.1)$$

Here, x represents the internal activation, $\lambda = 0.98$, α is the self-recurrent excitatory connection, $F(x) = x/(1+x)$, for $x > 0$ represents the output activation function. $I_i(t)$ represents the external input at time step t to unit i. Units in each layer compete for activation, which is governed by the within-layer inhibition parameter β. Each unit receives inhibition from every other unit in the same layer. The activation of each unit (only in the memory layer) is supplemented with zero-mean Gaussian noise ξ, with

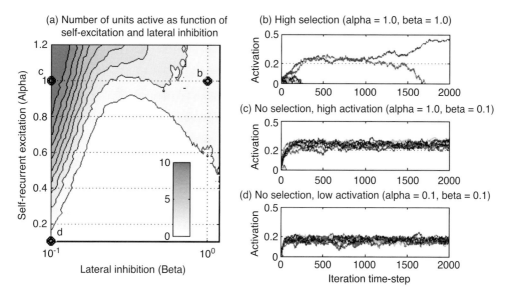

Figure 8.3 Profiles of the influence of the self-recurrency and lateral inhibition parameters on the activation of ten activated units. (a) Two-dimensional contour map of the number of activated units (at 2000 iteration time steps). The values for the lateral inhibition are on a logarithmic scale. The three dots are parameter combinations that were used in the activation trajectories to illustrate the model dynamics. (b) Activation trajectories for high selection. At first, two (out of ten) units are most active, followed by one unit increasing in activation; a selection has taken place. (c) Activation trajectories with low inhibition, but high activation leading to no selection, but all units being above a 0.2 threshold. (d) Activation trajectories with low inhibition and low activation, leading to no selection and all units being below a 0.2 threshold.

standard deviation σ. The parameter values vary between layers, but are chosen to minimise epiphenomological dynamics that may obscure the comparison between the CQ and RS mechanisms. For example, in order to compare the models, each model should be able to produce an output. If the connection between the activation and selection layer is too weak, the CQ model, but not the RS model, produces an output; if the response suppression is too weak, the RS model, but not the CQ model, produces an output. Each layer can be interpreted as representing a set of brain areas that have been implicated in memory activation, memory selection, and action selection.

Figure 8.3 shows the influence of the parameters α and β on the activation of the representations, which eventually govern the overall system behaviour. Figure 8.3a shows a variety of values for α and β, the average number of representations (out of 10, $I_i = 0.33$ for all) that are still activated above a fixed threshold (0.2, as used in previous work) after 2000 iterations over 100 simulation runs ($\sigma = 0.1$). Figure 8.3b–d show for three points from the Figure 8.3a, the corresponding activation trajectories. As can be seen, increasing the self-recurrent excitation will increase the number of representations that are still active above the threshold at the end of the simulation. However, this is only true for low levels of inhibition, as an intermediate level of inhibition dampens the overall activation, putting an upper bound to the total number of activated representations. With high inhibition, the system goes into a winner-takes-all selection mode.

8.4.1.1   Activation layer

The activation layer contains representations of the words that are to be recalled. The memory representations may already be in an active state (they are in the short-term buffer; Davelaar *et al.*, 2005) or are (re)activated by a cue, which could be a category name (semantic cue, as in a verbal fluency task) or a contextual reference (episodic cue, as in a list memory task). In this chapter, only cued activations are considered. The cue activates the first ten items in the memory layer range from 0.28 to 0.37 (0.01 difference between units). The activated representations compete weakly with each other. In the simulations, zero-mean Gaussian noise is added to the activations of the memory units ($\alpha = 0$, $\beta = 0.1$, $\sigma = 0.1$).

8.4.1.2   Selection layer

The selection layer (modelled after Usher and McClelland, 2001) contains representations that receive weighted input, $W_{ms}F(x)$, from those in the activation layer, where W_{ms} represents the connection weight between the activation and the selection layer. The activated representations compete strongly, ($\beta = 1.0$), with each other, and have moderate, ($\alpha = 1.0$), self-connections. Both the activation and selection layers could be implemented in pre-frontal areas, such as the VLPFC (Badre *et al*, 2005).

8.4.1.3   Output layer

The output layer contains representations that receive weighted input, $W_{so}H[F(x),0.4]$, from those in the selection layer, with $W_{so} = 2.0$ and $H[F(x),0.4] = 1$, when $F(x) > 0.4$, 0 otherwise. The units are inert with no dynamics other than activation decay after a unit in the selection layer has provided a pulse to the output layer. This allows for obtaining an exact point in time in which a response is initiated. The connection between the selection and the output layer represents the 'direct pathway' or the 'selection pathway' (Gurney *et al.*, 2001) in the basal ganglia.

8.4.1.4   Inhibition layer

The inhibition layer contains representations that receive input, $H[F(x),0.4]$, from those in the selection layer. To maximise the influence of the inhibition layer on the retrieval dynamics and thereby make the whole system sensitive to differences related to the RS and CQ mechanisms only, units in the inhibition layer have strong self-excitation and do not inhibit each other ($\alpha = 2.0$, $\beta = 0$). This implements a form of output buffer in which all selected items are maintained throughout the retrieval phase and prevents perseverations and repetitions. The neural substrate of the inhibition layer is assumed to include subcortical areas of the basal ganglia that are in the 'indirect' or 'control' pathway. In addition, the self-recurrent connection may be interpreted as including cortical projections to the subthalamic nucleus. Recent work by Frank (2006) and Frank, Sherman and Scheres (Chapter 13, this volume) suggests that a critical function of the

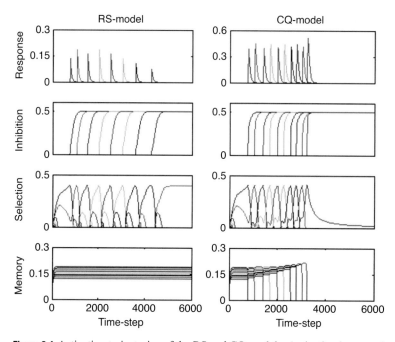

Figure 8.4 Activation trajectories of the RS and CQ models. Activation between layers goes from 'memory' to 'selection' to 'output', with 'inhibition' suppressing the activation at either the 'memory' (CQ model) or the 'selection' (RS model) layer. The RS model does not produce all responses (eight spikes in the output layer), whereas the CQ model does. Note also that the activation in the memory layer for the CQ model shows the signature of the CQ mechanism (after an output the corresponding trace is inhibited, which causes an increase in activation for the remaining traces). See plate section for colour version.

subthalamic nucleus is to prevent responding (too early). Bogacz (2007) and Davelaar (2009) further addressed the optimality of this inhibition mechanism.

8.4.2   Study 1: RS versus CQ mechanisms

Here the RS and CQ models are compared and analysed. The first simulation shows the qualitative behaviour of the two models. This is followed by a comparative analysis using novel computational techniques.

8.4.2.1   Simulation 1: RS versus CQ

In the first simulation, the weighted output of the inhibition layer, $W_{inh}F(x)$, is sent to the selection layer or the memory layer to implement the RS and CQ models, respectively. Figure 8.4 shows a noiseless simulation of both implementations. As can be seen, of the ten activated representations in the memory layer, only eight produce a response in the RS model, whereas all produce a response in the CQ model. Figure 8.5a presents a comparison of the first recall latency and the subsequent IRTs for both noiseless simulations. The results are striking. The RS model shows increasing IRTs throughout

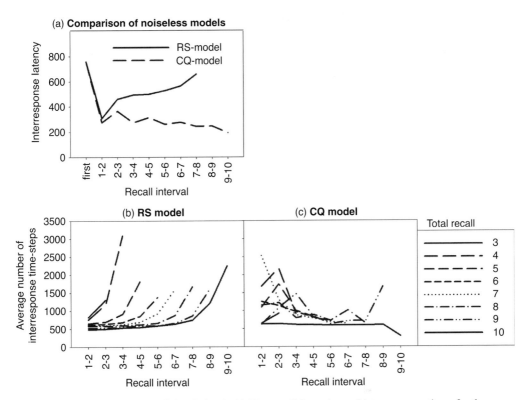

Figure 8.5 Results of simulation 1. (a) First recall latencies and interresponse times for the noiseless RS and CQ models. Note the increase in IRT for the RS model and the decrease in IRT for the CQ model. (b) IRTs as a function of total recall and recall interval for the RS model. (c) IRTs as a function of total recall and recall interval for the CQ model.

the retrieval phase, whereas the CQ model shows a gradual decrease in IRTs. The RS model produces increased IRTs because with each response the responsible unit in the activation layer continues to send activation to the corresponding unit in the selection layer. As this unit is inhibited, the next highest unit will win the competition, but as it receives less activation, it takes longer to reach the response threshold. This continues throughout the recall phase, leading to ever-increasing IRTs. The CQ model, however, reduces the number of activated units in the activation layer, thereby reducing the competition in the selection layer. With less competition, the units in the selection layer can more readily reach the response threshold, resulting in ever-decreasing IRTs.

The models were run with noise ($\sigma = 0.1$) in the activation layer. To obtain a wide range of total recall, 1000 simulations were run with $W_{ms} = [1.4 : 2.0, \text{step } 0.1]$, which is justified under the assumption that the activations of the memory representations are modulated by attentional (Usher and Davelaar, 2002) or motivational factors. Despite this range, the CQ model produced all ten responses in 99.2% of the simulations. Figures 8.5b and c show the IRTs as a function of the total recall and the recall interval for the RS and CQ models, respectively. These figures mimic the noiseless results in

Figure 8.5a. Human behavioural data are in accordance with the results of the RS model (e.g., Murdock and Okada, 1970).

8.4.2.2   Comparative analysis

Four model implementations are compared. The RS and the CQ model differ in the locus of the post-response suppression; for each model, we consider this suppression remaining throughout the remainder of the retrieval phase or gradually decaying. The analysis addresses the question of how central a particular pattern, in this case the slope of the IRT profile, is to a particular model and thereby provides a general answer to what type of implementation of sequential retrieval captures existing data on IRT profiles in a free recall paradigm best. Note that all four implementations exhibit sequential behaviour and are compared to data from memory experiments. Different results may be obtained if the models are compared against data from motor planning.

The models are compared using Parameter Space Partitioning (PSP; Pitt *et al.*, 2006). This procedure involves identifying a particular set of patterns and going through the multidimensional parameter space in search of those patterns (for more details, see Pitt *et al.*, 2006). The PSP procedure selects a set of parameters and evaluates the model's prediction (or pattern). The algorithm works such that it samples from each pattern at least once and uniformly, yielding an estimate of the size of the parameter space that is occupied by a particular pattern.

PSP was used on the four models (CQ and RS, with and without gradual decay of inhibition) to address whether and how much the slope of the IRT function is influenced by (1) the structural differences between the models, (2) the presence/absence of decaying inhibition, and (3) four chosen parameters. These parameters were chosen because initial explorations by hand showed that these parameters mattered most in the simulations. These parameters were the connection weight between the activation layer and the selection layer, W_{ms}, the self-recurrency of the unit in the selection layer, α, the lateral inhibition between all pairs in the selection layer, β, and the threshold, θ, above which a response is made. In the models with decaying inhibition, the self-recurrency of the units in the inhibition layer was reduced to 1.2, which was shown to be a compromise between obtaining noticeable reactivation while preventing too many repetitions (perseverations). The models are named RS^0 and CQ^0 for those without decaying inhibition, and $RS^\triangle$ and $CQ^\triangle$ for those with decaying inhibition.

Procedure

Step 0: Explore all models by hand and define a parameter boundary and an initial set of parameters. The parameter vector used for the initial parameters was $P_0 = [W_{ms}; \alpha; \beta; \theta] = [2.0; 1.0; 1.0; 0.4]$. The boundaries were set to $W_{ms} = [1.2 : 2.2]$, $\alpha = [0.8 : 2.0]$, $\beta = [0.2 : 2.0]$, and $\theta = [0.3 : 0.5]$.

Step 1: Patterns were defined by the slope of the IRT-function and the number of items reported within a simulation run of 6000 iterations. This yields 2 (slope > 0, slope ≤ 0) $\times$ 8 (3 through 10 outputs) + (no output or less than 3 outputs) = 17 patterns. PSP was applied to the noiseless models (the procedure is limited to nonstochastic simulation runs) with the initial set of parameters, P_0, and default values. All models produced all

Table 8.1 Result of the PSP algorithm under steps 1 and 2. The percentages indicate the amount of the valid space (where the model produces slopes for the IRT function) and the percentage of that space that contains the pattern of positive slopes. Step 1 results are taken over all total output (eight data points). Step 2 results are averaged across 17 PSP runs with standard deviations in brackets.

		Model			
		Without decay		With decay	
PSP run		RS^0	CQ°	RS^Δ	CQ^Δ
Step 1	Valid	54.9%	32.2%	17.2%	28.7%
	Slope > 0	85.0%	38.0%	83.9%	78.9%
Step 2	Valid	56.2% (3.6%)	37.8% (3.3%)	25.9% (2.6%)	34.2% (3.8%)
	Slope > 0	89.1% (5.8%)	42.5% (5.9%)	91.4% (7.4%)	77.3% (5.7%)

Table 8.2 Total number of parameter sets obtained in step 2 for each model against each possible pattern.

	Model			
	Without decay		With decay	
	RS^0	CQ°	RS^Δ	CQ^Δ
Invalid	34,357	43,409	49,980	43,878
Valid (slope <= 0)	22,498	36,861	16,377	17,966
Valid (slope > 0)	43,640	37,567	51,989	44,676

17 patterns. Calculated log(volume) of the region of all possible patterns occupied by a certain pattern favoured the RS models, as measured with the number of times that the log(volume) is greater for the positive slope for a given total output ($RS^0 - 8/8$; $CQ^0 - 4/8$; $RS^\Delta - 8/8$; $CQ^\Delta - 3/8$). This step produced additional parameter sets, one for each of the 17 patterns.

Step 2: Parameter sets that were obtained under step 1 were used as initial parameters in a further search through parameter space. This guarantees that all regions will be sampled. To speed up the simulations, the number of patterns was reduced to 3 (slope > 0, slope $\leq$ 0, no output or less than 3 outputs). All unique combinations of parameters and the corresponding pattern were stored for further analysis.

The averaged log(volume) was informative. Table 8.1 shows that there is great consistency across the two steps. The RS models do generally better than the CQ models, but this difference is greatly attenuated when a decaying of response suppression is implemented (for all comparisons, p < 0.001). The central thesis that when it comes to modelling IRTs, RS is preferred over CQ, is further supported by the parameter sets stored for each model. Table 8.2 shows the number of parameter sets for each model against each pattern. Again it can be observed that a positive slope is more central to the RS than to the CQ model, and that with decay of response suppression implemented this difference decreases.

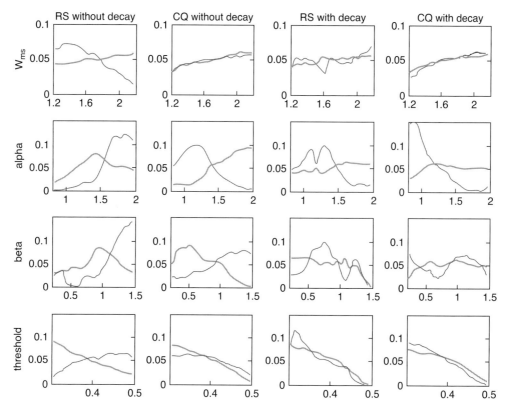

Figure 8.6 Normalised relative frequency distributions for each of the four parameters and for each of the four models. From top to bottom: W_{ms}, α, β, and threshold. The thick lines represent the distribution of the parameter values (shown on the x-axes) for which the corresponding model produced and IRT function with slope > 0. The thin lines represent the distribution of the parameter values for which the corresponding model produced and IRT function with slope ≤ 0. A uniform distribution would be $y = 0.05$. Note the strong influence of the self-recurrency (α) and lateral inhibition (β) parameters, and that models implementing decaying response suppression (the two right columns) are less sensitive (flat line) to the values of the α and β parameters than the models that do not implement a decaying response suppression (two left columns).

Figure 8.6 shows the normalised distributions of relative frequencies for each model, for the valid patterns and for each of the four parameters. A uniform distribution would be a horizontal line with $y = 0.05$. The strength between the activation and selection layers does not affect the slope of the IRT function. Only the RS^0 model tends to be somewhat affected by this parameter. The same holds for the threshold parameter. The self-recurrency and the lateral inhibition in the selection layer greatly affect the slope of the IRT-function, depending on the model. For RS^0, positively sloped IRT functions have intermediate values of α and β, whereas for negatively sloped IRT functions the values of α and β are large. For CQ^0, positively sloped IRT functions have high α and low β (suggesting low selection), whereas for negatively sloped IRT-functions α is low and β is large (suggesting high selection). For RS^Δ, positively sloped IRT functions

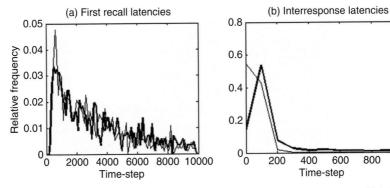

Figure 8.7 Results of simulation 2. Comparison of small (thin line) and large (thick line) memory set sizes. (a) First recall latency distributions. The two distributions overlap considerably. (b) IRT distributions.

have undetermined values of α and β, whereas for negatively sloped IRT functions the values of α and β are small. Finally, for CQ^{Δ}, positively sloped IRT functions have undetermined values of α and β, whereas negatively sloped IRT-functions have low values of α and high values for β (suggesting high selection).

In summary, the values for α and β seem to suggest that the CQ models tend to settle into high or low mode of selection producing negatively or positively sloped IRT functions, respectively, whereas RS models consistently keep the same mode of selection. These mode preferences are attenuated with decaying response suppression.

8.4.3   Study 2: extant data and the RS model

Study 1 supports the view that the RS model captures the IRT profiles best. In the following study, the RS model is further tested on its ability to capture data reported in the extant literature.

8.4.3.1   Simulation 2: setsize effects

Rohrer and colleagues (Rohrer, 1996, 2002; Rohrer and Wixted, 1994; Rohrer *et al.*, 1995, 1999; Wixted and Rohrer, 1993) have shown that the distribution of recall latencies reflect the size of the memory set, which could be utilised to identify loci for memory deficits in patient populations. To this end, 1000 simulations of the RS model were run with 5 or 15 memory units being activated (the 5 highest activated units were used in both setsizes, therefore any effect on first recall latencies can only be attributed to setsize). Inhibition in the selection layer was lowered to $\beta = 0.8$ and $W_{ms} = 4.0$. As can be seen in Figure 8.7, the RS model is sensitive to differences in setsize (average recall: 0.918 and 0.307, for setsize 5 and 15, respectively). In particular, the model is slower when the memory set is larger. The reason for this is that with larger setsize, more items activate units in the activation layer and therefore in the selection layer. The overall increase in competing representations leads to a slower rise in activation for each of the units in the selection layer. This continues throughout the recall phase, leading also to longer IRTs.

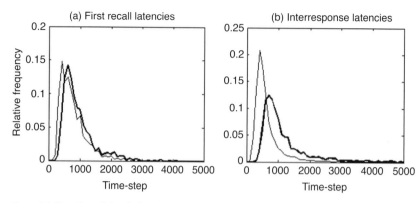

Figure 8.8 Results of simulation 3. Comparison of normal selection threshold (thin line) and high selection threshold (representing Huntington's disease; thick line). (a) First recall latency distributions. The mean recall latency is slower for the HD simulation. (b) IRT distributions for normal and HD simulation.

For the first recall latencies, the average latency was 3164 time steps with size = 5 and 3456 time steps with size = 15; for the IRT, 99 time steps with size = 5, 603 time steps with size = 15. The RS model not only captures the IRT profile, but is also sensitive to the size of the memory set, thereby providing computational validation of the theoretical analyses of Wixted and Rohrer (1994).

8.4.3.2   **Simulation 3: Alzheimer's dementia versus Huntington's disease**
Patients with AD suffer from increased loss of neural tissue that represents long-term memory (see for example, Fleischman and Gabrieli, 1999). This includes aspects of episodic and semantic memory. As in memory retrieval tasks, recall latencies reflect the size of the memory set, patients with AD are faster in retrieving items, but have a lower total recall. Simulation 2 showed the effect of setsize and is not repeated here. HD is caused by a loss of striatal neurons, resulting in a decreased output to the thalamus. In the model, HD would affect the selection layer and is approximated by increasing the selection threshold, which slows down the retrieval process without affecting the memory set.

The RS model with selection $\beta = 1.0$ and $W_{ms} = 2.0$ was used (10 items; 1000 runs) with the difference that the selection threshold was increased from 0.40 to 0.44. As can be seen in Figure 8.8, the HD simulation is indeed slower in retrieving items. For the first recall latencies, the average latency was 991 time steps (HD) compared to 825 time steps (baseline); for the IRT, 1262 time steps (HD) compared to 700 time steps (baseline). This contrasts the results of patients with AD (setsize effect).

8.5   Discussion

The aim of this chapter is to compare two commonly used mechanisms of sequential memory retrieval and evaluate their ability to capture the IRTs in free recall. A generic model is used in which the two mechanisms are implemented. Simulations revealed that the RS mechanism provides a better overall qualitative match to the published data on retrieval latencies in a free recall paradigm than the CQ mechanism. A comparative analysis of four model implementations (RS_Δ, CQ^Δ, RS^0, and CQ^0) revealed that the RS models produce a positive slope of the IRT function more often than the CQ models, and that this difference between RS and CQ models is smaller if the response suppression decays gradually during the retrieval phase. This latter mechanism makes the CQ^Δ model (CQ with gradual decay of suppression) more similar to the RS models (RS^0 and RS^Δ). The RS mechanism has subsequently been tested on its sensitivity to the size of the activated memory set and its success is promising for further research in the specific neural implementation of the mechanism. The use of recall distributions has been shown to provide a better understanding of the memory deficits in AD and HD (Section 8.4.3) and resolve theoretical debates that have focused mainly on total recall as the dependent variable. The RS model captures the differences in recall latency distributions between patients with AD or HD. The important utility of IRT analyses in this domain justifies further developments and analyses of the computational architecture to quantitatively account for the neuropsychological data.

8.5.1   Implications for dynamical models of memory

The CQ mechanism has had great impact on the memory literature, but the simulations show that for profiles of IRTs in free recall, the mechanism does not fare well compared to the RS mechanism unless additional assumptions are in place. Even though the evaluation between the two types of models in simulation 1 may imply that CQ models are inappropriate for free recall, this does not invalidate CQ models. In fact, given the neurophysiological support for CQ dynamics, it is conceivable that CQ dynamics may play a dominant role at the response level and less so at the memory level. Note that the successes of CQ models are found in tasks that require execution of a well-learned motor program, whether it is drawing geometric shapes (Averbeck, *et al.*, 2002), or pronouncing words (Hartley and Houghton, 1996). As such, the use of CQ dynamics may be more related to the unpacking of chunks, where the content of chunks could be words (as in serial recall), movements (as in typing or spelling; Glasspool and Houghton, 2005; Hartley and Houghton, 1996), or even other chunks (as in planning; Cooper and Shallice, 2000). Within the literature on serial recall, not much emphasis has been placed on retrieval latencies (but see Farrell and Lewandowsky, 2004; Kahana and Jacobs, 2000). Nevertheless, in a production system, Anderson and Matessa (1997) explicitly modelled the IRTs as the unpacking of chunks, with equal time needed for each item within a chunk and with additional time to move from one to the other chunk. In a follow-up paper (Anderson, *et al.*, 1998), some aspects of free recall were modelled, but not retrieval latencies.

An important assumption of some CQ models is that after a response it made, the representation leading to an overt response is inhibited. This response suppression decays gradually over time, leading to reselection. Despite this critical feature (i.e., decay of response suppression), the neurophysiological data that supported competitive queuing in general (Averbeck, *et al.*, 2002) does not show this pattern. Although repetitions in movements in making geometric shapes are unlikely, decay of response suppression seems not to be needed to account for repetition errors in serial recall (Botvinick and Plaut, 2006; Farrell and Lewandowsky, 2002) and is even directly contested empirically (Duncan and Lewandowsky, 2005).

Recent work on recall memory has incorporated new theoretical approaches to working memory (Davelaar *et al.*, 2005, 2006). In this research, the content of working memory was defined as the activated part of long-term memory (e.g., Cowan, 2001) and the modelling work was focused on the encoding of information in episodic memory. In that work, episodic memory is the matrix of connection weights between a contextual system (related to the medial-temporal lobe) and the cortical long-term memory system. In these models of free recall, the retrieval process was approximated by a selection and recovery phase, akin to that of global memory models. The dynamical model of retrieval presented here provides the back-end to those previous models of encoding.

8.5.2   Implications for dynamical models of sequential selection

As mentioned in the introduction, studying free recall may be a more useful paradigm than serial recall to study the properties of sequential retrieval from memory, as serial recall places an external constraint on the inherent selection mechanism. However, under the assumption that this is indeed the case, the question then arises of how the inherent selection mechanism is influenced by this external constraint of output order. In other words, assuming that an RS mechanism underlies all kinds of sequential behaviour, how does the need for a particular correct serial order affect the operations of the selection? A partial answer to this is revealed by a closer look at how the slope of the RS models is affected by the parameters (see Figure 8.6). In free recall, a positive slope of the IRT-function is observed, whereas a negative slope is observed for serial performance such as typing (Salthouse, 1986). To capture a negative slope (i.e., ever faster responding) in the RS^0 model, the higher self-recurrency would normally lead to more items becoming active, but the higher lateral inhibition prevents this (together with the lower weight from the activation layer to the selection layer). With every retrieved item (in the selection layer) being inhibited after reaching a threshold, the item next highest in activation shoots up. As the overall competition within the selection layer decreases during the retrieval phase, the IRT between successive retrievals becomes shorter. The same dynamics happens in the RS^Δ model, where because of the gradual decay of response suppression, the overall selection mechanism needs to be liberal and with a low response threshold. Interestingly, the amount of self-recurrency is also lower.

In a computational study of response selection, Usher and Davelaar (2002) proposed that the parameters for self-recurrency and lateral inhibition in a selection layer are modulated by norepinephrine (NE) in a positive manner (both parameters are positively correlated with the level of NE). Applied here, the hypothesis is that the instruction to perform in a particular ordered sequence leads to a modulation in NE, which translates into a higher or lower self-recurrency and lateral inhibition in the selection layer and thereby producing an observable negative or positive slope in the IRT function of actions, respectively. Note that the covariation between self-recurrency and lateral inhibition as function of the IRT-slope is negative for the CQ models, critically distinguishing the CQ and RS models on their reliance on these two parameters. Further extensions incorporating noise and a consideration of other types of behaviour (e.g., error profiles) are needed.

8.5.3   Relation to other psychological domains

The evaluation of the memory retrieval dynamics could inform other domains within psychology, such as decision making and neuropsychological assessment. Recent work in the field of decision making incorporates aspects of memory theories (e.g., Dougherty, *et al.*, 1999; Thomas *et al.*, 2008). For example, when a physician is generating a number of hypotheses about a possible diagnosis, the information about the symptoms is used to cue the memory system and search the activated part of memory to produce a number of likely diagnoses. This type of research could benefit from a deeper understanding of how the retrieval dynamics are affected by such variables as the number of possible hypotheses (search set), motivation of the physician (focus of attention for selection), and dual-task situation (affects the retrieval speed).

In the domain of neuropsychological assessment, a recent study (Scahill *et al.*, 2005) showed that current episodic memory tasks fail to differentially diagnose patients with AD from patients with semantic dementia (SD, a progressive neurodegeneration of the temporal lobe, characterised by loss of semantic memory). It is not certain yet whether episodic memory tasks may contribute in the differential diagnosis. Rohrer *et al.* (1999) argued that recall latencies contain information that separates patients with AD from patients with HD. The search for alternative (and additional) methods of differentiating between these two groups of patients can be facilitated by neurocomputational models of the kind presented here in which certain components have a clear neurological counterpart. Using simulations of lesions, they can create informed predictions to guide development of more sensitive tests. This type of modelling extends beyond the measures related to sequential retrieval and combined with other dynamical models of memory may prove to be of high value to clinicians.

8.5.4   Conclusion

This chapter compared two mechanisms by which simultaneously activated representations produce actions (here the recall of memoranda) in a sequential manner. Although these two mechanisms have been used in a variety of models, they have not been compared directly to each other before. By examining the dynamics of sequential selection through retrieval latencies, it has been shown that sampling-with-replacement captured human memory retrieval better than sampling-without-replacement. Both are further improved by including dynamics of response suppression that gradually fades. This evaluation provides the cognitive modeller with a tool with which to choose the components of a selection mechanism and provides insights into the internal dynamics of a chosen implementation by addressing the patterns it produces given a certain parameter space. Finally, the analyses provide a handle to understand qualitative differences in sequential behaviour through global modulation of critical parameters, which require further evaluation from empirical and computational studies in humans and animals.

Acknowledgements

The author would like to thank Michael Dougherty and Isaiah Harbison for stimulating discussions on memory retrieval and Joanna Bryson for critical comments. Substantial parts of the simulation work were conducted while the author was at the University of Maryland, College Park and University of California, San Diego.

References

Anderson, J. R., D. Bothell, C. Lebiere, and M. Matessa (1998). An integrated theory of list memory. *J. Mem. Lang.* **38**: 341–80.

Anderson, J. R. and M. Matessa (1997). A production system theory of serial memory. *Psychol. Rev.* **104**: 728–48.

Averbeck, B. B., M. V. Chafee, D. A. Crowe, and A. P. Georgopoulos (2002). Parallel processing of serial movements in prefrontal cortex. *Proc. Nat. Acad. Sci.* **99**: 13172–7.

Badre, D., R. A. Poldrack, E. J. Pare-Blagoev, R. Z. Insler, and D. A. Wagner (2005). Dissociable controlled retrieval and generalized selection mechanisms in ventrolateral prefrontal cortex. *Neuron* **47** 907–18.

Bogacz, R. (2007). Optimal decision-making theories: linking neurobiology with behaviour. *Trends Cogn. Sci.* **11**: 118–25.

Botvinick, M. M. and D. C. Plaut (2006). Short-term memory for serial order: a recurrent neural network model. *Psychol. Rev.* **113**: 201–33.

Brown, G. D. A., T. Preece, and C. Hulme (2000). Oscillator-based memory for serial order. *Psychol. Rev.* **107**: 127–81.

Burgess, N. and G. J. Hitch (1999). Memory for serial order: a network model of the phonological loop and its timing. *Psychol. Rev.* **106**: 551–81.

Cooper, R. and T. Shallice (2000). Contention scheduling and the control of routine activities. *Cogn. Neuropsychol.* **17**: 297–338.

Cowan, N. (2001). The magical number 4 in short-term memory: a reconsideration of mental storage capacity. *Behav. Brain Sci.* **24**: 87–185.

Davelaar, E. J. (2009). Conflict-monitoring and (meta)cognitive control. In *Connectionist models of behaviour and cognition II*, ed. J. Mayor, N. Ruh, and K. Plunkett. Singapore: WorldScientific, pp. 241–52.

Davelaar, E. J., Y. Goshen-Gottstein, A. Ashkenazi, H. J. Haarmann, and M. Usher (2005). The demise of short-term memory revisited: empirical and computational investigations of recency effects. *Psychol. Rev.* **112**: 3–42.

Davelaar, E. J., H. J. Haarmann, Y. Goshen-Gottstein, and M. Usher (2006). Semantic similarity dissociates short- from long-term recency: testing a neurocomputational model of list memory. *Mem. Cogn.* **34**: 323–34.

Dougherty, M. R. P., C. F. Gettys, and E. E. Ogden (1999). MINERVA-DM: a memory processes model for judgments of likelihood. *Psychol. Rev.* **106**: 180–209.

Duncan, M. and S. Lewandowsky (2005). The time course of response suppression: no evidence for a gradual release from inhibition. *Memory* **13**: 236–46.

Farrell, S. and S. Lewandowsky (2002). An endogenous distributed model of ordering in serial recall. *Psychon. B. Rev.* **9**: 59–79.

Farrell, S. and S. Lewandowsky (2004). Modelling transposition latencies: constraints for theories of serial order memory. *J. Mem. Lang.* **51**: 115–35.

Fleischman, D. A. and J. Gabrieli (1999). Long-term memory in Alzheimer's disease. *Curr. Opin. Neurobiol.* **9**: 240–44.

Frank, M. J. (2006). Hold your horses: a dynamic computational model for the subthalamic nucleus in decision making. *Neural Networks* **19**: 1120–36.

Glasspool, D. W. (2005). Modelling serial order in behaviour: evidence from performance slips. In *Connectionist Model in Cognitive Psychology*, ed. G. Houghton. Hove: Psychology Press, pp. 241–70.

Glasspool, D. W. and G. Houghton (2005). Serial order and consonant-vowel structure in a graphemic output buffer model. *Brain Lang.* **94**: 304–30.

Gronlund, S. D. and R. M. Shiffrin (1986). Retrieval strategies in recall of natural categories and categorized lists. *J. Psychol. Learn.* **12**: 550–61.

Grossberg, S. (1978a). Behavioral contrast in short-term memory: serial binary memory models or parallel continuous memory models? *J. Math. Psychol.* **17**: 199–219.

Grossberg, S. (1978b). A theory of human memory: self-organization and performance of sensory-motor codes, maps, and plans. In *Progress in theoretical biology*. Vol. 5, ed. R. Rosen and F. Snell. New York: Academic Press, pp. 233–374.

Gurney, K., T. J. Prescott, and P. Redgrave (2001). A computational model of action selection in the basal ganglia. I. A new functional anatomy. *Biol. Cybern.* **84**: 401–10.

Hartley, T. and G. Houghton, (1996). A linguistically constrained model of short-term memory for words and nonwords. *J. Mem. Lang.* **35**: 1–31.

Henson, R. N. A. (1998). Short-term memory for serial order: the start-end model. *Cognitive Psychol.* **36**: 73–137.

Henson, R. N. A., D. G. Norris, M. P. A. Page, and A. D. Baddeley (1996). Unchained memory: error patterns rule out chaining model of immediate serial recall. *Q. J. Exp. Psychol.* **49**: 80–115.

Hintzman, D. L. (1984). MINERVA 2: A simulation model of human memory. *Behav. Res. Meth. Ins. C.* **16**: 96–101.

Houghton, G. (1990). The problem of serial order: a neural network model of sequence learning and recall. In *Current Research in Natural Language Generation*, ed. R. Dale, C. Mellish, and M. Zock. London: Academic Press, pp. 287–318.

Kahana, M. J. and J. Jacobs (2000). Interresponse times in serial recall: effects of intraserial repetition. *J. Exp. Psychol. Learn.* **26**: 1188–97.

Murdock, B. B. (1982). A theory for the storage and retrieval of item and associative information. *Psychol. Rev.* **89**: 609–26.

Murdock, B. B. and R. Okada (1970). Interresponse times in single-trial free recall. *J. Exp. Psychol.* **86**: 263–7.

Page, M. P. A. and R. N. A. Henson (2001). Computational models of short-term memory: modeling serial recall of verbal material. In *Working Memory in Perspective*, ed. J. Andrade. Hove, UK: Psychology Press, pp. 177–98.

Page, M. P. A. and D. Norris (1998). The primacy model: a new model of immediate serial recall. *Psychol. Rev.* **105**: 761–81.

Patterson, K. E., R. H. Meltzer, and G. Mandler (1971). Inter-response times in categorized free recall. *J. Verb. Learn. Verb. Be.* **10**: 417–26.

Pitt, M. A., W. Kim, D. J. Navarro, and J. I. Myung (2006). Global model analysis by parameter space partitioning. *Psychol. Rev.* **113**: 57–83.

Raaijmakers, J. G. W. and R. M. Shiffrin (1980). SAM: a theory of probabilistic search of associative memory. In *The Psychology of Learning and Motivation*, Vol. 14, ed. G. Bower. New York: Academic Press.

Raaijmakers, J. G. W. and R. M. Shiffrin (1981). Search of associative memory. *Psychol. Rev.* **88**: 93–134.

Rohrer, D. (1996). On the relative and absolute strength of a memory trace. *Mem. Cogn.* **24**: 188–202.

Rohrer, D. (2002). The breadth of memory search. *Memory* **10**: 291–301.

Rohrer, D., D. P. Salmon, J. T. Wixted, and J. S. Paulsen (1999). The disparate effects of Alzheimer's disease and Huntington's disease on semantic memory. *Neuropsychology* **13**: 381–8.

Rohrer, D. and J. T. Wixted (1994). An analysis of latency and interresponse time in free recall. *Mem. Cogn.* **22**: 511–24.

Rohrer, D., J. T. Wixted, D. P. Salmon, and N. Butters (1995). Retrieval from semantic memory and its implications for Alzheimer's disease. *J. Psychol. Learn.* **21**: 1127–39.

Salthouse, T. A. (1986). Perceptual, cognitive, and motoric aspects of transcription typing. *Psychol. Bull.* **99**: 303–19.

Scahill, V. L., J. R. Hodges, and K. S. Graham (2005). Can episodic memory tasks differentiate semantic dementia from Alzheimer's disease? *Neurocase* **11**: 441–51.

Thomas, R. P., M. R. Dougherty, A. Sprenger, and J. I. Harbison (2008). Diagnostic hypothesis generation and human judgment. *Psychol. Rev.*, **115**: 115–85.

Usher, M. and E. J. Davelaar (2002). Neuromodulation of decision and response selection. *Neural Networks* **15**: 635–45.

Usher, M. and J. L. McClelland (2001). The time course of perceptual choice: the leaky, competing accumulator model. *Psychol. Rev.* **108**: 550–92.

Wixted, J. T. and D. Rohrer (1993). Proactive interference and the dynamics of free recall. *J. Psychol. Learn.* **19**: 1024–39.

Wixted, J. T. and D. Rohrer (1994). Analysing the dynamics of free recall: an integrative review of the empirical literature. *Psychon. Bull. Rev.* **1**: 89–106.

Part II

Computational neuroscience models

9 Introduction to Part II: computational neuroscience models

Tony J. Prescott, Joanna J. Bryson, and Anil K. Seth

A central and largely unsolved problem in the brain sciences is to understand the functional architecture of the vertebrate nervous system. Many questions about this architecture revolve around the issue of action selection. Because it is a fundamental property of neurons to be selective with regard to the patterns of input activity to which they respond, claims that particular brain subsystems are specifically or preferentially involved in the selection of action, as distinct to other aspects of control, must meet more stringent requirements (see below). It is also by no means inevitable that the functional decomposition of the brain will contain specialist action-selection mechanisms (see Seth, this volume). Appropriate behavioural switching could be a global property of nervous system function, and of its embedding in a body and environment, that cannot be attributed to specific subcomponents of brain architecture. In other words, it is plausible that an animal may 'flip' from one integrated pattern of behavioural output to another without some identifiable internal 'switch' being thrown. On the other hand, theoretical arguments can be presented, based for instance on the benefits that accrue from modularity (Bryson, 2005; Prescott *et al.*, 1999; Wagner and Altenberg, 1996), to suggest that biological control systems may include specialised action-selection components. Hence, one important debate in this field is whether there are specialised mechanisms for action selection in animal nervous systems, and, if so, where these might be found (see also Prescott, 2007, for an evolutionary perspective on this question).

9.1 Neural substrates for action selection in cortico-basal ganglia loops

Redgrave *et al.* (1999) have proposed that, to be considered as a candidate action-selection mechanism, a neural subsystem should exhibit the following properties. First, it should have inputs that carry information about both internal and external cues relevant to decision making. Second, there should be some internal mechanism that allows calculation of the urgency or 'salience' that should be attached to each available action. Third, there should be mechanisms that allow for the resolution of conflicts between competing actions based on their relative salience. Finally, the outputs of the system should be configured so as to allow the expression of winning actions whilst disallowing

Modelling Natural Action Selection, eds. Anil K. Seth, Tony J. Prescott and Joanna J. Bryson.
Published by Cambridge University Press. © Cambridge University Press 2012.

losers. There is now a growing consensus in the neuroscience literature that the *basal ganglia* – a group of functionally related structures found in the mid- and forebrain of all vertebrates – meet these criteria and therefore may represent an important neural action-selection substrate.

A key characteristic of the basal ganglia is its connectivity, in the form of multiple parallel loops, with both cortical and subcortical systems involved in either the control of movement, planning, or in the sequencing of thought. Houk (this volume) characterises these loops as 'distributed processing modules' implementing an action-selection function and contrast them with loops via the cerebellum, whose complementary role is to refine and amplify selected commands. The idea of cortico-basal ganglia loops as a substrate for action selection is a consistent theme in the computational neuroscience models presented in this book (Chambers *et al.*, this volume; Cisek, this volume; Frank *et al.*, this volume; Hazy *et al.*, this volume; Stafford and Gurney, this volume). However, there are also important differences in emphasis, and in the precise functional characterisation of the role of the basal ganglia, among these contributions. For instance, Hazy *et al.* and Frank *et al.* share a common starting point in adopting a model of basal ganglia function that stresses the differential role of two intrinsic basal ganglia pathways – one monosynaptic (sometimes termed the 'direct' pathway) that inhibits basal ganglia output structures, and another disynaptic (or 'indirect') that has a net-excitatory effect on outputs. According to these authors, the first pathway provides a 'go' signal that allows (gates) a desired movement by suppressing basal ganglia inhibition of target structures, while the second pathway is 'no-go', preventing the performance of an undesired movement. The same pathways (along with others) are also represented in the Stafford and Gurney and Chambers *et al.* models, however these authors emphasise the synergistic operation of intrinsic basal ganglia mechanisms that results in an appropriate balance of basal ganglia output to both winning and losing channels. Whilst the differences between these alternative accounts can seem relatively subtle, the fact that they are fully specified computationally means that they have the capacity to generate different predictions that can be investigated and tested against empirical data (Gurney *et al.*, 2004).

A significant focus of current debate is on the balance between intrinsic basal ganglia mechanisms and extrinsic mechanisms elsewhere in the brain in deciding what actions are selected. For Cisek (this volume), the selection of visually guided reaching movements within the primate fronto-parietal cortex depends largely upon intra-cortical mechanisms, inhibitory and excitatory, with the basal ganglia and prefrontal cortex acting to bias this selection process. Beginning with the traditional distinction between the dorsal ('where') and ventral ('what') cortical processing streams, Cisek argues that the dorsal stream contains specialised substreams each configured to meet the needs of alternative forms of action. At any one moment, several action plans may be active, triggered by the opportunities afforded by the current task or environment context. This view emphasises that the specification of action, that is the computation of the parameters of movement, can occur alongside the selection of action and possibly within the same neural substrate. Chambers *et al.* (this volume) address a similar theme but from a rather different perspective. Their contribution begins with the observation that sensorimotor systems in the primate brain are typically embedded in positive feedback loops that have the beneficial effect of integrating sensory information over time (thereby mitigating the effects of noise) and decoupling response size from the strength of sensory evidence. However, a distributed control architecture consisting of multiple positive feedback loops cannot be left to operate unchecked. Within this architecture the basal ganglia can be seen as an arbitrator that uses the mechanism of disinhibition to regulate the accumulation of evidence within loops.

Houk *et al.* (this volume) describe two empirical studies whose inspiration has also been modelling of the neural substrate for action selection in primates. These studies illustrate the interplay between analytic and synthetic approaches in the brain sciences, where biological investigations, predicated on existing models, generate data that match key predictions while raising new questions for modellers to address. As larger-scale models are developed that encompass both cortical and subcortical mechanisms (e.g., Hazy *et al.*, this volume; Frank *et al.*, this volume), the dynamics of the interactions between these selective processes at different levels of the neuraxis (nervous system architecture) will become better understood. For instance, in mammals, and particularly in primates, basal ganglia loops involving the pre-frontal cortex (PFC) have long been identified with a general role in executive function (see e.g., Miller and Cohen, 2001). For Hazy *et al.* (this volume) loops through the PFC provide modulation of working memory representations by taking advantage of a similar circuitry to that which, in more posterior loops, allows the selection of actions. These authors argue that the microanatomy of the PFC suggests the presence of multiple (perhaps 20 000 in humans) local neuronal groups, or 'stripes', that could provide the substrate for encoding independent working memories. In their computational model (see also O'Reilly and Frank, 2006), intrinsic, recurrent excitatory connections within each simulated stripe allow active representations to be maintained, whilst disinhibition, via a basal ganglia loop, can bring about the rapid updating of a specific representation. Learning occurs as the result of a dopamine-based reinforcement learning rule. In their chapter, Hazy *et al.* propose two new extensions to this architecture. First, that basal ganglia loops involving the deeper layers of the PFC allow gating of the effects of working memory representations on processing elsewhere in the brain, and, second, that phasic noradrenaline release plays a role in regulating the balance between exploitation of learnt strategies and exploration of new alternatives.

9.2   The decomposition of control for behavioural sequencing

The problem of action selection is often not a matter of making the best one-off decision, but of generating appropriate behavioural sequences whose net consequence is to achieve some desirable, but longer-term outcome. In ethology (see Seth, this volume), neuroscience and psychology (see Botvinick, this volume), robotics (Bryson, 2000; Crabbe this volume), and machine learning (e.g., Barto and Mahadevan, 2003), it has often been argued that behavioural sequences have a natural hierarchical decomposition. That is, that action selection is best organised to take place at multiple levels of abstraction from choosing among high-level objectives (e.g., whether to eat, drink, or rest) through to selecting among alternative movements that could serve the same specific, immediate goal (e.g., which grasp to use in picking up a cup).

Botvinick (this volume), presents an alternative perspective on this topic by arguing that behaviour that might appear to be hierarchically organised might be best implemented by a processing framework that does not have a hierarchical decomposition. To motivate this proposal, Botvinick describes a connectionist model of sequence learning based on Elman's (1990) recurrent neural network architecture. When required to learn the task of 'making a cup of coffee' – which can be decomposed as a series of subtasks each containing a number of elementary actions – the network achieves this goal without representing the hierarchical nature of the problem in an explicit way. Botvinick argues that this non-hierarchical solution shows a context sensitivity and ability to take advantage of structural overlap between tasks that is also characteristic of natural sequential behaviour. The challenge of sequencing is not limited only to the generation of explicit behaviour: recall from Part I that Davelaar presents a model of sequencing of memory retrieval which has important clinical implications in accounting for patterns of memory loss in Alzheimer's and Huntington's diseases.

9.3   Subcortical substrates for action selection

The cortico-basal ganglia loops that are the focus of much of the research described above are known to exist alongside loops connecting the basal ganglia to a wide range of subcortical structures involved in sensorimotor coordination (McHaffie *et al.*, 2005). The evolution of mammals saw a substantial increase in the role of the forebrain in action specification and control (Butler and Hodos, 1996) largely supplementing, rather than replacing, the sensorimotor functionality of these systems lower down the neuraxis. This complex layered architecture provides multiple levels of sensorimotor competence (Prescott *et al.*, 1999), and the option to choose between subcortical systems that provide a rapid response to immediate contingencies, and cortical systems that provide sophisticated adjudication between alternatives, taking greater account of context, past experiences, and likely future opportunities (McHaffie *et al.*, 2005). Key structures such as the sub-thalamic nucleus, which appears to provide a global, inhibitory 'hold your horses' signal (see Frank *et al.* this volume), may have evolved, at least in part, in order to regulate this trade-off between speed and sophistication of action selection.

Evidence from decerebrate and altricial animals, and from surgical interventions in patients with Parkinson's disease, suggests the presence of a brainstem substrate for action selection. Specifically, Humphries *et al.* (this volume), argue that a centralised structure, the medial reticular formation (MRF), fits the Redgrave *et al.* (1999) criteria for an action selection mechanism. The identification of the MRF with a possible action selection role has a long history that includes one of the first, if not *the* first, computational neuroscience models (Kilmer *et al.*, 1969). Based upon the most recent anatomical data, Humphries *et al.* (2006) previously described a structural model of the MRF intrinsic architecture which suggests that it is configured at the neuronal level as a 'small-world network' (Watts and Strogatz, 1998) – implying properties such as rapid cross-network synchronisation, consistent stabilisation, and persistent activity that could be useful for the representation and resolution of action selection competitions. In their chapter, Humphries *et al.* show that the intrinsic organisation of the MRF connectivity may have evolved to minimise connection length for a characteristic pattern of network configuration that can be described as a series of stacked 'clusters'. These authors then set out a computational model that explores alternative hypotheses concerning the possible functional organisation of the MRF, concluding that an architecture in which the output of each cluster represents a subcomponent of a complete behaviour appears most consistent with available evidence.

9.4   Disorders of action selection: clinical implications of action selection modelling

As the above discussion suggests, and as already exemplified by Davelaar (this volume), modelling approaches to the understanding of natural action selection can give useful insights in circumstances where the normal flow of integrated behaviour becomes disrupted as a consequence of damage or disease. A cluster of neurological conditions that includes Parkinson's disease (PD), schizophrenia, Huntington's disease, Tourette's syndrome, attention deficit/hyperactivity disorder (ADHD), and obsessive–compulsive disorder, can be linked to the same cortico-basal ganglia circuits that have been identified above as key substrates for the selection of action. Computational models of these substrates therefore have the potential to provide improved explanations for how these disorders arise and why particular patterns of symptoms are observed, and to serve as vehicles in which to investigate possible avenues for treatment.

Building on a broad platform of earlier modelling work investigating motor control and decision making in intact basal ganglia loops, Frank *et al.* (this volume) explore the functional consequences of model manipulations that simulate specific types of brain damage or abnormality thought to underlie PD, decision making deficits in patients with frontal cortex damage, and ADHD. For instance, with respect to PD, Frank *et al.* present a unifying computational hypothesis – reduced dynamic range in dopaminergic modulation of the basal ganglia – that explains a range of motor and cognitive deficits seen in this disease. On the basis of their model, Frank *et al.* were also able to make predictions about the effects of dopamine medications on learning that were later verified experimentally, and to make suggestions about the likely impact of deep brain stimulation (a surgical treatment for PD) on cognitive processes. The relevance of computational neuroscience models for understanding brain disorders involving action selection is also considered by Houk *et al.* (this volume), focusing particularly on schizophrenia. Like Frank *et al.*, these authors emphasise that success in understanding these complex neurological disorders will most likely require models at multiple levels of analysis from biophysically detailed models of cellular processes through to systems-level models, of the type we have focused on in this volume, that can link neurophysiological systems to observable behaviour.

9.5   Perceptual selection in decision making

The final chapter in this part highlights the notion, previously encountered in Part I, that action selection can be mediated not only by motor control systems but also by perceptual systems Stafford and Gurney (this volume) focus on the Stroop task, in which subjects have to name the ink colour of letter strings that spell out the name of a (congruent or incongruent) colour. Previously, Cohen *et al.* (1990) showed that a version of the leaky competing accumulator (LCA) model (see Bogacz *et al.*, this volume) could account for the basic Stroop phenomenon. Stafford and Gurney show that by introducing a response selection method based on an existing model of the basal ganglia (Gurney *et al.*, 2001), additional empirical data can be accounted for, making certain cognitive interpretations of the Stroop result (e.g., speed of processing) less likely. This study serves to demonstrate the convergence of themes between Part I and Part II of this book, showing how models incorporating relevant neuroanatomy can usefully extend those based primarily on computational principles.

References

Barto, A. G. and S. Mahadevan, (2003). Recent advances in hierarchical reinforcement learning. *Discrete Event Dyn. S.* **13**(4): 341–79.

Bryson, J. (2000). Cross-paradigm analysis of autonomous agent architecture. *J. Exp. Theor. Artif. In.* **12**(2): 165–189.

Bryson, J. J. (2005). Modular representations of cognitive phenomena in AI, psychology, and neuroscience. In *Visions of Mind: Architectures of Cognition and Affect*, ed. D. N. Davis. Hershey, PA: Idea Group Publishing, pp. 66–89.

Butler, A. B., and W. Hodos (1996). *Comparative Vertebrate Neuroanatomy*. New York: Wiley-Liss.

Cohen, J. D., K. Dunbar, and J. L. McClelland (1990). On the control of automatic processes: a parallel distributed processing account of the Stroop effect. *Psychol. Rev.* **97**(3): 332–61.

Elman, J. (1990). Finding structure in time. *Cogn. Sci.* **14**: 179–211.

Gurney, K., T. J. Prescott, and P. Redgrave (2001). A computational model of action selection in the basal ganglia. I. A new functional anatomy. *Biol. Cybern.* **84**(6): 401–10.

Gurney, K., T. J. Prescott, J. Wickens, and P. Redgrave (2004). Computational models of the basal ganglia: from membranes to robots. *Trends Neurosci.* **27**: 453–9.

Humphries, M. D., K. Gurney, and T. J. Prescott (2006). The brainstem reticular formation is a small-world, not scale-free, network. *Proc. Soc. Roy. Soc. B. Biol. Sci.* **273**(1585): 503–11.

Kilmer, W. L., McCulloch, W. S., and Blum, J. (1969). A model of the vertebrate central command system. *Int. J. Man. Mach. Stud.* **1**: 279–309.

McHaffie, J. G., T. R. Stanford, B. E. Stein, V. Coizet, and P. Redgrave (2005). Subcortical loops through the basal ganglia. *Trends Neurosci.* **28**(8): 401–407.

Miller, E. K. and J. D. Cohen (2001). An integrative theory of prefrontal cortex function. *Annu. Rev. Neurosci.* **27**: 167–202.

O'Reilly, R. C. and M. J. Frank (2006). Making working memory work: a computational model of learning in the prefrontal cortex and basal ganglia. *Neural Computation* **18**: 283–328.

Prescott, T. J. (2007). Forced moves or good tricks? Landmarks in the evolution of neural mechanisms for action selection. *Adapt. Behav.* **15**: 9–31.

Prescott, T. J., P. Redgrave, and K. N. Gurney (1999). Layered control architectures in robots and vertebrates. *Adapt. Behav.* **7**(1): 99–127.

Redgrave, P., T. Prescott, and K. N. Gurney (1999). The basal ganglia: a vertebrate solution to the selection problem? *Neuroscience* **89**: 1009–23.

Wagner, G. P. and L. Altenberg (1996). Perspective: complex adaptations and the evolution of evolvability. *Evolution* **50**(3): 967–76.

Watts, D. J. and S. H. Strogatz (1998). Collective dynamics of 'small-world' networks. *Nature* **393**: 440–2.

10 Action selection and refinement in subcortical loops through basal ganglia and cerebellum

James C. Houk

Summary

Subcortical loops through the basal ganglia and cerebellum form computationally powerful distributed processing modules (DPMs). This chapter relates the computational features of a DPM's loop through the basal ganglia to experimental results for two kinds of natural action selection. First, data from both monkeys and humans in a step-tracking task were used to decipher the neural mechanisms that underlie the detection of movement errors leading to selection of corrective movements called submovements. Second, functional brain imaging of human subjects during a serial-order recall task was used to study brain activity associated with decoding a sequence of actions from information held in working memory. Our DPM-based model assists in the interpretation of puzzling data from both of these experiments. These analyses lead to a broad discussion of the DPM concept and how it relates to neuroscience, modularity, engineering, evolution, mathematical recursion, agent-based modelling, Bayesian computations, and brain disorders. The loops through basal ganglia and cerebellum profit from exceptional combinations of unique cellular properties together with advantageous neural circuitry. Their modular organisation means that DPMs regulate pattern formation in multiple areas of the cerebral cortex, thus initiating and refining different kinds of action (or thought), depending on the area of the brain. We then use our findings to formulate a novel model of the etiology of schizophrenia.

10.1 Introduction

The higher order circuitry of the brain is comprised of a large-scale network of distributed processing modules (DPMs). Each of approximately 100 cerebral cortical areas is individually regulated by relatively private loops through subcortical structures, particularly through the basal ganglia and cerebellum (Houk, 2005; Houk and Wise, 1995; Kelly and Strick, 2003, 2004). These DPMs have powerful computational architectures as summarised in Figure 10.1. Each DPM receives cortico-cortical input vectors from approximately seven other DPMs (although only two are shown in Figure 10.1). (The

Modelling Natural Action Selection, eds. Anil K. Seth, Tony J. Prescott and Joanna J. Bryson.
Published by Cambridge University Press. © Cambridge University Press 2012.

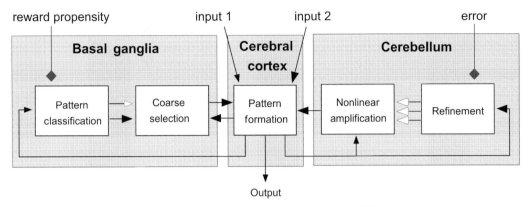

Figure 10.1 Schematic of a Distributed Processing Module (DPM). Relatively private loops through basal ganglia (BG) and cerebellum (CB) regulate the output vector transmitted by each module. In this manner, responses to input vectors by circuits within each area of cerebral cortex become elaborated by more sophisticated processing steps in BG and CB. Net excitatory pathways are shown with black arrowheads, net inhibitory pathways are shown with white arrowheads, and diamonds signify neuromodulatory and training inputs. Modified from Houk (2005).

estimate of seven derives from Felleman and Van Essen, 1991.) The final outcome of all of the computations in a given DPM is a spatiotemporal pattern of activity in the module's output vector, representing the activity in its set of cortical output neurons. This output is sent as input to other DPMs, or to the brainstem or spinal cord. In this manner, arrays of DPMs form large-scale networks that function in combination to control behaviour, or thought. The reader should consult Houk (2005) for a detailed description of this architecture and a justification of its capacity to control both actions and thoughts. The brief overview of functional operations in loops through basal ganglia (BG) and cerebellum (CB) given in the next two paragraphs is a summary that applies to the selection and initiation of movement commands that control discrete actions.

A DPM's loop through BG is thought to regulate action selection (Gurney *et al.*, 2001; Houk, 2001; 2005; Houk and Wise, 1995; Redgrave *et al.*, 1999). The label 'Coarse Selection' is used in Figure 10.1 in recognition of the fact that BG output neurons recorded during a task comprised of multiple options typically do not select one unique action. Instead they code for a small set of potential actions, for example, forearm rotations with different amplitudes, velocities, and directions of movement as opposed to a unique movement (Gdowski *et al.*, 2007). In spite of this qualification, coarse action selection poses a very difficult problem for a subject in a natural setting. While in my office, I have to decide whether I will pick up a writing instrument, type on my keyboard, scratch my chin, or walk to the kitchen to fetch a beverage (and think of all the other potential actions). On the input side of the BG loop in Figure 10.1, the 'Pattern Classification' operation receives a huge vector of neural signals from one area of cerebral cortex (and functionally adjacent areas) plus a reward propensity signal from dopamine neurons in the midbrain. The cortical input is highly diverse in both qualitative and quantitative dimensions, providing a challenging computational problem for pattern classification. The reward signal produces a short-term attentional modulation of useful neuronal responses (Nicola *et al.*, 2000) plus a long-term consolidation of the synaptic weights that promoted them (Houk, 2005). In this manner, a diversity of events in a diversity of contexts can be classified with respect to their relevance and saliency. According to most contemporary models (reviewed in Houk, 2007), bursts of medium spiny neurons in the striatum, via a direct pathway through BG, disinhibit their targets in the thalamus, allowing thalamo-cortical loops to initiate tentative patterns of activity that represent coarse selections of appropriate actions. There are also mechanisms, via less direct pathways through BG, for inhibiting the selection of patterns that would represent poor choices in action selection as discussed in Gurney *et al.* (2001) and Houk and Wise (1995).

While a small set of potential patterns is being coarsely selected by a BG loop, a pair of loops (Figure 10.1) through the CB amplify and sculpt this preliminary activation into a refined output vector (Houk and Mugnaini, 2003). The 'Nonlinear Amplification' step is implemented by a positive-feedback loop through the cerebellar nucleus. Regenerative positive feedback causes 'Nonlinear Amplification' that includes an induction of bistability in individual modules and multistability in the network (Wang, Dam, *et al.*, 2008). Bistability creates a behavioural threshold for the initiation of an action command while positive feedback amplifies the command's intensity, duration, and spatial extent (Houk *et al.*, 1993). Selective restraint of this amplification process and sculpting it into an accurate action command is implemented by the 'Refinement' operation, mediated by Purkinje cells in the cerebellar cortex, considered to be the site of the brain's most powerful neuronal architecture for resolving difficult control problems (Houk and Mugnaini, 2003; Houk and Wise, 1995; Raymond *et al.*, 1996). The cerebellar cortex is well suited for this important refinement operation.

In the present chapter, we relate the computational features of a DPM's loop through BG to experimental results for two kinds of natural action selection. First, mechanisms fostering the coarse selection and initiation of corrective submovements will be inferred from microelectrode recordings and behavioural analyses in monkeys and from functional brain imaging in humans. Second, functional imaging during a serial order recall task will be used to study human brain activity during the selection of sequential actions from working memory. Our DPM-based model assists in the interpretation of puzzling data from both categories of experiments. We come to posit that the many loops through the BG each regulate the pattern formation required for coarse action selection in a given area of cerebral cortex. This operation leads to the initiation of different kinds of action (or thought) mediated by different areas of the cerebral cortex.

10.2   Selection and initiation of corrective submovements

Tangential velocity traces of hand movements in primate reaching tasks display multiple peaks, a phenomenon that has been well-known since Woodworth's seminal paper in 1899. However, the cause of these irregularities is still under debate. The traditional view has held that multiple peaks in velocity can be attributed to the use of overlapping

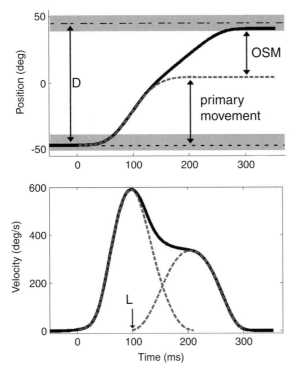

Figure 10.2 Movement error correction by discrete submovements. This example shows the decomposition of a hand movement into a primary movement and an OSM (overlapping submovement). When the primary movement misses the target, the OSM is generated predictively to correct the error. Note that the velocity trace shows an inflection that is detected as an OSM by the soft-symmetry algorithm. D is the target distance and L is the latency of the OSM. Modified from Fishbach *et al.* (2007).

submovements (OSMs) to correct reaching errors. More recent theories suggest that the same effect can be attributed to a continuous control system that is subject to delays and nonlinearity (Bhushan and Shadmehr, 1999; Kawato *et al.*, 1992; Shadmehr and Mussa-Ivaldi, 1994; Sternad and Schaal, 1999). Whatever the underlying mechanisms, it can be difficult to detect the occurrences of OSMs in rapid movement trials. Several years ago we described a novel soft-symmetry algorithm that uses higher derivatives (velocity, acceleration, jerk, and snap) of movement traces for detecting OSMs (Fishbach *et al.*, 2005). Instead of insisting on perfectly symmetric trajectories, as in Novak *et al.* (2000), soft-symmetry relaxes this constraint by a small degree. These algorithms allow single behavioural trials to be decomposed into their component parts, as illustrated in Figure 10.2. This permits the statistical analyses of submovement behavioural features that are exploited in the next section. Single trial analysis also facilitates interesting comparisons with the activity patterns of individual neurons.

Figure 10.3 shows examples of two movements (blue traces) along with simultaneously recorded firing patterns (green spikes on top) of two neurons in the primary motor cortex (M1). The first example (Figure 10.3a) is a primary movement followed by a delayed

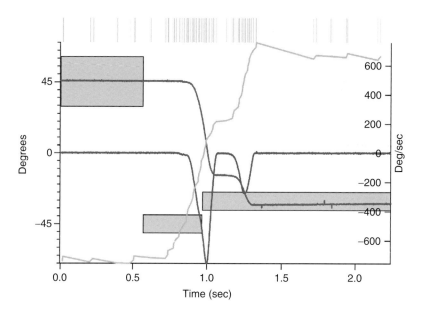

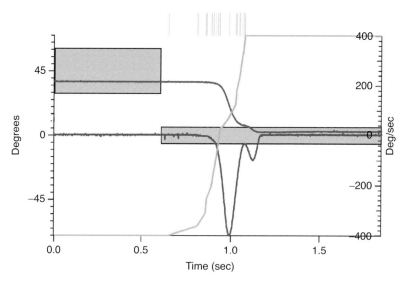

Figure 10.3 Segmented movements of a monkey and associated bursts of discharge in primary motor cortex. The monkey turned a rotating handle to move a cursor horizontally on a screen (blue trace = position; red trace = velocity) to acquire a target (shaded boxes). (a) The firing pattern of a motor cortical neuron during a trial that contains a delayed submovement. (b) The firing pattern of another motor cortical cell during a trial that contains an overlapping submovement. Each motor cortical neuron shows two bursts of discharge, which are marked by upward deflections in the green baseline-rate normalised cumulative sum (CUSUM) traces. Taken from Houk *et al.* (2007). See plate section for colour version.

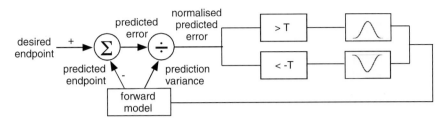

Figure 10.4 The NPE (Normalised Predictive Error) model of how corrective submovements are generated. Vision provides the information about the desired endpoint, which can be updated as rapidly as 180 ms when a visual perturbation is introduced at movement onset (Fishbach *et al.*, 2007). The NPE model uses a type of forward model to compute the predicted endpoint based on both efference copy and sensory input, and it computes the prediction variance based on past experience. The normalised predicted error (Z-score) must exceed a threshold value T in order to initiate a corrective submovement. The executed submovement follows an approximately bell-shaped velocity profile. Taken from Houk *et al.* (2007).

submovement (DSM), marked by the two downward deflections of the red velocity trace. The second example (Figure 10.3b) is a primary movement with an overlapping submovement (OSM). In this task, the monkey turns a rotating handle to move a cursor horizontally on a screen to acquire a target. The motor cortical neurons fire bursts of discharge that precede both the primary movements and the corrective submovements. The green CUSUM traces clearly mark each burst with an upward deflection that is proportional to the number of spikes in the burst. (CUSUM means baseline-rate normalised cumulative sum histogram (cf. Gibson *et al.*, 1985).) The first burst is large and occurs prior to the primary movement. The second burst is smaller and precedes the delayed submovement (DSM) in Figure 10.3a and the overlapping submovement (OSM) in Figure 10.3b. Both primary movements and corrective submovements appear to be controlled by the motor cortex.

10.2.1   Abstract model of how corrective submovements are generated

Statistical analyses of behavioural features of rapid primary movements and their corrective submovements revealed a recurrent pattern in the organisation of fast and accurate primate reaching (Fishbach *et al.*, 2007). OSM onset times show appreciable variability and are highly correlated with the normalised amplitude of the primary movement. We hypothesised that this submovement initiation pattern is incompatible with a continuous model of movement control and that it fits a particular discrete model of movement control particularly well. According to this model, a correction is initiated when the normalised predicted error (NPE) exceeds a threshold value T. Figure 10.4 illustrates the NPE model. Note that predicted error applies to the ongoing trial, whereas prediction variance is computed over the subject's past experience with similar trials. These two factors, current error (also called *likelihood*) and prediction variance (related to the *prior*, as in prior knowledge), are the cornerstones of Bayesian models of decision making (Koerding, 2007).

We tested the NPE model against alternative control models using mechanistic implementations of simulated movements (Barringer *et al.*, 2008). The output of each control model tested was fed into a fixed model of the neuromuscular system in order to generate statistical movement data for comparison between models and with animal behaviour. Amplitude-dependent noise was added to the pulse phase of the simulated command and no noise was added to the step phase. A simple mass-spring model with linear damping did not permit a clear distinction to be seen between a movement's endpoint, which exhibited variance as a consequence of motor command variance, and the system's equilibrium position, which showed no variance. Substituting fractional power damping for linear damping overcame that problem. Fractional power damping (proportional to velocity raised to the fifth power) has been used in previous modelling studies to capture the basic nonlinearity of the neuromuscular system (Barto *et al.*, 1999; Houk *et al.*, 2002; Karniel and Inbar, 1999; Wang, Dam, *et al.*, 2008); it seems to be very important for effective damping in the control of rapid movements (Barto *et al.*, 1999) and explains the relationship between amplitude, velocity, and duration of rapid human movements (Karniel and Inbar, 1999).

Continuous control policies in general do not account for the large range of submovement onset times found in the animal data analysed by Fishbach *et al.* (2007). In contrast, the use of a discrete control policy explained both the large range and the linear increase in submovement onset times as the normalised amplitude of the primary movement increased. All of the discrete control processes that we tested issued corrective movements that improved accuracy, and most of them shortened the duration of movement. However, the NPE policy outperformed, in terms of speed and accuracy (see Novak *et al.*, 2002 for a discussion of speed–accuracy trade-off), a suite of other similar discrete policies for online error correction. Furthermore this policy resulted in trajectories that were qualitatively similar to primate reaching movements. Our findings are consistent with the hypothesis that both the NPE model and actual primate reaching behaviour display performance that is essentially optimal.

The NPE controller relies on prediction of the endpoint of the primary movement to decide when to issue corrective motor commands. The predictions plotted in Figure 10.5 were calculated using the soft-symmetry algorithm. This component of the NPE model yielded distributions and levels of accuracy similar to the monkey data. Variability was largest at s_1, the first snap extrema, diminished a little at j_1, the first jerk extrema, diminished appreciably at a_1, the first acceleration extrema, and became very small at v_1, the first velocity extrema. These plots illustrate how NPE accuracy increases as the movement progresses. In essence, the NPE model computes the statistical significance of an error, and waits until that measure goes above a threshold value T before initiating a movement correction.

10.2.2   Neural mechanisms

Our human functional brain imaging results (Tunik *et al.*, 2009) document an important role for a BG loop through the putamen in deciding when and how a movement should be corrected. During event-related fMRI, subjects moved a cursor to capture targets

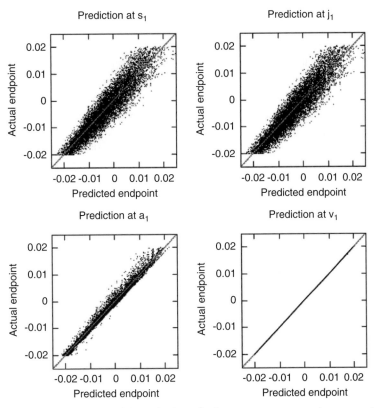

Figure 10.5 Predictions of the endpoints of primary movements can become quite accurate soon after movement onset. The soft-symmetry algorithm was used to predict endpoints at several points (the first snap extrema s_1, the first jerk extrema j_1, the first acceleration extrema a_1, the first velocity extrema v_1) along a recorded trajectory. Actual endpoints were derived from entire trajectories. Modified from Barringer *et al.* (2008).

presented at varying movement amplitudes. Movements were performed in a rehearsed null and a novel viscous (25% random trials) torque field. Movement error feedback was provided after each trial. The viscous field invoked significantly larger error at the end of the primary movement. Subjects compensated by producing more corrections than they had in the null condition. Corrective submovements were appropriately scaled such that terminal error was similar between the two conditions. A task contrast comparing activation in all movement conditions with rest was huge and included all of the sensorimotor regions (e.g., motor, premotor, parietal, cerebellar, basal ganglia). It was used as a mask to limit our search volume in the brain. Parametric analysis identified two regions where the BOLD (Blood Oxygen Level Dependent) signal correlated with the number of submovements per trial: a cerebellar region similar to the one seen in the task contrast and the contralateral dorsal putamen. A separate parametric analysis identified brain regions where activity correlated with movement amplitude. This identified the same cerebellar region as above, bilateral parietal cortex, and left primary motor and premotor cortex. Our data indicate that the BG and CB play complementary roles in

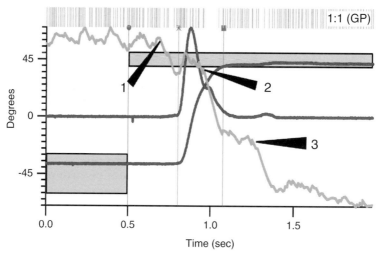

Figure 10.6 Activity during a single trial of an internal segment of globus pallidus (GPi) neuron. In this task the monkey turns a rotating handle to move a cursor horizontally on a screen (blue trace = position; red trace = velocity) to acquire a target (blue boxes). The baseline-rate normalised cumulative sum histogram (CUSUM) for the neuron (green trace) shows three downward deflections marking three pauses in the high tonic discharge rate in this GPi neuron. The first pause (arrow 1) is small and occurs prior to the primary movement; the second and third pauses are stronger and are associated with tiny corrective submovements (arrows 2 and 3). Modified from Houk *et al.* (2007). See plate section for colour version.

regulating ongoing actions when precise updating is required. The BG play a key role in contextually based motor decision making, i.e., for deciding if and when to correct a given movement by initiating corrective submovements, and the CB is more generally involved in amplifying and refining the command signals to specify movements with different amplitudes, velocities, and directions.

Our single cell recordings in monkeys (Roy *et al.*, 2008) demonstrated that BG output is appropriate for initiating corrective submovements. Since output cells in the internal segment of the globus pallidus (GPi) project, via thalamus, to many different areas in the cerebral cortex, neurons need to be sampled from the region of GPi that projects to the primary motor cortex (Roy *et al.*, 2003). The sampled neurons should also be ones that are well related to the task. Figure 10.6 is an example from our ongoing work that meets both of these criteria.

Figure 10.6 illustrates the typical high spontaneous discharge rate of BG output neurons. Firing rate is modulated in association with both the primary movement and with an overlapping submovement (OSM) and a delayed submovement (DSM) that occurred in this particular trial (see the red velocity trace in Figure 10.6 and compare this neuron with the motor cortical neuron illustrated in Figure 10.3). The CUSUM (green trace) clearly shows three pauses in the high tonic firing rate. Pause 1 is small and occurs prior to the large primary movement; pauses 2 and 3 precede tiny corrective submovements. Figure 9 in Houk *et al.* (2007) demonstrates the reliability of these single cell properties across trials. Note that the pauses corresponding to the corrective submovements are as strong or stronger than the pause for the primary movement, even though the corrections that they apparently control are typically much smaller than is the primary movement. These discrepant amplitude relationships in the firing rate data are puzzling. Motor cortex units show smaller bursts for the small corrective movements than for the larger primary movements (Figure 10.3). In the next section we describe a model of knowledge transfer that appears to explain this result.

10.2.3   Interpretation of the puzzling firing rate data

The DPM model of voluntary movement control, learning, and memory (Houk, 2010) posits that practice in a task allows regularly rehearsed processing steps to be exported from the BG and/or CB to the area of cerebral cortex to which the channel projects (Houk, 2005; Houk and Wise, 1995; Hua and Houk, 1997; Novak *et al.*, 2003; see also Pasupathy and Miller, 2005). The loop through BG is specialised for early learning based on reinforcement, particularly in the striatum where synaptic inputs to spiny neurons are reinforced by reward prediction signals sent by dopamine neurons. In contrast, learning in the cerebral cortex is specialised for learning from practice (Merzenich *et al.*, 1996). The inputs from BG (and CB) force cortical neurons to rehearse their responses over repeated practice trials. This causes a strengthening of synaptic inputs that fire at the same time as the neuron is forced to fire. This process of 'fire together–wire together' effectively allows knowledge stored in BG (and CB) synapses to migrate to synapses in the cerebral cortex. The result is that responses become faster and more accurate.

   The process of selecting an appropriate primary movement can be exported to the motor cortex because the small set of primary movements is rehearsed in every trial. In contrast, corrective submovements vary substantially from trial to trial, as described earlier, so nothing regular is rehearsed. This model of knowledge transfer from the basal ganglia to the cerebral cortex is supported by recordings from striatal neurons in rats during a lever pressing task (Carelli *et al.*, 1997) and by combined recordings of single cell activity from the striatum and frontal cortex (Pasupathy and Miller, 2005; see also Brasted and Wise, 2004). It is also supported by Frank's (2005) simulations of dopamine modulation in the basal ganglia and by functional brain imaging data (Toni *et al.*, 2002).

10.2.4   Integrative control of hand movement and on-line error correction

The above account deals mainly with cortical–basal ganglionic loops whereas most DPMs also have loops through cerebellum. Regarding the latter, presently we know most about signal processing in the loop between CB and M1, the primary motor cortex (Houk and Mugnaini, 2003). There are actually two loops in each cortical–cerebellar module. The one through the cerebellar nucleus is predominately excitatory and is responsible for the high firing rates of voluntary movement commands (Holdefer *et al.*, 2005). This is the 'Nonlinear Amplification' block in Figure 10.1 – positive feedback appears to be responsible for the amplification. The longer loop through cerebellar cortex uses the strong inhibitory output from Purkinje cells to restrain the positive feedback and, most importantly, to set the fixed points of this attractor network (Houk and Mugnaini, 2003).

How do cortical–basal ganglionic and cortical–cerebellar modules work together? Figure 10.6 shows an example of a GPi neuron in the basal ganglia helping to select a primary movement and subsequent submovements in a tracking task. As mentioned above, three pauses in firing are marked by arrows in Figure 10.6. These pauses should provoke disinhibitions of the M1 neurons to which the GPi neuron, via the thalamus, projects, thus facilitating bursts of discharge to promote a primary movement and one or more corrective submovements. Each of these bursts would also need to be amplified and refined by the cerebellum. Amplification in intensity and time would serve to generate any given element of the M1 output vector in Figure 10.1, and spatial amplification would recruit the large population of M1 neurons (additional elements of that vector) that are required to produce a movement (Georgopoulos, 1995). The cerebellar cortex would then use its large multifaceted input to restrain and refine the entire M1 output vector, shaping it into a composite motor command regulating the direction, velocity, and duration of a primary movement, and of the subsequent corrective submovements that home in on the target. Figure 10.3 shows examples of two elements in that output vector.

What might be the relationship between the abstract operations in Figure 10.4 and the neurophysiological operations outlined in Figure 10.1? It does not necessarily follow that the nervous system breaks down its processing steps into a stage of forward modelling, followed by a stage of error prediction, followed by a normalisation based on past experience. Spiny neurons on the input side of the loop through BG receive a huge input vector from the cortex and are probably capable of a powerful neuromodulated pattern classification operation. This neurobiological step might be capable of computing signals reflecting elements of the normalised predicted error directly in one operation. We believe that this single step explanation is an attractive possibility that warrants empirical investigation, perhaps based on single cell recordings from BG output neurons. Recall our earlier suggestion that the output of a BG loop does not select unique individual actions (Gdowski et al., 2007). Instead, it appears to select coarsely a set of approximate actions, which we designate a ballpark action. This ballpark needs to be amplified and refined in order to produce an accurate movement.

The $\pm$T thresholds for triggering initial activity in one of the two alternative motor command pathways in Figure 10.4 maps well onto the bistable properties of the CB modules that were analysed in Wang, Dam, et al. (2008). Individual CB modules are microscopic loops between motor cortex and the cerebellar nucleus. Positive feedback around any given loop gives rise to bistability, and transitions between quiescent and active states require a threshold activity level that is defined by a separatrix between these opposing states. An antagonistic pair of modules would model the $\pm$T channels in Figure 10.4. Expanding these ideas into the real-world case of a choice among some large number N of alternative actions can probably be accommodated by introducing N modules into the reciprocity model, an idea that is elaborated on in Section 10.4.2.

Convergence upon a precise choice for a movement or submovement command appears to be controlled by Purkinje cell activity in the cerebellar cortex (Houk and

Mugnaini, 2003). As mentioned before, Purkinje cell activity sets the fixed points of the attractor network. Purkinje cells need to pause and burst in order to program and control the timing and on-state intensities of the composite motor commands that are sent to the limb neuromuscular system. These control operations by the cerebellar cortex give rise to the bell-shaped trajectories of the resultant limb movements. Initial learning and later adaptation is guided by the error signals that are transmitted via climbing fibres.

Note that the present view of how BG and CB loops function is strongly based upon neuroscience, particularly neuroanatomical and neurophysiological findings. Others have based their views and their models on analogy with engineering principles. A prominent example of the latter can be found in Smith and Shadmehr (2005), who observed different motor deficits in patients with a BG disorder (Huntington's disease) versus those with CB degeneration. Huntington's patients adjust poorly to unexpected perturbations of ongoing movements and to deviations from an optimal or desired movement trajectory. CB patients, in contrast, adjust their ongoing movements more or less normally, but are poor at adapting to errors made during previous movements, unlike the Huntington's patients. According to the engineering-based interpretations of Smith and Shadmehr, BG loops control on-line error corrections and CB loops update internal models. More specifically, they maintain that BG loops monitor movement progress and produce real-time responses to errors, whereas CB loops update an internal representation of the physical dynamics of the limb (adaptive adjustment of a 'forward model') and they update a sensorimotor map that transforms the desired limb state into motor commands that produce that state (by adaptively adjusting an 'inverse-dynamics model'). The interpretations of Smith and Shadmehr (2005) would lead to the conclusion that BG loops are solely responsible for corrective submovements, with CB loops playing a completely different role, updating internal models. Although we accept the empirical findings reported by Smith and Shadmehr, we interpret the data very differently. In our view, both BG and CB loops participate in within-movement, on-line error correction in addition to movement-to-movement updating, and the operations of both BG and CB loops involve something like 'forward models', such as those illustrated for the NPE model in Figure 10.4. In large measure, our contrasting view results from using neuroscience rather than engineering concepts. So, when we say that CB loops use 'something like' forward models, we mean that the CB uses direct adaptive control to alter ongoing motor commands (Barto *et al.*, 1999), rather than a physically instantiated 'internal model'. The brain does not have specific regions and/or synapses for building 'forward' models as opposed to 'inverse' models or, for that matter, 'internal models' of any sort. According to neuroscientific principles, the brain's processors merely compute the required output signals, without any need to instantiate internal models, and they do so for both primary movements and for corrective submovements (Novak, 2001).

During the course of sensorimotor learning, the cerebral cortex, BG and CB work in parallel but unique ways (Doya 1999; Houk, 2010; Houk and Wise, 1995; Lu *et al.*, 1998). The loop through the basal ganglia learns to use coarse action selection to discover ballpark actions that are appropriate in a given context (Houk, 2005), utilising reinforcement learning (Sutton and Barto, 1998). The loop through the CB learns to refine these coarse action selections through a simplified form of supervised learning

(Berthier *et al.*, 1993). The cerebral cortex, being regulated by input from both BG and CB, learns through practice to perform these operations faster and more accurately, utilising unsupervised Hebbian learning (Bliss and Collingridge, 1993; Hua and Houk, 1997; Merzenich *et al.*, 1996). The result of these diverse forms of learning is summarised in Houk (2010) and has been simulated in robots by Doya (1999).

10.3   Serial order processing

Tasks in which lists of items are presented, after which the subject is required to recall the items in the same order in which they were presented, require serial order processing and sequential action selection from working memory. Immediate serial order recall has been broadly studied in the cognitive domain (Botvinick and Plaut, 2006). In this section, we utilise a task dubbed 'Replicate' (Houk *et al.*, 2007), which displays many standard patterns of serial recall behaviour, but which also can be conveniently applied across research modalities and, in particular, across species. Benchmark properties of serial order recall include: (1) a graded decline in recall accuracy with sequence length, (2) transposition gradients reflecting a tendency for items to be recalled at serial positions near to their original positions, (3) item similarity effects including (a) a tendency for items to be recalled near the item where they originally appeared, (b) a tendency for sequences of more similar items to be recalled less accurately than sequences of less similar items (Botvinick and Plaut 2006).

10.3.1   The Replicate task

In Replicate, K targets are presented on an N × N grid of squares in a randomised sequence, and the subjects are required to remember their positions and serial order over a brief delay. The subjects are then cued to use a joystick to move a cursor to the K positions in the same order in which they were originally presented. The phase of target presentation requires the setting up of a working memory representation, which must be sustained through the delay period and then decoded in order to produce correct joystick movements; we thus refer to the three phases of the task as the encoding, maintenance, and decoding phases.

Human behavioural studies with Replicate confirmed that the task generates several standard patterns of recall behaviour (Houk *et al.*, 2007). A total of 32 Replicate trials were performed, eight at each of four sequence lengths (3–6 for half the subjects, 4–7 for the other half). Each trial was initiated by the subject using the joystick to move a cursor into the central tile in a 5 × 5 grid. A target sequence then appeared, with each target location illuminated for a total of 500 ms. Following a 10 s delay, the joystick cursor changed colour, cuing the subject to replicate the target sequence, returning to the central tile when finished. A maximum of 3 s was allotted for identification of each location. Our error analysis demonstrated that the Replicate task yields the typical visual memory span of 4–5 items, and that errors frequently involve (1) transpositions of items located near to one another in the sequence and/or (2) substitution of a location target with a nearby location in the grid. These results demonstrate that Replicate has several benchmark properties of serial order recall that have been studied with lists of more cognitive items such as objects or words (Botvinick and Plaut, 2006). In a monkey subject, studies of recall performance in a 3×3 Replicate with K = 3 or 4 items demonstrated a number of important parallels with human immediate serial order recall (Botvinick et al., 2009). This finding is consistent with a single mechanism for serial order processing being shared across primate species.

10.3.2   Functional neuroimaging (fMRI) of Replicate in human subjects

For our brain imaging study (Houk et al., 2007), we employed a control task dubbed 'Chase'. In Chase, a sequence of location cues appears just as in Replicate, but subjects use the joystick to track these cues immediately as they appear. Chase involves similar stimulus and response sequences to Replicate, but eliminates the working memory component.

Brain fMRI activity of subjects performing 4×4 Replicate with K = 3 items utilised two primary BOLD contrasts. An 'Execute' contrast was made between the period of sensory guided joystick movements in the Chase task and a rest period. This contrast was designed to show the neural correlates of motor execution. A 'Decode' contrast was made between the memory guided movement period of the Replicate task and the sensory guided movement period of the Chase task. This contrast was designed to reveal the neural correlates of the decoding process while simultaneously controlling for BOLD activity related to pure motor execution. Whole brain Echo Planar Imaging data (24 6-mm slices, TR = 2000 ms) were collected from ten subjects, and a partial-brain scanning protocol focusing on the BG (12 6-mm slices, TR = 1000 ms) was used for nine subjects.

In the participants who provided whole-brain data, the Decoding network included the right dorsolateral prefrontal cortex, the left dorsal premotor area, bilateral superior parietal lobules, left primary motor cortex, right inferior parietal cortex, and portions of CB. The Execution network included left primary motor and dorsal premotor cortex, left putamen, and right cerebellar cortex.

The partial-brain imaging protocol provided better sensitivity to changes within the striatum of the basal ganglia. The differential BOLD activity in the caudate nucleus and putamen were strikingly different for the Execute and Decode contrasts (Figure 10.7). A significant increase in activity was found in the putamen for Execute, whereas a significant decrease in activity was found in the caudate nucleus for Decode. The deactivation, representing a statistically significant decrease in blood flow in the caudate during the decoding operation, was puzzling. Brain processing is believed to require increased synaptic activity, which recruits increased metabolism and blood flow, as detected by an increase in BOLD signal (Logothetis, 2002).

Decreases in BOLD are considered mysterious (Gusnard and Raichle, 2001) and are usually explained by greater synaptic processing in the control task as opposed to the main task. In our Decode contrast, this could happen if the caudate were actively engaged in the sensory-guided control task Chase, due to the presence of visual targets

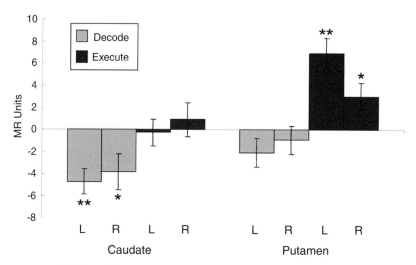

Figure 10.7 Differential BOLD activity in the right and left head of the caudate and putamen for the Decode (gray), and Execute (black) contrasts. Error bars indicate standard error. Single asterisk (*) indicates a significant difference (t(8) ≥ 2.36, p < 0.05) while double asterisks (**) indicate a highly significant difference (t(8) ≥ 4.16, p < 0.01). A significant decrease in activity was found in the caudate nucleus for decoding, whereas a significant increase in activity was found in the putamen for execution. Deactivation, representing a statistically significant decrease in blood flow in the caudate for the Decode contrast, was surprising. Taken from Houk *et al.* (2007).

for each movement of the joystick. However, Figure 10.7 indicates that the caudate is not particularly active in the Execute contrast. The statistically significant decrease in BOLD for the Decode contrast seems to need a better explanation.

10.3.3   Action selection in the loop through the basal ganglia

Although many authors have suggested that the loop through the basal ganglia plays an important role in action selection, there are diverse views concerning the mechanism by which this might occur. Most authors agree that action selection occurs in the input nucleus of the BG loop, namely the striatum (but see Rubchinsky *et al.*, 2003). There are diverse views about the mechanisms for preventing actions; they will not be discussed here.

The dorsal part of the striatum, the neostriatum, is comprised of two divisions, the caudate nucleus and the putamen. The principal neurons of both caudate and putamen, the medium spiny neurons, are inhibitory GABAergic projection neurons. They emit an elaborate array of collaterals to neighbouring spiny neurons before they project to output stages of the BG, namely to either the globus pallidus or substantia nigra pars reticulata. The drawing in Figure 10.8a shows schematically two of these spiny neurons receiving excitatory input from the cortex. Spiny neurons have collaterals that inhibit each other and give rise to an inhibitory feedback network entirely within the neostriatum. This local feedback network mediates a competitive pattern classification

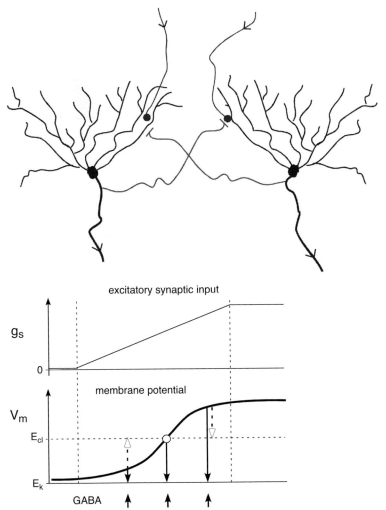

excitatory synaptic input

g_s

0

membrane potential

V_m

E_{cl}

E_k

GABA

Figure 10.8 Competitive pattern classification between spiny neurons in the neostriatum.
(a) Illustration of dendrites (above), soma, and projection axons (below) of two spiny neurons.
Two synaptic inputs from the cerebral cortex are shown. Two inhibitory collaterals are shown in
the middle. Note that one collateral inhibits a dendrite directly to mediate postsynaptic inhibition,
whereas the other one inhibits a presynaptic terminal to mediate presynaptic inhibition.
(b) Schematic illustration of why competition mediated by presynaptic inhibition is more
effective than competition mediated by postsynaptic inhibition. The time plots show net
excitatory synaptic input (g_s) from cortex (top) and membrane potential (V_m) of a spiny neuron
(bottom) as the cortical input slowly increases (between the two vertical dashed lines). In the
absence of synaptic input, V_m is near the potassium equilibrium potential E_K. As synaptic input
g_s increases, V_m moves in the positive direction in a sigmoidal fashion (typical of a down-state to
up-state transition). The arrows at the bottom indicate times of GABA release from inhibitory
collaterals. Open and dashed arrows illustrate how postsynaptic inhibition actually depolarises
(excites) spiny neurons that are in the down state and only mediates shunting inhibition when V_m
is at the chloride equilibrium potential E_{Cl}. Closed and solid arrows show that presynaptic
inhibition always decreases membrane potential (inhibits) and therefore is qualitatively more
effective than postsynaptic inhibition. Taken from Houk *et al.* (2007).

operation. Collateral inhibition is deemed an effective mechanism for competition by some authors (Plenz, 2003) and ineffective by others, the latter believing that feedforward inhibition regulates the pattern classification operation (Tepper *et al.*, 2004). Beiser and Houk (1998) modelled both mechanisms and found that both worked, but the inhibitory feedback network worked more effectively than the feedforward network.

What had not been considered before the report by Houk *et al.* (2007) is the possibility that the inhibitory feedback network relies on presynaptic, as opposed to postsynaptic, inhibition. This is surprising since presynaptic inhibition of cortical input to the neostriatum has been demonstrated electrophysiologically (Calabresi *et al.*, 1991; Nisenbaum *et al.*, 1993) and morphologically (Lacey *et al.*, 2005). Indeed, the operation of a presynaptic mechanism for collateral inhibition could also explain the mysterious fMRI BOLD deactivation that we found in caudate for the Decode contrast (Figure 10.7). Synaptic input is believed to be a strong contributor to BOLD signals (Arbib *et al.*, 2000; Logothetis, 2002). Since presynaptic inhibition would decrease synaptic input, that could explain the deactivation for the caudate. The activation seen for putamen presumably results from a greater dependence on postsynaptic inhibition.

10.3.4   Model of competitive pattern classification

Presynaptic inhibition should give rise to a computationally powerful mechanism for pattern classification. Beiser and Houk (1998) found that, since the equilibrium potential for postsynaptic GABAergic inhibition (E_{Cl} in Figure 10.8b) is between the down and up state of spiny neurons, this mechanism for mediating competition between neighbouring spiny neurons is quite sensitive to spontaneous membrane potential and to model parameters. It performed better than feedforward inhibition, but it was not optimal. Presynaptic inhibition has no equilibrium potential – it just reduces the synaptic input regardless of the membrane potential of the spiny neuron (Figure 10.8b). This presynaptic advantage reflects a qualitative principled effect that should be robust to parameter selection.

In Houk *et al.* (2007) we modelled a minimal network of recurrent loops from cortex through basal ganglia and back to cortex that encodes the serial order of two visual cues, A and B (Figure 10.9). The reader is referred to the 'Implementation details' posted in the Electronic Appendix of that article. Recurrent loops in the direct pathway through the prefrontal (PF) cortex, caudate (CD) nucleus, GPi, and thalamus (T) were used to encode two visual cues, A and B. Computational units AB and BA are labelled for the sequence they respond to best, whereas Ax (Bx) is activated by A (B) independent of its serial order. Prefrontal cortex projections are excitatory, with synaptic weights represented by dot sizes. Caudate spiny units are interconnected by inhibitory collaterals to form a competitive network. Via their projections, CD units are inhibitory to GPi units. The high spontaneous activity of GPi units provides a tonic inhibitory background to the thalamus, and inhibition of this background activity provokes a disinhibition of thalamic units. Rebound activity of thalamic units starts positive feedback and sustained activity in the reciprocal excitatory pathway between the thalamus and cortex. This would initiate activity in the loop through CB but that additional feature was not included in the present model.

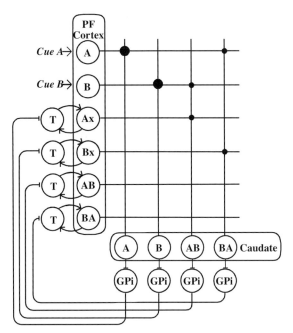

Figure 10.9 Serial order encoding network. Recurrent loops in the direct pathway through the prefrontal (PF) cortex, caudate (CD) nucleus, globus pallidus pars internus (GPi), and thalamus (T) are used to encode two visual cues, A and B. Computational units AB and BA are labelled for the sequence they respond to best; Ax (Bx) is activated by A (B) independent of its serial order. Prefrontal cortex projections are excitatory, with synaptic weights represented by dot sizes. Caudate spiny units are interconnected by inhibitory collaterals to form a competitive pattern classification network. Caudate units are inhibitory to GPi units, which in turn inhibit thalamic units. This disinhibition activates thalamic units and interconnected PF cortex units. The loop is completed by reciprocal excitatory connections between the thalamus and cortex, which are responsible for the model's working memory. The loop performs a recursion-like operation. Taken from Houk *et al.* (2007).

Medium spiny neurons were simulated (Houk *et al.*, 2007) using a minimal biophysical model (Gruber *et al.*, 2003) to which we added excitatory and postsynaptic inhibitory conductance inputs. Presynaptic inhibition was modelled by dynamically decreasing the excitatory synaptic weights of the input from the PF cortex. The GPi–T–PF loop was abstractly modelled based upon the Beiser and Houk model (1998) with a sigmoidal function to transform membrane potentials into firing rates. The network was instantiated using either no inhibition, presynaptic inhibition, or postsynaptic inhibition in the caudate, and the model was then subjected to noise.

Presynaptic inhibition yielded improved noise tolerance and decreased energy requirements compared with postsynaptic inhibition. When the network was subjected to noisy inputs, the misclassification rate without inhibition was 54.6% but fell to 24.1% for postsynaptic inhibition and 19.4% for presynaptic inhibition (a 4.8% decrease with presynaptic versus postsynaptic inhibition, $p < 0.001$). Presynaptic inhibition also decreased the summed magnitude of synaptic activity in caudate from 118 to 98 (a difference of

−16.9%, p < 0.001). The decreased excitatory synaptic activity in the presence of presynaptic inhibition can account for the reduced fMRI BOLD signal seen in caudate during the decoding contrast (Figure 10.7). In summary, presynaptic inhibition yields improved pattern classification while also explaining the puzzling decrease in fMRI BOLD.

10.3.5   Pattern classification in phylogeny

Complex social relations, intelligence, and language depend critically on the brain's capacity for serial order processing. Lashley (1951) postulated that the brain analyses and controls serial order by creating and using a spatial pattern of neural activity, which he equated to a thought. The execution of sequential actions based on a thought requires translation of spatial patterns into a sequence of actions in the time domain. The translation process is analogous to the application of syntax in language.

Even relatively simple thoughts, such as the working memory of a target sequence in the Replicate task, require that quite complicated spatial patterns be encoded. In the 3×3 task studied behaviourally in a monkey with K = 3 or 4 items, there are 336 or 1680 possible sequences. In the task that was imaged, 4×4 Replicate with K = 3 items, there are 3360 possible sequences. The 5×5 task that was studied behaviourally in humans requires more than 5 million spatial patterns for 5 item sequences, which approximates the spatial working memory capacity of human subjects.

The pattern classification operation in the DPM model (Figure 10.1) faces an incredibly difficult task. It needs to classify up to 5 million different spatial patterns of cortical activity. Although our simulation model greatly simplified the complexity of the task, it clearly demonstrated that pattern classification profits from competition mediated by collateral inhibition between spiny neurons. The simulation also demonstrated that performance is superior when competition is mediated by presynaptic inhibition as opposed to postsynaptic inhibition.

Furthermore, these simulation results offered an explanation for a puzzling imaging result. The decrease in BOLD seen in the caudate indicated that decreased synaptic activity occurred under conditions when caudate neurons were actively engaged in the decoding operation. This was explained by using presynaptic inhibition to mediate competitive pattern classification in the model. But why instead was an increase in BOLD observed in the putamen in association with execution? We believe this observation relates to phylogeny. The DPM that operates on working memories via a loop from dorsolateral prefrontal cortex (dl-PFC) through the caudate nucleus (Kelly and Strick, 2004) is phylogenetically newer than the loop through the putamen to and from primary motor cortex (the M1-DPM). Preuss (1995) reviewed the phylogeny of prefrontal cortex and concluded that this frontal region is likely to be unique to primates; for an update of this discussion, see Wise (2008). The phylogenetically older M1-DPM generates the voluntary motor commands that control each individual movement whether or not it belongs to a sequence.

This phylogenetic hypothesis fits well with our simulation finding that performance is superior when competition is mediated by presynaptic inhibition as opposed to postsynaptic inhibition. Since presynaptic inhibition in the striatum is mediated by GABAb receptors, it is quite relevant that GABAb receptor binding sites are found at an extremely high density in the caudate nucleus of the monkey (Bowery *et al.*, 1999), but in unremarkable density in the rat (Bowery *et al.*, 1987). This combined morphological evidence from the same laboratory supports the hypothesis that a predominance of presynaptic inhibition of cortical input to the neostriatum is phylogenetically more recent than is a predominance of postsynaptic inhibition. The above logic fits well with our contention that presynaptic inhibition is favoured in the phylogenetically newer loop between dl-PFC and caudate, as opposed to postsynaptic inhibition in the loop between M1 and putamen. Furthermore, this can explain why we found a BOLD deactivation in the caudate associated with decoding along with a BOLD activation in putamen associated with execution.

In summary, we postulate that a superior mechanism for competitive pattern classification in the striatum evolved in primates, and that this adaptation is expressed late in ontogeny, shortly after the development of the BG loop with motor cortex. In Subsection 10.4.3.1 this concept is used to propose a potential phenotype of schizophrenia.

10.4   Discussion

The model of action selection presented in this chapter was motivated by the existence of powerful computational features in subcortical loops that interface with multiple areas of the cerebral cortex (Houk, 2005; Introduction). A given area of cerebral cortex together with its loops through BG and cerebellum CB form a DPM. The consistency of their neuronal architecture suggests that DPMs have generic signal processing functions. Our current model of these generic functions was enunciated in Section 10.2. In Section 10.3 we focused on an application of the DPM concept to the combined cognitive and motor problems faced by tasks that require serial order processing. The emphasis was on additional features in phylogenetically newer loops through BG. In the present section, an attempt is made to integrate and expand upon the concepts emphasised in the previous sections of this chapter. But first, a summary is in order.

A DPM's loop through BG is particularly important in action selection. The Coarse Selection stage shown on the left in Figure 10.1 relies on input from an elegant Pattern Classification operation that takes place in the striatal layer of a DPM's loop through BG. Computationally powerful pattern classification derives from several unique features of striatal medium spiny neurons (Houk, 2005). These features include: (1) a high convergence ratio (Kincaid *et al.*, 1998) that presents nearly 20 000 different cortical inputs to any given spiny neuron, (2) a three-factor learning rule that uses reward-predicting training signals from dopamine neurons to consolidate long-term potentiation (LTP) learning (Houk *et al.*, 1995), (3) a dopamine-mediated attentional neuromodulatory factor (Nicola *et al.*, 2000) that induces bistability and nonlinear amplification in spiny neurons (Gruber *et al.*, 2003), and (4) competition among spiny neurons mediated by presynaptic and postsynaptic collateral inhibition (Figure 10.8; Houk *et al.*, 2007; Plenz, 2003).

If the pattern classification stage is so elegant, why does this operation only result in a Coarse Selection? We believe this is because loops through BG have evolved to accommodate the most difficult choices vertebrates face in a natural setting (cf. Prescott, 2005). Natural settings pose truly a multitude of options that depend on intricate motivations as well as on complex planning of strategies. There are so many different things that one could decide to do, a further narrowing down of possibilities needs to be made in loops through the CB. It is true that most experiments are not designed to explore many different options. For example, the Go/No Go choice, which has been used to great advantage in many studies of the BG (see Chapters 12 and 15), is a very simple decision. In our studies of fast and accurate movements (Section 10.2), we were fortunate to have the inherent noise of the motor system create the necessity of options for a multitude of submovement possibilities in each direction of motion. This evidently brought out the need for assistance from the loop through CB in the final choice, deciding which microscopic modules, and how much of each for how long, to use. These results suggest that the loop through BG can express its coarse selection as a crude basin of attraction in the loop between motor cortex and cerebellar nucleus. The cerebellar cortex then selects precise fixed points for that attractor basin in order to make the ultimate decision more accurately. Such shared decision making appears to be an elegant hardware solution to the immense difficulty of tasks in a natural setting. Note that many tasks designed for experimental work may not pose sufficient challenge to demonstrably engage the CB stage of action selection and refinement.

The issues addressed in Section 10.3 of this chapter challenged action selection in a different manner. The emphasis was not upon precision of action, but rather on the neuroscientific mechanisms that mediate competitive pattern classification in the striatum. Presynaptic inhibition was found to be more effective than postsynaptic inhibition for pattern classification. The results also led to the hypothesis that one or more genetic mutations in primates promoted presynaptic inhibition in the BG loops that interface with the prefrontal cortex (Section 10.3.5). These loops would then be better able to tackle complex tasks that often require serial order processing. Ohta and Gunji (2006) documented superior computational capabilities when the architecture of a simple recurrent network included presynaptic inhibition.

10.4.1   Serial order processing, basal ganglia loops and recursion

Beiser and Houk (1998) used a neurobiologically realistic model of the loop between dl-PFC and BG to study serial order processing computationally. They concluded that the model's capacity for encoding the serial order of events (whether sensory, motor or cognitive) results from three computational features that combine in a cooperative manner: (1) pattern classification within the caudate nucleus of the striatum, (2) working memory of the outcome of pattern classification, (3) a recursion-like operation brought about because the BG loop deposits the working memory of prior classifications into an updated input vector to the caudate from dl-PFC. The updated vector represents not only current events but also events that occurred in the past, which function as temporal context. Whereas earlier in this chapter we focused on feature (1), the mechanism for pattern classification in the striatum, this section focuses on feature (3), the mathematical operation called recursion. Note that the recursion-like operation that is implemented by a single DPM is limited by feature (2), namely the working memory capacity of a single module, which has been estimated as $\sim 7 \pm 2$ (Miller, 1956).

Speaking more generally, Chomsky and his colleagues (Hauser *et al.*, 2002) consider recursion as a very powerful computational operation that underlies the rich, expressive, and open-ended power of human language (also see Elman, 2004). The recursion-like operation in a DPM can be defined as an ability to use the results of one pattern classification operation to update the spatial pattern that provides the input for the next pattern classification operation. This property gives each cortical–basal ganglionic loop the capacity for serial order processing using a recursion-like operation. However, this example does not include all of the properties of recursion.

What property of mathematical recursion does a DPM lack? According to the computational view, recursion is a method of defining functions in which the function being defined is used within its own definition. Computing such a function can be done through the use of subroutines that call themselves. As pointed out in Houk (2005), the capacity to execute the same sequence of computational steps appears to be reproduced about a hundred times across the cerebral cortex, once in each DPM. The ability to hold a computational result in working memory while calling upon, through cortical–cortical connectivity, another DPM to perform a different computation and report back, is quite analogous to a subroutine call. An example discussed further in Houk (2005) is the decoding of a serial order working memory into a sequence of individual movements during serial order recall. Think of this as analogous to the translation of a thought into a sequence of words (a phrase or a sentence), or as phonological processing. (Note that the rhyming task we analysed in Booth *et al.* (2007) engaged loops through BG and CB, even though the task was a simple choice decision that did not require recursion.) To summarise the above discussion, arrays of DPMs appear to be well suited to doing limited recursion using their generic signal processing operations.

Now let us review some neuroscientific issues. As discussed above, anatomically demonstrated projections that loop back to the same area of cortex from which they derive (Kelly and Strick, 2004) allow individual cortical–basal ganglionic modules to perform a recursion-like operation (Beiser and Houk, 1998). Presynaptic inhibition probably improves this operation both in phylogeny and in ontogeny (Section 10.3.5). Next consider that long-term memories of serial order could be stored in cortico-cortical synapses or in the synapses between cortical neurons and striatal spiny neurons. The latter storage mechanism is thought to have a larger memory capacity for salient information (Houk and Wise, 1995). Furthermore, the recall from a large repertoire of previously learned sequences stored in cortico-striatal synapses should also be efficient because cortical–basal ganglionic modules implement parallel searches through a vast repertoire of past experiences stored in the synapses of spiny neurons. Although a storage site in cortico-cortical synapses is thought to have a smaller memory capacity, its advantage is that after long periods of practice it can consolidate a motor memory that allows exceptionally rapid and accurate responses (Matsuzaka *et al.*, 2007). However, the memory consolidated is a specialised computation, as opposed to the generic one implemented by a DPM. Note also that the affordance competition ideas discussed by Cisek in Chapter 11 are likely to apply to these consolidated cortical memories.

The important points in this section are that (1) individual DPMs have a simple recursion-like capability that is limited by its working memory capacity, and (2) a network of DPMs is capable of performing better versions of recursion, limited by the number of DPMs in the brain. Given the large expansion of the cerebral cortex and its associated DPMs during human evolution, these ideas may help to explain *universal grammar* (Hauser *et al.*, 2002) as an emergent property of large arrays of DPMs. A DPM-based model of language needs to be developed to test this idea.

10.4.2   Networks of DPMs and agent-based modelling

A DPM can be thought of as an agent with its own properties and actions. This is useful because the cerebral network as a whole can then be considered as a multi-agent system. Each DPM would receive different inputs and thus compute different outputs, even though the information processing operations of all of the agents would be the same. Agent-based modelling (ABM) could then be used to systematically test the collective effects of individual action selection operations. The power of this method is the topic of Bryson *et al.*'s chapter in this book. The authors state that an ABM's utility to science should be measured (1) by its explanatory ability and (2) by its ability to improve itself.

We have already seen that the DPM architecture explains many features of the neuroscience of movement and serial order processing. Interestingly, this modular architecture also explains an important scaling feature of brain anatomy. In Section 10.2.4, it was pointed out that the M1-DPM is comprised of an array of microscopic modules that individually have essentially the same computational architecture as the entire M1-DPM module. Here we use the term 'mesoscopic' to denote the DPM scale of modularity. Somewhat like Freeman (2000), by this term we mean a larger scale than microscopic. The real-world case of a choice among some very large number N of alternative microscopic modules and elemental motor commands could be accommodated by utilising a mesoscopic network of N microscopic modules in the reciprocity model. We have already explored a network of eight modules and found it capable of making realistic planar movements (Wang, Dam, *et al.*, 2008), which is not trivial because it solves a classic problem in motor control called the redundancy problem. We used more microscopic modules than actually needed to move in 2D space.

In Section 10.2, we noted that the prior and the likelihood in Bayesian models of decision theory (see Berniker *et al.*, this volume) map quite well onto the two main factors of the normalised predictive error (NPE) model. Each (mesoscopic) module in the DPM architecture may thus be considered a neurobiological implementation of a Bayesian decision-making agent. Each such decision maker receives uncertain information and makes decisions based on local rules. Conceptualising the brain as a network of DPM agents, one might systematically compare behaviour and neural activities assuming the interplay of coupled Bayesian agents. This approach promises to reveal interesting links between normative models which ask how computations could be performed optimally and implementational models which ask how interactions across loops in DPM agents give rise to efficient motor behaviour.

A natural way to test the explanatory ability of the DPM-as-an-agent concept is to explore the ability of a small network of DPMs to interact with an apparatus (the ABM's environment) to perform the Replicate task. A starting hypothesis might be that three DPMs are sufficient to perform the task. One would be needed to encode the serial order of successive visual stimuli into a distributed working memory of target sequence (resembling a thought in the psychological sense). A second would be needed to compute a motor plan by successively decoding the working memory into a specification of the next movement in the sequence (Fraser *et al.*, 2008). A third DPM would be needed to generate the set of motor commands that execute any given action, the key-presses. The latter vector should mimic the spatiotemporal dynamics of voluntary motor commands in M1, the primary motor cortex (Georgopoulos, 1995).

The whole brain functional imaging results described in Section 10.3.2 and in Fraser *et al.* (2008) reveal a large network of brain areas, larger than the hypothetical network of DPMs suggested above. An ABM model would be a good way to explore the dynamics and parameter spaces that give rise to optimal solutions.

We have also demonstrated that the DPM concept is capable of improving itself. Section 10.3 described a mysterious BOLD decrease and explained it as a mutation in primates that favoured a presynaptic mechanism for competitive pattern classification in the striatum. There is ample room in this agent-based model for additional improvements, which should be greatly facilitated by the inherent linkages of the DPM framework to cellular, molecular, and systems-level neuroscience.

10.4.3   Understanding action selection deficits in brain disorders

Neurological and psychiatric disorders often impair our capacity for action selection. Computational models of these decision-making processes offer a useful approach for investigating the etiology of a particular disease and for exploring potential treatments of the deficits. To facilitate this, it is helpful if the model is capable of bridging from molecular processes to cellular neurophysiology to systems neurophysiology to behaviour. This was one of the motivations for developing the DPM model of mind agents (Houk, 2005).

In Chapter 15, Frank and colleagues make good use of computational models to relate Parkinson's disease and attention deficit hyperactivity disorders (ADHD) to action selection deficits in a diverse range of tasks. Since serial order processing challenges the capacity for action selection, one additional task worth consideration is the serial order recall task Replicate that was described in Section 10.3 of the present chapter. Subjects are asked to recall sequences of K spatial targets in the same order in which they are presented. Patients suffering from schizophrenia show prominent deficits: whereas normal subjects have no difficulty recalling K = 1–4 targets, patients make huge errors for K = 3 or 4 (Fraser *et al.*, 2004). Based on the Beiser–Houk (1998) model of loops through BG, the authors concluded that the deficit is likely to arise in the caudate nucleus, a BG site where spiny neurons compete with each other in action selection

(Figure 10.8a), as discussed in Section 10.3. In fact, the caudate nucleus does undergo a progressive deformation in schizophrenia patients (Wang, Mamah, *et al.*, 2008).

The model of competitive pattern classification presented in Section 10.3 might assist further analysis of these schizophrenia findings. Simulating normal subjects, we found that presynaptic inhibition, in addition to out-performing postsynaptic inhibition, also explained the mysterious decrease in BOLD signal in the caudate nucleus (Figure 10.7). If patients suffer from a deficit in presynaptic inhibition, the caudate BOLD decrease in the Decode contrast should be attenuated or even reversed. This prediction could be tested by imaging the Replicate task in schizophrenia patients.

10.4.3.1   A model of the etiology of schizophrenia

The above ideas and concepts promote inquiry concerning the origin of schizophrenia. A central paradox of schizophrenia is that a condition which is considered to be genetic in origin survives in the population in spite of a fecundity disadvantage. The magnitude of the latter is such that any genetic predisposition should be eliminated from the population within a few generations. Instead, since the incidence of schizophrenia remains steady at 1–2%, one can conclude that there is an accompanying genetic advantage (Huxley *et al.*, 1964). In analysing this issue, Kuttner *et al.* (1967) offered three advantageous functions that might accompany the inheritance of schizophrenia: (1) a capacity for complex social relations, (2) intelligence, and (3) language. Crow and colleagues have made a strong case for an evolutionary link between the origin of language and the etiology of schizophrenia (Berlim *et al.*, 2003; Crow, 1997). Their hypothesis is consistent with the prominent deficit in competitive pattern classification in schizophrenia mentioned above – language contains abundant examples of serial order processing.

Earlier we suggested that the presynaptic mechanism for competitive pattern classification in the striatum is defective in schizophrenia. Since $GABA_B$ receptors mediate presynaptic inhibition in the striatum, it is reasonable to search the literature for genetic evidence relevant to this hypothesis. In fact, there is a modified expression of the $GABA_B$ receptor in schizophrenia (Enna and Bowery, 2004). This implicates the modified $GABA_BR1$ gene on chromosome 6p21.3 (Martin *et al.*, 2001) as a major contributor to schizophrenia. It is interesting that Matthysse *et al.* (2004) reported a linkage of eye tracking disorder, one of the best known traits associated with schizophrenia, to 6p21.1, which is very close to the locus for $GABA_BR1$ (*GABBR1*).

Since the inheritance of schizophrenia is multigenic (Freedman *et al.*, 2001), the gene identified by Freedman, Leonard and collaborators (*CHRNA7*) is also strongly implicated, a gene that codes the expression of the alpha-7 nicotinic receptor. This receptor is prevalent in many of the loops between the cerebral cortex and the cerebellar nuclei (Breese *et al.*, 1997). Altered transmission in these loops is thought to contribute to the cognitive dysmetria of schizophrenia (Andreasen, 1999).

How can the model presented here help us to understand the survival of genes responsible for schizophrenia? Our model suggests that superior action selection in the Replicate task results from competitive pattern classification mediated by presynaptic, as opposed to postsynaptic, inhibition of excitatory input to the neostriatum from the cerebral cortex. Based on the above, it seems reasonable to postulate that presynaptic inhibition in the caudate nucleus depends on GABBR1. This could explain the genetic advantage. However, schizophrenia patients apparently suffer from defective pattern classification in caudate (Fraser *et al.*, 2004) – how could that happen? A genetic polymorphism in *GABBR1* with a minor allele frequency that reduces the strength of presynaptic inhibition in the striatum might explain why loss of reproductive fitness does not eliminate the disease (Crow's (1997) paradox). In Section 10.3.5, we suggested that the mechanism for competition in the striatum evolved in primates from mainly postsynaptic inhibition to mainly presynaptic inhibition, and that this mutation is expressed late in ontogeny, shortly after the development of the BG loop with motor cortex. If the mutation that fortified *GABBR1* occurred in primates, the genetic polymorphism mentioned above could explain Crow's paradox.

Maternal immune activation also increases the risk for schizophrenia (Patterson, 2007). Anti-IL-6 injection in pregnant mice causes schizophrenia-like deficits in adult offspring. The cytokine interleukin-6 (IL-6) is critical for mediating both behavioural and transcriptional changes in the offspring (Smith *et al.*, 2007). How might immune activation combine with specific models of genetic abnormalities in order to explain schizophrenia?

As mentioned earlier, the Freedman–Leonard model posits a genetic variation that affects alpha7-nicotinic receptor function. This variation is present in several families at risk for schizophrenia (Martin *et al.*, 2001) and is linked to impaired prepulse inhibition (PPI) of auditory responses in schizophrenia. In rats, Borrell *et al.* (2002) demonstrated that prenatal immune challenge induces PPI deficit, and that the deficit occurs later in life, mimicking patient findings. Furthermore, female rats manifest this disruption somewhat later than male rats, which also resembles the known sex differences in human patients. They attributed the deficits to abnormalities in BG where cellular changes were found, for example, in the nucleus accumbens.

We suggest instead, or in addition, that impaired PPI could be a failure in the motor system's link to and from the cerebellum. Results from the Patterson laboratory show that maternal immune activation causes a loss of Purkinje cells in the CB (Shi *et al.*, 2009). Results from the Mugnaini laboratory show similar anomalies produced by administration to pregnant dams of drugs interfering with DNA synthesis (Sekerkova *et al.*, 2004). These interventions interfere with gene activation and silencing programs at embryonic days coinciding with peak production of Purkinje cells. The loss and displacement of cerebellar Purkinje cells during development is a marker for the malfunction of a potent inhibitory circuit that includes cerebellar nucleus and numerous motor nuclei. Thus, subcortical loops through CB could mediate PPI and might underlie its deficit in schizophrenia.

We have recently noted (Houk *et al.*, 2009) that other *GABA* receptor genes are located only 5–6 megabases centromeric to *CHRNA7* and mapped within the linkage. This locus contains an imprinted cluster of genes including *GABRB3* and *GABRA5* (Stefan *et al.*, 2005), which are highly expressed in hippocampus and amygdala of mice (Lein *et al.*, 2006). *GABRB3* is paternally imprinted but its maternal allelic expression could be increased in response to maternal infection, making it a potential epigenetic–genetic candidate gene for schizophrenia. Prominent interconnections exist between hippocampus and CB that could be part of an arousal reaction representing an emotional response (Newman and Reza, 1979). Hyperactivity of this loop because of Purkinje cell abnormalities during development, perhaps augmented by hippocampal GABA abnormalities, might help to explain the positive signs of schizophrenia.

The overall hypothesis proposed here is that genetic variations in GABA and alpha7-nicotinic receptors combined with maternal immune activation could explain the occurrence of schizophrenia in some families. We further hypothesise that the occurrences of schizophrenia in other families may be related to deficits in the same subcortical neural circuitry caused by alternative genetic variations that interfere with these circuit functions. A DPM model that included loops through hippocampus might elucidate underlying mechanisms. For perspective, the reader is referred to a recent thoughtful review of the neurobiology of mental health (Siddique, 2007).

10.5   Summary

We posit that both on-line error correction and serial order recall are prime examples of natural action selection. They appear to use analogous mechanisms for signal processing in their respective distributed processing modules (DPMs). Agent-based models comprised of networks of DPMs may provide a useful substrate for studying complex behaviours and for exploring the underlying dynamics of the mind. Such simulations might help us to understand the etiology and treatment of schizophrenia, Parkinson's disease, ADHD, and other psychiatric and neurological diseases.

Acknowledgements

This multimodal research was made possible by grants NS44837 and P01-NS44383 from the National Institute of Neurological Disorders and Stroke. We are grateful to numerous colleagues for providing many helpful comments and suggestions. Special thanks go to Steven Wise for thoroughly reviewing the entire manuscript, to Andrew Barto and Bob Scheidt for critical review of Section 10.2, to Konrad Körding for helpful comments on Section 10.4.2, and to Tony Prescott for suggestions throughout. Enrico Mugnaini provided extensive useful discussion of Section 10.4.3.

References

Andreasen, N.C. (1999). A unitary model of schizophrenia: Bleuler's 'fragmented phrene' as schizencephaly. *Arch. Gen. Psychiatry* **56**: 781–7.

Arbib, M. A., A. Billard, M. Iacoboni, and E. Oztop (2000). Synthetic brain imaging: grasping, mirror neurons and imitation. *Neural. Netw.* **13**(8–9): 975–97.

Barringer, C., A. G. Barto, and J. C. Houk (2008). Simulated reaching supports the Normalized Predicted Error (NPE) discrete control hypothesis for on-line error correction of voluntary movements. *Society for Neuroscience.* November 2008, Washington DC.

Barto, A.G., A. H. Fagg, N. Sitkoff, and J. C. Houk (1999). A cerebellar model of timing and prediction in the control of reaching. *Neural Comput.* **11**: 565–594.

Beiser, D. G. and J. C. Houk (1998). Model of cortical-basal ganglionic processing: encoding the serial order of sensory events. *J. Neurophysiol.* **79**: 3168–88.

Berlim, M. T., B. S. Mattevi, P. Belmonte-de-Abreu, and T. J. Crow (2003). The etiology of schizophrenia and the origin of language: Overview of a theory. *Compr. Psychiat.* **44**: 7–14.

Berthier, N. E., S. P. Singh, A. G. Barto, and J. C. Houk (1993). Distributed representation of limb motor programs in arrays of adjustable pattern generators. *J. Cogn. Neurosci.* **5**: 56–78.

Bhushan, N. and R. Shadmehr (1999). Evidence for a forward dynamics model in human adaptive motor control. *In Advances in Neural Processing Systems*, Vol. 11, ed. M. S. Kearns, S. A. Solla, and D. A. Cohn. Cambridge, MA: MIT Press, pp. 3–9.

Bliss T. V. P. and G. L. Collingridge (1993). A synaptic model of memory: long-term potentiation in the hippocampus. *Nature* **361**: 31–9.

Booth, J. R., L. Wood, D. Lu, J. C. Houk, and T. Bitan (2007). The role of the basal ganglia and cerebellum in language processing. *Brain Res.* **1133**(1): 136–44.

Borrell, J., J. M. Vela, A. Arevalo-Martin, E. Molina-Holgado, and C. Guaza (2002). Prenatal immune challenge disrupts sensorimotor gating in adult rats. Implications for the etiopathogenesis of schizophrenia. *Neuropsychopharmacology* **26**(2): 204–15.

Botvinick, M. M. and D. C. Plaut (2006). Short-term memory for serial order: a recurrent neural network model. *Psychol. Rev.* **113**: 201–33.

Botvinick, M. M., J. Wang, E. Cowan, *et al.* (2009). An analysis of immediate serial recall performance in a Macaque. *Anim. Cogn. doi* **10**: 1007/s10071–009–0226.

Bowery, N. G., A. L. Hudson, and G. W. Price (1987). GABAA and GABAB receptor site distribution in the rat central nervous system. *Neuroscience* **20**(2): 365–83.

Bowery, N. G., K. Parry, G. Goodrich, I. Illinsky, and K. Kultas-Illinsky (1999). Distribution of GABA(B) binding sites in the thalamus and basal ganglia of the rhesus monkey (*Macaca mulatta*). *Neuropharmacology* **38**(11): 1675–82.

Brasted, P. J. and S. P. Wise (2004). Comparison of learning-related neuronal activity in the dorsal premotor cortex and striatum. *Eur. J. Neurosci.* **19**: 721–40.

Breese, C. R., C. Adams, J. Logel, *et al.* (1997). Comparison of the regional expression of nicotinic acetylcholine receptor α7 mRNA and [125I]-α-Bungarotoxin binding in human postmortem brain. *J. Comp. Neurol.* **387**: 385–398.

Calabresi, P., N. B. Mercuri, M. DeMurtas, and G. Bernardi (1991). Involvement of GABA systems in feedback regulation of glutamate- and GABA-mediated synaptic potentials in rat neostriatum. *J. Physiol.* **440**: 581–99.

Carelli, R. M., M. Wolske, and M. O. West (1997). Loss of lever press-related firing of rat striatal forelimb neurons after repeated sessions in a lever pressing task. *J. Neurosci.* **17**(5): 1804–14.

Crow, T. J. (1997). Is schizophrenia the price that *Homo sapiens* pays for language? *Schizophr. Res.* **28**(2–3): 127–41.

Doya, K. (1999). What are the computations of the cerebellum, the basal ganglia and the cerebral cortex? *Neural Networks* **12**: 961–74.

Elman, J. L. (2004). An alternative view of the mental lexicon. *Trends Cogn. Sci.* **8**: 301–306.

Enna, S. J. and N. G. Bowery (2004). GABAb receptor alterations as indicators of physiological and pharmacological function. *Biochem. Pharma.* **68**: 1541–8.

Felleman, D. J. and D. C. Van Essen (1991). Distributed hierarchical processing in the primate cerebral cortex. *Cereb. Cortex* **1**(1): 1–47.

Fishbach, A., S. A. Roy, C. Bastianen, L. E. Miller, and J. C. Houk (2005). Kinematic properties of on-line error corrections in the monkey. *Exp. Br. Res.* **164**: 442–57.

Fishbach, A., S. A. Roy, C. Bastianen, L. E. Miller, and J. C. Houk (2007). Deciding when and how to correct a movement: discrete submovements as a decision making process. *Exp. Br. Res.* **177**: 45–63.

Frank, M. J. (2005). Dynamic dopamine modulation in the basal ganglia: a neurocomputational account of cognitive deficits in medicated and nonmedicated Parkinsonism. *J. Cogn. Neurosci.* **17**: 51–72.

Fraser, D., S. Park, G. Clark, D. Yohanna, and J. C. Houk (2004). Spatial serial order processing in schizophrenia. *Schizophr. Res.* **70**(2–3): 203–13.

Fraser D., P. Reber, T. Parrish, *et al.* (2008). Cortical neural correlates of serial order recall: cognitive and motor decoding. *Society for Neuroscience 38th Annual Meeting*, November 2008, program ID# 484.28

Freedman, R., S. Leonard, A. Oliney, *et al.* (2001). Evidence for the multigenic inheritance of schizophrenia. *Am. J. Med. Gen.* **105**: 794–800.

Freeman, W. J. (2000). Mesoscopic neurodynamics: from neuron to brain. *J. Physiol. Paris* **94**(5–6): 303–22.

Gdowski, M. J., L. E. Miller, C. Bastianen, E. K. Nenonene, and J. C. Houk (2007). Signaling patterns of globus pallidus internal segment neurons during forearm rotation. *Brain Res.* **1155**: 56–69.

Georgopoulos, A. P. (1995). Motor cortex and cognitive processing. In *The Cognitive Neurosciences*, ed. M. S. Gazzaniga. Cambridge, MA: MIT Press, pp 507–517.

Gibson, A. R., J. C. Houk, and N. J. Kohlerman (1985). Relation between red nucleus discharge and movement parameters in trained macaque monkeys. *J. Physiol. (Lond.)* **358**: 551.

Gruber, A. J., S. A. Solla, D. J. Surmeier, and J. C. Houk (2003). Modulation of striatal single units by expected reward: a spiny neuron model displaying dopamine-induced bistability. *J. Neurophys.* **90**: 1095–114.

Gurney, K., T. J. Prescott, and P. Redgrave (2001). A computational model of action selection in the basal ganglia. I. A new functional anatomy. *Biol. Cybern.* **84**: 401–410.

Gusnard, D. A. and M. E. Raichle (2001) Searching for a baseline: functional imaging and the resting human brain. *Nature Rev. Neurosci.* **2**: 685–94.

Hauser, M. D., N. Chomsky, and W. T. Fitch (2002). The faculty of language: what it is, who has it, and how did it evolve. *Science* **298**: 1569–79.

Holdefer, R. N., J. C. Houk, and L. E. Miller (2005). Movement-related discharge in the cerebellar nuclei persists after local injections of GABA-A antagonists. *J. Neurophysiol.* **93**(1): 35–43.

Houk, J. C. (2001). Neurophysiology of frontal-subcortical loops. In *Frontal-Subcortical Circuits in Psychiatry and Neurology*, ed. D. G. Lichter and J. L. Cummings. New York: Guilford Publications, pp. 92–113.

Houk, J. C. (2005). Agents of the mind. *Biol. Cybern.* **92**: 427–37.

Houk J. C. (2007). Models of basal ganglia. *Scholarpedia*, p.22663. Available at http://www.scholarpedia.org/article/Models_of_Basal_Ganglia.

Houk, J. C. (2010). Voluntary movement: control, learning and memory. In *Encyclopedia of Behavioral Neuroscience*, ed. G. F. Koob, M. Le Moal, and R. F. Thompson. Oxford: Academic Press, pp. 455–8.

Houk, J. C., J. L. Adams, and A. G. Barto (1995). A model of how the basal ganglia generates and uses neural signals that predict reinforcement. In *Models of Information Processing in the Basal Ganglia*, ed. J. C. Houk, J. L. Davis, and D. G. Beiser. Cambridge, MA: MIT Press, pp. 249–74.

Houk, J. C., C. Bastianen, D. Fansler, *et al.* (2007). Action selection in subcortical loops through the basal ganglia and cerebellum. *Phil. Trans. R. Soc. B.* **362**: 1573–83.

Houk, J. C., A. H. Fagg, and A. G. Barto (2002). Fractional power damping model of joint motion. In *Progress in Motor Control: Structure–Function Relations in Voluntary Movements*, Vol. 2, ed. C. A. Wrisberg and M. Latash. Champaign, IL: Human Kinetics, pp. 147–78.

Houk, J. C., J. Keifer, and A. G. Barto (1993). Distributed motor commands in the limb premotor network. *Trends Neurosci.* **16**: 27–33.

Houk, J. C. and E. Mugnaini (2003). Cerebellum. In *Fundamental Neuroscience*, ed. L. R. Squire *et al.* Oxford: Academic Press, pp. 841–72.

Houk J. C., E. Mugnaini, and E. Redei (2009). Maternal immune activation in combination with allelic variations of imprinted genes may explain the etiology of schizophrenia. *Soc. Neurosci. Abst.* #2009-S-17652-SfN (745.16).

Houk, J. C. and S. P. Wise (1995). Distributed modular architectures linking basal ganglia, cerebellum, and cerebral cortex: their role in planning and controlling action. *Cerebral Cortex* **5**: 95–110.

Hua S. E. and J. C. Houk (1997). Cerebellar guidance of premotor network development and sensorimotor learning. *Learn. Mem.* **4**: 63–76.

Huxley, J., E. Mayr, H. Osmond, and A. Hoffer (1964) Schizophrenia as a genetic morphism. *Nature* **204**: 220–1.

Karniel, A. and G. F. Inbar (1999). The use of a nonlinear muscle model in explaining the relationship between duration, amplitude, and peak velocity of human rapid movements. *J. Motor Behav.* **31**(3): 203–206.

Kawato, M., M. Katayama, H. Gomi, and Y. Koike (1992). Coordinated arm movements: Virtual trajectory control hypothesis and learning inverse models. *International Symposium on Information Sciences*, Iizuka Kyusyuu, Japan.

Kelly, R. M. and P. L. Strick (2003). Cerebellar loops with motor cortex and prefrontal cortex of a nonhuman primate. *J. Neurosci.* **23**: 8432–44.

Kelly, R. M. and P. L. Strick (2004). Macro-architecture of basal ganglia loops with the cerebral cortex: use of rabies virus to reveal multisynaptic circuits. *Prog. Brain Res.* **143**: 449–59.

Kincaid, A. E., T. Zheng, and C. J. Wilson (1998). Connectivity and convergence of single corticostriatal axons. *J. Neurosci.* **18**(12): 4722–31.

Koerding, K. (2007). Decision theory: what 'should' the nervous system do? *Science* **318**(5850): 606–10.

Kuttner, R. E., A. B. Lorincz, and D. A. Swan (1967). The schizophrenia gene and social evolution. *Psychol. Rep.* **20**: 407–12.

Lacey, C. J., J. Boyes, O. Gerlach, *et al.* (2005). GABAb receptors at glutamatergic synapses in the rat striatum. *Neuroscience* **136**: 1083–95.

Lashley, K. S. (1951). The problem of serial order in behavior. In *Cerebral Mechanisms in Behavior*, ed. L. A. Jeffres. New York: John Wiley and Sons, Inc., pp. 112–36.

Lein, E. S., M. J. Hawrylycz, N. Ao, *et al.* (2006). Genome-wide atlas of gene expression in the adult mouse brain. *Nature* **445**(7124): 168–76.

Logothetis, N. (2002). The neural basis of the blood-oxygen-level-dependent functional magnetic resonance imaging signal. *Phil. Trans. R. Soc. Lond. B* **357**: 1003–1037.

Lu, X., O. Hikosaka, and S. Miyachi (1998). Role of monkey cerebellar nuclei in skill for sequential movement. *J. Neurophysiol.* **79**: 2245–54.

Martin, S. C., S. J. Russek, and D. H. Farb (2001). Human GABAbR genomic structure: evidence for splice variants in GABAbR1 but not GABAbR2. *Gene* **278**: 63–79.

Matsuzaka, Y., N. Picard, and P. L. Strick (2007). Skill representation in the primary motor cortex after long-term practice. *J. Neurophysiol.* **97**(2): 1819–32.

Matthysse, S., P. S. Holzman, J. F. Gusella, *et al.* (2004). Linkage of eye movement dysfunction to chromosome 6p in schizophrenia: additional evidence. *Am. J. Med. Genet. B Neuropsychiatr. Genet.* **128**(1): 30–6.

Merzenich, M., B. Wright, W. Jenkins, *et al.* (1996). Cortical plasticity underlying perceptual, motor, and cognitive skill development: implications for neurorehabilitation. *Cold Spring Harb. Symp. Quant. Biol.* **61**: 1–8.

Miller, G. A. (1956). The magical number seven, plus or minus two: some limits to our capacity for processing information. *J. Exp. Psychol.* **41**: 329–35.

Newman, P. P. and H. Reza (1979). Functional relationships between the hippocampus and the cerebellum: an electrophysiological study of the cat. *J. Physiol.* **287**: 405–26.

Nicola, S. M., J. Surmeier, and R. C. Malenka (2000). Dopaminergic modulation of neuronal excitability in the striatum and nucleus accumbens. *Annu. Rev. Neurosci.* **23**: 185–215.

Nisenbaum, E. S., T. W. Berger, and A. A. Grace (1993). Depression of glutamatergic and GABAergic synaptic responses in striatal spiny neurons by stimulation of presynaptic GABA-B receptors. *Synapse* **14**(3): 221–42.

Novak, K. E. (2001). Neural control of discrete movement segments/the role of the cerebellum in the control and learning of movements. *Doctoral thesis in Biomedical Engineering*. Evanston, Northwestern University.

Novak K. E., L. E. Miller, and J. C. Houk (2000). Kinematic properties of rapid hand movements in knob turning task. *Exp. Brain Res.* **132**(4): 419–33.

Novak, K. E., L. E. Miller, and J. C. Houk (2002). The use of overlapping submovements in the control of rapid hand movements. *Exp. Brain Res.* **144**: 351–64.

Novak, K. E., L. E. Miller, and J. C. Houk (2003). Features of motor performance that drive adaptation in rapid hand movements. *Exp. Brain Res.* **148**: 388–400.

Ohta, H. and Y. P. Gunji (2006). Recurrent neural network architecture with pre-synaptic inhibition for incremental learning. *Neural Networks* **19**(8): 1106–19.

Pasupathy, A. and E. K. Miller (2005). Different time courses of learning-related activity in the prefrontal cortex and striatum. *Nature* **433**(7028): 873–6.

Patterson, P. H. (2007). Neuroscience. Maternal effects on schizophrenia risk. *Science* **318**(5850): 576–7.

Plenz, D. (2003). When inhibition goes incognito: feedback interaction between spiny projection neurons in striatal function. *TINS* **26**: 14427–32.

Prescott, T. J. (2005). Forced moves or good tricks in design space? Great moments in the evolution of the neural substrate for action selection. *Adapt. Behav.* **15**(1): 9–31.

Preuss, T. M. (1995). Do rats have prefrontal cortex? The Rose–Woolsey–Akert program reconsidered. *J. Cogn. Neurosci.* **7**(1): 1–24.

Raymond, J. L., S. G. Lisberger, and M. D. Mauk (1996). The cerebellum: a neuronal learning machine? *Science* **272**: 1126–31.

Redgrave, P., T. J. Prescott, and K. Gurney (1999). The basal ganglia: a vertebrate solution to the selection problem? *Neuroscience* **89**(4): 1009–23.

Roy, S. A., C. Bastianen, E. Nenonene, *et al.* (2003). Neural correlates of corrective submovement formation in the basal ganglia and motor cortex. *Society for the Neural Control of Movement Abstracts.*

Roy S., E. Tunik, C. Bastianen, *et al.* (2008). Firing patterns of GPi neurons associated with primary movements and corrective submovements. *Society for Neuroscience*, November 2008, Washington D.C.

Rubchinsky, L. L., N. Kopel, and K. A. Sigvardt (2003). Modeling facilitation and inhibition of competing motor programs in basal ganglia subthalamic nucleus–pallidal circuits. *PNAS* **100**: 14427–32.

Sekerkova, G., E. Ilijic, and E. Mugnaini (2004). Bromodeoxyuridine administered during neurogenesis of the projection neurons causes cerebellar defects in rat. *J. Comp. Neurol.* **470**(3): 221–39.

Shadmehr, R. and F. A. Mussa-Ivaldi (1994). Adaptive representation of dynamics during learning of a motor task. *J. Neurosci.* **14**(5 Pt 2): 3208–24.

Shi, L., S. E. Smith, N. Malkova, *et al.* (2009). Activation of the maternal immune system alters cerebellar development in the offspring. *Brain Behav. Immun.* **23**(1): 116–23.

Siddique, T. (2007). Neurobiology of mental health. *Pak. J. Neurol. Sci.* **2**(4): 230–4.

Smith, S. E., J. Li, K. Garbett, K. Mirnics, and P. H. Patterson (2007). Maternal immune activation alters fetal brain development through interleukin-6. *J. Neurosci.* **27**(40): 10695–702.

Smith, M. A. and R. Shadmehr (2005). Intact ability to learn internal models of arm dynamics in Huntington's disease but not cerebellar degeneration. *J. Neurophysiol.* **93**(5): 2809–21.

Stefan, M., K. C. Claiborn, E. Stasiek, *et al.* (2005). Genetic mapping of putative Chrna7 and Luzp2 neuronal transcriptional enhancers due to impact of a transgene-insertion and 6.8 Mb deletion in a mouse model of Prader–Willi and Angelman syndromes. *BMC Genomics* **6**: 157.

Sternad, D. and S. Schaal (1999). Segmentation of endpoint trajectories does not imply segmented control. *Exp. Brain Res.* **124**(1): 118–36.

Sutton, R. S. and A. G. Barto (1998). *Reinforcement Learning: An Introduction.* Cambridge, MA: MIT Press.

Tepper, J. M., T. Koos, and C. J. Wilson (2004). GABAergic microcircuits in the neostriatum. *Trends Neurosci.* **27**(11): 662–9.

Toni, I., J. Rowe, K. E. Stephan, and R. E. Passingham (2002). Changes of cortico-striatal effective connectivity during visuomotor learning. *Cerebral Cortex* **12**: 1040–1047.

Tunik, E., J. C. Houk, and S. T. Grafton (2009). Basal ganglia contribution to the initiation of corrective submovements. *Neuroimage* **47**: 1757–66.

Wang, J., G. Dam, S. Yildirim, *et al.* (2008). Reciprocity between the cerebellum and the cerebral cortex: nonlinear dynamics in microscopic modules for generating voluntary motor commands. *Complexity* **14**(2): 29–45.

Wang, L., D. Mamah, M. P. Harms, *et al.* (2008). Progressive deformation of deep brain nuclei and hippocampal-amygdala formation in schizophrenia. *Biol. Psychiatry* **64**(12): 1060–8.

Wise, S. P. (2008) Forward frontal fields: phylogeny and fundamental function. *Trends Neurosci.* **31**: 599–608.

Woodworth, R. S. (1899). The accuracy of voluntary movement. *Psychol. Rev.* **3**(2): 1–114.

11 Cortical mechanisms of action selection: the affordance competition hypothesis[1]

Paul Cisek

Summary

At every moment, the natural world presents animals with two fundamental pragmatic problems: selection between actions that are currently possible, and specification of the parameters or metrics of those actions. It is commonly suggested that the brain addresses these by first constructing representations of the world on which to build knowledge and make a decision, and then by computing and executing an action plan. However, neurophysiological data argues against this serial viewpoint. In contrast, it is proposed here that the brain processes sensory information to specify, in parallel, several potential actions that are currently available. These potential actions compete against each other for further processing, while information is collected to bias that competition until a single response is selected. The hypothesis suggests that the dorsal visual system specifies actions which compete against each other within the fronto-parietal cortex, while a variety of biasing influences are provided by prefrontal regions and the basal ganglia. A computational model is described which illustrates how that competition may take place in the cerebral cortex. Simulations of the model capture qualitative features of neurophysiological data and reproduce various behavioural phenomena.

11.1 Introduction

At every moment, the natural environment presents animals with many opportunities and demands for action. The presence of food offers an opportunity to satiate hunger, while the appearance of a predator demands caution or evasion. An animal cannot perform all of these behaviours at the same time because they often share the same effectors (you only have two hands; you can only transport yourself in one direction at a time, etc.). Thus, one fundamental issue faced by every behaving creature is the question of action *selection*. That question must be resolved, in part, by using external sensory

---

[1] This chapter is a new version of an earlier publication (Cisek, 2007) which appeared in *Philosophical Transactions of the Royal Society B*. The present version expands upon that earlier article with some discussion of recent experimental results.

Modelling Natural Action Selection, eds. Anil K. Seth, Tony J. Prescott and Joanna J. Bryson.
Published by Cambridge University Press. © Cambridge University Press 2012.

information about objects in the world, and in part, by using internal information about current behavioural needs.

Furthermore, the animal must tailor the actions it performs to the environment in which it is situated. Grasping a fruit requires accurate guidance of the hand to the location of the fruit, while evading a predator requires one to move in an unobstructed direction that leads away from the threat. The *specification* of the parameters of actions is a second fundamental issue faced by behaving creatures. Specification of actions also must use sensory information from the environment. In particular, it requires information about the spatial relationships among objects and surfaces in the world, represented in a coordinate frame relative to the orientation and configuration of the animal's body.

Traditional cognitive theories propose that these two questions are resolved in a serial manner, that we select 'what to do' before specifying 'how to do it'. According to this view, the perceptual system first collects sensory information to build an internal descriptive representation of objects in the external world (Marr, 1982). Next, this information is used along with representations of current needs and memories of past experience to make judgements and decide upon a course of action (Johnson-Laird, 1988; Newell and Simon, 1972; Shafir and Tversky, 1995). The resulting plan is then used to generate a desired trajectory for movement which is finally realised through muscular contraction (Keele, 1968; Miller *et al.*, 1960). In other words, the brain first builds knowledge about the world using representations which are independent of actions, and this knowledge is later used to make decisions, compute an action plan, and finally execute a movement.

However, studies of the cerebral cortex have encountered difficulties in interpreting neural activity in terms of distinct perceptual, cognitive, or motor systems. For example, visual processing diverges in the cortex into separate systems sensitive to object identity and spatial location (Ungerleider and Mishkin, 1982), with no single representation of the world (Stein, 1992), leading to the question of how these disparate systems are bound together to form a unified percept (Cisek and Turgeon, 1999; von der Malsburg, 1996). Cells in the posterior parietal cortex appear to reflect a mixture of sensory (Andersen, 1995; Colby and Goldberg, 1999), motor (Snyder *et al.*, 1997), and cognitive information (Platt and Glimcher, 1999), leading to persistent debates on their functional role. A recent review of data on the parietal cortex has suggested that 'current hypotheses concerning parietal function may not be the actual dimensions along which the parietal lobes are functionally organised; on this view, what we are lacking is a conceptual advance that leads us to test better hypotheses' (Culham and Kanwisher, 2001, pp. 159–60). In other words, perhaps the concepts of separate perceptual, cognitive, and motor systems, which theoretical neuroscience inherits from cognitive psychology, are not appropriate for bridging neural data with behaviour.

Even stronger concerns regarding cognitive psychology's suitability as a bridging framework are raised by considerations of evolutionary history (Hendriks-Jansen, 1996; Sterelny, 1989). Brain evolution is strikingly conservative and major features of modern neural organisation can be seen in the humble *Haikouichthys*, a primitive jawless fish that lived during the early Cambrian epoch over 520 million years ago (Shu *et al.*, 2003). Since the development of the telencephalon, the basic outline of the vertebrate nervous system has been strongly conserved throughout its phylogenetic history (Butler and Hodos, 2005; Holland and Holland, 1999; Katz and Harris-Warrick, 1999). The basic topology of neural circuitry is analogous across very diverse species (Karten, 1969) and even recently elaborated structures such as the mammalian neocortex have homologues among non-mammalian species (Medina and Reiner, 2000). Although the idea that brain evolution consists of new structures being added on top of old structures (e.g., the 'Triune Brain'; MacLean, 1973) is still popular among non-specialists, it has been rejected in recent decades of comparative neuroanatomical work (Butler and Hodos, 2005; Deacon, 1990). Brain evolution consists of the differentiation and specialisation of existing structures (Krubitzer and Kaas, 2005), shifts in existing axonal projection patterns (Deacon, 1990), and modifications of developmental 'morphogenetic fields' (Gilbert *et al.*, 1996), not through the addition of new structures. Thus, the basic anatomical and functional organisation of the primate brain reflects an ancient architecture which was well-established by the time of the earliest terrestrial tetrapods. This architecture could not have been designed to serve the needs of higher cognitive abilities, which did not exist, but must have been laid down so as to best address the needs of simple, interactive behaviour.

An emphasis on the brain's role in interactive behaviour is by no means novel. Similar ideas have for a long time been central to theories in ethology (Ewert *et al.*, 2001; Hinde, 1966), and have recently led to several new viewpoints on cognition (Adams and Mele, 1989; Beer, 2000; Clark, 1997; Núñez and Freeman, 2000; Thelen *et al.*, 2001), and interactive behaviour (Brooks, 1991; Hendriks-Jansen, 1996; Prescott *et al.*, 1999; Seth, 2007). All of these are similar to several lines of thought that are much older (Ashby, 1965; Gibson, 1979; Maturana and Varela, 1980; Mead, 1938; Merleau-Ponty, 1945; Powers, 1973) in some cases by over a hundred years (Bergson, 1896; Dewey, 1896; Jackson, 1884). Most of these viewpoints emphasise the pragmatic aspects of behaviour (Gibson, 1979; Millikan, 1989; Piaget, 1967), a theme that underlies several proposals regarding representation (Dretske, 1981; Gallese, 2000; Hommel *et al.*, 2001), memory (Ballard *et al.*, 1995; Glenberg, 1997), and visual consciousness (O'Regan and Noë, 2001). Here, it is proposed that these views, which emphasise the brain's role in controlling behaviour in real time (Cisek, 1999), provide a better basis for interpreting neurophysiological data than the traditional framework of cognitive psychology (Cisek, 2001).

Continuous interaction with the world often does not allow one to stop to think or to collect information and build a complete knowledge of one's surroundings. To survive in a hostile environment, one must be ready to act at short notice, releasing into execution actions which are at least partially prepared. These are the fundamental demands which shaped brain evolution. They motivate animals to process sensory information in an action-dependent manner, to build representations of the potential actions which the environment currently affords. In other words, the perception of a given natural setting may involve not only representations which capture information about the identity of objects in the setting, but also representations which specify the parameters of possible actions that can be taken (Cisek, 2001; Fadiga *et al.*, 2000; Gibson, 1979). With a set of such potential actions partially specified, the animal is ready to quickly perform actions if circumstances demand. In essence, it is possible that the nervous system addresses the questions of specification ('how to do it') *before* performing selection ('what to do'). Indeed, for continuous interactive behaviour, it may be best to perform both specification and selection processes at all times, to enable continuous adjustment to the changing world.

The proposal made here is that *the processes of action selection and specification occur simultaneously*, and continue even during overt performance of movements. That is, sensory information arriving from the world is continuously used to specify several currently available potential actions, while other kinds of information are collected to select from among these the one that will be released into overt execution at a given moment (Cisek, 2001; Cisek and Kalaska, 2005; Fagg and Arbib, 1998; Glimcher, 2001; Gold and Shadlen, 2001; Kalaska *et al.*, 1998; Kim and Shadlen, 1999; Platt, 2002). From this perspective, behaviour is viewed as a constant competition between internal representations of conflicting demands and opportunities, of the potential actions that Gibson (1979) termed 'affordances'. Hence, the framework presented here is called the 'affordance competition' hypothesis.

It is not proposed that complete action plans are prepared for all of the possible actions that one might take at a given moment. First, only actions which are *currently* available are specified in this manner. Second, many possible actions are eliminated from processing by selective attention mechanisms which limit the sensory information that is transformed into representations of action. Finally, complete action planning is not proposed even for the final selected action. Even in cases of highly practiced behaviours, no complete pre-planned motor program or entire desired trajectory appears to be prepared (Cisek, 2005; Kalaska *et al.*, 1998,).

11.2   The affordance competition hypothesis

The view of behaviour as a competition between actions has been common in studies of animal behaviour and the interpretation of subcortical circuits (Ewert, 1997; Ewert *et al.*, 2001; Prescott *et al.*, 1999). However, it is more rarely used to explain the activity of cerebral cortical regions, perhaps due to an assumption that the cortex is a new structure concerned with new, cognitive functions. However, as discussed above, that assumption is not justified. The organisation of the cerebral cortex has been conserved for a long time, motivating one to interpret it, like subcortical circuits, in terms of interactive behaviour. Figure 11.1 outlines a proposal on how the affordance competition hypothesis may be used to interpret neural data from the primate cerebral cortex during visually guided behaviour.

The visual system is organised into two parallel processing pathways: an occipito-temporal 'ventral stream' in which cells are sensitive to information about the identity of objects, and an occipito-parietal 'dorsal stream' in which cells are sensitive to spatial information (Ungerleider and Mishkin, 1982). From the traditional cognitive perspective, the ventral stream builds a representation of 'what' is in the environment, while the dorsal stream builds a representation of 'where' things are. However, the dorsal stream does

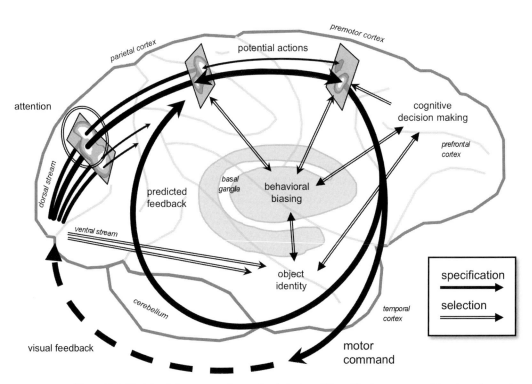

Figure 11.1 Sketch of the proposed neural substrates of the affordance competition hypothesis, in the context of visually guided movement. The primate brain is shown, emphasising the cerebral cortex, cerebellum, and basal ganglia. Filled dark arrows represent processes of action specification, which begin in the visual cortex and proceed rightward across the parietal lobe, transforming visual information into representations of potential actions. Polygons represent three neural populations along this route: (1) The leftmost represents the encoding of potential visual targets, modulated by attentional selection; (2) The middle represents potential actions encoded in parietal cortex; (3) The rightmost represents activity in premotor regions. Each population is depicted as a map of neural activity, with activity peaks corresponding to the lightest regions. As the action specification occurs across the fronto-parietal cortex, distinct potential actions compete for further processing. This competition is biased by input from the basal ganglia and prefrontal cortical regions which collect information for action selection (double-line arrows). This biasing influences the competition in a number of loci, and because of reciprocal connectivity, these influences are reflected over a large portion of the cerebral cortex. The final selected action is released into execution and causes both overt feedback through the environment (dashed black arrow) and internal predictive feedback through the cerebellum.

not appear to contain any unified representation of the space around us, but rather diverges into a number of substreams each specialised toward the needs of different kinds of actions (Andersen *et al.*, 1997; Colby and Goldberg, 1999; Matelli and Luppino, 2001; Stein, 1992; Wise *et al.*, 1997). For example, the lateral intraparietal area (LIP) is concerned with the control of gaze (Snyder *et al.*, 2000b; Snyder *et al.*, 1997), represents space in a body-centred reference frame (Snyder *et al.*, 1998b), and is strongly interconnected with parts of the oculomotor system including the frontal eye fields (FEF) and the superior colliculus (Paré and Wurtz, 2001). In contrast, the medial intraparietal area (MIP) is involved in arm reaching actions (Cui and Andersen, 2007; Ferraina and Bianchi, 1994; Kalaska and Crammond, 1995; Pesaran *et al.*, 2008; Scherberger and Andersen, 2007; Snyder *et al.*, 1997), represents target locations with respect to the current hand location (Buneo *et al.*, 2002; Graziano *et al.*, 2000), and is interconnected with frontal regions involved in reaching, such as the dorsal premotor cortex (PMd) (Johnson *et al.*, 1996; Marconi *et al.*, 2001). The anterior intraparietal area (AIP) is involved in grasping (Baumann *et al.*, 2009), is sensitive to object size and orientation, and is interconnected with the grasp-related ventral premotor cortex (PMv) (Nakamura *et al.* 2001; Rizzolatti and Luppino, 2001).

These observations are consistent with the proposal that the major role of the dorsal visual stream is not to build a unified representation of the world, but rather to mediate various visually guided actions (Goodale and Milner, 1992). It may therefore be part of the system for action specification (Cisek, 2001; Cisek and Turgeon, 1999; Fagg and Arbib, 1998; Kalaska *et al.*, 1998; Passingham and Toni, 2001), processing visual information to specify potential actions of various kinds: LIP cells specify potential saccade targets; MIP cells specify possible directions for reaching, etc. Furthermore, the dorsal stream represents not only a single unique movement that has already been selected, but rather offers a variety of options to choose from, including multiple saccade targets (Kusunoki *et al.*, 2000; Platt and Glimcher, 1997) as well as multiple reaching movements (Cisek *et al.*, 2004). It does not, of course, represent all possible movements. As one proceeds further along the dorsal stream, one finds an increasing influence of attentional modulation, with information from particular regions of interest enhanced while information from other regions is suppressed (Desimone and Duncan, 1995; Treue, 2001). The result is that the parietal representation of external space becomes increasingly sparse as one moves away from the striate cortex (Gottlieb *et al.*, 1998). In other words, only the most promising targets for movements make it so far as to be represented in the parietal cortex. From this perspective, the phenomenon of selective attention is seen as an early mechanism for action selection (Allport, 1987; Neumann, 1990; Tipper *et al.*, 1998; Tipper *et al.*, 1992), reducing the volume of information that is transformed into action-related representations.

As mentioned, parietal cortical areas are strongly and reciprocally interconnected with frontal regions involved in movement control. LIP is interconnected with FEF, MIP with PMd and primary motor cortex (M1), AIP with ventral premotor cortex (PMv), etc. (Matelli and Luppino, 2001). As a result, the fronto-parietal system may be viewed as a set of loops spanning over the central sulcus, each processing information related to a different aspect of movement (Jones *et al.*, 1978; Marconi *et al.*, 2001; Pandya and Kuypers, 1969). If these regions are involved in representing potential actions, as assumed here, then they appear to do so in tandem. For example, potential reaching actions are represented together by both MIP and PMd (Cisek and Kalaska, 2005; Cisek *et al.*, 2004). It is proposed that the competition between potential actions plays out in large part within this reciprocally interconnected fronto-parietal system. Within each cortical area, cells with different movement preferences mutually inhibit each other, creating competition between distinct potential actions. This competition is biased by excitatory input from a variety of sources, including both cortical and subcortical regions.

The influence of all of these biasing factors modulates the activity in frontal and parietal neurons, with information favouring a given action causing activity related to that action to increase, while information against an action causes it to decrease.

Indeed, neurophysiological evidence for the modulation of fronto-parietal activity by 'decision factors' is very strong. For example, recent studies of decision making show that LIP activity correlates not only with sensory and motor variables, but also with decision variables such as expected utility (Platt and Glimcher, 1999), local income (Sugrue et al., 2004), hazard rate (Janssen and Shadlen, 2005), relative subjective desirability (Dorris and Glimcher, 2004), and log-likelihood estimates (Yang and Shadlen, 2007). More generally, variables traditionally considered as sensory, cognitive, or motor, appear to be mixed in the activity of individual cells in many regions, including prefrontal cortex (Constantinidis et al., 2001; Hoshi et al., 2000), premotor cortex (Cisek and Kalaska, 2005; Romo et al., 2004), FEF (Coe et al., 2002; Gold and Shadlen, 2000; Thompson et al., 1996), LIP (Coe et al., 2002; Platt and Glimcher, 1997; Shadlen and Newsome, 2001), and the superior colliculus (Basso and Wurtz, 1998; Horwitz et al., 2004). Such mixing of variables is difficult to interpret from the perspective of distinctions between sensory, motor, and cognitive systems, and it has led to persistent debates about the functional role of specific cortical regions. For example, some studies have shown that neurons in area LIP respond only to stimuli which capture attention, leading to its interpretation as a 'salience map' (Bisley and Goldberg, 2003; Colby and Goldberg, 1999; Kusunoki et al., 2000). However, other studies have shown that these activities are stronger when the stimulus serves as the target of a saccade (as opposed to a reach), leading to the interpretation of LIP as a representation of intended saccades (Snyder et al., 1997, 1998a, 2000a). These competing interpretations have been the subject of a long and vibrant debate. However, from the perspective of the affordance competition hypothesis, both interpretations are correct: neural activity in fronto-parietal regions correlates with sensory and motor variables because it is involved in the specification of potential actions using sensory information, and it is modulated by decision variables (including salience/attention) because competition between potential actions is influenced by various sources of biasing inputs.

There are many potential sources from which biasing inputs might originate. Because action selection is a fundamental problem faced by even the most primitive of vertebrates, it likely involves neural structures which developed very early and have been conserved in evolution. A promising candidate is the basal ganglia (Frank et al., this volume; Hazy et al., this volume; Kalivas and Nakamura, 1999; Leblois et al. 2006; Mink, 1996; Redgrave et al., 1999), which are strongly interconnected with specific cortical areas (Alexander and Crutcher, 1990a; Middleton and Strick, 2000) and exhibit activity that is related both to movement parameters (Alexander and Crutcher, 1990b, 1990c) and decision variables such as reward (Schultz et al., 2000) and expectation (Lauwereyns et al., 2002). However, it is also likely that action selection involves brain structures which have become particularly developed in recent evolution, such as the prefrontal cortex of primates. The prefrontal cortex is strongly implicated in decision making (Bechara et al., 1998; Fuster et al., 2000; Kim and Shadlen, 1999; Miller, 2000; Rowe et al., 2000; Tanji and Hoshi, 2001), which may be viewed as an aspect of advanced action selection. Neurons in the dorsolateral prefrontal cortex (DLPFC) are sensitive to various combinations of stimulus features, and this sensitivity is always related to the particular demands of the task at hand (di Pellegrino and Wise, 1991; Hoshi *et al.*, 1998; Kim and Shadlen, 1999; Quintana and Fuster, 1999; Rainer *et al.*, 1998). Prefrontal decisions appear to evolve through the collection of 'votes' for categorically selecting one action over others, as demonstrated by studies of saccade target and reach target selection (Kim and Shadlen, 1999; Tanji and Hoshi, 2001). Of course, the prefrontal cortex is not a homogeneous system but a diverse collection of specialised regions, including some which appear to be involved in aspects of working memory (Bechara *et al.*, 1998; Fuster and Alexander, 1971; Petrides, 2000; Rowe *et al.*, 2000). Here, we include only a very simplified account of one particular subregion of PFC, the DLPFC.

What role might the ventral visual stream play within the functional architecture of Figure 11.1? Cell responses in the anterior inferotemporal (IT) cortex are sensitive to features of a currently viewed stimulus (Desimone *et al.*, 1984; Tanaka *et al.*, 1991), and to the behavioural context in which that stimulus is presented (Eskandar *et al.*, 1992). These results have been taken to implicate IT in object recognition. However, it may also serve a more humble role. Studies of animal behaviour over the last hundred years have shown that many kinds of behaviours are elicited by simple combinations of particular stimulus features, what ethologists referred to as 'sign stimuli' (Hinde, 1966; Tinbergen, 1950). Neural responses in IT cortex are compatible with a putative role in sign stimulus detection, which could serve as a front-end input to action selection via direct projections from temporal cortex to prefrontal regions (Saleem *et al.*, 2000). Thus, an early role of what is now the ventral stream may have been the detection of the stimulus combinations that were relevant for selection of actions in a particular behavioural context, and this may have eventually evolved into the sophisticated object recognition ability of modern mammals.

In the view schematised by Figure 11.1, specification and selection processes operate in parallel. As an animal interacts with its world, sensorimotor processing in the dorsal stream is continuously fine-tuning an ongoing action even while it continues to build egocentric representations of alternative potential actions that could be performed. Meanwhile, selection mechanisms vote for which of those actions progress furthest in sensorimotor processing and whether the animal will switch behaviour from its ongoing task to a new one which might become more immediately relevant. For example, while a monkey is feeding on some fruit that is within reach, its parietal system can continue to represent nearby branches as potential escape routes in case its ventral stream detects evidence that a leopard has appeared.

Although during natural behaviour the processes of specification and selection will occur simultaneously, we can still make predictions about what would happen if an animal endowed with such a parallel architecture was placed in a neurophysiological laboratory. In this highly controlled setting, time is broken up into discrete trials, each starting with the presentation of a stimulus and ending with the production of a response. What would the architecture of Figure 11.1 predict about the time-course of neural events?

When the stimulus is first presented, we should expect an initial fast feedforward sweep of activity along the dorsal stream, crudely representing the potential actions that are most directly specified by the stimulus. Indeed, Schmolesky *et al.* (1998) showed that responses to simple visual flashes appear very quickly throughout the dorsal visual system, and engage putatively motor-related areas like FEF in as little as 50 ms. This is significantly *earlier* than some visual areas such as V2 and V4. In general, even within the visual system neural activation does not appear to follow a serial sequence from 'early' to 'late' areas (Paradiso, 2002). In a reaching task, population activity in PMd discriminates the direction of the cue within 50 ms of its appearance (Cisek and Kalaska, 2005). These fast responses are not purely visual, as they reflect the context within which the stimulus is presented. For example, they reflect whether the monkey expects to see one or two stimuli (Cisek and Kalaska, 2005), reflect anticipatory biases or priors (Coe *et al.*, 2002; Takikawa *et al.*, 2002), and can be entirely absent if the monkey already knows what action to take and can ignore the stimulus altogether (Crammond and Kalaska, 2000). In short, these phenomena are compatible with the notion of a fast dorsal specification system that quickly uses visual information to specify the potential actions most consistently associated with a given stimulus. The speed of that system also allows us to quickly adjust ongoing movements to perturbations (Day and Lyon, 2000; Desmurget *et al.*, 1999).

After the initial options are quickly specified, we expect that slower selection processes will begin to sculpt the neural activity patterns by introducing a variety of task-relevant biasing factors. Indeed, extrastriate visual areas MT and 7a respond to a stimulus in about 50 ms, but begin to reflect the influence of attention in 100–120 ms (Constantinidis and Steinmetz, 2001; Treue, 2001). FEF neurons respond to the onset of a stimulus in 50 ms (Schmolesky *et al.*, 1998), but detect the singleton of a visual-search array with a median of about 100 ms and discriminate pro- versus anti-saccades in about 120 ms (Sato and Schall, 2003). LIP neurons respond to stimulus onset in about 50 ms and discriminate targets from distractors in 138 ms (Thomas and Pare, 2007). Neurons in the dorsal premotor cortex respond to a visual cue in 50 ms but begin to predict the monkey's choice in 110–130 ms (Cisek and Kalaska, 2005).

A recent study by Ledberg and colleagues (2007) provides an overall picture of the time-course observed in all of the experiments described above. These authors simultaneously recorded local field potentials (LFPs) from up to 15 cerebral cortical regions of monkeys performing a conditional Go/NoGo task. Because LFPs are believed to reflect the summed dendritic input to an area, they are an excellent measure of processing onset latency. Through an elegant experimental design, Ledberg and colleagues were able to detect the first neural events that responded to the presence of a stimulus, those which discriminated its identity, as well as those predicting the monkey's chosen response. In agreement with earlier studies (cf. Schmolesky *et al.*, 1998), they observed a fast feedforward sweep of stimulus onset-related activity appearing within 50–70 ms in striate and extrastriate cortex, and 55–80 ms in FEF and premotor cortex. Discrimination of different stimulus categories occurred later, within about 100 ms of onset in prestriate areas and 200 ms in prefrontal sites. The Go/NoGo decision appeared about 150 ms after stimulus onset, nearly simultaneously within a diverse mosaic of cortical sites including prestriate, inferotemporal, parietal, premotor, and prefrontal areas. In summary, when behaviour is experimentally isolated in the laboratory, the continuous and parallel processes critical for interaction appear as two waves of acti-vation: an early wave crudely specifying a menu of options, and a second wave that discriminates between them about 120–150 ms after stimulus onset (Ledberg *et al.*, 2007). In summary, it appears that the brain can very quickly specify multiple potential actions within its fast fronto-parietal sensorimotor control system, but it takes approxi-mately 150 ms to integrate information sufficiently in order to make a decision between them.

11.3   A computational model of reaching decisions

The broad concepts outlined in the previous section can be translated into more concrete and testable hypotheses through a mathematical model of the neural processes which may implement action specification and selection in the mammalian cerebral cortex. A model of the cortical mechanisms which specify reaching movements and select between them has been described by Cisek (2006) and it is summarised briefly here.

Figure 11.2a illustrates the circuit model and suggests how its elements may corre-spond to specific cortical regions. Because the model focuses on visually guided reaching actions, it includes some of the main cortical regions involved in reaching behaviour, such as the posterior parietal cortex (PPC), PMd, M1, and prefrontal cortex (PFC). These were chosen as a subset of the complete distributed circuits for reaching control, sufficient to demonstrate a few central concepts. Other relevant regions not currently modelled are the supplementary motor areas, somatosensory cortex, and many subcor-tical structures including the basal ganglia, red nucleus, etc. The input to the model consists of visual information about target direction and a signal triggering movement onset (GO signal), and the output is the direction of movement. The control of the overt movement is not simulated here (for compatible models of execution, see Bullock *et al.*, 1998; Bullock and Grossberg, 1988; Cisek *et al.*, 1998; Houk *et al.*, 1993; Kettner *et al.*, 1993; McIntyre and Bizzi, 1993).

In the model, each neural population was implemented as a set of 90 mean-rate leaky-integrator neurons, each of which is broadly tuned to a particular direction of movement. All of the weights are fixed to resemble the known anatomical connections between the modelled regions. Within each population, neurons with similar tuning excite each other while neurons with dissimilar tuning inhibit each other. Between populations, neurons with similar tuning excite each other through reciprocal topological connections. Noise is added to all neural activities. See Cisek (2006) for details of the model's implementation.

In the model, neural populations do not encode a unique value of a movement param-eter (such as a single direction in space) but can represent an entire distribution of potential values of movement parameters (e.g., many possible directions represented simultaneously). This proposal is related to the attention model of Tipper *et al.* (2000), the 'decision field' theory of Erlhagen and Schöner (2002), and the 'Bayesian cod-ing' hypothesis (Dayan and Abbott, 2001; Knill and Pouget, 2004; Sanger, 2003). It suggests that given a population of cells, each with a preferred value of a particular movement parameter, one can interpret the activity across the population as something

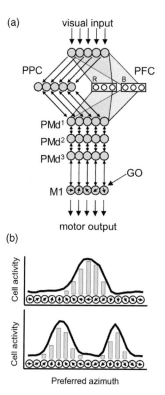

Figure 11.2 Computational model described in Cisek (2006). (a) Each neural layer is depicted by a set of circles representing cells with different preferences for a movement parameter (e.g., direction). Thin arrows represent topographic connections (in most cases reciprocal) between layers involved in action specification. Grey polygons represent the input to and from prefrontal cortex, which is divided into two subpopulations each preferring a different stimulus colour. These projections are also topographic, but with much lower spatial resolution. Visual inputs are presented to the input layer, and the GO signal gates activity in primary motor cortex. Abbreviations: PPC: posterior parietal cortex; PFC: prefrontal cortex; PMd: dorsal premotor cortex; M1: primary motor cortex. (b) Each population consists of cells with different preferred directions, and their pattern of activity can represent one potential reach direction (top) or several potential directions simultaneously (bottom).

akin to a probability density function of potential values of that parameter. Sometimes, the population may encode a range of contiguous values defining a single action, and at other times, several distinct and mutually exclusive potential actions can be represented simultaneously as distinct peaks of activity in the population (Figure 11.2b). The strength of the activity associated with a particular value of the parameter reflects the likelihood that the final action will have that value, and it is influenced by a variety of factors including salience, expected reward, estimates of probability, etc. This hypothesis predicts that activity in the population is correlated with many decision variables, as observed in the frontal (Coe *et al.*, 2002; Gold and Shadlen, 2000; Hoshi *et al.*, 2000; Kim and Shadlen, 1999; Roesch and Olson, 2004; Romo *et al.*, 2004) and parietal cortex

(Coe *et al.*, 2002; Dorris and Glimcher, 2004; Glimcher, 2003; Janssen and Shadlen, 2005; Platt and Glimcher, 1999; Shadlen and Newsome, 2001; Sugrue *et al.*, 2004).

The model suggests that sensory information in the dorsal visual stream is used to specify the spatial parameters of *several* currently available potential actions in parallel. These potential actions are represented simultaneously in frontal and parietal cortical regions, appearing as distinct peaks of activity in the neural populations involved in sensorimotor processing (Cisek and Kalaska, 2005; Cisek *et al.*, 2004; Platt and Glimcher, 1997; Figure 11.2b). Whenever multiple peaks appear simultaneously within a single frontal or parietal cortical region, they compete against each other through mutual inhibition. This is related to the biased competition mechanism in theories of visual attention (Boynton, 2005; Desimone, 1998). To state it briefly, cells with similar parameter preferences excite each other while cells with different preferences inhibit each other. This basic mechanism can explain a variety of neural phenomena, such as the inverse relationship between the number of options and neural activity associated with each (Basso and Wurtz, 1998; Cisek and Kalaska, 2005), narrowing of tuning functions with multiple options (Cisek and Kalaska, 2005), and relative coding of decision variables (Roesch and Olson, 2004).

Because neural activities are noisy, competition between distinct peaks of activity cannot follow a simple 'winner-take-all' rule or random fluctuations would determine the winner each time, rendering informed decision making impossible. To prevent this, small differences in levels of activity should be ignored by the system. However, if activity associated with a given choice becomes sufficiently strong, it should be allowed to suppress its opponents and conclusively win the competition. In other words, there should be a threshold of activity above which a particular peak is selected as the final response choice. This is consistent with sequential sampling models of decision making (Bogacz *et al.*, 2006; Mazurek *et al.*, 2003; Reddi *et al.*, 2003; Smith and Ratcliff, 2004; Usher and McClelland, 2001) which propose that decisions are made when neural activity reaches some threshold. In the model, this threshold emerges from the nonlinear dynamics between competing populations of cells (Cisek, 2006; Grossberg, 1973).

Finally, the model suggests that the competition which occurs between potential actions represented in the fronto-parietal system is biased by a variety of influences from other regions, including the basal ganglia (Brown *et al.*, 2004; Leblois *et al.*, 2006; Redgrave *et al.*, 1999) and PFC (Miller, 2000; Tanji and Hoshi, 2001) which accumulate evidence for each particular choice (Figure Figure 11.1). Here, only the influence of PFC is modelled, although it is likely that basal ganglia projections play a significant role in action selection (Frank *et al.*, this volume; Hazy *et al.*, this volume; Houk *et al.*, this volume; Stafford and Gurney, this volume). Several studies have shown that some cells in the lateral PFC are sensitive to conjunctions of relevant sensory and cognitive information (Miller, 2000; Rainer *et al.*, 1998; Tanji and Hoshi, 2001; White and Wise, 1999), and that they gradually accumulate evidence over time (Kim and Shadlen, 1999). Many studies have suggested that the orbitofrontal cortex and the basal ganglia provide signals which predict the reward associated with a given response (Schultz *et al.*, 2000), which could also serve as input to bias the fronto-parietal competition.

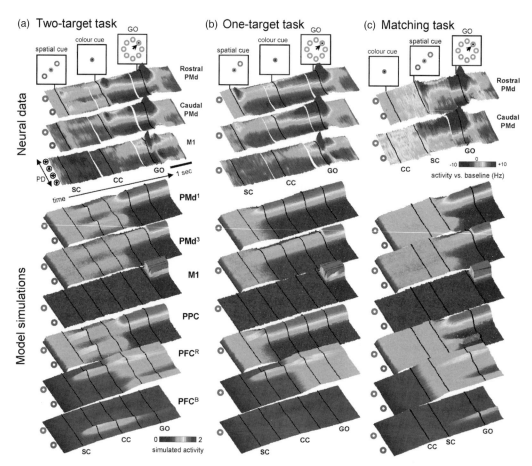

Figure 11.3 Comparison between neural activity and model simulations in three kinds of tasks. (a) Two-target task. During the spatial cue (SC), two possible targets are presented, one red and one blue. During the colour cue (CC), the centre indicates which of these is the correct target. The GO signal instructs the monkey to begin the movement. Neural data (Cisek and Kalaska, 2005) is shown from three sets of neurons: rostral PMd, caudal PMd, and primary motor cortex (M1). In each, neural activity is depicted as a 3D surface in which time runs from left to right and cells are sorted by their preferred direction along the left edge. Circles indicate the locations of the two targets. Simulated model activities are depicted in the same format, where black lines indicate behavioural events (spatial cue on, spatial cue off, colour cue on, colour cue off, GO). (b) One-target task, same format. (c) Matching task, same format. See plate section for colour version.

The operation of the model can be most easily understood in the context of a particular task. For example, Figure 11.3a shows a reach-decision task in which the correct target was indicated through a sequence of cues: during the spatial-cue period (SC), two possible targets were presented, and during a subsequent colour-cue period (CC), one of these was designated as the correct target. In the model, the appearance of the spatial cue causes activity in two groups of cells in PPC, each tuned to one of the targets. Mutual excitation between nearby cells creates distinct peaks of activity, which compete against each other through the inhibitory interactions between cells with different preferred directions. Because of the topographic projections between PPC and PMd, two peaks appear in PMd as well, although they are weaker in the lower PMd layers (compare layers PMd^1 and PMd^3). These two peaks continue to be active and to compete against each other even after the targets vanish, due to the positive feedback between layers. At the same time, activity accumulates in the PFC cells selective for the particular location–colour conjunctions. The colour cue is simulated as uniform excitation to all PFC cells preferring the given colour (in this case, PFC^R), and it pushes that group of PFC cells toward stronger activity than the other. This causes the competition in PMd to become unbalanced, and one peak increases its activity while the other is suppressed. In the model, this is equivalent to a decision. Finally, once the GO signal is given, activity is allowed to flow from PMd^3 into M1, and the peak of the M1 activity is taken to define the initial direction of the movement.

The simulation reproduces many features of neural activity recorded from the dorsal premotor and primary motor cortex of a monkey performing the same reach-decision task (Cisek and Kalaska, 2005). As shown in Figure 11.3a, PMd cells tuned to both spatial targets were active during the SC, and then during the CC, one of these became more strongly active (predicting the monkey's choice), while the other was suppressed. Note how the activity was weaker while both options were present, consistent with the hypothesis that the two groups of cells exert an inhibitory influence on each other. As in the model, these phenomena were seen more strongly in the rostral part of PMd than in the caudal part. The model also exhibits sustained activity ('working memory') because after the targets are removed (second black line in the simulation images) target information is maintained in both the PPC and PMd (Figure 11.3a and b).

Figure 11.3c shows a variation of the task in which the CC is presented before the SC. In this case, no directionally tuned activity appears in PMd during the colour-cue period, and after the spatial targets are presented there is sustained activity corresponding only to the correct target. Thus, the neural activity is determined not by the sensory properties of the stimulus (which are the same as in Figure 11.3a) but by the movement information specified by the stimulus. However, note that immediately after the SC, there is a brief burst toward the incorrect target, in both the neurons in rostral PMd and in the PMd^1 population in the model (Figure 11.3c). One might be tempted to classify this as a pure 'sensory' response. However, at least in the model, this burst is more correctly described as a brief representation of a potential action, aborted quickly in light of the prior information provided by the colour cue. Again, this is seen most strongly in the rostral part of PMd, in both the data and the model.

Figure 11.4 shows some predictions about the context-dependent timing of cortical responses. As discussed above, studies on the timing of attentional and decisional processes suggest that action selection occurs in 120–150 ms after stimulus presentation in a distributed network of regions (Cisek and Kalaska, 2005; Constantinidis and Steinmetz, 2001; Ledberg *et al.*, 2007; Sato and Schall, 2003; Thomas and Pare, 2007; Treue, 2001). This is compatible with the model, but we can make a further prediction. While the distributions of latencies should be similar across cortical regions, we predict that they are not identical, and that they will follow a specific context-dependent trend. In particular,

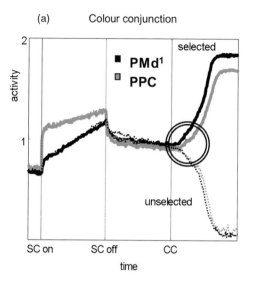

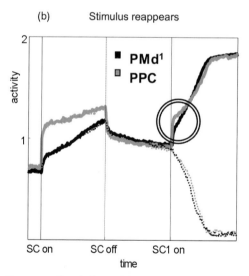

Figure 11.4 Simulations of the context-dependent order of neural activation. (a) Simulation of the standard two-target task (in which the decision is made on the basis of a colour conjunction rule). Black lines show the time course of the average activity of two groups of PMd[1] cells – cells tuned to the selected target (thick line) and cells tuned to the unselected target (thin dotted line). Grey lines show the activity of PPC cells tuned to the selected (thick line) and unselected targets (thin dotted line). Vertical lines indicate the time of SC onset, SC offset, and CC onset. The double circle emphasises the first activity which reflects the decision made by the network, which appears in PMd prior to PPC. (b) Simulation of a task in which instead of a colour cue, the decision is made when one of the target stimuli reappears at the time marked as 'SC1 on'. In this situation, the decision is reflected first in PPC, before it appears in PMd (note the activity emphasised by the double circle).

consider the case when a decision is made on the basis of cognitive information, such as a learned colour cue (as in the two-target task described above). Because such cues are collected by prefrontal regions which project into rostral PMd, the bias introduced by the cue will begin to unbalance the PMd competition directly, which will then in turn (through fronto-parietal connections) cause the PPC competition to become unbalanced. Therefore, a decision made on the basis of such cognitive cues will first be expressed in frontal cortex and then, a very short time later, in parietal regions. This is indeed what was observed during neural recordings in the two-target task, which showed that PMd neurons tended to reflect the decision about 80 ms before PPC neurons (Cisek *et al.*, 2004). This phenomenon is simulated in Figure 11.4a. In particular, note that just after the colour cue is presented (circle) the neural activity tuned to the selected target begins to diverge from the activity tuned to the unselected target first in PMd (black lines), and then shortly afterwards in PPC (gray lines).

In contrast, consider a situation in which the decision is made on the basis of a more direct sensory signal, such as the reappearance of one of the targets. This information will first be available in parietal cortex, and will cause the PPC competition to become unbalanced, which will then in turn unbalance the PMd competition. Therefore, a decision made on the basis of the reappearance of a stimulus will first be expressed in parietal cortex and then very soon after appear in PMd. Figure 11.4b simulates this phenomenon. Note that just after the target reappears (circle), the activity in PPC (gray lines) reflects this event slightly before the activity in PMd (black lines).

Although such conditions have not been directly tested in neurophysiological recording experiments, the model predicts that the sequence by which decision-related activity spreads across the cerebral cortex is dependent upon the nature of the information which guides the choice that is made.

Recent neurophysiological studies have supported these predictions. For example, when monkeys perform pop-out visual search, neural activity in LIP reflects the choice before FEF and PFC, but if the task involves conjunction search then it is FEF and PFC which reflect the choice before LIP (Buschman and Miller, 2007). Assumptions about expected actions (priors) influence activity in SEF before FEF and LIP (Coe *et al.*, 2002; Pesaran *et al.*, 2008). Interestingly, in a Go/NoGo task in which monkeys made decisions on the basis of cognitive rules, activity predicting the response appeared in PMd *even before PFC*, which presumably processes the rule information (Wallis and Miller, 2003). It is as if, at least in that kind of task, a decision may be *influenced* by noisy neural votes arriving in part from PFC but is *determined* by a consensus that is reached in PMd.

In addition to reproducing qualitative features of neural activity during various action selection tasks, the model produces important psychophysical results on the spatial and temporal characteristics of human motor decisions. For example, it is well-known that reaction times in choice-tasks increase with the number of possible choices. This can be explained by the model (see Figure 11.5a), because the activity associated with each option is reduced as the number of options is increased (compare model PMd activity in Figure 11.3a versus Figure 11.3b), and it therefore takes longer for the activity to reach the decision threshold. Furthermore, it has also been shown that reaction time is not only determined by the number of targets but also by their spatial configuration. For example,

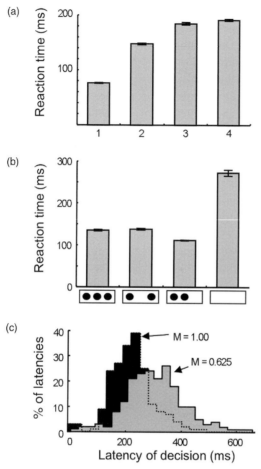

Figure 11.5 Latency effects. (a) Simulated reaction time during tasks with one, two, three, or four targets presented for 1.3 s, followed by a single correct target for 0.1 s, followed by the GO signal. Reaction times were calculated as first time after the GO signal that any neuron in the M1 population exceeded an activity threshold of 1.5. The mean and standard error are shown for N = 300 replications in each condition. (b) Simulated reaction time when cues are presented for 0.8 s followed by a single target for 0.3 s prior to the GO. The bars show mean ± s.e. of reaction time in four conditions: when three cues are presented 80° apart, two cues 160° apart, two cues 80° apart, or no cue at all. N = 100 in each condition. (c) Distributions of decision latency computed during simulations (each with two targets) using a CC cue of different magnitudes. The decision latency was calculated as the time between the CC cue and the first time any PMd[3] cell activity exceeded 0.75. N = 200 for each condition.

Bock and Eversheim (2000) showed that reaction time in a reaching task is similar with two or five targets as long as they subtend the same spatial angle, but shorter if two targets are closer together. This finding is difficult to account for with models in which the options are represented by discrete groups of neurons, but is easily reproduced in a model such as the present one, in which movements are specified by a continuous population (see Figure 11.5b). The model also reproduces the important finding that reducing the

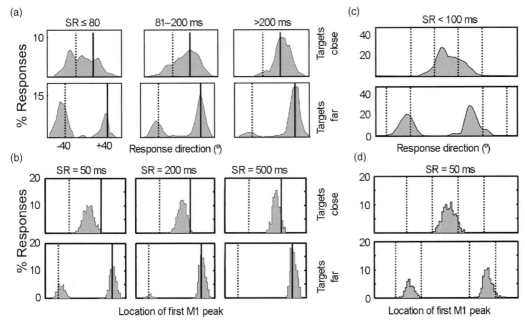

Figure 11.6 Data and simulation of the timed response paradigms of Ghez *et al.* (1997) and Favilla (1997). (a) Behavioural data from the Ghez *et al.* (1997) task. Each panel shows the distribution of initial directions of force production with respect to two targets (vertical lines). Data is aligned such that the correct target (solid line) is on the right. Different distributions are reported for different delays between target identification and movement onset, and for different angular separations between the targets. (b) Simulations of the Ghez *et al.* (1997) task. Each panel shows the distribution of initial directions, calculated as the preferred direction of the first M1 cell whose activity exceeded a threshold of 1.75. (c) Behavioural data from the Favilla (1997) task, in which four targets are shown either all 30° apart or grouped into two pairs that are far apart. Same format as (a). (d) Simulations of the Favilla (1997) task, same format as (b).

quality of evidence for a given choice, makes reaction times longer and more broadly distributed. The model produces this (see Figure 11.5c), through the same mechanism proposed by other models which involve a gradual accumulation to threshold: that with weaker evidence, the rate of accumulation is slower and the threshold is reached later in time, and therefore variability in accumulation rate produces broader distributions of reaction times (Carpenter and Williams, 1995; Ratcliff *et al.*, 2003; Smith and Ratcliff, 2004).

The model also explains several observations on the spatial features of movements made in the presence of multiple choices. For example, Ghez and colleagues (1997) showed that when subjects are forced to make choices quickly, they move to targets randomly if they are spaced further than 60° apart ('discrete mode'), and in-between them if the targets are close together ('continuous mode'), as shown in Figure 11.6a. The model reproduces all of these results (Figure 11.6b). When two targets are far apart, they create multiple competing peaks of activity in the PMd–PPC populations, and the decision is determined by which peak happens to fluctuate higher when the signal to move is given. However, if the targets are close together, then their two corresponding peaks merge into one because of the positive feedback between cells with similar parameter preferences (a similar explanation has been proposed by Erlhagen and Schöner, 2002). In a related experiment, Favilla (1997) demonstrated that the discrete and continuous modes can occur at the same time when four targets are grouped into two pairs that are far apart but each of which consists of two targets close together (see Figure 11.6c). This is also reproduced by the model (Figure 11.6d) (except for an additional central bias exhibited by human subjects). With four targets, peaks corresponding to targets within each pair merge together and then the two resulting peaks compete and are selected discretely.

11.4   Discussion

This chapter describes a theoretical framework called the 'affordance competition hypothesis', which suggests that behaviour involves a constant competition between currently available opportunities and demands for action. It is based on the idea that the brain's basic functional architecture evolved to mediate real-time interaction with the world, which requires animals to continuously specify potential actions and to select between them. This framework is used to interpret neural data from the primate cerebral cortex, suggesting explanations for a number of important neurophysiological phenomena. A computational model is presented to illustrate the basic ideas of the hypothesis and to suggest how neural populations in the cerebral cortex may implement a competition between representations of potential actions.

  The model presented above shares a number of features with existing models of decision making. For example, it is similar to a class of models called 'sequential sampling models' (Bogacz *et al.*, 2006; Mazurek *et al.*, 2003; Reddi *et al.*, 2003; Roe *et al.*, 2001; Smith and Ratcliff, 2004; Usher and McClelland, 2001), which propose that decisions are made by accumulating information for a given choice until it reaches some threshold. In some models, the evidence is accumulated by a single process (e.g., Smith and Ratcliff, 2004), in some it is collected by separate processes which independently race toward the threshold (Reddi *et al.*, 2003; Roe *et al.*, 2001), and in some the independent accumulators inhibit each other (Usher and McClelland, 2001). Some models separate the decision process into serial stages (e.g., Mazurek *et al.*, 2003), and in some it occurs when a single population exhibits a transition from biased competition to binary choice (Machens *et al.*, 2005; Wang, 2002). While the present model shares similarities with these, it extends their scope in an important way. In all of the models of decision making described above, the choices are predefined and represented by distinct populations, one per choice. In contrast, the present model suggests that the choices themselves emerge within a population of cells whose activity represents the probability density function of potential movements. In other words, the model describes the mechanism by which the choices are defined using spatial information. In this sense, it is related to the models of Erlhagen and Schöner (2002) and Tipper *et al.* (2000), which also discuss continuous specification of movement parameters within a distributed representation. To summarise, the present model may be seen as combining three lines of thought: (1) sequential sampling models of accumulation of evidence to a threshold; (2) models of a phase transition from encoding options to binary choice behaviour (Cisek, 2006); and (3) models of action specification within a distributed population. It also suggests a plausible manner in which these concepts can be used to interpret neural data in specific cortical regions.

The model presented here makes a number of predictions which distinguish it from many other models of decision making. First, it focuses on decisions about actions (as opposed to sensory discrimination) and suggests that these are made within the very same neural circuits that control the execution of those actions. These circuits are distributed among a large set of brain regions. In the case of visually guided reaching, decisions are made within the fronto-parietal circuit that includes both PMd and parietal area MIP. In the specific mathematical formulation described above, the competition between actions uses information from PFC, but the decision first appears in PMd, in agreement with data (Wallis and Miller, 2003). However, the broader framework of the affordance competition hypothesis does not impose any rigid temporal sequence in which decisions appear in the fronto-parietal system. Each population in the network is proposed to involve competitive interactions, and biasing influences can modulate that competition in different places. Because cortico-cortical connections are bi-directional, if a decision begins to emerge in one region then it will propagate outward to other regions. For example, decisions based on sensory features such as stimulus salience may first appear in parietal cortex and then influence frontal activity. In contrast, decisions based on abstract rules may first be expressed in frontal regions and propagate backward to PPC. Thus, decisions are proposed to emerge as a 'distributed consensus' which is reached when a competition between representations of potential actions is unbalanced by the accumulation of evidence in favour of a given choice.

Although the mathematical model presented here is similar in some ways to previous models of decision making, it is based on a somewhat unusual theoretical foundation. The affordance competition hypothesis, illustrated schematically in Figure 11.1, differs in several important ways from the cognitive neuroscience frameworks within which models of decision making are usually developed. Importantly, it lacks the traditional emphasis on explicit representations which capture knowledge about the world. For example, the activity in the dorsal stream and the fronto-parietal system is not proposed to encode a representation of objects in space, or a representation of motor plans, or cognitive variables such as expected value. Instead, it implements a particular, functionally motivated mixture of all of these variables. From a traditional perspective, such activity appears surprising because it does not have any of the expected properties of a sensory, cognitive, or motor representation. It does not capture knowledge about the world in the explicit descriptive sense expected from cognitive theories, and has proven difficult to interpret from that perspective (see above). However, from the perspective of affordance competition, mixtures of sensory information with motor plans and cognitive biases make perfect sense. Their functional role is not to describe the world, but to mediate adaptive interaction with the world.

In summary, instead of viewing the functional architecture of behaviour as serial stages of representation, we view it as a set of competing sensorimotor loops. This is by no means a novel proposal. It is related to several theories which describe behaviour as

(a)

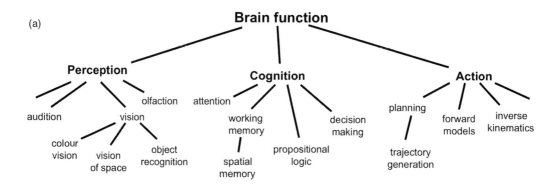

(b)

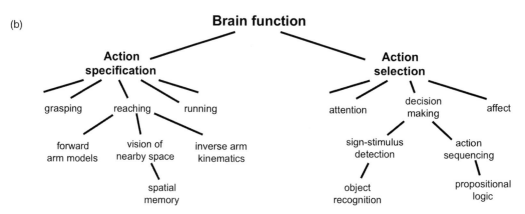

Figure 11.7 Two possible conceptual taxonomies of neural processes. (a) The taxonomy implied by classical cognitive science, in which brain functions are classified as belonging to perceptual, cognitive, or action systems. (b) An alternative taxonomy, in which brain functions are classified as processes aiding either action specification or action selection.

a competition between actions (Ewert *et al.*, 2001; Hendriks-Jansen, 1996; Kornblum *et al.*, 1990; Prescott *et al.*, 1999; Toates, 1998), and as discussed above, to a number of philosophical proposals made throughout the last hundred years. The present discussion is an attempt to unify these and related ideas with a growing body of neurophysiological data. It is suggested that a great deal of neural activity in the cerebral cortex can be interpreted from the perspective of a competition between potential movements more easily than in terms of traditional distinctions between perception, cognition, and action (Cisek, 2001). It is not suggested that distinctions between perceptual, cognitive, and motor processes be discarded entirely (they are certainly appropriate for interpreting primary sensory and motor regions), but only that other conceptual distinctions may be better suited to understanding central regions.

Figure 11.7 provides a schematic of the conceptual differences between the affordance competition hypothesis and the traditional frameworks of cognitive neuroscience. Traditional frameworks tend to view brain function as consisting of three basic classes of neural processes (see Figure 11.7a): *perceptual systems*, which take sensory information and construct internal representations of the world (e.g., Marr, 1982); *cognitive systems*, which use that representation along with memories of past experience to build knowledge, form judgments, and make decisions about the world (Johnson-Laird, 1988; Newell and Simon, 1972; Shafir and Tversky, 1995); and *action systems*, which implement the decisions through planning and execution of movements (Keele, 1968; Miller *et al.*, 1960). Each of these broad classes can be subdivided into subclasses. For example, perception includes different modalities such as vision, which can be subdivided further into object recognition, spatial vision, etc. Likewise, cognition includes processes such as working memory storage and retrieval, decision making, etc. These conceptual classes and subclasses are used to define research specialties, categorise scientific journals, and to interpret the functional role of specific brain regions.

Here, a different taxonomy of concepts is proposed (Figure 11.7b). Brain function is seen as fundamentally serving the needs of interactive behaviour, which involves two classes of processes: *action specification processes*, which use sensory information to define potential actions and guide their execution on-line; and *action selection processes*, which help to select which potential action will be performed at a given moment. Each of these can be subdivided further. For example, action specification can be divided into the specification of different kinds of actions, such as reaching, which involves spatial vision, inverse kinematics, etc. Action selection includes processes, such as visual attention, which select information on the basis of sensory properties, as well as decision making, which selects potential actions on the basis of more abstract rules. Note that many of the same concepts appear within both taxonomies, albeit in a different context. For example, vision of space is seen as closely related to object recognition in Figure 11.7a, but in Figure 11.7b they are thought of as contributing to very different behavioural abilities.

It is proposed here that the taxonomy of Figure 11.7b may be better suited to interpreting neural activity in many brain regions because it more closely reflects the basic organisation of the nervous system. Several aspects of brain anatomy are reflected in Figure 11.7b, such as the distinction between tectal and striatal circuits, dorsal and ventral visual streams, and the divergence of parietal processing toward different kinds of actions (of course, the specification and selection systems are not completely separate: as described above, mechanisms for action selection must influence activity related to specification at many loci of sensorimotor processing throughout the dorsal stream). Furthermore, one may view the relationships between the conceptual classes and subclasses in Figure 11.7b as reflecting, at least to some extent, the phylogenetic relationships between them. For example, one can speculate that processes such as 'object recognition' evolved as specialisations of older mechanisms of decision making which did not explicitly represent the identity of objects but simply detected particular features, called 'sign stimuli' (Hinde, 1966; Tinbergen, 1950). A classification of concepts which aims to reflect their phylogenetic relationships is important because the conservative nature of neural evolution motivates us to view all brain functions as modifications of ancestral mechanisms. Abilities such as sophisticated cognitive decision making did not appear from thin air, complete with appropriate anatomical connections and a full developmental schedule. They evolved within an ancestral context of real-time, interactive behaviour. Viewed from this perspective, even the advanced cognitive abilities of higher primates can be understood as serving the fundamental goal of all brain activity – to endow organisms with the ability to interact with their environment in adaptive ways.

Acknowledgements

The author wishes to thank Andrea Green and Steve Wise for helpful comments on various versions of this chapter. This work was supported by the New Emerging Teams grant NET-54000 from the Canadian Institutes of Health Research.

References

Adams, F. and A. Mele (1989). The role of intention in intentional action. *Can. J. Phil.* **19**: 511–31.

Alexander, G. E. and M. D. Crutcher (1990a). Functional architecture of basal ganglia circuits: neural substrates of parallel processing. *TINS* **13**(7): 266–71.

Alexander, G. E. and M. D. Crutcher (1990b). Neural representations of the target (goal) of visually guided arm movements in three motor areas of the monkey. *J. Neurophysiol.* **64**(1): 164–78.

Alexander, G. E. and M. D. Crutcher (1990c). Preparation for movement: Neural representations of intended direction in three motor areas of the monkey. *J. Neurophysiol.* **64**(1): 133–50.

Allport, D. A. (1987). Selection for action: some behavioral and neurophysiological considerations of attention and action. In *Perspectives on Perception and Action*, ed. H. Heuer and A. F. Sanders. Hillsdale, NJ: Lawrence Erlbaum Associates, pp. 395–419.

Andersen, R. A. (1995). Encoding of intention and spatial location in the posterior parietal cortex. *Cereb. Cortex* **5**: 457–69.

Andersen, R. A., L. H. Snyder, D. C. Bradley, and J. Xing (1997). Multimodal representation of space in the posterior parietal cortex and its use in planning movements. *Annu. Rev. Neurosci.* **20**: 303–30.

Ashby, W. R. (1965). *Design for a Brain: The Origin of Adaptive Behaviour*. London: Chapman and Hall.

Ballard, D. H., M. M. Hayhoe, and J. B. Pelz (1995). Memory representations in natural tasks. *J. Cognitive Neurosci.* **7**(1): 66–80.

Basso, M.A. and R. H. Wurtz (1998). Modulation of neuronal activity in superior colliculus by changes in target probability. *J. Neurosci.* **18**(18): 7519–34.

Baumann, M. A., M. C. Fluet, and H. Scherberger (2009). Context-specific grasp movement representation in the macaque anterior intraparietal area. *J. Neurosci.* **29**(20): 6436–48.

Bechara, A., H. Damasio, D. Tranel, and S. W. Anderson (1998). Dissociation of working memory from decision making within the human prefrontal cortex. *J. Neurosci.* **18**(1): 428–37.

Beer, R. D. (2000). Dynamical approaches to cognitive science. *Trends. Cogn. Sci.* **4**(3): 91–9.

Bergson, H. (1896). *Matter and Memory*, New York: Macmillan.

Bisley, J. W. and M. E. Goldberg (2003). Neuronal activity in the lateral intraparietal area and spatial attention. *Science* **299**(5603): 81–6.

Bock, O. and Eversheim, U. (2000). The mechanisms of movement preparation: a precuing study. *Behav. Brain Res.* **108**(1): 85–90.

Bogacz, R., E. Brown, J. Moehlis, P. Holmes, and J. D. Cohen (2006). The physics of optimal decision making: a formal analysis of models of performance in two-alternative forced-choice tasks. *Psychol. Rev.* **113**(4): 700–65.

Boynton, G. M. (2005). Attention and visual perception. *Curr. Opin. Neurobiol.* **15**(4): 465–9.

Brooks, R. (1991) Intelligence without representation. *Artif. Intell.* **47**: 139–59.

Brown, J. W., D. Bullock, and S. Grossberg (2004). How laminar frontal cortex and basal ganglia circuits interact to control planned and reactive saccades. *Neural Netw.* **17**(4): 471–510.

Bullock, D., P. Cisek, and S. Grossberg (1998). Cortical networks for control of voluntary arm movements under variable force conditions. *Cereb. Cortex* **8**: 48–62.

Bullock, D. and S. Grossberg (1988). Neural dynamics of planned arm movements: emergent invariants and speed-accuracy properties during trajectory formation. *Psychol. Rev.* **95**(1): 49–90.

Buneo, C. A., M. R. Jarvis, A. P. Batista, and R. A. Andersen (2002). Direct visuomotor transformations for reaching. *Nature* **416**(6881): 632–6.

Buschman, T. J. and E. K. Miller (2007). Top-down versus bottom-up control of attention in the prefrontal and posterior parietal cortices. *Science* **315**(5820): 1860–2.

Butler, A. B. and W. Hodos (2005). *Comparative Vertebrate Neuroanatomy: Evolution and Adaptation*, New York: Wiley-Liss.

Carpenter, R. H. and M. L. Williams (1995). Neural computation of log likelihood in control of saccadic eye movements. *Nature* **377**(6544): 59–62.

Cisek, P. (1999). Beyond the computer metaphor: behaviour as interaction. *J. Consciousness Stud.* **6**(11–12): 125–42.

Cisek, P. (2001). Embodiment is all in the head. *Behav. Brain Sci.* **24**(1): 36–8.

Cisek, P. (2005). Neural representations of motor plans, desired trajectories, and controlled objects. *Cogn. Process.* **6**: 15–24.

Cisek, P. (2006). Integrated neural processes for defining potential actions and deciding between them: a computational model. *J. Neurosci.* **26**(38): 9761–70.

Cisek, P. (2007). Cortical mechanisms of action selection: the affordance competition hypothesis. *Phil. Trans. Roy. Soc. B. Biol. Sci.* **362**(1485): 1585–99.

Cisek, P., S. Grossberg, and D. Bullock (1998). A cortico-spinal model of reaching and proprioception under multiple task constraints. *J. Cogn. Neurosci.* **10**(4): 425–44.

Cisek, P. and J. F. Kalaska (2005). Neural correlates of reaching decisions in dorsal premotor cortex: specification of multiple direction choices and final selection of action. *Neuron* **45**(5): 801–14.

Cisek, P., N. Michaud, and J. F. Kalaska (2004). Integration of motor planning and sensory feedback in area 5. Program No. 655.13. Neuroscience Meeting Planner. San Diego, CA: Society for Neuroscience.

Cisek, P. and M. Turgeon (1999). 'Binding through the fovea', a tale of perception in the service of action. *Psyche* **5**(34).

Clark, A. (1997). *Being There: Putting Brain, Body, and World Together Again*. Cambridge, MA: MIT Press.

Coe, B., K. Tomihara, M. Matsuzawa, and O. Hikosaka (2002). Visual and anticipatory bias in three cortical eye fields of the monkey during an adaptive decision-making task. *J. Neurosci.* **22**(12): 5081–90.

Colby, C. L. and M. E. Goldberg (1999). Space and attention in parietal cortex. *Annu. Rev. Neurosci.* **22**: 319–49.

Constantinidis, C., M. N. Franowicz, and P. S. Goldman-Rakic (2001). The sensory nature of mnemonic representation in the primate prefrontal cortex. *Nat. Neurosci.* **4**(3): 311–6.

Constantinidis, C. and M. A. Steinmetz (2001). Neuronal responses in area 7a to multiple-stimulus displays: I. neurons encode the location of the salient stimulus. *Cereb. Cortex* **11**(7): 581–91.

Crammond, D. J. and J. F. Kalaska (2000). Prior information in motor and premotor cortex: activity during the delay period and effect on pre-movement activity. *J. Neurophysiol.* **84**(2): 986–1005.

Cui, H. and R. A. Andersen (2007). Posterior parietal cortex encodes autonomously selected motor plans. *Neuron* **56**(3): 552–9.

Culham, J. C. and N. G. Kanwisher (2001). Neuroimaging of cognitive functions in human parietal cortex. *Curr. Opin. Neurobiol.* **11**(2): 157–63.

Day, B. L. and I. N. Lyon (2000). Voluntary modification of automatic arm movements evoked by motion of a visual target. *Exp. Brain Res.* **130**(2): 159–68.

Dayan P. and L. F. Abbott (2001). *Theoretical Neuroscience*. Cambridge, MA: MIT Press.

Deacon, T. W. (1990). Rethinking mammalian brain evolution. *Amer. Zool.* **30**: 629–705.

Desimone, R. (1998). Visual attention mediated by biased competition in extrastriate visual cortex. *Philos. Trans. R. Soc. Lond B Biol. Sci.* **353**(1373): 1245–55.

Desimone, R., T. D. Albright, C. G. Gross, and C. Bruce (1984). Stimulus-selective properties of inferior temporal neurons in the macaque. *J. Neurosci.* **4**(8): 2051–62.

Desimone, R. and J. Duncan (1995). Neural mechanisms of selective visual attention. *Annu. Rev. Neurosci.* **18**: 193–222.

Desmurget, M., C. M. Epstein, R. S. Turner, *et al.* (1999). Role of the posterior parietal cortex in updating reaching movements to a visual target. *Nat. Neurosci.* **2**(6): 563–7.

Dewey, J. (1896). The reflex arc concept in psychology. *Psychol. Rev.* **3**(4): 357–70.

di Pellegrino, G. and S. P. Wise (1991). A neurophysiological comparison of three distinct regions of the primate frontal lobe. *Brain* **114**: 951–78.

Dorris, M. C. and P. W. Glimcher (2004). Activity in posterior parietal cortex is correlated with the relative subjective desirability of action. *Neuron* **44**(2): 365–78.

Dretske, F. (1981). *Knowledge and the Flow of Information*. Oxford: Blackwell.

Erlhagen, W. and G. Schöner (2002). Dynamic field theory of movement preparation. *Psychol. Rev.* **109**(3): 545–72.

Eskandar, E. N., B. J. Richmond, and L. M. Optican (1992). Role of inferior temporal neurons in visual memory. I. Temporal encoding of information about visual images, recalled images, and behavioral context. *J. Neurophysiol.* **68**(4): 1277–95.

Ewert, J-P. (1997). Neural correlates of key stimulus and releasing mechanism: a case study and two concepts. *TINS* **20**(8): 332–9.

Ewert, J-P., H. Buxbaum-Conradi, F. Dreisvogt, *et al.* (2001). Neural modulation of visuomotor functions underlying prey-catching behaviour in anurans: perception, attention, motor performance, learning. *Comp. Biochem. Physiol. A* **128**(3): 417–60.

Fadiga, L., L. Fogassi, V. Gallese, and G. Rizzolatti (2000). Visuomotor neurons: ambiguity of the discharge or 'motor' perception? *Int. J. Psychophysiol.* **35**(2–3): 165–77.

Fagg, A. H. and M. A. Arbib (1998). Modeling parietal-premotor interactions in primate control of grasping. *Neural Networks* **11**(7–8): 1277–303.

Favilla, M. (1997). Reaching movements: concurrency of continuous and discrete programming. *Neuroreport* **8**(18): 3973–7.

Ferraina, S. and L. Bianchi (1994). Posterior parietal cortex: functional properties of neurons in area 5 during an instructed-delay reaching task within different parts of space. *Exp. Brain Res.* **99**(1):175–8.

Fuster, J. M. and G. E. Alexander (1971). Neuron activity related to short-term memory. *Science* **173**(997): 652–4.

Fuster, J. M., M. Bodner, and J. K. Kroger (2000). Cross-modal and cross-temporal association in neurons of frontal cortex. *Nature* **405**(6784): 347–51.

Gallese, V. (2000). The inner sense of action: agency and motor representations. *J. Consciousness Stud.* **7**(10): 23–40.

Ghez, C., M. Favilla, M. F. Ghilardi, *et al.* (1997). Discrete and continuous planning of hand movements and isometric force trajectories. *Exp. Brain Res.* **115**(2): 217–33.

Gibson, J. J. (1979). *The Ecological Approach to Visual Perception*. Boston, MA: Houghton Mifflin.

Gilbert, S. F., J. M. Opitz, and R. A. Raff (1996). Resynthesizing evolutionary and developmental biology. *Dev. Biol.* **173**(2): 357–72.

Glenberg, A. M. (1997). What memory is for. *Behav. Brain Sci.* **20**(1): 1–55.

Glimcher, P. W. (2001). Making choices: the neurophysiology of visual-saccadic decision making. *TINS* **24**(11): 654–9.

Glimcher, P. W. (2003). The neurobiology of visual-saccadic decision making. *Annu. Rev. Neurosci.* **26**: 133–79.

Gold, J. I. and M. N. Shadlen (2000). Representation of a perceptual decision in developing oculomotor commands. *Nature* **404**(6776): 390–4.

Gold, J. I. and M. N. Shadlen (2001). Neural computations that underlie decisions about sensory stimuli. *Trends Cogn. Sci.* **5**(1):10–16.

Goodale, M. A. and A. D. Milner (1992). Separate visual pathways for perception and action. *TINS* **15**(1): 20–25.

Gottlieb, J. P., M. Kusunoki, and M. E. Goldberg (1998). The representation of visual salience in monkey parietal cortex. *Nature* **391**(6666): 481–4.

Graziano, M. S. A., D. F. Cooke, and C. S. R. Taylor (2000). Coding the location of the arm by sight. *Science* **290**(5497): 1782–6.

Grossberg, S. (1973). Contour enhancement, short term memory, and constancies in reverberating neural networks. *Stud. Appl. Math.* **52**: 213–57.

Hendriks-Jansen, H. (1996). *Catching Ourselves in the Act: Situated Activity, Interactive Emergence, Evolution, and Human Thought*. Cambridge, MA: MIT Press.

Hinde, R. A. (1966). *Animal Behaviour: A Synthesis of Ethology and Comparative Psychology*. New York: McGraw-Hill Book Company.

Holland, L. Z. and N. D. Holland (1999). Chordate origins of the vertebrate central nervous system. *Curr. Opin. Neurobiol.* **9**(5): 596–602.

Hommel, B., J. Müsseler, G. Aschersleben, and W. Prinz (2001). The theory of event coding (TEC): a framework for perception and action planning. *Behav. Brain Sci.* **24**(5): 849–937.

Horwitz, G. D., A. P. Batista, and W. T. Newsome (2004). Representation of an abstract perceptual decision in macaque superior colliculus. *J. Neurophysiol.* **91**(5): 2281–96.

Hoshi, E., K. Shima, and J. Tanji (1998). Task-dependent selectivity of movement-related neuronal activity in the primate prefrontal cortex. *J. Neurophysiol.* **80**(6): 3392–7.

Hoshi, E., K. Shima, and J. Tanji (2000). Neuronal activity in the primate prefrontal cortex in the process of motor selection based on two behavioral rules. *J. Neurophysiol.* **83**(4): 2355–73.

Houk, J. C., J. Keifer, and A. G. Barto (1993). Distributed motor commands in the limb premotor network. *TINS* **16**(1): 27–33.

Jackson, J. H. (1884 [1958]). Evolution and dissolution of the nervous system. In *Selected writings of John Hughlings Jackson*, ed. J Taylor. London: Staples Press, pp. 45–75.

Janssen, P. and M. N. Shadlen (2005). A representation of the hazard rate of elapsed time in macaque area LIP. *Nat. Neurosci.* **8**(2): 234–41.

Johnson, P. B., S. Ferraina, L. Bianchi, and R. Caminiti (1996). Cortical networks for visual reaching: physiological and anatomical organization of frontal and parietal arm regions. *Cereb. Cortex* **6**(2):102–19.

Johnson-Laird, P. N. (1988). *The Computer and the Mind: An Introduction to Cognitive Science.* Cambridge, MA: Harvard University Press.

Jones, E. G., J. D. Coulter, and H. C. Hendry (1978). Intracortical connectivity of achitectonic fields in the somatic sensory, motor and parietal cortex of monkeys. *J. Comp. Neurol.* **181**: 291–348.

Kalaska, J. F. and D. J. Crammond (1995). Deciding not to GO: Neuronal correlates of response selection in a GO/NOGO task in primate premotor and parietal cortex. *Cereb. Cortex* **5**: 410–28.

Kalaska, J. F., L. E. Sergio, and P. Cisek (1998). Cortical control of whole-arm motor tasks. In *Sensory Guidance of Movement, Novartis Foundation Symposium #218*, ed. M. Glickstein. Chichester, UK: John Wiley and Sons, pp. 176–201.

Kalivas, P. W. and M. Nakamura (1999). Neural systems for behavioral activation and reward. *Curr. Opin. Neurobiol.* **9**(2): 223–7.

Karten, H. J. (1969). The organization of the avian telencephalon and some speculations on the phylogeny of the amniote telencephalon. *Ann. N.Y. Acad. Sci.* **167**(1): 164–79.

Katz, P. S. and R. M. Harris-Warrick (1999). The evolution of neuronal circuits underlying species-specific behavior. *Curr. Opin. Neurobiol.* **9**(5): 628–33.

Keele, S. W. (1968). Movement control in skilled motor performance. *Psychol. Bull.* **70**: 387–403.

Kettner, R. E., J. K. Marcario, and N. L. Port (1993). A neural network model of cortical activity during reaching. *J. Cogn. Neurosci.* **5**(1):14–33.

Kim, J-N. and M. N. Shadlen (1999). Neural correlates of a decision in the dorsolateral prefrontal cortex of the macaque. *Nat. Neurosci.* **2**(2):176–85.

Knill, D. C. and A. Pouget (2004). The Bayesian brain: the role of uncertainty in neural coding and computation. *Trends Neurosci.* **27**(12): 712–9.

Kornblum, S., T. Hasbroucq, and A. Osman (1990). Dimensional overlap: cognitive basis for stimulus-response compatibility – a model and taxonomy. *Psychol. Rev.* **97**(2): 253–70.

Krubitzer, L. and J. Kaas (2005). The evolution of the neocortex in mammals: how is phenotypic diversity generated? *Curr. Opin. Neurobiol.* **15**(4): 444–53.

Kusunoki, M., J. Gottlieb, and M. E. Goldberg (2000). The lateral intraparietal area as a salience map: the representation of abrupt onset, stimulus motion, and task relevance. *Vision Res.* **40**(10–12): 1459–68.

Lauwereyns, J., K. Watanabe, B. Coe, and O. Hikosaka (2002). A neural correlate of response bias in monkey caudate nucleus. *Nature* **418**(6896): 413–7.

Leblois, A., T. Boraud, W. Meissner, H. Bergman, and D. Hansel (2006). Competition between feedback loops underlies normal and pathological dynamics in the basal ganglia. *J. Neurosci.* **26**(13): 3567–83.

Ledberg, A., S. L. Bressler, M. Ding, R. Coppola, and R. Nakamura (2007). Large-scale visuo-motor integration in the cerebral cortex. *Cereb. Cortex* **17**(1): 44–62.

Machens, C. K., R. Romo, and C. D. Brody (2005). Flexible control of mutual inhibition: a neural model of two-interval discrimination. *Science* **307**(5712): 1121–4.

MacLean, P. D. (1973). *A Triune Concept of the Brain and Behaviour.* Toronto: University of Toronto Press.

Marconi, B., A. Genovesio, A. Battaglia-Mayer, *et al.* (2001). Eye–hand coordination during reaching. I. Anatomical relationships between parietal and frontal cortex. *Cereb. Cortex.* **11**(6): 513–27.

Marr, D. C. (1982). *Vision.* San Francisco: W. H. Freeman.

Matelli, M. and G. Luppino (2001). Parietofrontal circuits for action and space perception in the macaque monkey. *Neuroimage.* **14**(1 Pt 2):S27–S32.

Maturana, H. R. and F. J. Varela (1980). *Autopoiesis and Cognition: The Realization of the Living,* Boston, MA: D. Reidel.

Mazurek, M. E., J. D. Roitman, J. Ditterich, and M. N. Shadlen (2003). A role for neural integrators in perceptual decision making. *Cereb. Cortex* **13**(11): 1257–69.

McIntyre, J. and E. Bizzi (1993). Servo hypotheses for the biological control of movement. *J. Motor Behav.* **25**(3): 193–202.

Mead, G. H. (1938). *The Philosophy of the Act.* Chicago, IL: University of Chicago Press.

Medina, L. and A. Reiner (2000). Do birds possess homologues of mammalian primary visual, somatosensory and motor cortices? *TINS* **23**(1): 1–12.

Merleau-Ponty, M. (1945). *Phénoménologie de la perception.* Paris: Gallimard.

Middleton, F. A. and P. L. Strick (2000). Basal ganglia and cerebellar loops: motor and cognitive circuits. *Brain Res. Rev.* **31**(2–3): 236–50.

Miller, E. K. (2000). The prefrontal cortex and cognitive control. *Nature Rev. Neurosci.* **1**(1): 59–65.

Miller, G. A., E. Galanter, and K. H. Pribram (1960). *Plans and the Structure of Behavior.* New York: Holt, Rinehart and Winston, Inc.

Millikan, R. G. (1989). Biosemantics. *J. Philosophy* **86**(6): 281–97.

Mink, J. W. (1996). The basal ganglia: focused selection and inhibition of competing motor programs. *Prog. Neurobiol.* **50**(4): 381–425.

Nakamura, H., T. Kuroda, M. Wakita, *et al.* (2001). From three-dimensional space vision to prehensile hand movements: the lateral intraparietal area links the area V3A and the anterior intraparietal area in macaques. *J. Neurosci.* **21**(20): 8174–87.

Neumann, O. (1990). Visual attention and action. In *Relationships Between Perception and Action: Current Approaches,* ed. O Neumann and W Prinz. Berlin: Springer-Verlag, pp. 227–67.

Newell, A. and H. A. Simon (1972). *Human Problem Solving.* Englewood Cliffs, NJ: Prentice-Hall.

Núñez, R. and W. J. Freeman (2000). *Reclaiming Cognition: The Primacy of Action, Intention and Emotion.* Thorverton, UK: Imprint Academic.

O'Regan, J. K. and A. Noë (2001). A sensorimotor account of vision and visual consciousness. *Behav. Brain Sci.* **24**(5): 939–1011.

Pandya, D. N. and H. G. J. M. Kuypers (1969). Cortico-cortical connections in the rhesus monkey. *Brain Res.* **13**: 13–36.

Paradiso, M. A. (2002). Perceptual and neuronal correspondence in primary visual cortex. *Curr. Opin. Neurobiol.* **12**(2): 155–61.

Paré, M. and R. H. Wurtz (2001). Progression in neuronal processing for saccadic eye movements from parietal cortex area lip to superior colliculus. *J. Neurophysiol.* **85**(6): 2545–62.

Passingham, R. E. and I. Toni (2001). Contrasting the dorsal and ventral visual systems: guidance of movement versus decision making. *Neuroimage* **14**(1 Pt 2): S125–S131.

Pesaran, B., M. J. Nelson, and R. A. Andersen (2008). Free choice activates a decision circuit between frontal and parietal cortex. *Nature* **453**(7193): 406–9.

Petrides, M. (2000). The role of the mid-dorsolateral prefrontal cortex in working memory. *Exp. Brain Res.* **133**(1): 44–54.

Piaget, J. (1967). *Biologie et Connaissance: Essai sur les Relations Entre les Régulation Organiques et les Processus Cognitifs*. Paris: Editions Gallimard.

Platt, M. L. (2002). Neural correlates of decisions. *Curr. Opin. Neurobiol.* **12**(2): 141–8.

Platt, M. L. and P. W. Glimcher (1997). Responses of intraparietal neurons to saccadic targets and visual distractors. *J. Neurophysiol.* **78**(3): 1574–89.

Platt, M. L. and P. W. Glimcher (1999). Neural correlates of decision variables in parietal cortex. *Nature* **400**(6741): 233–8.

Powers, W. T. (1973). *Behavior: The Control of Perception*. New York: Aldine Publishing Company.

Prescott, T. J., P. Redgrave, and K. Gurney (1999). Layered control architectures in robots and vertebrates. *Adapt. Behav.* **7**: 99–127.

Quintana, J. and J. M. Fuster (1999). From perceptions to actions: temporal integrative functions of prefrontal and parietal neurons. *Cereb. Cortex* **9**(3): 213–21.

Rainer, G., W. F. Asaad, and E. K. Miller (1998). Selective representation of relevant information by neurons in the primate prefrontal cortex. *Nature* **363**(6885): 577–9.

Ratcliff, R., A. Cherian, and M. Segraves (2003). A comparison of macaque behavior and superior colliculus neuronal activity to predictions from models of two-choice decisions. *J. Neurophysiol.* **90**(3): 1392–407.

Reddi, B. A. J., K. N. Asrress, and R. H. S. Carpenter (2003). Accuracy, information, and response time in a saccadic decision task. *J. Neurophysiol.* **90**(5): 3538–46.

Redgrave, P., T. J. Prescott, and K. Gurney (1999). The basal ganglia: a vertebrate solution to the selection problem? *Neuroscience* **89**(4): 1009–23.

Rizzolatti, G. and G. Luppino (2001). The cortical motor system. *Neuron* **31**(6): 889–901.

Roe, R. M., J. R. Busemeyer, and J. T. Townsend (2001). Multialternative decision field theory: a dynamic connectionist model of decision making. *Psychol. Rev.* **108**(2): 370–92.

Roesch, M. R. and C. R. Olson (2004). Neuronal activity related to reward value and motivation in primate frontal cortex. *Science* **304**(5668): 307–10.

Romo, R., A. Hernandez, and A. Zainos (2004). Neuronal correlates of a perceptual decision in ventral premotor cortex. *Neuron* **41**(1): 165–73.

Rowe, J. B., I. Toni, O. Josephs, R. S. Frackowiak, and R. E. Passingham (2000). The prefrontal cortex: response selection or maintenance within working memory? *Science* **288**(5471): 1656–60.

Saleem, K. S., W. Suzuki, K. Tanaka, and T. Hashikawa (2000). Connections between anterior inferotemporal cortex and superior temporal sulcus regions in the macaque monkey. *J. Neurosci.* **20**(13): 5083–101.

Sanger, T. D. (2003). Neural population codes. *Curr. Opin. Neurobiol.* **13**(2): 238–49.

Sato, T. R. and J. D. Schall (2003). Effects of stimulus-response compatibility on neural selection in frontal eye field. *Neuron* **38**(4): 637–48.

Scherberger, H. and R. A. Andersen (2007). Target selection signals for arm reaching in the posterior parietal cortex. *J. Neurosci.* **27**(8): 2001–12.

Schmolesky, M. T., Y. Wang, D. P. Hanes, *et al.* (1998). Signal timing across the macaque visual system. *J. Neurophysiol.* **79**(6): 3272–8.

Schultz, W., L. Tremblay, and J. R. Hollerman (2000). Reward processing in primate orbitofrontal cortex and basal ganglia. *Cereb. Cortex* **10**(3): 272–84.

Seth, A. K. (2007). The ecology of action selection: insights from artificial life. *Philos. Trans. R. Soc. Lond B Biol. Sci.* **362**(1485): 1545–58.

Shadlen, M. N. and W. T. Newsome (2001). Neural basis of a perceptual decision in the parietal cortex (area lip) of the rhesus monkey. *J. Neurophysiol.* **86**(4): 1916–36.

Shafir, E. and A. Tversky (1995). Decision making. In *Thinking: An Invitation to Cognitive Science*, ed. E. E. Smith and D. N. Osherson. Cambridge, MA: MIT Press, pp. 77–100.

Shu, D. G., S. C. Morris, J. Han, *et al.* (2003). Head and backbone of the Early Cambrian vertebrate *Haikouichthys. Nature* **421**(6922): 526–9.

Smith, P. L. and R. Ratcliff (2004). Psychology and neurobiology of simple decisions. *Trends Neurosci.* **27**(3): 161–8.

Snyder, L. H., A. P. Batista, and R. A. Andersen (1997). Coding of intention in the posterior parietal cortex. *Nature* **386**:167–70.

Snyder, L. H., A. P. Batista, and R. A. Andersen (1998a). Change in motor plan, without a change in the spatial locus of attention, modulates activity in posterior parietal cortex. *J. Neurophysiol.* **79**(5): 2814–9.

Snyder, L. H., A. P. Batista, and R. A. Andersen (2000a). Intention-related activity in the posterior parietal cortex: a review. *Vision Res.* **40**(10–12): 1433–41.

Snyder, L. H., A. P. Batista, and R. A. Andersen (2000b). Saccade-related activity in the parietal reach region. *J. Neurophysiol.* **83**(2):1099–102.

Snyder, L. H., K. L. Grieve, P. Brotchie, and R. A. Andersen (1998b). Separate body- and world-referenced representations of visual space in parietal cortex. *Nature* **394**(6696): 887–91.

Stein, J. F. (1992). The representation of egocentric space in the posterior parietal cortex. *Behav. Brain Sci.* **15**: 691–700.

Sterelny, K. (1989). Computational functional psychology: problems and prospects. In *Computers, Brains, and Minds*, ed. P. Slezak and W. R. Albury. Dordrecht: Kluwer Academic Publishers, pp. 71–93.

Sugrue, L. P., G. S. Corrado, and W. T. Newsome (2004). Matching behavior and the representation of value in the parietal cortex. *Science* **304**(5678): 1782–7.

Takikawa, Y., R. Kawagoe, and O. Hikosaka (2002). Reward-dependent spatial selectivity of anticipatory activity in monkey caudate neurons. *J. Neurophysiol.* **87**(1): 508–15.

Tanaka, K., H-A. Saito, Y. Fukada, and M. Moriya (1991). Coding visual images of objects in the inferotemporal cortex of the macaque monkey. *J. Neurophysiol.* **66**(1): 170–89.

Tanji, J. and E. Hoshi (2001). Behavioral planning in the prefrontal cortex. *Curr. Opin. Neurobiol.* **11**(2): 164–70.

Thelen, E., G. Schöner, C. Scheier, and L. B. Smith (2001). The dynamics of embodiment: a field theory of infant perseverative reaching. *Behav. Brain Sci.* **24**(1): 1–34.

Thomas, N. W. and M. Pare (2007). Temporal processing of saccade targets in parietal cortex area LIP during visual search. *J. Neurophysiol.* **97**(1): 942–7.

Thompson, K. G., D. P. Hanes, N. P. Bichot, and J. D. Schall (1996). Perceptual and motor processing stages identified in the activity of macaque frontal eye field neurons during visual search. *J. Neurophysiol.* **76**(6): 4040–55.

Tinbergen, N. (1950). The hierarchical organisation of nervous mechanisms underlying instinctive behavior. *Symp. Soc. Exp. Biol.* **4**: 305–12.

Tipper, S. P., L. A. Howard, and G. Houghton (1998). Action-based mechanisms of attention. *Phil. Trans. R. Soc. Lond. B* **353**(1373): 1385–93.

Tipper, S. P., L. A. Howard, and G. Houghton (2000). Behavioural consequences of selection from neural population codes. In *Control of Cognitive Processes: Attention and Performance XVIII*, ed. S. Monsell and J. Driver. Cambridge, MA: MIT Press, pp. 223–45.

Tipper, S. P., C. Lortie and G. C. Baylis (1992). Selective reaching: evidence for action-centered attention. *J. Exp. Psychol. Human* **18**(4): 891–905.

Toates, F. (1998). The interaction of cognitive and stimulus-response processes in the control of behaviour. *Neurosci. Biobehav. R.* **22**(1): 59–83.

Treue, S. (2001). Neural correlates of attention in primate visual cortex. *Trends Neurosci.* **24**(5): 295–300.

Ungerleider, L. G. and M. Mishkin (1982). Two cortical visual systems. In *Analysis of Visual Behavior*, Vol. 18, ed. D. J. Ingle, M. A. Goodale, R. J. W. Mansfield. Cambridge, MA: MIT Press, pp. 549–86.

Usher, M. and J. L. McClelland (2001). The time course of perceptual choice: the leaky, competing accumulator model. *Psychol. Rev.* **108**(3): 550–92.

von der Malsburg, C. (1996). The binding problem of neural networks. In *The Mind-Brain Continuum: Sensory Processes*, Vol. 7, ed. R. Llinás and P. S. Churchland. Cambridge, MA: MIT Press, pp. 131–46.

Wallis, J. D. and E. K. Miller (2003). From rule to response: neuronal processes in the premotor and prefrontal cortex. *J. Neurophysiol.* **90**(3): 1790–806.

Wang, X. J. (2002). Probabilistic decision making by slow reverberation in cortical circuits. *Neuron* **36**(5): 955–68.

White, I. M. and S. P. Wise (1999). Rule-dependent neuronal activity in the prefrontal cortex. *Exp. Brain Res.* **126**(3): 315–35.

Wise, S. P., D. Boussaoud, P. B. Johnson, and R. Caminiti (1997). Premotor and parietal cortex: corticocortical connectivity and combinatorial computations. *Annu. Rev. Neurosci.* **20**: 25–42.

Yang, T. and M. N. Shadlen (2007). Probabilistic reasoning by neurons. *Nature* **447**(7148): 1075–80.

12 Toward an executive without a homunculus: computational models of the prefrontal cortex/basal ganglia system

Thomas E. Hazy, Michael J. Frank, and Randall C. O'Reilly

Summary

The prefrontal cortex (PFC) has long been thought to serve as an 'executive' that controls the selection of actions, and cognitive functions more generally. However, the mechanistic basis of this executive function has not been clearly specified, often amounting to a homunculus. This chapter reviews recent attempts to deconstruct this homunculus by elucidating the precise computational and neural mechanisms underlying the executive functions of the PFC. The overall approach builds upon existing mechanistic models of the basal ganglia (BG) and frontal systems known to play a critical role in motor control and action selection, where the BG provide a 'Go' versus 'NoGo' modulation of frontal action representations. In our model, the BG modulate working memory representations in prefrontal areas to support more abstract executive functions. We have developed a computational model of this system that is capable of developing human-like performance on working memory and executive control tasks through trial-and-error learning. This learning is based on reinforcement learning mechanisms associated with the midbrain dopaminergic system and its activation via the BG and amygdala. Finally, we briefly describe various empirical tests of this framework.

12.1 Introduction

There is widespread agreement that some regions of the brain play a larger role in controlling our overall behaviour than others, with a strong consensus that the prefrontal cortex (PFC) is a 'central executive' (e.g., Baddeley, 1986; Christoff et al., 2009; Conway et al., 2005; Duncan, 2001; Koechlin and Summerfield, 2007; Miller and Cohen, 2001; Shallice, 1988). However, this central executive label raises many more questions than it answers. How does the PFC know what actions or plans to select? How does experience influence the PFC? How do the specific neural properties of the PFC enable this kind of function, and how do these differ from those in other, non-executive areas?

Modelling Natural Action Selection, eds. Anil K. Seth, Tony J. Prescott and Joanna J. Bryson.
Published by Cambridge University Press. © Cambridge University Press 2012.

Without answers to these kinds of questions, the notion of a central executive is tanta-mount to positing a homunculus (small man) living inside the PFC and controlling our actions.

This chapter reviews ongoing research attempting to characterise the computational and neural mechanisms by which the prefrontal cortex guides cognition and behaviour. We see these mechanisms as an evolutionary extension of the same frontal cortical and basal ganglia (BG) mechanisms involved in the motor control system, which are relatively better characterised and do not have the same degree of mysterious executive function associated with them. In this motor domain, the basal ganglia modulate frontal motor representations, by providing 'Go versus 'NoGo' signals that reflect the prior reward history of actions (Berns and Sejnowski, 1998; Cisek, 2007; Cisek, this volume; Dominey *et al.*, 1995; Houk, this volume; Houk and Wise, 1995; Houk *et al.*, 2007; Mink, 1996; Wickens, 1993; Wickens *et al.*, 1995). In the PFC, the basal ganglia can similarly provide Go/NoGo modulation controlling the maintenance of more abstract PFC working memory representations, which in turn guide behaviour and cognition (Frank *et al.*, 2001; Frank *et al.*, 2007c; Frank *et al.*, this volume; Hazy *et al.*, 2006; Hazy *et al.*, 2007; O'Reilly, 2006; O'Reilly and Frank, 2006). These PFC represen-tations include plans, goals, task-relevant sensory stimuli, partial products of ongoing processing, etc.

We have identified six core functional demands that collectively serve to define the fundamental nature of prefrontal cortical function from a neuro-mechanistic perspective. Further, whereas our initial focus was on the mechanisms by which the BG–PFC system learns when to update and maintain information in working memory (Frank *et al.*, 2001; Hazy *et al.*, 2006; O'Reilly and Frank, 2006), here we extend the model to include an *output gating* mechanism that can determine which of a subset among multiple parallel active representations should be currently used to guide action selection (similar to the model of Brown *et al.*, 2004). Interestingly, the same BG mechanisms that can drive the selection of when to update PFC working memory representations can also be used (in parallel circuits) to select which of the already maintained PFC representations should be actually be used to guide behaviour.

This chapter has two goals: to describe (1) the latest version of our prefrontal cortex, basal ganglia working memory (PBWM) model, including two important extensions recently added, and (2) our ongoing attempt to model several key working memory tasks in a single instantiation of the model. The chapter's overall organisation follows accordingly: we first describe the PBWM computational model and how it relates work-ing memory with motor control and action selection. (We see working memory as the fundamental mechanism underlying executive function generally.) In elucidating our model, we place special emphasis on six key functional demands underlying working memory. We then describe two new extensions to the model, output gating and a mech-anism for dealing with the exploration/exploitation trade-off in learning (Aston-Jones and Cohen, 2005). Finally, we outline a research trajectory to simulate an increasing number of the most important task paradigms of working memory and executive func-tion in a single instantiation of a comprehensive model built around the core PBWM mechanisms.

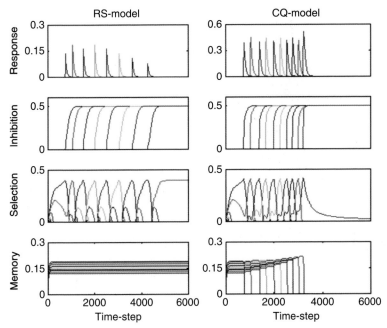

Figure 8.4 Activation trajectories of the RS and CQ models. Activation between layers goes from 'memory' to 'selection' to 'output', with 'inhibition' suppressing the activation at either the 'memory' (CQ model) or the 'selection' (RS model) layer. The RS model does not produce all responses (eight spikes in the output layer), whereas the CQ model does. Note also that the activation in the memory layer for the CQ model shows the signature of the CQ mechanism (after an output the corresponding trace is inhibited, which causes an increase in activation for the remaining traces).

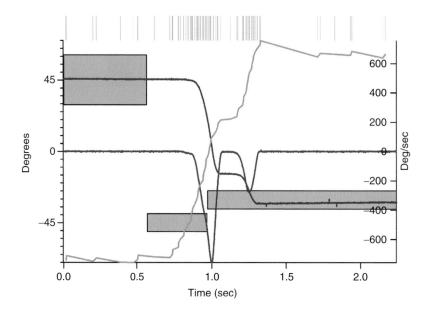

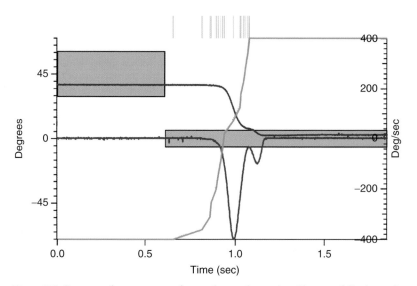

Figure 10.3 Segmented movements of a monkey and associated bursts of discharge in primary motor cortex. The monkey turned a rotating handle to move a cursor horizontally on a screen (blue trace = position; red trace = velocity) to acquire a target (shaded boxes). (a) The firing pattern of a motor cortical neuron during a trial that contains a delayed submovement. (b) The firing pattern of another motor cortical cell during a trial that contains an overlapping submovement. Each motor cortical neuron shows two bursts of discharge, which are marked by upward deflections in the green baseline-rate normalised cumulative sum (CUSUM) traces. Taken from Houk *et al.* (2007).

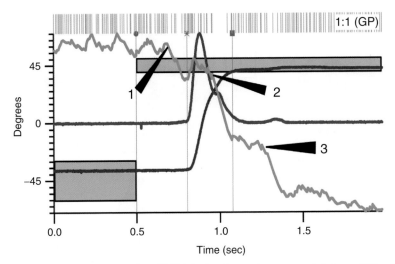

Figure 10.6 Activity during a single trial of an internal segment of globus pallidus (GPi) neuron. In this task the monkey turns a rotating handle to move a cursor horizontally on a screen (blue trace = position; red trace = velocity) to acquire a target (blue boxes). The baseline-rate normalised cumulative sum histogram (CUSUM) for the neuron (green trace) shows three downward deflections marking three pauses in the high tonic discharge rate in this GPi neuron. The first pause (arrow 1) is small and occurs prior to the primary movement; the second and third pauses are stronger and are associated with tiny corrective submovements (arrows 2 and 3). Modified from Houk *et al.* (2007).

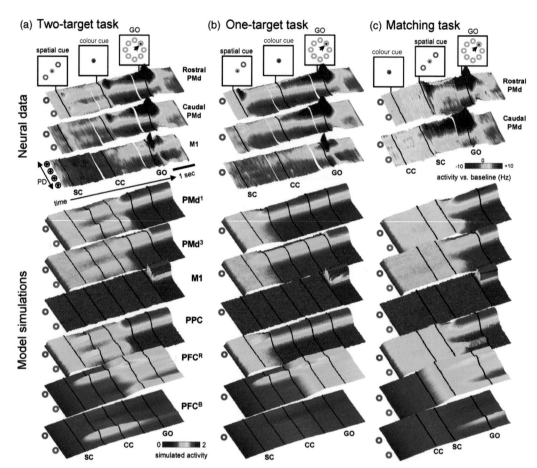

Figure 11.3 Comparison between neural activity and model simulations in three kinds of tasks. (a) Two-target task. During the spatial cue (SC), two possible targets are presented, one red and one blue. During the colour cue (CC), the centre indicates which of these is the correct target. The GO signal instructs the monkey to begin the movement. Neural data (Cisek and Kalaska, 2005) is shown from three sets of neurons: rostral PMd, caudal PMd, and primary motor cortex (M1). In each, neural activity is depicted as a 3D coloured surface in which time runs from left to right and cells are sorted by their preferred direction along the left edge. Coloured circles indicate the locations of the two targets. Simulated model activities are depicted in the same format, where black lines indicate behavioural events (spatial cue on, spatial cue off, colour cue on, colour cue off, GO). (b) One-target task, same format. (c) Matching task, same format.

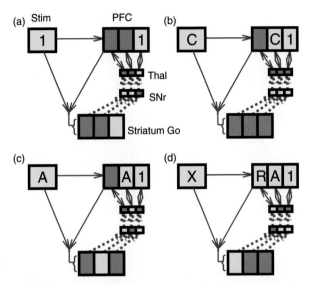

Figure 12.5 Illustration of how basal ganglia maintenance gating of different prefrontal cortex (PFC) stripes can solve the 1–2-AX task (light shading = active; dark = not active). Only three stripes are shown for clarity; we have estimated elsewhere there may actually be in the order of 20 000 stripes in the human frontal cortex (Frank *et al.*, 2001). (a) The 1 task is gated into an anterior PFC stripe because a corresponding striatal stripe fired Go. (b) The distractor C fails to fire striatal Go neurons, so it will not be maintained; however, it does elicit transient PFC activity. Note that the 1 persists because of gating-induced robust maintenance. (c) The A is gated in to a separate stripe. (d) A right keypress motor action is activated based on X input plus maintained PFC context.

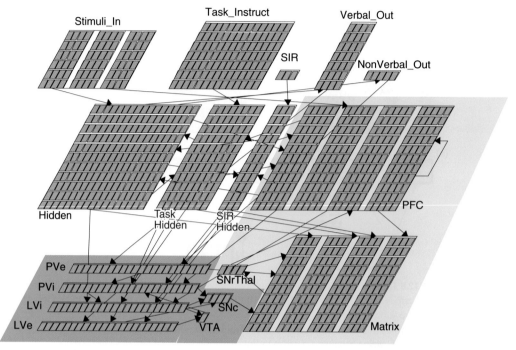

Figure 12.7 Overall structure of the MT model. Similar to our other PBWM models, the input/output layers are at the top-left of the diagram. The prefrontal cortex (PFC) and basal ganglia (BG) layers are at the bottom-right. The PVLV learning algorithm layers are in the lower left hand corner (highlighted in darker grey), and the full PBWM component also includes the BG (Matrix, SNrThal) and PFC on the right hand side (highlighted in lighter grey). Depending on the particular task, single or multiple featured stimuli are presented in one or more 'slots' in the Stimuli_In layer, along with task instructions in the Task_Instruct and SIR (store, ignore, recall) layers. Based on these inputs, plus context provided by PFC input, the Hidden layer determines the correct output in verbal or nonverbal form, or both. The shown model has four 'stripes' reflected in the four subgroups of the PFC and Matrix (striatal matrisomes) layers, and the four units of the SNc and SNrThal layers. SNc = substantia nigra, pars compacta; SNrThal = abstracted layer reflecting direct and indirect pathways via substantia nigra, pars reticulata and thalamus; VTA = ventral tegmental area; PVe = primary value (PV) excitatory, external reward; PVi = primary value inhibitory (anatomically associated with patch/striosomes of ventral striatum); LVi = learned value (LV) inhibitory (same anatomical locus); and LVe = learned value, excitatory (anatomically associated with the central nucleus of the amygdala).

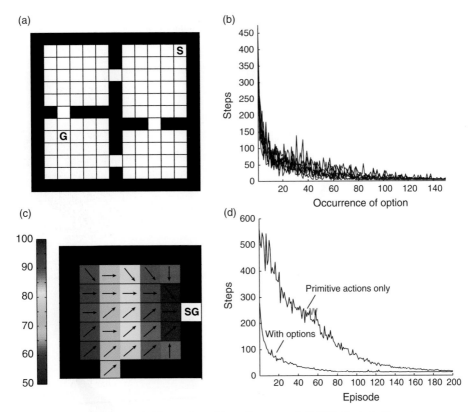

Figure 13.4 (a) The rooms problem, adapted from Sutton *et al.* (1999). *S*: start; *G*: goal.
(b) Learning curves for the eight doorway options, plotted over the first 150 occurrences of each (mean over 100 simulation runs). See Appendix A for simulation details. (c) The upper left room from panel A, illustrating the policy learned by one doorway option. Arrows indicate the primitive action selected most frequently in each state. SG: option subgoal. Colours indicate the option-specific value for each state. (d) Learning curves indicating solution times, i.e., number of primitive steps to goal, on the problem illustrated in panel a (mean over 100 simulation runs). Upper data series: performance when only primitive actions were included. Lower series: performance when both primitive actions and doorway options were included. Policies for doorway options were established through earlier training (see Chapter 13, Appendix A).

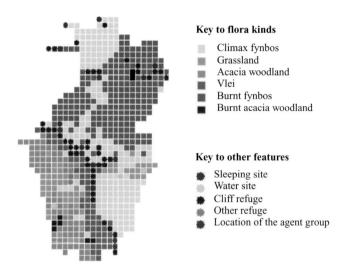

Figure 20.1 Graphical output from the simulator showing the habitat types and distributions.

Key to flora kinds

Climax fynbos
Grassland
Acacia woodland
Vlei
Burnt fynbos
Burnt acacia woodland

Key to other features

Sleeping site
Water site
Cliff refuge
Other refuge
Location of the agent group

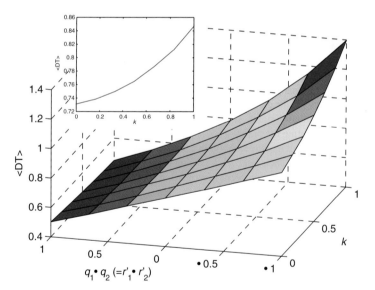

Figure 22.5 Results from numerical simulation of the *A. mellifera* direct-switching model. When decay $k > 0$, decision making is more strongly affected by the difference in discovery rates and recruitment rates from the home nest ($q_1 - q_2$ and $r'_1 - r'_2$); if these differences are in favour of the superior alternative site (site 1), then decision time can be reduced by increasing k, however if the differences favour the inferior alternative then increasing k increases decision time. Inset: if all differences are equally likely then mean decision time (y-axis) is minimised when k (x-axis) equals zero.

12.2   The PBWM model of working memory

Based on our cumulative work on a wide variety of working memory tasks, we have identified a core set of six functional demands, enumerated below, that are required by tasks involving working memory and executive function. Taken together, these functional demands provide a basic set of constraints for our biologically based PBWM model. Regarding the relationship between working memory and executive function, we see the former as providing the fundamental process that underlies executive function generally. Briefly, we believe it is the rapid and selective pattern of updating of PFC stripes (largely under control of the basal ganglia) that results in the emergent set of phenomena we recognise as executive function. The 1–2-AX task, which is an extension of the widely studied AX version of the continuous performance task (AX-CPT), provides a nice demonstration of these information-processing demands on the working memory/executive function system.

The AX-CPT is a standard working memory task that has been extensively studied in humans (Braver and Cohen, 2000; Braver et al., 1999; Cohen et al., 1997b; Frank and O'Reilly, 2006). The subject is presented with sequential letter stimuli (A, X, B, Y), and is asked to detect the specific sequence of an A followed on the very next event by an X, by pushing the target (right) button. All other combinations (A-Y, B-X, B-Y) should be responded to with a non-target (left) button push. This task requires a relatively simple form of working memory, where the prior stimulus must be maintained over a delay until the next stimulus appears, so that the subject can discriminate the target from non-target sequences. This is the kind of activation-based working memory that has often been observed, for example, in electrophysiological studies of working memory in monkeys (e.g., Funahashi et al., 1989; Fuster and Alexander, 1971; Kubota and Niki, 1971; Miller et al., 1996; Miyashita and Chang, 1988).

In the 1–2 extension of the AX-CPT task (1–2-AX; Figure 12.1; Dayan, 2007; Frank et al., 2001; O'Reilly and Frank, 2006), the target sequence varies depending on prior *task demand* stimuli (a 1 or 2). Specifically, if the subject last saw a 1, then the target sequence is A-X. However, if the subject last saw a 2, then the target sequence is B-Y. Thus, the task demand stimuli define an *outer loop* of active maintenance (maintenance of task demands) within which there can be any number of inner loops of active maintenance for the A-X level sequences.

12.2.1   Six key functional demands for working memory

Using the 1–2-AX task as a concrete example, six key functional demands placed upon the working memory system can be identified:

1. *Rapid updating:* The working memory system should be able to rapidly encode and maintain new information as it occurs. In the 1–2-AX task, as each relevant stimulus is presented, it must be rapidly encoded in working memory.
2. *Robust maintenance:* Information that remains relevant should be maintained in the face of the interference from ongoing processing or other stimulus inputs. In the

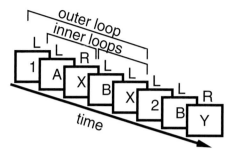

Figure 12.1 The 1–2-AX task. Stimuli (in boxes) are presented one at a time in a sequence and the subject is required to press either a left or right key (L, R; no boxes) after each stimulus. Correct responses are the right key (R) to a target sequence of two stimuli, or a left key (L) otherwise (cue only; wrong sequence). Target sequences are determined as follows: If the subject last saw a 1, then the target sequence is an A followed by an X. If a 2 was last seen, then the target is a B followed by a Y. Distractor stimuli (e.g., 3, C, Z) may also be presented at any point, but are to be ignored (no response). Thus, the maintenance of the task stimuli (1 or 2) constitutes a temporal outer-loop around multiple inner-loop memory updates required to detect the target sequence. See text for a more detailed explanation.

1–2-AX task, the task demand stimuli (1 or 2) in the outer loop must be maintained in the face of the interference from ongoing processing of inner loop stimuli and irrelevant distractors. Also, a specific A or B must also be maintained for the duration of each inner loop.

3. *Multiple, separate working memory representations:* To maintain the outer loop stimuli (1 or 2) while updating the inner loop stimuli (A or B), these two sets of representations must be distinct within the PFC (i.e., they must not be in direct mutual competition with one another, such that only one such representation could be active at a time).

4. *Selective updating:* Only some elements of working memory should be updated at any given time, while others are maintained. For example, in the inner loop, A or B should be updated while the task demand stimulus (1 or 2) is maintained.

5. *Independent output-gating for top-down biasing of processing:* For working memory representations to achieve controlled processing, they must be able to bias (control) processing elsewhere in the brain – and at the appropriate time. For example, whichever outer loop stimulus (1 or 2) is relevant at a given time must bias processing in the PFC/BG system itself, to condition responses and working memory updates as a function of the current target sequence.

6. *Learning what and when to gate:* Underlying all successful working memory task performance is the need to learn when to gate appropriately – both gating 'in' for maintenance and 'out' for biasing elsewhere in the processing stream. This is a particularly challenging problem in the maintenance case because the benefits of having gated something in are typically only available later in time (e.g., encoding the 1 task demand stimulus only affects overt behaviour and error-feedback later when confronted with an A-X sequence).

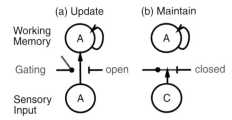

(a) Update   (b) Maintain

Working
Memory

Gating   ⊢— open   ⊢— closed

Sensory
Input

Figure 12.2 Illustration of active maintenance gating. When the gate is open, sensory input can rapidly update working memory (e.g., encoding the cue item A in the 1–2-AX task), but when it is closed, it cannot, thereby preventing other distracting information (e.g., distractor C) from interfering with the maintenance of previously stored information.

Earlier computational work has instantiated and validated several aspects of this overall theory, including the graded nature of controlled processing (Cohen *et al.*, 1990); the ability of PFC representations to bias subsequent processing (Cohen and Servan-Schreiber, 1992); the role of PFC in active maintenance (Braver *et al.*, 1995); and the ability of the BG to update PFC working memory representations (Frank *et al.*, 2001). Most recently, we have been focused on elucidating the mechanisms of the PFC/BG system, and most specifically, how it can learn to do what it has to do to support working memory.

The six functional demands described above have been published previously in more basic form (Hazy *et al.*, 2006). Here we modify them in a significant way to reflect a newly recognised demand for an independent *output-gating* mechanism (incorporated primarily into demand 5). This new demand is necessarily separate and distinct from the previously described maintenance-gating mechanism (O'Reilly and Frank, 2006). The motivation for such a demand, and our proposed mechanism will be elaborated upon below.

12.2.2   Dynamic updating via basal ganglia gating

One of the main implications of the above functional demands is that the first two functional demands (rapid updating versus robust maintenance) are in direct conflict with each other when viewed in terms of standard neural processing mechanisms. This motivates the need for a dynamic gating mechanism to switch between these two modes of operation (Anderson *et al.*, 2004; Ashby *et al.*, 1998; Balleine and Dickinson, 1998; Braver and Cohen, 2000; Cohen *et al.*, 1997a; Cohen *et al.*, 2002; Dayan, 2007, 2008; Frank *et al.*, 2001; Hochreiter and Schmidhuber, 1997; Jilk *et al.*, 2008; Klein *et al.*, 2007; Moustafa *et al.*, 2008; O'Reilly and Frank, 2006; O'Reilly and Munakata, 2000; O'Reilly *et al.*, 1999; Pauli *et al.*, 2009, 2010; Redgrave *et al.*, 1999; Todd *et al.*, 2008). When the gate is open, working memory can get updated by incoming stimulus information; when it is closed, currently active working memory representations are robustly maintained even in the face of potential interference as from intervening distractor stimuli (Figure 12.2).

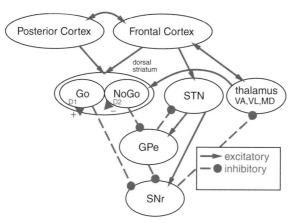

Figure 12.3 The basal ganglia are interconnected with the frontal cortex through a series of parallel loops, each of the form shown. Working backward from the thalamus, which is bidirectionally excitatory with frontal cortex, the SNr (substantia nigra pars reticulata) is tonically active and inhibiting this excitatory circuit. When direct pathway 'Go' neurons in dorsal striatum fire, they inhibit the SNr, and thus disinhibit the frontal cortex, producing a gating-like modulation that we argue triggers the update of working memory representations in prefrontal cortex. The indirect pathway 'NoGo' neurons of dorsal striatum counteract this effect by inhibiting the inhibitory GPe (globus pallidus, external segment). The STN (subthalamic nucleus) provides an additional dynamic background of inhibition (NoGo) by exciting the SNr.

A central tenet of the PBWM model is that the basal ganglia provide the dynamic gating mechanism for information maintained via sustained activation in the PFC, just as the BG are thought to 'gate' action selection in the motor areas of the frontal cortex. In the motor system, the basal ganglia are interconnected with frontal cortex through a series of parallel loops (Figure 12.3). When direct pathway 'Go' neurons in dorsal striatum fire, they inhibit the substantia nigra pars reticulata (SNr), and thus disinhibit the frontal cortex, producing a gating-like modulation that triggers the 'release' of one action, out of many, competing pre-activated actions. In like manner, we argue that the BG works with the PFC to trigger the updating of working memory representations in the PFC. The indirect pathway 'NoGo' neurons of dorsal striatum counteract this effect by inhibiting the inhibitory globus pallidus, external segment (GPe). The subthalamic nucleus (STN) provides an additional dynamic background of inhibition (NoGo) by exciting the SNr (see Frank, 2006; Frank *et al.*, 2007a for computational advantages of this global NoGo signal for action selection). As reviewed in Frank *et al.* (2001), this idea is consistent with a wide range of empirical data and other computational models that have been developed largely in the domain of motor control, but also for working memory as well (e.g., Berns and Sejnowski, 1998; Cisek, 2007; Cisek, this volume; Dominey *et al.*, 1995; Houk, this volume; Houk and Wise, 1995; Houk *et al.*, 2007; Wickens *et al.*, 1995). Our ideas regarding just how the PFC and BG might accomplish this complex coordination in support of working memory and executive function are outlined below, along with a brief description of the specific biologically plausible computational mechanisms that our PBWM model uses to instantiate them. New to this latest version of the model is the addition of an output gating mechanism (demand 5), which leverages the same BG/PFC circuitry and Go/NoGo modulation (Brown *et al.*, 2004).

1. *Rapid updating* occurs when direct pathway spiny neurons in the dorsal striatum fire (*Go* units). Go firing directly inhibits the SNr, and releases its tonic inhibition of the thalamus. This thalamic disinhibition enables, but does not directly cause (i.e., gates), a loop of excitation into the corresponding PFC 'stripe' (see *Multiple, separate working memory representations*, below). The effect of this net excitation is to toggle the state of bistable currents in the PFC neurons. Striatal Go neurons in the direct pathway are in competition (downstream in the SNr, if not actually in the striatum; Mink, 1996; Wickens, 1993) with a corresponding *NoGo* (indirect) pathway that promotes *greater* inhibition of thalamic neurons, thereby working to block gating.

2. *Robust maintenance* occurs via two intrinsic PFC mechanisms: (a) recurrent excitatory connectivity (e.g., O'Reilly *et al.*, 1999; Zipser, 1991), and (b) bistability (Durstewitz and Seamans, 2002; Durstewitz *et al.*, 1999, 2000; Lisman *et al.*, 1999; Seamans and Yang, 2004; Wang, 1999), the latter of which is toggled between a maintenance state and a non-maintenance state by the Go gating signal from the BG. [For an interesting variation on this basic theme, see Prescott *et al.*, 2006, for an account that places much of the burden of active maintenance in the motor domain (so called *behavioural persistence*) in the basal ganglia themselves, rather than in the frontal cortex as we would emphasise. It may be that both areas serve as substrates for active maintenance in both domains (motor and cognitive), or it may be that the BG play more of a role in behavioural persistence, while the PFC is the substrate of active maintenance for more cognitive (working memory) functions. Future work will be necessary to sort these issues out.]

3. *Multiple, separate working representations* are possible because of the 'striped' micro-anatomy of the PFC, which is characterised by small, relatively isolated groups of interconnected neurons, thereby preventing undue interference between representations in different (even nearby) stripes (Levitt *et al.*, 1993; Pucak *et al.*, 1997). We think of these frontal cortical stripes as being functionally similar to – and roughly the same size as – the well described hypercolumns of the visual cortex. Finally, we have estimated elsewhere there may be in the order of 20 000 such stripes in the human frontal cortex (Frank *et al.*, 2001), with progressively fewer in lower species as one goes backward down the phylogenetic tree. Thus, the pure quantity of stripes present in the frontal cortex may be an important variable in determining cognitive abilities, an idea we explore briefly in the final section.

4. *Selective updating* occurs because of the existence of independently updatable parallel loops of connectivity through different areas of the basal ganglia and frontal cortex (Alexander *et al.*, 1986; Graybiel and Kimura, 1995; Middleton and Strick, 2000). We hypothesise that these loops are selective to the relatively fine-grained level of the anatomical stripes in PFC. This stripe-based gating architecture has an important advantage over the *global* nature of a purely dopamine-based gating signal (e.g., Braver and Cohen, 2000; Rougier and O'Reilly, 2002; Tanaka, 2002), which appears computationally inadequate for supporting a selective updating function by itself.

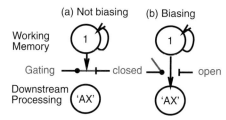

Figure 12.4 Illustration of output gating showing a single outer-loop stripe biasing (not biasing) inner loop processing. When the gate is open, actively maintained representations in the outer loop stripe can bias processing in the inner loop stripes, so as to attend to the A-X target sequence, but when the output-gate is closed, it cannot. Instead, active representations in another outer-loop stripe (not shown) might be exerting an influence (e.g., 2–B-Y). This output-gating process learns and functions largely independently of the maintenance gating system (Figure 12.2).

5. *Independent output-gating for top-down biasing of processing* occurs via output-gated projections from actively maintained representations in PFC to relevant areas throughout the brain (Figure 12.4), most typically the posterior cortex, but also the hippocampus and the PFC/BG itself (Cohen and Servan-Schreiber, 1992; Fuster, 1989). New here is the recognition that access to biasing influence should operate only *when appropriate* and not at other times indiscriminately. We adopt the hypothesis that this output-gating function is accomplished by means of the unique laminar frontal cortical column architecture and its specific connectivity pattern with the BG and thalamus (Brown *et al.*, 2004). Briefly, deep, output-generating laminae of the PFC (particularly lamina Vb) display thresholded behaviour so that these layers do not fire until a threshold is reached via a specific BG-gated thalamic input signal. In effect, output-gating is the same mechanism as the motor gating that the BG is typically described as performing (e.g., Frank, 2005; Gurney *et al.*, 2001; Houk, this volume; Houk *et al.*, 1995, 2007; Humphries *et al.*, this volume; Mink, 1996).

6. *Learning what and when to gate* (for both maintenance and output) is accomplished by a dopamine-based reinforcement-learning mechanism that is capable of providing temporally appropriate learning signals to train gating update activity in the striatal Go and NoGo synapses (Frank, 2005; O'Reilly and Frank, 2006); this learning occurs in parallel for maintenance and for output. Thus, each striatal medium spiny neuron (MSN) develops its own unique pattern of connection weights enabling separate Go versus NoGo decisions in each stripe.

Figure 12.5 shows how the BG-mediated selective gating mechanism can enable basic performance of the 1–2-AX task. When a task demand stimulus is presented (e.g., 1), a BG gating signal (i.e., a Go signal) must be activated to enable a particular PFC stripe to gate in and retain this information (panel a), and no stripe (or NoGo firing) should be activated for a distractor such as C (Panel b). A *different* stripe must be gated for the subsequent cue stimulus A (panel c). When the X stimulus is presented, the combination of this stimulus representation plus the maintained PFC working memory representations is sufficient to trigger a target response R (panel d).

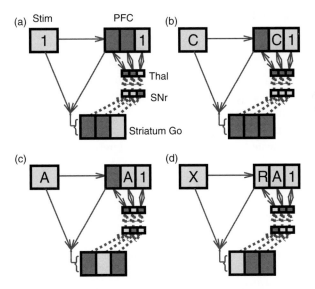

Figure 12.5 Illustration of how basal ganglia maintenance gating of different prefrontal cortex (PFC) stripes can solve the 1–2-AX task (light shading = active; dark = not active). Only three stripes are shown for clarity; we have estimated elsewhere there may actually be in the order of 20 000 stripes in the human frontal cortex (Frank *et al.*, 2001). (a) The 1 task is gated into an anterior PFC stripe because a corresponding striatal stripe fired Go. (b) The distractor C fails to fire striatal Go neurons, so it will not be maintained; however, it does elicit transient PFC activity. Note that the 1 persists because of gating-induced robust maintenance. (c) The A is gated in to a separate stripe. (d) A right keypress motor action is activated based on X input plus maintained PFC context. See plate section for colour version.

The need for an output-gating mechanism can be motivated by considering a situation where a motor plan is being formulated. For example, you might be planning a sequence of steps (e.g., picking up a set of plates, condiments, and other items sitting on the table after dinner), and need to figure out the best order to execute these steps. As you are juggling the possible orderings in your mind, you do not want to actually execute those actions. Thus, the maintenance-gating function is enabling the updating of different action plan representations, while the output gates remain closed to prevent actual actions from being executed based on these plans. Then, once the plan is ready to execute, the output-gating mechanism fire Go signals for each step of the plan in order. This coordination between maintenance and output gating can apply to more abstract cognitive operations in addition to concrete motor actions.

In addition, even situations that may appear to only require output-gating often require a maintenance-gating step as well. For example, in the motor domain (where output gating is synonymous with motor action gating), there are many cases where a motor plan must first be selected and maintained even for a few hundreds of milliseconds, and this could benefit from maintenance gating. Thus, the clear implication of this overall formulation is that both output gating and maintenance gating apply equally well to the action selection and working memory domains.

12.2.3   Learning when to gate in the BG

Of all the aspects of our model that purport to deconstruct the homunculus, learning when to gate is clearly the most critical. For any model, either the explicit knowledge of when to update working memory must be programmed in by the model's designer or, somehow, a model must learn it on its own, relying only on its training experience as it interacts with any primitive built-in biases and constraints (much like the architectural and/or parametric constraints discovered by evolution). That is, without such a learning mechanism, our model would have to resort to some kind of intelligent homunculus to control gating.

Our approach for simulating how the BG learns to update task-relevant versus irrelevant working memory information builds on prior work showing how the same basic mechanism can bring about the learning of the appropriate selection of motor responses. Specifically, the BG are thought to learn to facilitate the selection of the most appropriate response, while suppressing all other competing responses (Mink, 1996). In our models, the BG learn the distinction between good and bad responses via changes in dopamine firing in response to reward signals during positive and negative reinforcement (Frank, 2005). The net effect is that increases in DA enhance BG Go firing and learning via simulated D1 receptors, whereas decreases in dopamine during negative reinforcement have the opposite effect, enhancing NoGo firing and learning via simulated D2 receptors. This functionality enables the BG system to learn to discriminate between subtly different reinforcement values of alternative responses (Frank, 2005), and is consistent with several lines of biological and behavioural evidence (for review see Frank and O'Reilly, 2006). This direct modulation of Go versus NoGo actions in BG can train the output-gating mechanism in our model, which is functionally the same as a motor control gating mechanism.

A similar logic applies to training maintenance gating: increases in dopamine reinforce BG Go firing to gate information into working memory that contributes to better performance at later time steps, while decreases in dopamine allow the model to learn that a current working memory state is contributing to poor performance (Figure 12.5). In this manner, the BG eventually come to gate in information that is task-relevant, because maintenance of this information over time leads to adaptive behaviour and reinforced responses. Conversely, the system learns to ignore distracting information, because its maintenance will interfere with that of task-relevant information and therefore lead to poor performance. The overall PBWM model of the role of the PFC and BG in working memory makes a number of further predictions, several of which have been validated empirically (Frank *et al.*, 2004; Frank and O'Reilly, 2006; Frank *et al.*, 2007c, this volume; Waltz *et al.*, 2007).

From a computational perspective, maintenance gating also requires very specific mechanisms to deal with the *temporal credit assignment problem*. The benefits of having encoded a given piece of information into prefrontal working memory are typically only available later in time (e.g., encoding the 1 task demand stimulus can only really help later (in terms of getting an actual reward) when confronted with an A-X sequence).

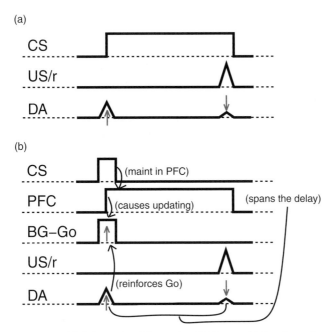

Figure 12.6 (a) Schematic of dopamine (DA) neural firing for an input stimulus (input, e.g., a tone) that reliably predicts a subsequent reward (unconditioned stimulus US/r). Initially, DA fires at the point of reward, but then over repeated trials learns to fire at the onset of the stimulus. (b) This DA firing pattern can solve the temporal credit assignment problem for prefrontal cortex (PFC) active maintenance. Here, the PFC maintains the transient input stimulus (initially by chance), leading to reward. As the DA system learns, it can predict subsequent reward at stimulus onset, by virtue of PFC 'bridging the gap' (in place of a sustained input). DA firing at stimulus onset reinforces the firing of basal ganglia Go neurons, which drive updating in PFC.

Thus, the problem is to know which prior events were critical for subsequent good (or bad) performance.

The firing patterns of midbrain dopamine (DA) neurons (ventral tegmental area, VTA; substantia nigra pars compacta, SNc; both strongly innervated by the BG) exhibit the properties necessary to solve the temporal credit assignment problem, because they learn to fire for stimuli that predict subsequent rewards (e.g., Schultz, 1998; Schultz *et al.*, 1993). This property is illustrated in schematic form in Figure 12.6a for a simple Pavlovian conditioning paradigm, where a stimulus (e.g., a tone) predicts a subsequent reward. Figure 12.6b shows how this predictive DA firing can reinforce BG Go firing to gate in and subsequently maintain a stimulus, when such maintenance leads to subsequent reward. Specifically, the DA firing can move discretely from the time of a reward to the onset of a stimulus that, if maintained in the PFC, leads to the subsequent delivery of this reward. Because this DA firing occurs at the time when the stimulus comes on, it is well timed to facilitate the storage of this stimulus in PFC. In our model, this occurs by reinforcing the connections between the stimulus and the Go gating neurons in the striatum, which then cause updating of PFC to maintain the stimulus.

The apparently predictive nature of DA firing has most often been explained in terms of the temporal differences (TD) reinforcement learning mechanism (Contreras-Vidal and Schultz, 1999; Houk *et al.*, 1995; Joel *et al.*, 2002; Montague *et al.*, 1997; Schultz *et al.*, 1995; Sutton, 1988; Sutton and Barto, 1998; Suri *et al.*, 2001). However, extensive exploration and analysis of these models has led us to develop a somewhat different account, which moves away from the explicit prediction framework upon which TD is based (Hazy *et al.*, 2010; O'Reilly and Frank, 2006; O'Reilly *et al.*, 2007). Our alternative learning mechanism, called PVLV (primary value and learned value) involves two separable but interdependent learning mechanisms, each of which is essentially a simple delta-rule or Rescorla–Wagner mechanism (Rescorla and Wagner, 1972; Widrow and Hoff, 1960). This PVLV mechanism shares several features in common with the model of Brown *et al.* (1999).

Further details of the PBWM model and PVLV learning mechanism are beyond the scope of this chapter but the basic results are that the resulting model can learn complex working memory tasks such as the 1–2-AX task based purely on trial-and-error experience with the task.

12.2.4   Empirical tests of the model

As previously noted, much evidence supports the role of the PFC in active maintenance during working memory tasks and for the existence of at least two mechanisms (recurrent connectivity and bistability) that could support it (e.g., Durstewitz *et al.*, 2000; Lisman *et al.*, 1999; Wang, 1999; Zipser, 1991). Bistability is of particular empirical relevance to the PBWM model, since it provides a viable candidate for the 'toggling' process required by PBWM. In addition, considerable evidence supports the existence of a 'striped' micro-anatomy in the PFC (Levitt *et al.*, 1993; Pucak *et al.*, 1997).

With regard to the more novel aspects of the model, some evidence is available to suggest there is a 'striped' micro-architecture within the well documented striato-cortical loops, that is there may be a more finely granular micro-anatomical functional organisation within the striatal matrix compartment (matrisomes) (Flaherty and Graybiel, 1993; Holt *et al.*, 1997), and that this finely granular functional organisation may be preserved in the striatal projections to the pallidum (Flaherty and Graybiel, 1993). The PBWM model makes an explicit, verifiable claim that such micro-anatomical fine structure ought to exist, another strong prediction of the model.

With regard to the issue of whether or not the basal ganglia can specifically trigger the toggling process of active maintenance in the PFC, a prominent feature of the PBWM model, accumulating evidence from our group supports this prediction in Parkinson's patients (Frank *et al.*, 2004), in normals on dopaminergic agents (Frank and O'Reilly, 2006), in attention deficit/hyperactivity disorder (ADHD) patients (Frank *et al.*, 2007b) and, most recently, in schizophrenia patients (Waltz *et al.*, 2007). These studies have also supported the hypothesis that it is the differential effect of phasic DA burst-firing on Go and NoGo MSNs in the striatum that is critical to learning when to gate, another important component of the PBWM model.

12.3   Simulating multiple WM tasks in a single model

The PBWM model is complex, as might be expected considering the complexity of the phenomena it is meant to explain. Nonetheless, it is still far from a complete account and we continue to refine and extend it. Accordingly, it makes sense to continue to look for more and better ways to constrain the performance of the model by subjecting it to increasingly stringent tests. One strategy that we have employed successfully in the past with both our hippocampal and posterior cortical models is to apply them to a progressively wider range of relevant phenomena. To the extent that the same basic model can account for a progressively wider range of data, it provides confidence that the model is capturing some critical core elements of cognitive function. The virtues of this general approach have been forcefully argued by Newell (1990).

For these reasons, one of our goals is to be able to simulate an increasingly wider range of working memory and executive tasks using a *single* instantiation of the PBWM model. This research builds upon earlier work simulating many of the paradigmatic tasks thought to be characteristic of working memory and executive function, including: the Stroop effect (Cohen *et al.*, 1990; Herd *et al.*, 2006; O'Reilly and Munakata, 2000; Stafford and Gurney, 2007), the AX-CPT (Braver *et al.*, 1995), the 1–2-AX (O'Reilly and Frank, 2006), the Wisconsin card sort task (WCST) (Rougier and O'Reilly, 2002), the intradimensional/extradimensional (ID/ED) dynamic categorisation task (O'Reilly *et al.*, 2002), and the Eriksen flanker task (Bogacz and Cohen, 2004; Cohen *et al.*, 1992; Yeung *et al.*, 2004). In addition to these already modelled tasks, we also plan to simulate additional tasks not yet modelled by us: the ABCA/ABBA task (Miller *et al.*, 1996), serial recall (phonological loop) (Burgess and Hitch, 1999), Sternberg task (Sternberg, 1966), and the N-Back task (Braver *et al.*, 1997).

The earlier successful efforts have all used different models of varying levels of sophistication and complexity, thus motivating the current goal of consolidating the results onto a single comprehensive model. Although easily stated, this is far from a trivial undertaking. In the first place, models constructed to perform one task may have design features or parameters that work against good performance in other tasks. Thus, even getting the *same* model to perform multiple tasks *independently* is a significant challenge. Obviously, the problem will only get more difficult as one attempts to implement multiple tasks in a single instantiation due to the additional complication of cross-training interference.

12.3.1   The full MT model

To simulate a progressively wider range of working memory/executive function tasks using a *single* instantiation of a *single* model, we have developed the MT (multitask) model, a complex environment instantiation of the PBWM. Figure 12.7 shows the MT (multitask) model, with input/output layers appearing at the top of the network, posterior cortical 'hidden' layers and PFC layer in the middle, and BG/midbrain areas for learning and gating of PFC at the bottom. The input/output representations were designed to

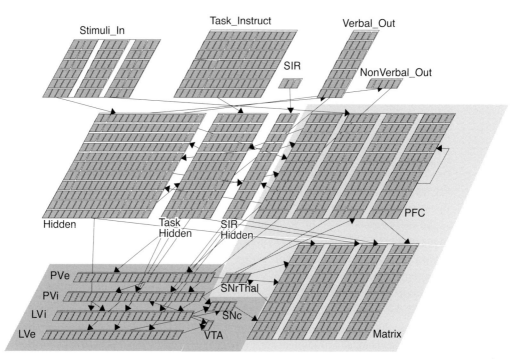

Figure 12.7 Overall structure of the MT model. Similar to our other PBWM models, the input/output layers are at the top-left of the diagram. The prefrontal cortex (PFC) and basal ganglia (BG) layers are at the bottom-right. The PVLV learning algorithm layers are in the lower left hand corner (highlighted in darker grey), and the full PBWM component also includes the BG (Matrix, SNrThal) and PFC on the right hand side (highlighted in lighter grey). Depending on the particular task, single or multiple featured stimuli are presented in one or more 'slots' in the Stimuli.In layer, along with task instructions in the Task_Instruct and SIR (store, ignore, recall) layers. Based on these inputs, plus context provided by PFC input, the Hidden layer determines the correct output in verbal or nonverbal form, or both. The shown model has four 'stripes' reflected in the four subgroups of the PFC and Matrix (striatal matrisomes) layers, and the four units of the SNc and SNrThal layers. SNc = substantia nigra, pars compacta; SNrThal = abstracted layer reflecting direct and indirect pathways via substantia nigra, pars reticulata and thalamus; VTA = ventral tegmental area; PVe = primary value (PV) excitatory, external reward; PVi = primary value inhibitory (anatomically associated with patch/striosomes of ventral striatum); LVi = learned value (LV) inhibitory (same anatomical locus); and LVe = learned value, excitatory (anatomically associated with the central nucleus of the amygdala). See plate section for colour version.

accommodate the vagaries of each individual task in a way that achieves a high level of surface validity.

The perceptual input representations in the MT model (Figure 12.8) assume a high level of perceptual preprocessing, such that different stimulus items ('objects') are represented with consistent and unique activity patterns. We encode three separate (orthogonal) stimulus dimensions: object identity, colour, and size, and we also provide three spatial locations in which a given object may appear. The task instruction layer tells the network what to do with the input stimuli, including the overall task and any more

Size:	Small	Medium	Large	X-Large
Colour:	Black	White	Red	Green
Object:	Circle	Square	Triangle	Diamond
	'Red'	'Green'	1	2
	A	B	X	Y

Figure 12.8 Perceptual input features, organised along three separate dimensions. Three separate locations of these features are provided as input to the network.

specific pieces of information that might be required (e.g., whether to do word reading or colour naming in the Stroop task). We have also included a subcategory of instruction inputs in the form of the store/ignore/recall (SIR) layer, which can be used to provide explicit working memory update signals that are encoded in a variety of different ways in different tasks, and may also be present via implicit timing signals via the cerebellum (e.g., Ivry, 1996; Mauk and Buonomano, 2004). The outputs include both verbal and non-verbal responses, the latter including button presses and pointing to locations.

The PFC is bidirectionally connected to all relevant high-level processing layers (sensory input, task hidden, central hidden, and output), and its associated BG layers receive from all of these layers as well to provide control over the learning and execution of the dynamic gating signals. Note that the shown PFC/BG system has four stripes, with each stripe representing a selectively updatable component of working memory. More stripes facilitate faster learning, but result in a larger, more computationally costly model, so the exact number of stripes is a matter of pragmatic optimisation in the model (in the brain, we estimate that many thousands of stripes are present).

When sensory inputs are presented, activation flows throughout the network in a bidirectional manner, so that internal posterior cortical 'hidden' layers are affected by both these bottom-input and maintained top-down activations in the PFC. In the Leabra algorithm that we use (see electronic supplementary material in Hazy *et al.*, 2007, for details), individual units are modelled as point neurons, with simulated ion channels contributing to a membrane potential, which is in turn passed through a thresholded nonlinear activation function to obtain a continuous instantaneous spike rate output that is communicated to other units. The inhibitory conductances are efficiently computed according to a k-winners-take-all algorithm (kWTA), which ensures that no more than some percentage (typically between 15–25%) of units within a layer are active at a time.

Outside of the BG system, learning occurs as a result of both Hebbian and error-driven mechanisms, with the error-driven learning computed in a biologically plausible fashion based on the GeneRec learning algorithm (O'Reilly, 1996). The learning mechanisms for the BG components (PVLV algorithm) were as described earlier.

12.3.2 Recent progress: the task contingency-shifting paradox in the WCST

Over several iterations of the MT model (incorporating progressively improving versions of PBWM), various versions have successfully replicated key results of a set of core tasks, including the Stroop, AX-CPT, and 1–2-AX, in addition to a set of more primitive component tasks (e.g., naming, matching, and comparing stimulus features, dimensions, and locations) that had been included in another, earlier model – the cross task generalisation model (Rougier *et al.*, 2005). This prior version was also able to do a version of the Wisconsin Card Sort task (WCST), using a simple, direct model of PFC gating that did not place particularly strong learning demands on the network. Most recently, a single instantiation of the current MT model has been trained to perform four separate tasks (AX-CPT, Erikson, Stroop, one-back version of n-back), switching between tasks with little difficulty based only on a task instruction cue indicating which task is currently relevant.

In moving to the more sophisticated current version, however, one that places more stringent learning demands on the model, we found that we ran into a new computational issue when uninstructed changes in task contingency occur, as in the WCST. This prompted a further modification to the core PBWM model (in addition to the output gating mechanism described earlier). Recall that in the WCST, subjects are required to place cards displaying multidimensional stimuli into piles according to which feature matches a relevant dimension that is not explicitly stated. The relevant dimension is kept constant over blocks of several trials, but is changed periodically without any signal – the only feedback the subject receives is whether their most recent response was correct or incorrect. This uncued change in environmental contingency presented a kind of paradox for earlier versions of PBWM, prompting the extension described below.

When task-contingencies change and the model makes errors, this results in phasic dopamine dips, which in our model depress Go (direct) pathway firing in the striatum, and enhance NoGo firing. In the maintenance gating mechanism, NoGo firing prevents updating and causes whatever was being maintained in the PFC working memory to continue to be maintained. But, this is the exact opposite of what needs to happen now that the model is making errors. Normally, this is not a problem when cues are provided in the environment since the Go/NoGo system can easily learn to use those cues to trigger a Go (update) signal. The problem is when the contingencies change *without warning*.

A potential solution to this problem comes from mechanisms that address the exploration/exploitation trade-off in reinforcement learning (Aston-Jones and Cohen, 2005). This trade-off arises when an agent is faced with either continuing to exploit the strategies that have worked well in the past, or exploring new strategies that might work better. At the point when errors are made, this decision becomes critical: do you just need to work harder at the current strategy, or give up and try something else? Based on a wide range of data, Aston-Jones and Cohen (2005) argue that neural systems in the anterior cingulate cortex (ACC) and locus coeruleus (LC) provide a means for dealing with this situation. Specifically, when some errors are made in the context of overall good performance, the system responds by working harder at the current strategy, as a result of phasic-mode noradrenaline released by the LC in precise time-lock with subsequent motor actions, under descending control of the ACC. However, as errors mount or are very strongly unexpected, the system switches to a fast-tonic mode that overwhelms extant phasic (time-locked) signals and supports greater exploration of alternative strategies.

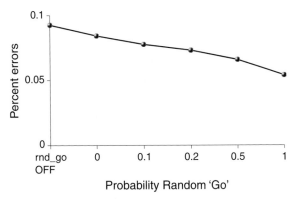

Figure 12.9 Performance on WCST as a function of the probability of firing an exploratory random Go when an error has been made after a threshold number of correct responses in a row (5), even when another stripe is already firing Go. A greater probability of random Go firing results in better performance, consistent with the idea that this error-driven modulation of exploratory behaviour is critical, as predicted by models of the noradrenaline system.

As a simple proxy for this set of mechanisms, the PBWM model now triggers random BG Go firing (causing exploration) when some threshold number of errors have been encountered after some number of correct responses in a row have been made (typically 5). In addition, this random Go firing is modulated by whether other Go firing is currently taking place. If no other stripes are firing Go, then it is imperative that a Go fire, to drive updating. If other stripes are firing Go, then in principle these could do appropriate updating of the PFC, and cause the network to adopt a new strategy or rule. However, we have found that additional random Go firing even in this case leads to better overall performance in the model, in proportion to the probability of this random Go firing occurring (Figure 12.9). Finally, see Frank *et al.* (2007c) for simulations of LC dynamics in BG models of action selection and their potential implication for decision making in neurological disorders such as ADHD.

12.4   Conclusion and future model development

Although many theoretical models have been developed purporting to explain aspects of working memory and executive function, the mechanistic basis underlying them has remained inadequately described, often amounting to a homunculus. In this chapter, we have reviewed some of the progress being made by our group and others in attempting to deconstruct this implicit homunculus by elucidating the precise computational and neural mechanisms underlying them, particularly the role of the PFC and basal ganglia. We are currently applying a comprehensive version of our PBWM model to a range of different working memory tasks to strongly test the cognitive neuroscience validity of the model. For example, the model can be used to explore roles of the individual neural systems involved by perturbing parameters to simulate development, aging, pharmacological manipulations, and neurological dysfunction, and it promises to be extensible to a broad array of other relevant manifestations of working memory and executive function. In addition to the basic goal of simulating all of these tasks with a single model, we think this overall approach will facilitate the exploration of many fundamental questions about the nature and origins of cognitive control, and intelligence more generally. Five of the key research directions we are currently pursuing – or plan to pursue in the near future – are described briefly below.

1. *Understanding the interaction between the specific architectural features of the PBWM model and the breadth of the training experience, as is characteristic of human development.* Perhaps the greatest mystery in cognitive processing is where all the 'smarts' come from to control the system in a task-appropriate manner (e.g., Chatham *et al.*, 2009; Dayan, 2007; O'Reilly and Munakata, 2000). How is it that people quickly adapt to performing certain novel cognitive tasks, when it can take monkeys months of highly focused training to learn those very same tasks? How much of this difference is due to nature (e.g., neuro-anatomical differences) versus nurture (training experience). A key hypothesis to be tested is that our model can be made to learn complex tasks significantly faster after being pre-trained on simpler, relevant ones, a result which would weigh towards a nurture-heavy explanation. Along another (not explicitly modelling) vein, an interesting empirical question might be whether one can demonstrate interspecific differences in performance between non-human primate species in these tasks (in addition to the obvious differences with humans), and to try to map these to things such as the gross number of frontal cortical stripes present in a species, or in differences in organisational structure. If we are successful in making progress towards these goals, it would represent a critical qualitative step forward in the modelling of human-like intelligence.

2. *The question of how the PFC is functionally organised is also prominent in the literature, and remains largely unresolved.* We think the path of research described here can shed considerable light on this issue as well. For example, how much of the increase in cognitive capability seen as one moves up the phylogenetic tree can be accounted for by a simple increase in the number of frontal lobe 'stripes' (a largely quantitative difference), versus how much is driven by new organisational changes, i.e., new functional specialisation (a more qualitative difference)? We would predict that both are probably important. Furthermore, we would expect that new organisational changes are probably relatively rare and that a specialised organisation in the PFC to support recursion (as exemplified in the 1–2-AX task) is probably limited to only a very few nesting levels given our notoriously limited recursive abilities. Previously, we and others have proposed that the anterior–posterior (and perhaps dorsal–ventral) axis of the PFC might be organised along a gradient from abstract to concrete, respectively (Badre and D'Esposito, 2009; Badre *et al.*, 2009; Botvinick *et al.*, 2009; Bunge *et al.*, 2009; Christoff and Gabrieli, 2000; Christoff *et al.*, 2009; Koechlin and Summerfield, 2007; O'Reilly and Munakata, 2000; O'Reilly *et al.*, 2002; Pauli *et al.*, 2009, 2010; Reynolds and O'Reilly, 2009; Sakagami *et al.*, 2006; Tanji and Hoshi, 2008; Wise, 2008; Wood and Grafman, 2003).

One particular organisational bias suggested by the biology is to have only the more posterior areas of PFC connected (bidirectionally) with posterior cortical areas, while more anterior PFC areas connect only with these posterior PFC areas. Thus, anterior PFC areas might be able to serve as more abstract biasing inputs to more posterior PFC areas, which in turn bias more specific processing in the posterior cortex. Similarly, orbitofrontal areas are thought to maintain motivational states and reinforcement values to bias decision-making processes in BG and other frontal regions (Balleine and Dickinson, 1998; Frank and Claus, 2006; Pauli *et al.*, 2009, 2010; Stalnaker *et al.*, 2007).

3. *Understanding the human capacity for generativity may be one of the greatest challenges facing the field of 'higher-level' cognitive function.* We think that the mechanisms of the PBWM model, and in particular its ability to exhibit limited variable-binding functionality, may be critical steps along the way to such an understanding. Some preliminary work using an earlier version of our basic model provides reason to be optimistic regarding this overall approach. In simulations of the cross-task generalisation task cited earlier (XT; Rougier *et al.*, 2005), we explored the ability of training on one set of tasks to generalise (transfer) to other, related tasks. In general, the key to generalisation in a neural network is the formation of abstract (e.g., categorical) representations (Munakata and O'Reilly, 2003; O'Reilly and Munakata, 2000). We think this pattern of results reflects a general principle for why the PFC should develop more abstract representations than the posterior cortex, and thus facilitate flexible generalisation to novel environments: abstraction derives from the maintenance of stable representations over time, interacting with learning mechanisms that extract commonalities over varying inputs.

4. *Further development on the interactions between output-biasing and input-maintenance gating mechanisms in support of working memory and executive function, along with related interactions with the action selection/motor planning system.* For example, which compartments and/or subsets of MSNs in the striatum handle input versus output gating? A related issue is the direct role of dopamine effects in the PFC. In brief, we think that *phasic* dopamine effects may be most manifest in the BG, where they are critical for highly discriminative Go versus NoGo learning, whereas longer lasting *tonic* dopamine effects in the PFC may help support robust maintenance of working memory representations (Cohen *et al.*, 2002; Durstewitz *et al.*, 2000; Seamans and Yang, 2004; Tanaka, 2002). In addition, phasic DA bursts within PFC may still be important for dictating *when* to update, while the same signals within the BG modulate *what* to update (Frank and O'Reilly, 2006). In the model described here, these dopaminergic effects in the PFC were abstracted and subsumed by a simple intracellular maintenance current – but these currents are known to depend on a healthy level of dopamine.

5. *Exploration of the performance monitoring function to deal with uncued (dynamic) changes in environmental contingency, probably involving the ACC and LC as briefly touched on earlier.* As noted in the WCST example, uncued changes in environmental contingency present an important challenge for which a robust understanding is beginning to emerge (Aston-Jones and Cohen, 2005; Botvinick *et al.*, 2004; Brown

and Braver, 2005; Chatham *et al.*, 2009; Reynolds and O'Reilly, 2009). Incorporating more sophisticated versions of these mechanisms into the core PBWM model is another developmental trajectory for our work.

References

Alexander, G. E., M. R. DeLong, and P. L. Strick (1986). Parallel organization of functionally segregated circuits linking basal ganglia and cortex. *Annu. Rev. Neurosci.* **9**(05): 357–81.

Anderson, J. R., D. Bothell, M. D. Byrne, *et al.* (2004). An integrated theory of the mind. *Psychol. Rev.* **111**(4): 1036–60.

Ashby, F. G, L. A. Alfonso-Reese, A. U. Turken, and E. M. Waldron (1998). A neuropsychological theory of multiple systems in category learning. *Psychol. Rev.* **105**(3): 442–81.

Aston-Jones, G. and J. D. Cohen (2005). An integrative theory of locus coeruleus-norepinephrine function: adaptive gain and optimal performance. *Annu. Rev. Neurosci.* **28**(07): 403–50.

Baddeley, A. D. (1986). *Working Memory*. New York: Oxford University Press.

Badre, D. and M. D'Esposito (2009). Is the rostro-caudal axis of the frontal lobe hierarchical? *Nature reviews* **10**(9): 659–69.

Badre, D., J. Hoffman, J. Cooney, and M. D'Esposito (2009). Hierarchical cognitive control deficits following damage to the human frontal lobe. *Nature Neurosci.* **12**(4): 515–22.

Balleine, B. W. and A. Dickinson (1998). Goal-directed instrumental action: contingency and incentive learning and their cortical substrates. *Neuropharmacology* **37**(05): 407–19.

Berns, G. S. and T. J. Sejnowski (1998). A computational model of how the basal ganglia produces sequences. *J. Cogn. Neurosci.* **10**(December): 108–21.

Bogacz, R. and J. D. Cohen (2004). Parameterization of connectionist models. *Behav. Res. Meth. Inst. Comp.* **36**(4): 732–41.

Botvinick, M. M., J. D. Cohen, and C. S. Carter (2004). Conflict monitoring and anterior cingulate cortex: an update. *Trends Cogn. Sci.* **8**(12): 539–46.

Botvinick, M. M., Y. Niv, and A G. Barto (2009). Hierarchically organized behavior and its neural foundations: A reinforcement learning perspective. *Cognition* **113**(3): 262–80.

Braver, T. S., D. M. Barch, and J. D. Cohen (1999). Cognition and control in schizophrenia: a computational model of dopamine and prefrontal function. *Biol. Psych.* **46**(12): 312–28.

Braver, T. S. and J. D. Cohen (2000). On the control of control: the role of dopamine in regulating prefrontal function and working memory. In *Control of Cognitive Processes: Attention and Performance, XVIII*, ed. S. Monsell and J. Driver. Cambridge, MA: MIT Press, pp. 713–37.

Braver, T. S., J. D. Cohen, L. E. Nystrom, *et al.* (1997). A parametric study of frontal cortex involvement in human working memory. *NeuroImage* **5**(December): 49–62.

Braver, T. S., J. D. Cohen, and D. Servan-Schreiber (1995). A computational model of prefrontal cortex function. In *Advances in Neural Information Processing Systems*, ed. D. S. Touretzky, G. Tesauro, and T. K. Leen. Cambridge, MA: MIT Press, pp. 141–48.

Brown, J. W. and T. S. Braver (2005). Learned predictions of error likelihood in the anterior cingulate cortex. *Science* **307**(5712): 1118–21.

Brown, J., D. Bullock, and S. Grossberg (1999). How the basal ganglia use parallel excitatory and inhibitory learning pathways to selectively respond to unexpected rewarding cues. *J. Neurosci.* **19**(12): 10502–11.

Brown, J., D. Bullock, and S. Grossberg (2004). How laminar frontal cortex and basal ganglia circuits interact to control planned and reactive saccades. *Neural Networks*, **17**(04): 471–510.

Bunge, S. A., E. H. Helskog, and C. Wendelken (2009). Left, but not right, rostrolateral prefrontal cortex meets a stringent test of the relational integration hypothesis. *NeuroImage* **46**(1): 338–42.

Burgess, N. and G. J. Hitch (1999) Memory for serial order: a network model of the phonological loop and its timing. *Psychol. Rev.* **106**(December): 551–81.

Chatham, C. H., M. J. Frank, and Y. Munakata (2009). Pupillometric and behavioral markers of a developmental shift in the temporal dynamics of cognitive control. *Proc. Nat. Acad. Sci. USA* **106**(14): 5529–33.

Christoff, K. and J. D. E. Gabrieli (2000). The frontopolar cortex and human cognition: evidence for a rostrocaudal hierarchical organization within the human prefrontal cortex. *Psychobiology* **28**(January): 168–86.

Christoff, K., K. Keramatian, A. M. Gordon, R. Smith, and B. Mädler (2009). Prefrontal organization of cognitive control according to levels of abstraction. *Brain Res.* **1286**(Aug): 94–105.

Cisek, P. (2007). Cortical mechanisms of action selection: the affordance competition hypothesis. *Phil. Trans. Roy. Soc. B Biol. Sci.* **362**(1485): 1585–99.

Cohen, J. D., T. S. Braver, and J. W. Brown (2002). Computational perspectives on dopamine function in prefrontal cortex. *Curr. Opin. Neurobiol.* **12**(05): 223–29.

Cohen, J. D., T. S. Braver, and R. C. O'Reilly (1997a). A computational approach to prefrontal cortex, cognitive control and schizophrenia: recent developments and current challenges. *Phil. Trans. Roy. Soc. B. Biol. Sci.* **351**(04): 1515–27.

Cohen, J. D., K. Dunbar, and J. L. McClelland (1990). On the control of automatic processes: a parallel distributed processing model of the Stroop effect. *Psychol. Rev.* **97**(3): 332–61.

Cohen, J. D., W. M. Perlstein, T. S. Braver, *et al.* (1997b). Temporal dynamics of brain activity during a working memory task. *Nature* **386**(January): 604–608.

Cohen, J. D. and D. Servan-Schreiber (1992). Context, cortex, and dopamine: a connectionist approach to behavior and biology in schizophrenia. *Psychol. Rev.* **99**(04): 45–77.

Cohen, J. D., D. Servan-Schreiber, and J. L. McClelland (1992). A parallel distributed processing approach to auomaticity. *Am. J. Psychol.* **105**(January): 239–69.

Contreras-Vidal, J. L. and W. Schultz (1999). A predictive reinforcement model of dopamine neurons for learning approach behavior. *J. Comput. Neurosci.* **6**(08): 191–214.

Conway, A. R. A., M. J. Kane, and R. W. Engle (2005). Working memory capacity and its relation to general intelligence. *Trends Cogn. Sci.* **7**(12): 547–52.

Dayan, P. (2007). Bilinearity, rules, and prefrontal cortex. *Front. Comput. Neurosci.* **1**: 1, 10.3389/neuro.10.001.2007.

Dayan, P. (2008). Simple substrates for complex cognition. *Front. Comput. Neurosci.* **2**(2): 255.

Dominey, P., M. Arbib, and J-.P. Joseph (1995). A model of corticostriatal plasticity for learning oculomotor associations and sequences. *J. Cogn. Neurosci.* **7**(January): 311–36.

Duncan, J. (2001). An adaptive coding model of neural function in prefrontal cortex. *Nature Rev. Neurosci.* **2**(11): 820–9.

Durstewitz, D., M. Kelc, and O. Güntürkün (1999). A neurocomputational theory of the dopaminergic modulation of working memory functions. *J. Neurosci.* **19**(04): 2807.

Durstewitz, D. and J. K. Seamans (2002). The computational role of dopamine D1 receptors in working memory. *Neural networks* **15**(10): 561–72.

Durstewitz, D., J. K. Seamans, and T. J. Sejnowski (2000). Dopamine-mediated stabilization of delay-period activity in a network model of prefrontal cortex. *J. Neurophysiol.* **83**(04): 1733–50.

Flaherty, A. W. and A. M. Graybiel, (1993). Output architecture of the primate putamen. *J. Neurosci.* **13**(8): 3222–37.

Frank, M. J. (2005). Dynamic dopamine modulation in the basal ganglia: a neurocomputational account of cognitive deficits in medicated and nonmedicated Parkinsonism. *J. Cogn. Neurosci.* **17**(January): 51–72.

Frank, M. J. (2006). Hold your horses: a dynamic computational role for the subthalamic nucleus in decision making. *Neural Networks* **19**(10): 1120–36.

Frank, M. J. and Claus, E. D. (2006). Anatomy of a decision: striatoorbitofrontal interactions in reinforcement learning, decision making, and reversal. *Psychol. Rev.*, **113**(2): 300–326.

Frank, M. J., B. Loughry, and R. C. O'Reilly (2001). Interactions between the frontal cortex and basal ganglia in working memory: a computational model. *Cogn., Affect. Behav. Neurosci.* **1**(January): 137–60.

Frank, M. J. and R. C. O'Reilly (2006). A mechanistic account of striatal dopamine function in human cognition: psychopharmacological studies with cabergoline and haloperidol. *Behav. Neurosci.* **120**(06): 497–517.

Frank, M. J., J. Samanta, A. A. Moustafa, and S. J. Sherman (2007a). Hold your horses: impulsivity, deep brain stimulation, and medication in parkinsonism. *Science* **318**(11): 1309–12.

Frank, M. J., A. Santamaria, R. C. O'Reilly, and E. Willcutt (2007b). Testing computational models of dopamine and noradrenaline dysfunction in attention deficit/hyperactivity disorder. *Neuropsychopharmacol.* **32**(06): 1583–99.

Frank, M. J., A. Scheres, and S. J. Sherman (2007c). Understanding decision-making deficits in neurological conditions: insights from models of natural action selection. *Phil. Trans. Roy. Soc. B. Biol. Sci.* **362**(08): 1641–54.

Frank, M. J., L. C. Seeberger, and R. C. O'Reilly (2004). By carrot or by stick: cognitive reinforcement learning in Parkinsonism. *Science* **306**(January): 1940–3.

Funahashi, S., C. J. Bruce, and P. S. Goldman-Rakic (1989). Mnemonic coding of visual space in the monkey's dorsolateral prefrontal cortex. *J. Neurophysiol.* **61**(04): 331–49.

Fuster, J. M. (1989). *The Prefrontal Cortex: Anatomy, Physiology and Neuropsychology of the Frontal Lobe*. New York: Raven Press.

Fuster, J. M. and G. E. Alexander (1971). Neuron activity related to shortterm memory. *Science* **173**(January): 652–4.

Graybiel, A. M. and M. Kimura (1995). Adaptive neural networks in the basal ganglia. In *Models of Information Processing in the Basal Ganglia*, ed. J. C. Houk, J. L. Davis, and D. G. Beiser. Cambridge, MA: MIT Press, pp. 103–116.

Gurney, K., T. J. Prescott, and P. Redgrave (2001). A computational model of action selection in the basal ganglia. I. A new functional anatomy. *Biol. Cybern.* **84**(06): 401–410.

Hazy, T. E., M. J. Frank, J. Michael, and R. C. O'Reilly (2007). Towards an executive without a homunculus: computational models of the prefrontal cortex/basal ganglia system. *Phil. Trans. Roy. Soc. B. Biol. Sci.* **362**(1): 105–118.

Hazy, T. E., M. J. Frank, and R. C. O'Reilly (2006). Banishing the homunculus: Making working memory work. *Neuroscience* **139**(04): 105–118.

Hazy, T. E., M. J. Frank, and R. C. O'Reilly (2010). Neural mechanisms of acquired phasic dopamine responses in learning. *Neurosci. Biobehav. Rev.* **34**(5): 701–20.

Herd, S. A., M. T. Banich, and R. C. O'Reilly (2006). Neural mechanisms of cognitive control: an integrative model of Stroop task performance and FMRI data. *J. Cogn. Neurosci.* **18**(01): 22–32.

Hochreiter, S. and J. Schmidhuber (1997). Long short term memory. *Neural Comput.* **9**(January): 1735–80.

Holt, D. J., A. M. Graybiel, and C. B. Saper (1997). Neurochemical architecture of the human striatum. *J. Comp. Neurol.* **384**(1): 1–25.

Houk, J. C., Adams, J. L., and Barto, A. G. (1995). A model of how the basal ganglia generate and use neural signals that predict reinforcement. In *Models of Information Processing in the Basal, Ganglia* ed. J. C. Houk, J. L. Davis, and D. G. Beiser. Cambridge, MA: MIT Press, pp. 233–48.

Houk, J. C., C. Bastianen, D. Fansler, *et al.* (2007). Action selection and refinement in subcortical loops through basal ganglia and cerebellum. *Phil. Trans. Roy. Soc. B. Biol. Sci.* **362**(1485): 1573–83.

Houk, J. C. and Wise, S. P. (1995). Distributed modular architectures linking basal ganglia, cerebellum, and cerebral cortex: their role in planning and controlling action. *Cereb. Cortex* **5**(08): 95–110.

Ivry, R. (1996). The representation of temporal information in perception and motor control. *Curr. Opin. Neurobiol.* **6**(January): 851–7.

Jilk, D., C. Lebiere, R. C. O'Reilly, and J. Anderson (2008). SAL: an explicitly pluralistic cognitive architecture. *J. Exp. Theor. Artif. Intell.* **9**: 197–218.

Joel, D., Y. Niv, and E. Ruppin (2002). Actor-critic models of the basal ganglia: new anatomical and computational perspectives. *Neural Networks* **15**(10): 535–47.

Klein, T. A., J. Neumann, M. Reuter, *et al.* (2007). Genetically determined differences in learning from errors. *Science* **318**(5856): 1642–5.

Koechlin, E. and C. Summerfield (2007). An information theoretical approach to prefrontal executive function. *Trends Cogn. Sci.* **11**(6): 229–35.

Kubota, K. and H. Niki (1971). Prefrontal cortical unit activity and delayed alternation performance in monkeys. *J. Neurophysiol.* **34**(09): 337–47.

Levitt, J. B., D. A. Lewis, T. Yoshioka, and J. S. Lund (1993). Topography of pyramidal neuron intrinsic connections in macaque monkey prefrontal cortex (Areas 9 46). *J. Comp. Neurol.* **338**: 360–76.

Lisman, J. E., J. M. Fellous, and X. J. Wang (1999). A role for NMDA-receptor channels in working memory. *Nature Neurosci.* **1**(4): 273–5.

Mauk, M. D. and Buonomano, D. V. (2004) The neural basis of temporal processing. *Annu. Rev. Neurosci.* **27**(1): 307–340.

Middleton, F. A. and Strick, P. L. (2000). Basal ganglia output and cognition: evidence from anatomical, behavioral, and clinical studies. *Brain Cogn.* **42**(05): 183–200.

Miller, E. K. and J. D. Cohen (2001). An integrative theory of prefrontal cortex function. *Annu. Rev. Neurosci.* **24**: 167–202.

Miller, E. K., C. A. Erickson, and R. Desimone (1996). Neural mechanisms of visual working memory in prefontal cortex of the macaque. *J. Neurosci.* **16**(January): 5154.

Mink, J. W. (1996). The basal ganglia: focused selection and inhibition of competing motor programs. *Prog. Neurobiol.* **50**(03): 381–425.

Miyashita, Y. and H. S. Chang (1988). Neuronal correlate of pictorial short-term memory in the primate temporal cortex. *Nature*, **331**(03): 68–70.

Montague, P. R., P. Dayan, and T. J. Sejnowski (1997). A framework for mesencephalic dopamine systems based on predictive Hebbian learning. *J. Neurosci.* **16**(01): 1936–47.

Moustafa, A. A., M. X. Cohen, S. J. Sherman, and M. J. Frank (2008). A role for dopamine in temporal decision making and reward maximization in Parkinsonism. *J. Neurosci.* **28**(47): 12294–304.

Munakata, Y. and R. C. O'Reilly (2003). Developmental and computational neuroscience approaches to cognition: the case of generalization. *Cogn. Stud.* **10**(January): 76–92.

Newell, A. (1990). *Unified Theories of Cognition*. Cambridge, MA: Harvard University Press.

O'Reilly, R. C. (1996). Biologically plausible error-driven learning using local activation differences: the generalized recirculation algorithm. *Neural Comput.* **8**(5): 895–938.

O'Reilly, R. C. (2006). Biologically based computational models of high level cognition. *Science* **314**(10): 91–4.

O'Reilly, R. C., T. S. Braver, and J. D. Cohen (1999). A biologically based computational model of working memory. In *Models of Working Memory: Mechanisms of Active Maintenance and Executive Control*. ed. A. Miyake and P. Shah. New York: Cambridge University Press, pp. 375–411.

O'Reilly, R. C. and M. J. Frank (2006). Making working memory work: a computational model of learning in the prefrontal cortex and basal ganglia. *Neural Comput.* **18**: 283–328.

O'Reilly, R. C., M. J. Frank, T. E. Hazy, and B. Watz (2007). PVLV: The primary value and learned value Pavlovian learning algorithm. *Behav. Neurosci.* **121**(02): 31–49.

O'Reilly, R. C. and Y. Munakata (2000). *Computational Explorations in Cognitive Neuroscience: Understanding the Mind by Simulating the Brain*. Cambridge, MA: The MIT Press.

O'Reilly, R. C., D. C. Noelle, T. S. Braver, and J. D. Cohen (2002). Prefrontal cortex and dynamic categorization tasks: representational organization and neuromodulatory control. *Cereb. Cortex* **12**(02): 246–57.

Pauli, W. M., H. E. Atallah, and R. C. O'Reilly (2010). Integrating what and how/where with instrumental and Pavlovian learning: a biologically-based computational model. In *Cognition and Neuropsychology: International Perspectives on Psychological Science* (Volume 1), ed. P. A. Frensch and R. Schwarzer. Oxford: Psychology Press.

Pauli, W. M., T. E. Hazy, and R. C. O'Reilly (2009). Division of labor among multiple parallel cortico – basal ganglia – thalamic loops in Pavlovian and instrumental tasks: A biologically-based computational model. *Poster presented at the Multidisciplinary Symposium on Reinforcement Learning*.

Prescott, T. J., F. M. Montes, Gonzalez K. Gurney, M. D. Humphries, and P. Redgrave (2006). A robot model of the basal ganglia: behavior and intrinsic processing. *Neural Networks* **19**(1): 31–61.

Pucak, M. L., J. B .Levitt, J. S. Lund, and D. A. Lewis (1997). Patterns of intrinsic and associational circuitry in monkey prefrontal cortex. *J. Compar. Neurol.* **376**(03): 614–630.

Redgrave, P., T. J. Prescott, and K. Gurney (1999). The basal ganglia: a vertebrate solution to the selection problem? *Neuroscience* **89**(07): 1009.

Rescorla, R. A. and A. R. Wagner (1972). A theory of Pavlovian conditioning: variation in the effectiveness of reinforcement and non-reinforcement. In *Classical Conditioning II: Theory and Research*. ed. A. H. Black and W. F. Prokasy. *New York*: Appleton-Century-Crofts, pp. 64–99.

Reynolds, J. R. and R. C. O'Reilly (2009). Developing PFC representations using reinforcement learning. *Cognition*, **113**(5): 201–208.

Rougier, N. P., D. Noelle, T. S. Braver, J. D. Cohen, and R. C. O'Reilly (2005). Prefrontal cortex and the flexibility of cognitive control: rules without symbols. *Proc. Nat. Acad. Sci.* **102**(20): 7338–43.

Rougier, N. P., and O'Reilly, R. C. (2002). Learning representations in a gated prefrontal cortex model of dynamic task switching. *Cogn. Sci.* **26**(January): 503–20.

Sakagami, M., X. Pan, and B. Uttl (2006). Behavioral inhibition and prefrontal cortex in decision-making. *Neural Networks* **19**(8): 1255–65.

Schultz, W. (1998). Predictive reward signal of dopamine neurons. *J. Neurophysiol.* **80**(08): 1.

Schultz, W., P. Apicella, and T. Ljungberg (1993). Responses of monkey dopamine neurons to reward and conditioned stimuli during successive steps of learning a delayed response task. *J. Neurosci.* **13**(03): 900–913.

Schultz, W., R. Romo, T. Ljungberg, *et al.* (1995). Reward-related signals carried by dopamine neurons. In *Models of Information Processing in the Basal, Ganglia* ed. J. C. Houk, J. L. Davis, and D. G. Beiser, Cambridge, MA: MIT Press, pp. 233–48.

Seamans, J. K. and C. R. Yang (2004). The principal features and mechanisms of dopamine modulation in the prefrontal cortex. *Prog. Neurobiol.* **74**(09): 1–57.

Shallice, T. (1988) *From Neuropsychology to Mental Structure*. New York: Cambridge University Press.

Stafford, T. and K. N. Gurney (2007). Biologically constrained action selection improves cognitive control in a model of the Stroop task. *Phil. Trans. Roy. Soc. B. Biol. Sci.* **362**(1485): 1671–84.

Stalnaker, T. A., T. M. Franz, T. Singh, and G. Schoenbaum (2007). Basolateral amygdala lesions abolish orbitofrontal dependent reversal impairments. *Neuron* **54**(04): 51–8.

Sternberg, S. (1966). High speed scanning in human memory. *Science* **153**(January): 652–54.

Suri, R. E., J. Bargas, and M. A. Arbib (2001). Modeling functions of striatal dopamine modulation in learning and planning. *Neuroscience* **103**(04): 65–85.

Sutton, R. S. (1988). Learning to predict by the method of temporal differences. *Mach. Learn.* **3**(January): 9–44.

Sutton, R. S. and A. G. Barto (1998). *Reinforcement Learning: An Introduction*. Cambridge, MA: MIT Press.

Tanaka, S. (2002). Dopamine controls fundamental cognitive operations of multi-target spatial working memory. *Neural Networks* **15**(10): 573–82.

Tanji, J. and E. Hoshi (2008). Role of the lateral prefrontal cortex in executive behavioral control. *Physiol. Rev* **88**(1): 37–57.

Todd, M. T., Y. Niv, and J. D. Cohen (2008). Learning to use working memory in partially observable environments through dopaminergic reinforcement. In *Advances in Neural Information Processing Systems (NIPS) 21*, ed. D. Koller. Norwich, UK: Curran Associates.

Waltz, J. A., M. J. Frank, B. M. Robinson, and J. M. Gold (2007). Selective reinforcement learning deficits in schizophrenia support predictions from computational models of striatal-cortical dysfunction. *Biol. Psych.* **62**(09): 756–64.

Wang, X. J. (1999). Synaptic basis of cortical persistent activity: the importance of NMDA receptors to working memory. *J. Neurosci.* **19**(11): 9587.

Wickens, J. (1993). *A Theory of the Striatum*. Oxford: Pergamon Press.

Wickens, J. R., R. Kotter, and M. E. Alexander (1995). Effects of local connectivity on striatal function: simulation and analysis of a model. *Synapse*, **20**(January): 281–98.

Widrow, B. and M. E. Hoff (1960). Adaptive switching circuits. In *Institute of Radio Engineers, Western Electronic Show and Convention, Convention Record, Part 4* (January): 96–104.

Wise, S. P. (2008). Forward frontal fields: phylogeny and fundamental function. *Trends Neurosci.* **31**(12): 599–608.

Wood, J. N. and J. Grafman (2003). Human prefrontal cortex: processing and representational perspectives. *Nature Rev. Neurosci.* **4**(02): 139–47.

Yeung, N., M. M. Botvinick, and J. D. Cohen (2004). The neural basis of error detection: conflict monitoring and the error-related negativity. *Psychol. Rev.* **111**(4): 931–59.

Zipser, D. (1991). Recurrent network model of the neural mechanism of shortterm active memory. *Neural Comput.* **3**(January): 179–93.

13 Hierarchically organised behaviour and its neural foundations: a reinforcement-learning perspective[1]

Matthew M. Botvinick, Yael Niv, and Andrew G. Barto

Summary

Research on human and animal behaviour has long emphasised its hierarchical structure – the divisibility of ongoing behaviour into discrete tasks, which are comprised of subtask sequences, which in turn are built of simple actions. The hierarchical structure of behaviour has also been of enduring interest within neuroscience, where it has been widely considered to reflect prefrontal cortical functions. In this chapter, we re-examine behavioural hierarchy and its neural substrates from the point of view of recent developments in computational reinforcement learning. Specifically, we consider a set of approaches known collectively as *hierarchical reinforcement learning*, which extend the reinforcement learning paradigm by allowing the learning agent to aggregate actions into reusable subroutines or skills. A close look at the components of hierarchical reinforcement learning suggests how they might map onto neural structures, in particular regions within the dorsolateral and orbital prefrontal cortex. It also suggests specific ways in which hierarchical reinforcement learning might provide a complement to existing psychological models of hierarchically structured behaviour. A particularly important question that hierarchical reinforcement learning brings to the fore is that of how learning identifies new action routines that are likely to provide useful building blocks in solving a wide range of future problems. Here and at many other points, hierarchical reinforcement learning offers an appealing framework for investigating the computational and neural underpinnings of hierarchically structured behaviour.

In recent years, it has become increasingly common within both psychology and neuroscience to explore the applicability of ideas from machine learning. Indeed, one can now cite numerous instances where this strategy has been fruitful. Arguably, however, no area of machine learning has had as profound and sustained an impact on psychology and neuroscience as that of computational reinforcement learning (RL). The impact of RL was initially felt in research on classical and instrumental conditioning (Barto and Sutton, 1981; Sutton and Barto, 1990; Wickens *et al.*, 1995). Soon thereafter, its impact extended to research on midbrain dopaminergic function, where the temporal-difference learning

---

[1] This chapter is a revised version of an article originally published in *Cognition*, **113**(3), 262–280.

Modelling Natural Action Selection, eds. Anil K. Seth, Tony J. Prescott and Joanna J. Bryson. Published by Cambridge University Press. © Cambridge University Press 2012.

paradigm provided a framework for interpreting temporal profiles of dopaminergic activity (Barto, 1995; Houk *et al.*, 1995; Montague *et al.*, 1996; Schultz *et al.*, 1997). Subsequently, actor–critic architectures for RL have inspired new interpretations of functional divisions of labour within the basal ganglia and cerebral cortex (see Joel *et al.*, 2002, for a review), and RL-based accounts have been advanced to address issues as diverse as motor control (e.g., Miyamoto *et al.*, 2004), working memory (e.g., O'Reilly and Frank, 2006), performance monitoring (e.g., Holroyd and Coles, 2002), and the distinction between habitual and goal-directed behaviour (e.g., Daw *et al.*, 2005).

As ideas from RL permeate the fields of psychology and neuroscience, it is interesting to consider how RL research has continued to evolve within computer science. Here, attention has turned increasingly to factors that limit the applicability of RL. Perhaps foremost among these is the *scaling* problem. Unfortunately, basic RL methods do not cope well with large task domains, i.e., domains involving a large space of possible world states or a large set of possible actions. This limitation of RL has been little discussed within psychology and neuroscience, where RL has typically been applied to highly simplified learning situations. However, the scaling problem has direct implications for whether RL mechanisms can be plausibly applied to more complex behavioural contexts. Because such contexts would naturally include most scenarios animals and human beings face outside the laboratory, the scaling problem is clearly of relevance to students of behaviour and brain function.

A number of computational approaches have been developed to tackle the scaling problem. One increasingly influential approach involves the use of *temporal abstraction* (Barto and Mahadevan, 2003; Dietterich, 2000; Parr and Russell, 1998; Sutton *et al.*, 1999). Here, the basic RL framework is expanded to include temporally abstract actions, representations that group together a set of interrelated actions (for example, grasping a spoon, using it to scoop up some sugar, moving the spoon into position over a cup, and depositing the sugar), casting them as a single higher-level action or skill ('add sugar'). These new representations are described as temporal abstractions because they abstract over temporally extended, and potentially variable, sequences of lower-level steps. A number of other terms have been used as well, including 'skills', 'operators', 'macro-operators', and 'macro-actions'. In what follows, we will often refer to temporally abstract actions as *options*, following Sutton *et al.* (1999).

In most versions of RL that use temporal abstraction, it is assumed that options can be assembled into higher-level skills in a hierarchical arrangement. Thus, for example, an option for adding sugar might form part of other options for making coffee and tea. Given the importance of such hierarchical structures in work using temporal abstraction, this area of RL is customarily referred to as hierarchical reinforcement learning (HRL).

The emergence of HRL is an intriguing development from the points of view of psychology and neuroscience, where the idea of hierarchical structure in behaviour is familiar. In psychology, hierarchy has played a pivotal role in research on organised, goal-directed behaviour, from the pioneering work in this area (e.g., Estes, 1972; Lashley, 1951; Miller *et al*, 1960; Newell and Simon, 1963) through to the most recent studies (e.g., Anderson, 2004; Botvinick and Plaut, 2004; Schneider and Logan, 2006; Zacks *et al.*, 2007; and see Crabbe, this volume).

Behavioural hierarchy has also been of longstanding interest within neuroscience, where it has been considered to relate closely to prefrontal cortical function (Badre, 2008; Botvinick, 2008; Courtney et al., in press; Fuster, 1997; Koechlin et al., 2003; Wood and Grafman, 2003).

Thus, although HRL was not originally developed to address questions about human and animal behaviour, it is potentially of twofold relevance to psychology and neuroscience. First, HRL addresses a limitation of RL that would also be faced by any biological agent learning through RL-like mechanisms. The question thus naturally arises whether the brain might deal with this limitation in an analogous way. Second, the ideas at the heart of HRL resonate strongly with existing themes in psychology and neuroscience. The formal framework provided by HRL thus might provide leverage in thinking about the role of hierarchical structure in human and animal behaviour, and in particular how such structure might relate to behavioural and neuroscientific issues that have already been treated in terms of RL.

Our objective in this chapter is to consider HRL from these two perspectives. We begin, in the following section, by examining the scaling problem and considering how the use of temporal abstraction can help to ameliorate it. We then turn to HRL itself, detailing its representational and algorithmic assumptions. After establishing these, we discuss the potential implications of HRL for behavioural research. Here, we emphasise one fundamental computational issue that HRL brings into focus, which concerns the question of how reusable sets of skills might develop through learning. Finally, we consider the potential implications of HRL for interpreting neural function. To this end, we introduce a new actor–critic implementation of HRL, which makes explicit the computational requirements that HRL would pose for a neural implementation.

13.1   Temporal abstraction and the scaling problem

A key source of the scaling problem is the fact that an RL agent can learn to behave adaptively only by exploring its environment, trying out different courses of action in different situations or states of the environment, and sampling their consequences. As a result of this requirement, the time needed to arrive at a stable behavioural policy increases with both the number of different states in the environment and the number of available actions. In most contexts, the relationship between training time and the number of environmental states or actions is a positively accelerating function. Thus, as problem size increases, standard RL eventually becomes infeasible.

Numerous approaches have been adopted in machine learning to deal with the scaling problem. These include reducing the size of the state space by suppressing behaviourally irrelevant distinctions between states (state abstraction; see, e.g., Li and Walsh, 2006), and methods aimed at striking an optimal balance between exploration and exploitation of established knowledge (e.g., Kearns and Singh, 2002). HRL methods target the scaling problem by introducing temporally abstract actions (Barto and Mahadevan, 2003; Dietterich, 2000; Parr and Russell, 1998; Sutton et al., 1999). The defining characteristic of these abstract actions is that, rather than specifying a single 'primitive'

(a) 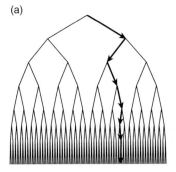   (b) 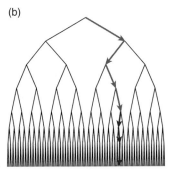   (c)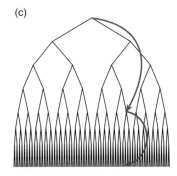

Figure 13.1 An illustration of how options can facilitate search. (a) A search tree with arrows indicating the pathway to a goal state. A specific sequence of seven independently selected actions is required to reach the goal. (b) The same tree and trajectory, the shading indicating that the first four and the last three actions have been aggregated into options. Here, the goal state is reached after only two independent choices (selection of the options). (c) Illustration of search using option models, which allow the ultimate consequences of an option to be forecast without requiring consideration of the lower-level steps that would be involved in executing the option.

action to execute, each abstract action instead specifies a whole *policy* to be followed, that is, a mapping from states to actions.[2] Once a temporally abstract action is initiated, execution of its policy continues until any member of a set of specified termination states is reached.[3] Thus, the selection of a temporally abstract action ultimately results in the execution of a sequence of primitive actions.

Adding temporal abstraction to RL can ease the scaling problem in two ways. The first way is through its impact on the exploration process. In order to see how this works, it is useful to picture the agent (i.e., the simulated human or animal) as searching a tree structure (Figure 13.1a). At the apex is a node representing the state occupied by the agent at the outset of exploration. Branching out from this node are links representing primitive actions, each leading to a node representing the state (and, possibly, reward) consequent on that action. Further action links project from each of these nodes, leading to their consequent states, and so forth. The agent's objective is to discover paths through the decision tree that lead to maximal accumulated rewards. However, the set of possible paths increases with the set of actions available to the agent, and with the number of reachable states. With increasing numbers of either it becomes progressively more difficult to discover, through exploration, the specific traversals of the tree that would maximise reward.

Temporally abstract actions can alleviate this problem by introducing *structure* into the exploration process. Specifically, the policies associated with temporally abstract actions can guide exploration down specific partial paths through the search tree, potentially allowing earlier discovery of high-value traversals. The principle is illustrated in Figures 13.1a and b. Discovering the pathway illustrated in Figure 13.1a using only primitive,

---

[2] An alternative term for temporal abstraction is thus *policy abstraction*.

[3] Some versions of HRL allow for options to be interrupted at points where another option or action is associated with a higher expected value. See, for example, Sutton *et al.* (1999).

one-step actions, would require a specific sequence of seven independent choices. This changes if the agent has acquired – say, through prior experience with related problems – two options corresponding to the differently shaded subsequences in Figure 13.1b. Equipped with these, the agent would only need to make two independent decisions to discover the overall trajectory, namely, select the two options. Here, options reduce the effective size of the search space, making it easier for the agent to discover an optimal trajectory.

The second, and closely related, way in which temporally abstract actions can ease the scaling problem is by allowing the agent to learn more efficiently from its experiences. Without temporal abstraction, learning to follow the trajectory illustrated in Figure 13.1a would involve adjusting parameters at seven separate decision-points. With predefined options (Figure 13.1b), policy learning is only required at two decision-points, the points at which the two options are to be selected. Thus, temporally abstract actions not only allow the agent to explore more efficiently, but also to make better use of its experiences.

Along with these advantages, there also comes a new computational burden. For in order to enjoy the benefits of temporal abstraction, the agent must have some way of *acquiring* a set of *useful* options. As we shall discuss, this requirement raises some of the most interesting issues in HRL, issues that also apply to human learning.

13.2   Hierarchical reinforcement learning

Having briefly discussed the motivation for incorporating temporal abstraction into RL, we now turn to a more direct description of how HRL operates. For simplicity, we focus on one specific implementation of HRL, the *options framework* described by Sutton *et al.* (1999). However, the points we shall emphasise are consistent with other versions of HRL as well (e.g., Dietterich, 2000; Parr and Russell, 1998; for an overview, see Barto and Mahadevan, 2003). Since one of our objectives is to explore potential neuroscientific correlates of HRL, we have implemented the options framework within an actor–critic architecture (defined below), allowing direct parallels to be drawn with previous work relating RL to functional neuroanatomy through the actor–critic framework.[4] In what follows, we provide an informal, tutorial-style overview of this implementation. Full technical details are presented in the Appendix A.

13.2.1   Fundamentals of RL: temporal difference learning in actor–critic models

RL problems comprise four elements: a set of world *states*; a set of *actions* available to the agent in each state; a *transition function*, which specifies the probability of transitioning from one state to another when performing each action; and a *reward function*, which indicates the amount of reward (or cost) associated with each such transition. Given

[4] For other work translating HRL into an actor–critic format, see Bhatnagara and Panigrahi (2006)

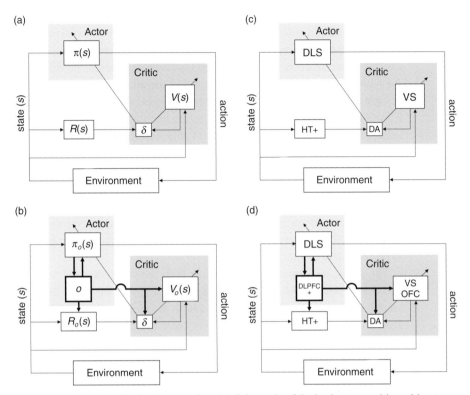

Figure 13.2 An actor–critic implementation. (a) Schematic of the basic actor–critic architecture. $R(s)$: reward function; $V(s)$: value function; δ: temporal difference prediction error; $\pi(s)$: policy, determined by action strengths W. (b) An actor–critic implementation of HRL. o: currently controlling option, $R_o(s)$: option-dependent reward function. $V_o(s)$: option-specific value functions; δ: temporal difference prediction error; $\pi_o(s)$: option-specific policies, determined by option-specific action/option strengths. (c) Putative neural correlates to components of the elements diagrammed in panel a. (d) Potential neural correlates to components of the elements diagrammed in panel c. Abbreviations: DA: dopamine; DLPFC: dorsolateral prefrontal cortex, plus other frontal structures potentially including premotor, supplementary motor and pre-supplementary motor cortices; DLS, dorsolateral striatum; HT+ : hypothalamus and other structures, potentially including the habenula, the pedunculopontine nucleus, and the superior colliculus; OFC: orbitofrontal cortex; VS, ventral striatum.

these elements, the objective for learning is to discover a policy, that is, a mapping from states to actions, that maximises cumulative long-term reward.[5]

In actor–critic implementations of RL, the learning agent is divided into two parts, an actor and a critic, as illustrated in Figure 13.2a (see, e.g., Barto *et al.*, 1983; Houk *et al.*, 1995; Joel *et al.*, 2002; Suri *et al.*, 2001). The *actor* selects actions according to a modifiable policy ($\pi(s)$ in Figure 13.2), which is based on a set of weighted associations

---

[5] It is often assumed that the utility attached to rewards decreases with the length of time it takes to obtain them, and in such cases the objective is to maximize the *discounted* long-term reward. Our implementation assumes such discounting. For simplicity, however, discounting is ignored in the main text.

from states to actions, often called *action strengths*. The *critic* maintains a *value function* ($V(s)$), associating each state with an estimate of the cumulative, long-term reward that can be expected subsequent to visiting that state. Importantly, both the action strengths and the value function must be learned based on experience with the environment. At the outset of learning, the value function and the actor's action strengths are initialised, for instance, uniformly or randomly, and the agent is placed in some initial state. The actor then selects an action, following a rule that favours high-strength actions but also allows for exploration (see Appendix A, Equation (A.1)). Once the resulting state is reached and its associated reward is collected, the critic computes a *temporal-difference prediction error* (denoted δ in Figure 13.2; see also Equation (A.2)). Here, the value that was attached to the previous state is treated as a prediction of (1) the reward that would be received in the successor state ($R(s)$), plus (2) the value attached to that successor state. A positive prediction error indicates that this prediction was too low, meaning that things turned out better than expected. Of course, things can also turn out worse than expected, yielding a negative prediction error.

The prediction error is used to update both the value attached to the previous state and the strength of the action that was selected in that state (see Equations (A.3) and (A.4)). A positive prediction error leads to an increase in the value of the previous state and the propensity to perform the chosen action at that state. A negative error leads to a reduction in these. After the appropriate adjustments, the agent selects a new action, a new state is reached, a new prediction error is computed, and so forth. As the agent explores its environment and this procedure is repeated, the critic's value function becomes progressively more accurate, and the actor's action strengths change so as to yield progressive improvements in behaviour, in terms of the amount of reward obtained.

13.2.2   Incorporating temporally abstract actions

The options framework supplements the set of single-step, primitive actions with a set of temporally abstract actions or options. An option is, in a sense, a 'mini-policy.' It is defined by an *initiation set*, indicating the states in which the option can be selected; a *termination function*, which specifies a set of states that will trigger termination of the option;[6] and an *option-specific policy*, mapping from states to actions (which now include other options).

Like primitive actions, options are associated with strengths, and on any timestep the actor may select either a primitive action or an option. Once an option is selected, actions are selected based on that option's policy until the option terminates. At that point, a prediction error for the option is computed. This error is defined as the difference between the value of the state where the option terminated and the value of the state where the option was initiated, plus whatever rewards were accrued during execution of the option (see Equation (A.6)). A positive prediction error indicates that things went better than expected since leaving the initiation state, and a negative prediction error means that things went worse. As in the case of primitive actions, the prediction error is

---

[6] The termination function may be probabilistic.

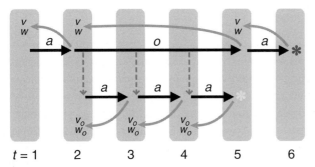

Figure 13.3 A schematic illustration of HRL dynamics. a, primitive actions; o, option. On the first timestep ($t = 1$), the agent executes a primitive action (forward arrow). Based on the consequent state (i.e., the state at $t = 2$), a prediction error δ is computed (arrow running from $t = 2$ to $t = 1$), and used to update the value (V) and action/option strengths (W) associated with the preceding state. At $t = 2$, the agent selects an option (long forward arrow), which remains active through $t = 5$. During this time, primitive actions are selected according to the option's policy (lower tier of forward arrows). A prediction error is computed after each (lower tier of curved arrows), and used to update the option-specific values (V_o) and action strengths (W_o) associated with the preceding state. These prediction errors, unlike those at the level above, take into account pseudo-reward received throughout the execution of the option (higher asterisk). Once the option's subgoal state is reached, the option is terminated. A prediction error is computed for the entire option (long curved arrow), and this is used to update the values and option strengths associated with the state in which the option was initiated. The agent then selects a new action at the top level, which yields external reward (lower asterisk). The prediction errors computed at the top level, but not at the level below, take this reward into account.

used to update the value associated with the initiation state, as well as the action strength associating the option with that state (see Equations (A.8) and (A.9); Figure 13.3).[7]

Implementing this new functionality requires several extensions to the actor–critic architecture, as illustrated in Figure 13.2b. First, the actor must maintain a representation of which option is currently in control of behaviour (o).[8] Second, because the agent's policy now varies depending on which option is in control, the actor must maintain a separate set of action strengths for each option ($\pi_o(s)$ in Figure 13.2b). Important changes are also required in the critic. Because prediction errors are computed when options terminate, the critic must receive input from the actor, telling it when such terminations occur (the arrow from o to δ). Finally, to be able to compute the prediction error at these points, the critic must also keep track of the amount of reward accumulated during each option's execution and the identity of the state in which the option was initiated (see Equations (A.6)–(A.9)).

---

[7] As discussed by Sutton *et al.* (1999), it is possible to update the value function based only on comparisons between states and their immediate successors. However, the relevant procedures, when combined with those involved in learning option-specific policies (as described later), require complicated bookkeeping and control operations for which neural correlates seem less plausible.

[8] If it is assumed that option policies can call other options, then the actor must also keep track of the entire set of active options and their calling relations.

13.2.3   Learning option policies

The description provided so far explains how the agent learns a top- or root-level policy, which determines what action or option to select when no option is currently in control of behaviour. We turn now to the question of how option-specific policies are learned.

In versions of the options framework that address such learning, it is often assumed that options are initially defined in terms of specific *subgoal* states. (The question of where these subgoals come from is an important one, which we address later.) It is further assumed that when an active option reaches its subgoal, the actions leading up to the subgoal are reinforced. To distinguish this reinforcing effect from the one associated with external rewards, subgoal attainment is said to yield *pseudo-reward* (Dietterich, 2000).

In order for subgoals and pseudo-reward to shape option policies, the critic in HRL must maintain not only its usual value function, but also a set of option-specific value functions ($V_o(s)$ in Figure 13.2b). As in ordinary RL, these value functions predict the cumulative long-term reward that will be received subsequent to occupation of a particular state. However, they are option-specific in the sense that they take into account the pseudo-reward that is associated with each option's subgoal state. A second reason that option-specific value functions are needed is that the reward (and pseudo-reward) that the agent will receive following any given state depends on the actions it will select. These depend, by definition, on the agent's policy, and under HRL the policy depends on which option is currently in control of behaviour. Thus, only an option-specific value function can accurately predict future rewards.

Despite the additions above, option-specific policies are learned in quite the usual way: on each step of an option's execution, a prediction error is computed based on the (option-specific) values of the states visited and the reward received (including pseudo-reward). This prediction error is then used to update the option's action strengths and the values attached to each state visited during the option (see Equations (A.6)–(A.9); Figure 13.3). With repeated cycles through this procedure, the option's policy evolves so as to guide behaviour, with increasing directness, toward the option's subgoals.

13.2.4   Illustrations of performance

To provide an illustration of HRL in action, we applied the preceding learning procedures to a toy 'rooms' problem introduced by Sutton *et al.* (1999). Here, the agent's task is to navigate through a set of rooms interconnected by doorways, in order to reach a goal state (Figure 13.4a). In each state, the agent can select any of eight deterministic primitive actions, each of which moves the agent to one of the adjacent squares (unless a wall prevents this movement). Additionally, within each room the agent can also select either of two options, each having one of the room's doors as its subgoal.

To illustrate the process of learning option-specific policies, the model was initially trained with only pseudo-rewards at the option subgoal states, i.e., without external reward. Figure 13.4b tracks the number of primitive actions each option required to reach its subgoal, showing that, through learning, this fell to a minimum over successive

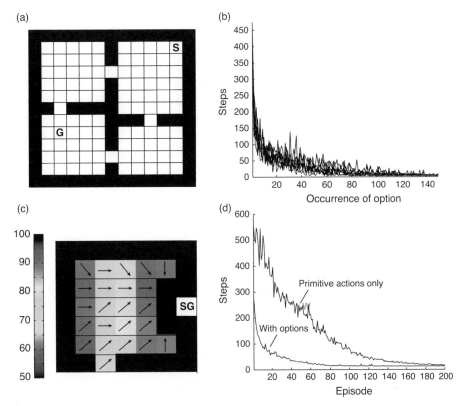

Figure 13.4 (a) The rooms problem, adapted from Sutton *et al.* (1999). *S*: start; *G*: goal.
(b) Learning curves for the eight doorway options, plotted over the first 150 occurrences of each
(mean over 100 simulation runs). See Appendix A for simulation details. (c) The upper left room
from panel A, illustrating the policy learned by one doorway option. Arrows indicate the
primitive action selected most frequently in each state. SG: option subgoal. Colours indicate the
option-specific value for each state. (d) Learning curves indicating solution times, i.e., number of
primitive steps to goal, on the problem illustrated in panel a (mean over 100 simulation runs).
Upper data series: performance when only primitive actions were included. Lower series:
performance when both primitive actions and doorway options were included. Policies for
doorway options were established through earlier training (see Appendix A). See plate section
for colour version.

executions of the option. Figure 13.4c illustrates the policy learned by one of the doorway
options, as well its option-specific value function.

A more fundamental point is illustrated in Figure 13.4d, which tracks the model's
performance after external rewards were introduced at the goal state *G*. The model
learns more rapidly to reach the goal state when both the doorway options and the eight
primitive actions are included[9] than when only the primitive actions are available. This

---

[9] As detailed in Appendix A, options were pre-trained, simulating transfer of knowledge from earlier experience. In this particular problem domain – although not necessarily in general – including options without
pre-training slows initial learning on the top-level problem, but later confers a benefit, allowing the agent to
converge on an optimal policy earlier than it does in the absence of options.

savings in training time reflects the impact of temporal abstraction on exploration and learning, as described in the previous section.

3.2.5   Other versions of HRL

As noted earlier, we based the foregoing overview of HRL on a particular implementation of HRL, the options framework (Sutton *et al.*, 1999). Although we continue to orient toward this paradigm throughout the rest of the chapter, it is important to bear in mind that there exist other versions of HRL, which differ from the options framework along a number of dimensions (see Barto and Mahadevan, 2003). The most highly developed among these are the HAM framework introduced by Parr and Russell (1998) and Dieterich's (1998, 2000) MAXQ framework. One aspect that distinguishes these two paradigms from the options framework is that they treat learning as a process occurring within a pre-established and partially fixed task/subtask hierarchy.[10] This approach has ramifications that further differentiate the HAM and MAXQ paradigms from the options framework, affecting, for example, the way that value functions are represented and how prediction errors are computed (see Barto and Mahadevan, 2003 for a detailed comparison among approaches).

We have chosen to focus on the options framework because the elements that it adds to standard RL are simpler and fewer in number than those added by other paradigms, and because in our opinion these new elements lend themselves more immediately to a neuroscientific interpretation. In Section 13.5, we consider several ways in which other HRL paradigms might lead to subtly different hypotheses and predictions. Nevertheless, we endeavour in what follows to concentrate on points that are broadly consistent with the full range of HRL implementations.

13.3   Behavioural implications

Having introduced the fundamentals of HRL, we turn now to a consideration of what their implications might be for behavioural and neuroscientific research. We begin with implications for psychology. As noted earlier, HRL treats a set of issues that have also been of longstanding interest to students of human and animal behaviour. HRL suggests a different way of framing some of these issues, and also brings to the fore some important questions that have so far received relatively little attention in behavioural research.

13.3.1   Relation to previous work in psychology

Lashley (1951) is typically credited with first asserting that the sequencing of low-level actions requires higher-level representations of task context. Since this point was

---

[10] Procedures for inducing the initial hierarchy from experience have been explored in MAXQ (see e.g., Mehta *et al.*, 2008), but this form of learning is treated as separate from the learning of policies over the hierarchy.

introduced, there has been extensive research into the nature and dynamics of such representations, much of which resonates with the idea of temporally abstract actions as found in HRL. Indeed, the concept of 'task representation', as it arises in much contemporary psychological work (e.g., Cohen *et al.*, 1990; Cooper and Shallice, 2000; Monsell, 2003), shares key features with the option construct. Both postulate a unitary representation that (1) can be selected or activated; (2) remains active for some period of time following its initial selection; (3) leads to the imposition of a specific stimulus-response mapping or policy; and (4) can participate in hierarchical relations with other representations of the same kind.

Despite this parallel, most psychological research on task representation has focused on issues different from those central to HRL. In recent work, the emphasis has often been on the dynamics of shifts from one task to another (e.g., Allport and Wylie, 2000; Logan, 2003; Monsell, 2003), or on competition between task sets (e.g., Monsell *et al.*, 2000; Pashler, 1994). Other studies have concentrated on cases where task representations function primarily to preserve information conveyed by transient cues (e.g., Cohen *et al.*, 1996; MacDonald *et al.*, 2000), a function not usually performed by options.

Among studies focusing on the issue of hierarchy, many have aimed at obtaining empirical evidence that human behaviour and its accompanying mental representations are in fact organised in a hierarchical fashion (e.g., Newtson, 1976; Zacks and Tversky, 2001). However, there have also been a series of theoretical proposals concerning the control structures underlying hierarchically organised behaviour (e.g., Arbib, 1985; Botvinick and Plaut, 2004; Cooper and Shallice, 2000; Dehaene and Changeux, 1997; Dell *et al.*, 1997; Estes, 1972; Grossberg, 1986; MacKay, 1987; Miller *et al.*, 1960; Rumelhart and Norman, 1982). The resemblance between these proposals and HRL mechanisms is variable. In most cases, for example, high-level task representations have been understood to send top-down activation directly to action representations, rather than to favour specific links from *stimuli* to responses, as in HRL (however, see Botvinick and Plaut, 2004; Ruh, 2007). Furthermore, in the vast majority of cases the focus has been on aspects of steady-state performance, such as reaction times and error patterns, rather than on the role of temporal abstraction in learning, the focus in HRL.

Having made this latter generalisation, it is also important to note several cases in which the role of task representations and hierarchical structure during learning have been directly considered. On the empirical side, there have been a number of studies examining the development of hierarchical structure in the behaviour of children (e.g., Bruner, 1973; Fischer, 1980; Greenfield and Schneider, 1977; Greenfield *et al.*, 1972). The general conclusion of such studies is that, over the course of childhood, behaviour shows a hierarchical development, according to which simple operations are gradually incorporated into larger wholes. The fit between this observation and the basic premises of HRL is, of course, clear.

The strongest parallels to HRL within psychology, however, are found in production-system based theories of cognition, in particular Soar (Lehman *et al.*, 1996) and ACT-R (Anderson, 2004). A key idea in both of these frameworks is that planning or problem solving can leverage *chunks*, 'if-then' rules that can trigger the execution of extended action sequences (Laird *et al.*, 1986; Lee and Taatgen, 2003; see also Hayes-Roth and

Hayes-Roth, 1979; Ward and Allport, 1987). Like temporally abstract actions in HRL, chunks can facilitate problem solving, increasing the speed and efficiency with which solutions are found. This function allows chunking to provide a natural account for the behavioural phenomenon of *positive transfer*, where improvements in problem-solving efficiency are observed on target problems when these are presented after prior exposure to structurally similar problems.

One factor that differentiates HRL from the Soar and ACT-R frameworks is its organisation around the single objective of reward maximisation. This aspect of HRL allows it to specify precisely what it means for hierarchically structured behaviour to be optimal, and this optimality criterion gives coherence to the learning and performance algorithms involved in HRL (even in cases – encountered regularly, in practice – where HRL does not yield perfect reward-maximising performance). In contrast, neither ACT-R nor Soar take reward maximisation as a central organising principle. ACT-R does include 'production utilities', which represent the probability that a given production will lead to achievement of the currently held goal (Anderson, 2004), a feature that resonates with the impact of pseudo-reward in HRL. And there have been recent efforts to integrate RL methods into the Soar framework (Nason and Laird, 2005). Notwithstanding these caveats, the centrality of reward maximisation in HRL remains distinctive. A countervailing strength of Soar, ACT-R, and related models is that they address a wide range of psychological issues – in particular, limitations in processing capacity – that are not addressed in existing formulations of HRL. The strengths of the two approaches thus appear to be complementary, and it is exciting to consider ways in which they might be integrated (see Nason and Laird, 2005, for some preliminary discussion along these lines).

13.3.2   Negative transfer

The previous section touched on the phenomenon of positive transfer, where established procedural knowledge facilitates the discovery of solutions to new problems. This phenomenon provides a direct point of contact between human behaviour and HRL, where, as demonstrated earlier, options arising from earlier experience can have the same facilitatory effect. However, the literature on transfer effects also highlights a contrary point that pertains equally to HRL, which is that in some circumstances pre-existing knowledge can hinder problem solving. Such *negative transfer* was most famously demonstrated by Luchins (1942), who found that human subjects were less successful at solving word problems when the subjects were first exposed to problems demanding a different solution strategy (see also Landrum, 2005; Rayman, 1982).

A direct analogue to negative transfer occurs in HRL when the temporally abstract actions available to the agent are not well suited to the learning problem. For illustration, consider the four-rooms problem described above (see Figure 13.4a). However, instead of the doorway options included in the earlier simulation, assume that the agent has a set of options whose subgoals are the states adjacent to the 'windows' marked in Figure 13.5a. Those options, which are not helpful in solving the problem of reaching the goal state G, cause the agent to spend time exploring suboptimal trajectories, with the

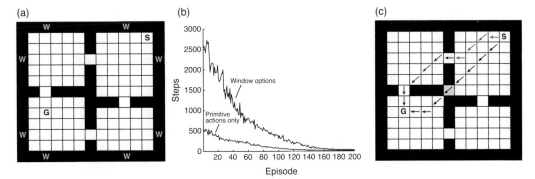

Figure 13.5 (a) The rooms problem from Figure 13.4, with 'windows' (*w*) defining option subgoals. (b) Learning curves for the problem illustrated in panel A. Lower data series: steps to goal over episodes with only primitive actions included (mean values over 100 simulation runs). Upper series: performance with both primitive actions and window options included. (c) Illustration of performance when a 'shortcut' is opened up between the upper right and lower left rooms (centre tile). Lower trajectory: path to goal most frequently taken after learning with only primitive actions included. Upper trajectory: path most frequently taken after learning with both primitive actions and doorway options. Black arrows indicate primitive actions selected by the root policy. Other arrows indicate primitive actions selected by two doorway options.

effect that learning is slowed overall (Figure 13.5b). A subtler but equally informative case is illustrated in Figure 13.5c. Here, the original doorway options are used, but now a new passageway has been opened up, providing a shortcut between the upper right and lower left rooms. When trained with primitive actions only, the agent learns to use this passage, finding the shortest path to the reward on 75% of training runs. However, when the original doorway options are also included, the agent learns to reach the goal only by way of the main doorways, eventually ignoring the passageway completely.[11]

These illustrations show that the impact of temporally abstract actions on learning and planning depends critically on which specific actions the agent has in its repertoire. This raises a pivotal question, which motivates a significant portion of current HRL research: by what means can a learning agent acquire temporally abstract actions that are likely to be useful in solving future problems, and avoid acquiring unhelpful ones? The existence of both positive and negative transfer in human performance indicates the relevance of this question to psychological theory as well. With this in mind, it is of interest to consider the range of answers that have been proposed in machine learning, and their potential relations to findings from behavioural science.

---

[11] Mean solution time over the last ten episodes from a total of 500 episodes, averaged over 100 simulation runs, was 11.79 with the doorway options (passageway state visited on 0% of episodes), compared with 9.73 with primitive actions only (passageway visited on 79% of episodes). Note that, given a certain set of assumptions, convergence on the optimal, shortest path, policy can be guaranteed in RL algorithms, including those involved in HRL. However, this is only strictly true under boundary conditions that involve extremely slow learning, due to a very slow transition from exploration to exploitation. Away from these extreme conditions, there is a marked tendency for HRL systems to 'satisfice', as illustrated in the passageway simulation.

13.3.3   The option discovery problem

One approach to the problem of discovering useful options has been to think of options as genetically specified, being shaped across generations by natural selection (Elfwing *et al.*, 2007; Houston *et al.*, this volume). Along these same lines, in empirical research, motor behaviour has often been characterised as building upon simple, innately specified components (e.g., Bruner, 1973). In some cases extended action sequences, such as grooming sequences in rodents, have been considered to be genetically specified (Aldridge and Berridge, 1998), functioning essentially as innate options.

While evolution seems likely to play an important role in providing the building blocks for animal and human behaviour, it is also clear that both animals and humans discover useful behavioural subroutines through learning (Conway and Christiansen, 2001; Fischer, 1980; Greenfield *et al.*, 1972). One proposal from HRL for how this might be accomplished is through analysis of externally rewarded action sequences. Here, as the agent explores a particular problem, or a series of interrelated problems, it keeps a record of states or subsequences that occur relatively frequently in trajectories that culminate in reward (McGovern, 2002; Pickett and Barto, 2002; Thrun and Scwhartz, 1995; see also Minton *et al.*, 1985; Yamada and Tsuji, 1989). These states and sequences pinpoint important 'bottlenecks' in the problem space – such as the doors in the rooms scenario discussed above – which are good candidates to become option subgoals. On the empirical side, this proposal appears consonant with work showing that humans, even very young children, can be extremely sensitive to the structure underlying repeating and systematically varying event sequences (Saffran *et al.*, 1996), a point that extends to hierarchical structure (Saffran and Wilson, 2003).

Another HRL approach to the option discovery problem involves analysing not trajectories through the problem space, but the problem space itself. Here, a graph is constructed to represent the relevant set of world states and the transitions that can be made among them through action. Graph partitioning methods are then used to identify states that constitute bottlenecks or access points within the graph, which are then designated as option subgoals (Mannor *et al.*, 2004; Menache *et al.*, 2002; Simsek *et al.*, 2005; see also Hengst, 2002; Jonsson and Barto, 2005). This set of approaches resonates with behavioural data showing that humans (including children) spontaneously generate causal representations from interactions with the world, and link these representations together into large-scale causal models (Gopnik *et al.*, 2004; Gopnik and Schulz, 2004; Sommerville and Woodward, 2005a; Sommerville and Woodward, 2005b). Whether such causal models are then applied toward the identification of useful subgoal states is an interesting question for empirical investigation.

Another approach within HRL takes the perspective that options can be formed during an analogue of a developmental period, without the need for any externally imposed tasks. Instead of learning from extrinsically provided rewards, the agent learns from intrinsic rewards generated by built-in mechanisms that identify subgoals – states or situations that have the property that skills capable of achieving them are likely to be useful in many different future tasks (Barto *et al.*, 2004; Singh *et al.*, 2005). One example of this approach assumes that certain action outcomes are unusually salient, and that the unexpected occurrence of these outcomes during exploratory behaviour triggers efforts to make them reoccur (and thus learning of options that treat these events as subgoals). More specifically, unexpected salient events are assumed to be intrinsically motivating. Singh *et al.* (2005) demonstrated how this mechanism can lead to the stepwise development of hierarchies of skills. The behaviour of the agent in their simulations bears an intriguing similarity to children's 'circular reactions', behaviour aimed at reproducing initially inadvertent action outcomes such as turning a light on and off (Fischer and Connell, 2003; Piaget, 1936 [1952]). Singh *et al.* (2005) pointed out the unexpected occurrence of a salient event is but one way to trigger intrinsic reward, with other possibilities suggested by the psychological literature (e.g., Berlyne, 1960; White, 1959) as well as earlier studies of internal rewards in the RL literature (e.g., Kaplan and Oudeyer, 2004; Schmidhuber, 1991). Oudeyer *et al.* (2007) provide an overview of much of this work.[12]

The intrinsic motivation approach to subgoal discovery in HRL dovetails with psychological theories suggesting that human behaviour is motivated by a drive toward exploration or toward mastery, independent of external reward (e.g., Berlyne, 1960; Harlow *et al.*, 1950; Ryan and Deci, 2000; White, 1959). Moreover, the idea that unanticipated events can engage reinforcement mechanisms is also consistent with neuroscientific findings. In particular, the same midbrain dopaminergic neurons that are thought to report a temporal-difference reward prediction error also respond to salient novel stimuli (Bunzeck and Duzel, 2006; Redgrave and Gurney, 2006; Schultz *et al.*, 1993).

When option discovery is viewed as a psychological problem, other possible mechanisms for option discovery are brought to mind, which go beyond those so far considered in HRL research. For example, Soar provides a highly detailed account of subgoal generation and chunk formation, according to which subgoals, and later chunks, are established in response to problem-solving impasses (Laird *et al.*, 1986; Lehman *et al.*, 1996). Another still richer source of useful subgoals might be provided by the social environment. For example, empirical work with both children and adults demonstrates that human observers spontaneously infer goals and subgoals from the behaviour of others (Gergely and Csibra, 2003; Meltzoff, 1995; Sommerville and Woodward, 2005a; Tenenbaum and Saxe, 2006; Woodward *et al.*, 2001). By this means, subgoals and associated action sequences could be gleaned both from deliberate demonstrations from parents, teachers, and others, and from the behaviour of unwitting models (Greenfield, 1984; Yan and Fischer, 2002). Indeed, it seems natural to think of much of education and child-rearing as involving the deliberate social transmission of useful action routines. Related to this idea is the technique of shaping, whereby training is provided on low-level tasks in preparation for training on more complex tasks. In recent work, Krueger and Dayan (2008) have offered a reinforcement learning account of shaping effects, which incorporates elements, such as subtask modularity, that parallel features of HRL.

---

[12] These studies, directed at facilitating the learning of environmental models, are also relevant to learning of option hierarchies.

13.4   Neuroscientific implications

In the above, we have suggested potential bi-directional links between HRL and research on learning and behaviour in humans and animals. We turn now to the potential implications of HRL for understanding neural function. To make these concrete, we will use the actor–critic formulation of HRL presented earlier. Previous work has already drawn parallels between the elements of the actor–critic framework and specific neuroanatomical structures. Situating HRL within the actor–critic framework thus facilitates the formation of hypotheses concerning how HRL might map onto functional neuroanatomy.[13]

Although accounts relating the actor–critic architecture to neural structures vary (see Joel *et al.*, 2002, for a review), one proposal has been to identify the actor with the dorsolateral striatum (DLS), and the critic with the ventral striatum (VS) and the mesolimbic dopaminergic system (see, e.g., Daw *et al.*, 2006; O'Doherty *et al.*, 2004; Figure 13.2c). Dopamine (DA), in particular, has been associated with the function of conveying reward prediction errors to both actor and critic (Barto, 1995; Montague *et al.*, 1996; Schultz *et al.*, 1997). In order to evaluate how HRL would modify this mapping, we will focus individually on the elements that HRL adds or modifies within the actor–critic framework, as introduced earlier. In the following two sections, we consider four key extensions, two relevant to the actor component, and two to the critic.

13.4.1   The actor in HRL: relation to prefrontal cortex

13.4.1.1   Extension 1: Support structure for temporally abstract actions
Under HRL, in addition to primitive actions, the actor must build in representations that identify specific temporally abstract actions or options. Using these, the actor must be able to keep track of which option is currently selected and in control of behaviour.

13.4.1.2   Potential neural correlates
This first extension to the actor–critic framework calls to mind functions commonly ascribed to the dorsolateral prefrontal cortex (DLPFC). The DLPFC has long been considered to house representations that guide temporally integrated, goal-directed behaviour (Fuster, 1997, 2004; Grafman, 2002; Petrides, 1995; Shallice and Burgess, 1991; Wood and Grafman, 2003). Recent work has refined this idea by demonstrating that DLPFC neurons play a direct role in representing *task sets*. Here, a single pattern of DLPFC activation serves to represent an entire mapping from stimuli to responses, i.e., a policy (Asaad *et al.*, 2000; Bunge, 2004; Hoshi *et al.*, 1998; Johnston and Everling, 2006; Rougier *et al.*, 2005; Shimamura, 2000; Wallis *et al.*, 2001; White, 1999). According to the guided activation theory proposed by Miller and Cohen (2001), prefrontal representations do not implement policies directly, but instead select among stimulus–response

---

[13] For different approaches to the mapping between HRL and neuroanatomy, see De Pisapia and Goddard (2003) and Zhou and Coggins (2002; 2004).

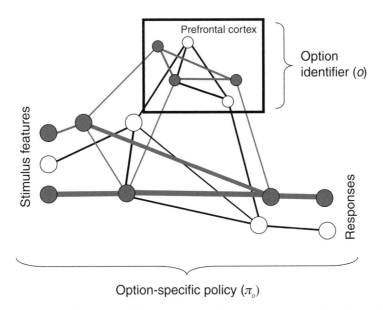

Figure 13.6 Illustration of the role of the prefrontal cortex, as postulated by guided activation theory (Miller and Cohen, 2001). Patterns of activation in prefrontal cortex (filled elements in the boxed region) effectively select among stimulus-response pathways lying elsewhere in the brain (lower area). Here, representations within the prefrontal cortex correspond to option identifiers in HRL, while the stimulus-response pathways selected correspond to option-specific policies. Figure adapted from Miller and Cohen (2001).

pathways implemented outside the prefrontal cortex (see also Cisek *et al.*, this volume). This division of labour fits well with the distinction in HRL between an option's identifier and the policy with which it is associated (Figure 13.6).

In addition to the DLPFC, there is evidence that other frontal areas may also carry representations of task set, including pre-supplementary motor area (pre-SMA; Rushworth *et al.*, 2004) and premotor cortex (PMC; Muhammad *et al.*, 2006; Wallis and Miller, 2003). Furthermore, like options in HRL, neurons in several frontal areas including DLPFC, pre-SMA, and supplementary motor area (SMA) have been shown to code for particular sequences of low-level actions (Averbeck and Lee, 2007; Bor *et al.*, 2003; Shima *et al.*, 2007; Shima and Tanji, 2000). Research on the frontal cortex also accords well with the stipulation in HRL that temporally abstract actions may organise into hierarchies, with the policy for one option (say, an option for making coffee) calling other, lower-level options (say, options for adding sugar or cream). This fits with numerous accounts suggesting that the frontal cortex serves to represent action at multiple, nested levels of temporal structure (Grafman, 2002; Sirigu *et al.*, 1995; Wood and Grafman, 2003; Zalla *et al.*, 2003), possibly in such a way that higher levels of structure are represented more anteriorly (Botvinick, 2008; Fuster, 2001, 2004; Haruno and Kawato, 2006; Koechlin *et al.*, 2003).

13.4.1.3   Extension 2: option-specific policies

In addition to its default, top-level policy, the actor in HRL must implement option-specific policies. Thus, the actor must carry a separate set of action strengths for each option.

13.4.1.4   Potential neural correlates

As noted earlier, it has been typical to draw a connection from the policy in standard RL to the DLS. For the DLS to implement the option-specific policies found in HRL, it would need to receive input from cortical regions representing options. It is thus relevant that such regions as the DLPFC, SMA, pre-SMA and PMC – areas potentially representing options – all project heavily to the DLS (Alexander *et al.*, 1986; Parent and Hazrati, 1995). Frank, O'Reilly and colleagues (Frank and Claus, 2006; O'Reilly and Frank, 2006; Rougier *et al.*, 2005) have put forth detailed computational models that show how frontal inputs to the striatum could switch among different stimulus-response pathways (see also Hazy *et al.* and Stafford and Gurney, this volume). Here, as in guided activation theory, temporally abstract action representations in frontal cortex select among alternative (i.e., option-specific) policies.

In order to support option-specific policies, the DLS would need to integrate information about the currently controlling option with information about the current environmental state, as is indicated by the arrows converging on the policy module in Figure 13.2b. This is consistent with neurophysiological data showing that some DLS neurons respond to stimuli in a way that varies with task context (Ravel *et al.*, 2006; see also Salinas, 2004). Other studies have shown that *action* representations within the DLS can also be task-dependent. For example, Aldridge and Berridge (1998) reported that, in rats, different DLS neurons fired in conjunction with simple grooming movements depending on whether those actions were performed in isolation or as part of a grooming sequence (see also Aldridge *et al.*, 2004; Graybiel, 1995, 1998; Lee *et al.*, 2006). This is consistent with the idea that option-specific policies (action strengths) might be implemented in the DLS, since this would imply that a particular motor behaviour, when performed in different task contexts, would be selected via different neural pathways.

Recall that, within HRL, policies are responsible for selecting not only primitive actions, but also for selecting options. Translated into neural terms, this would require the DLS to participate in the selection of options. This is consistent with data from Muhammad *et al.* (2006), who observed striatal activation that varied with task context (see also Graybiel, 1998). It is also consistent with the fact that the DLS projects heavily, via thalamic relays, to all of the frontal regions linked above with a role in representing options (Alexander *et al.*, 1986; Middleton and Strick, 2002).

Unlike the selection of primitive actions, the selection of options in HRL involves initiation, maintenance, and termination phases. At the neural level, the maintenance phase would be naturally supported within DLPFC, which has been extensively implicated in working memory function (Courtney *et al.*, 2011; D'Esposito, 2007; Postle, 2006). With regard to initiation and termination, it is intriguing that phasic activity has been observed, both within the DLS and in several areas of frontal cortex, at the boundaries of temporally extended action sequences (Fujii and Graybiel, 2003; Morris *et al.*, 2004; Zacks *et al.*, 2001). Since these boundaries correspond to points where new options would be selected, boundary-aligned activity in the DLS and frontal cortex is also consistent with a proposed role of the DLS in gating information into prefrontal working memory circuits (O'Reilly and Frank, 2006; Rougier *et al.*, 2005).

13.4.2   The critic in HRL: relation to orbitofrontal cortex

As noted earlier, HRL also requires two key extensions to the critic component of the actor–critic architecture.

13.4.2.1   Extension 3: Option-specific value functions

Under HRL, in addition to its top-level state-value function, the critic must also maintain a set of option-specific value functions. This is due to the fact that the value function indicates how well things are expected to go following arrival at a given state, which obviously depends on which actions the agent will select. Under HRL, the option that is currently in control of behaviour determines action selection, and also determines which actions will yield pseudo-reward. Thus, whenever an option is guiding behaviour, the value attached to a state must take the identity of that option into account.

13.4.2.2   Potential neural correlates

If there is a neural structure that computes something like option-specific state values, this structure would be expected to communicate closely with the VS, the region typically identified with the locus of state or state-action values in RL. However, the structure would also be expected to receive inputs from the portions of frontal cortex that we have identified as representing options. One brain region that meets both of these criteria is the orbitofrontal cortex (OFC), an area that has strong connections with both VS and DLPFC (Alexander *et al.*, 1990; Rolls, 2004). The idea that the OFC might participate in computing option-specific state values also fits well with the behaviour of individual neurons within this cortical region. OFC neurons have been extensively implicated in representing the reward value associated with environmental states (Rolls, 2004; Schultz *et al.*, 2000). However, other data suggests that OFC neurons can also be sensitive to shifts in response policy or task set (e.g., O'Doherty *et al.*, 2003). Critically, Schoenbaum *et al.* (1999) observed that OFC representations of event value changed in parallel with shifts in strategy, a finding that fits precisely with the idea that the OFC might represent option-specific state values.

13.4.2.3   Extension 4: Temporal scope of the prediction error

Moving from RL to HRL brings about an important alteration in the way that the prediction error is computed. Specifically, it changes the scope of the events that the prediction error addresses. In standard RL, the prediction error indicates whether things went better or worse than expected since the immediately preceding timestep. HRL, in addition, evaluates at the completion of an option whether things have gone better or worse than expected since the initiation of that option (see Figure 13.3). Thus, unlike standard RL, the prediction errors associated with options in HRL are framed around temporally extended events. Formally speaking, the HRL setting is no longer a Markov decision process, but rather a semi-Markov decision process (SMDP).

13.4.2.4   Potential neural correlates

This aspect of HRL resonates, once again, with data from the OFC. Note that, in order to evaluate whether things went better or worse than expected over the course of an entire option, the critic needs access, when an option terminates, to the reward prediction it made when the option was initially selected. This is consistent with the finding that within OFC, unlike some other areas, reward-predictive activity tends to be sustained, spanning temporally extended segments of task structure (Schultz *et al.*, 2000). Another relevant finding is that the response of OFC neurons to the receipt of primary rewards varies depending on the wait-time leading up to the reward (Roesch *et al.*, 2006; see Appendix A, Equation (A. 7)). This suggests, again, that the OFC interprets value within the context of temporally extended segments of behaviour.

The widened scope of the prediction error computation in HRL also resonates with work on midbrain DA function. In particular, Daw *et al.* (2003) suggested, based on midbrain responses to delayed rewards, that dopaminergic function is driven by representations that divide event sequences into temporally extended segments. In articulating this account, Daw *et al.* (2003) provided a formal analysis of DA function that draws on precisely the same principles of temporal abstraction that also provide the foundation for HRL, namely an SMDP framework.

In further examining the potential links between DA and HRL, it may be useful to consider recent work by O'Reilly and Frank (2006), which shows through computational modelling how DA might support learning in working memory circuits, supporting the performance of hierarchically organised, temporally extended tasks. This research addresses issues somewhat different from those that are central to HRL, focusing in particular upon tasks that require preservation of information conveyed by transient cues (a case treated in machine learning under the rubric of partially observable Markov decision problems). However, O'Reilly and colleagues have also begun to explore the application of similar mechanisms to the learning of abstract task representations (Rougier *et al.*, 2005). One interesting aspect of this latter work is its focus on cases where task-appropriate behaviour can be acquired through attending selectively to particular stimulus dimensions (e.g., colour or shape). This connects with some work in HRL, where the use of option-specific state representations have been explored (see, e.g., Dietterich, 2000; Jonsson and Barto, 2001). Characterising further the relationship between this approach within HRL and the computational work by Rougier and colleagues is an inviting area for further analysis.

13.5   Discussion

We have shown that recently developed HRL techniques have much in common with psychological accounts of hierarchically organised behaviour. Furthermore, through a new actor–critic implementation of HRL, we have suggested several points of contact between HRL and the neural substrates of decision making and hierarchical control. Before summing up, we briefly consider the relation of HRL to two further topics that have been at the focus of recent work on the control of action, and we enumerate some directions for further research.

13.5.1   Dual modes of action control

Work on animal and human behaviour suggests that instrumental actions arise from two modes of control, one built on established stimulus-response links or 'habits', and the other on prospective planning (Balleine and Dickinson, 1998). Daw *et al.* (2005) have mapped these modes of control onto RL constructs, characterising the former as relying on cached action values or strengths and model-free RL, and the latter as looking ahead based on an internal model relating actions to their likely effects, that is, model-based RL. Here we have cast HRL in terms of the cache-based system, both because this is most representative of existing work on HRL and because the principles of model-based search have not yet been as fully explored, either at the computational level or in terms of neural correlates. However, it is straightforward to incorporate temporal abstraction into model-based, prospective control. This is accomplished by assuming that each option is associated with an *option model*, a knowledge structure indicating the ultimate outcomes likely to result from selecting the option, the reward or cost likely to be accrued during its execution, and the amount of time this execution is likely to take (see Sutton *et al.*, 1999). Equipped with models of this kind, the agent can use them to look ahead, evaluating potential courses of action. Importantly, the search process can now 'skip over' potentially large sequences of primitive actions, effectively reducing the size of the search tree (Figure 13.1c; Hayes-Roth and Hayes-Roth, 1979; Kambhampati *et al.*, 1998; Marthi *et al.*, 2007). This kind of saltatory search process seems to fit well with everyday planning, which introspectively seems to operate at the level of temporally abstract actions ('Perhaps I should buy one of those new cell phones . . . Well, that would cost me a few hundred dollars . . . But if I bought one, I could use it to check my email . . . '). The idea of action models, in general, also fits well with work on motor control (e.g., Wolpert and Flanagan, 2001), which strongly suggests the involvement of predictive models in the guidance of bodily movements. Because option models encode the consequences of interventions, it is interesting to note that recent neuroimaging work has mapped representations of action outcome information in part to prefrontal cortex (Hamilton and Grafton, 2008), a region whose potential links with HRL we have already considered.

13.5.2   Strict versus quasi-hierarchical structure

Although human behaviour, like behaviour in HRL systems, is often hierarchically structured, there are also aspects of human behaviour that resist a strictly hierarchical account (Botvinick, 2007, 2008; Botvinick and Plaut, 2002, 2004, 2006). For example, naturalistic tasks exhibit a great deal of overlap or shared structure (Schank and Abelson, 1977), a point that is reflected in the errors or slips that occur in the performance of such tasks (Reason, 1992). Shared structure raises a problem because temporal abstractions have only a limited ability to exploit detailed patterns of overlap among tasks. Thus, using options (as they have so far been defined), it would be difficult to capture the overlap among tasks such as spreading jam on bread, spreading mustard on a hotdog, and spreading icing on a cake. Furthermore, execution of subtasks in everyday behaviour is highly context-sensitive, that is, the way in which a subtask is executed can depend on the larger task context in which it occurs (Agre, 1988). Context sensitivity raises the problem that different levels within a task hierarchy are no longer independent. For example, the subtask of picking up a pencil cannot be represented as a self-contained unit if the details of its execution (e.g., the rotation of the hand) depend on whether one is going to use the pencil to write or to erase (see Ansuini *et al.*, 2006). Significantly, related tensions between hierarchical compositionality and context-sensitivity have also been noted in work on HRL (Dietterich, 2000).

Botvinick and Plaut (2002, 2004, 2006) proposed a computational model of routine sequential behaviour that is sensitive to hierarchical task structure, but which also accommodates context-dependent subtask performance and overlap between tasks. That model, like the HRL model we have presented here, displays transfer effects when faced with new problems (Botvinick and Plaut, 2002). Furthermore, Ruh (2007) has demonstrated that the Botvinick and Plaut (2004) model can acquire target behaviours through RL. Understanding the relationship between this computational approach and HRL is an interesting challenge for further investigation.

13.5.3   Directions for further research

The idea that HRL algorithms may be relevant to understanding brain function and behaviour gives rise to a wide range of questions for experimental research. To begin with, almost all of the empirical parallels we have traced out in this chapter call for further experimental scrutiny. For example, although there is compelling evidence that dorsolateral PFC neurons represent task context, there is as of yet only indirect evidence (e.g., Badre, 2008; Zacks *et al.*, 2001) to support the idea that PFC neurons also code discretely for subtask segments in hierarchically structured tasks, as HRL would seem to require. Similarly, although there are established aspects of dopaminergic function that resonate with predictions from HRL, HRL also gives rise to predictions that would need to be tested through new experiments. In particular, the version of HRL we have focused on here predicts phasic dopaminergic discharge at subtask boundaries, scaling with the magnitude of option-level prediction errors.

In considering the coding of rewards, one particularly interesting question is whether there might exist a neural correlate of pseudo-reward. As detailed earlier, the options framework, like at least one other influential version of HRL (MAXQ, Dietterich, 2000), associates a separate reward function with each individual subtask representation. This pseudo-reward function is critical in shaping subtask-specific policies, directing action toward desirable subtask outcomes, i.e., subgoals. An obvious question is whether neural structures that are responsive to exogenous reward also respond to the attainment of subgoal states during the performance of hierarchically structured tasks (Ribas-Fernandes *et al.*, in press).

Having suggested this possibility, it is important to note that in the case of pseudo-reward, the framing of specific predictions requires consideration of differences between HRL implementations. Indeed, there exist versions of HRL, such as the HAM framework (Parr and Russell, 1998), that do not involve pseudo-reward at all, relying instead on a combination of ordinary, exogenous reward and fixed constraints to shape subtask policies. Another point on which HRL implementations differ, which may have implications for experimental predictions, is in the representation of the value function. Whereas the options framework, as we have discussed, maintains option-specific value functions, some other frameworks, including MAXQ (Andre and Russell, 2001, 2002; Dietterich, 2000), decompose these value functions into separate components, giving rise to slightly different learning algorithms. This difference may lead different HRL frameworks to make non-equivalent fine-grained predictions. For example, frameworks may vary in the prediction errors they would compute in a given domain, giving rise to divergent predictions concerning dopaminergic function. In sum, just as with non-hierarchical RL algorithms, any detailed investigation of HRL as a framework for interpreting neural function and behaviour will require some attention to algorithmic detail.

13.6   Conclusions

Computational RL has proved extremely useful to research on behaviour and brain function. Our aim here has been to explore whether HRL might prove similarly applicable. An initial motivation for considering this question derives from the fact that HRL addresses an inherent limitation of RL, the scaling problem, which would clearly be of relevance to any organism relying on RL-like learning mechanisms. Implementing HRL along the lines of the actor–critic framework, thereby bringing it into alignment with existing mappings between RL and neuroscience, reveals direct parallels between components of HRL and specific functional neuroanatomic structures, including the DLPFC and OFC. HRL suggests new ways of interpreting neural activity in these as well as several other regions. HRL also resonates strongly with issues in psychology, in particular with work on task representation and the control of hierarchically structured behaviour, adding to these a unifying normative perspective. Among the most important implications of HRL is the way in which it highlights the option discovery problem. Here, and on many other fronts, HRL appears to offer a potentially useful set of tools for further investigating the computational and neural basis of hierarchical structured behaviour.

Appendix A

We present here the details of our HRL implementation and the simulations briefly described in the main text. For clarity, we begin by describing our implementation of non-hierarchical RL, which was used in the simulations including only primitive actions. This will then be extended, in the next section, to the hierarchical case. All simulations were run using Matlab (The Mathworks, Natick, MA).

Basic actor–critic implementation

Task and representations

Following the standard RL approach (see Sutton and Barto, 1998), tasks were represented by four elements: a set of states S, a set of actions A, a reward function R assigning a real-valued number to every state transition, and a transition function T giving a new state for each pairing of a state with an action. In our simulations, S contained the set of location tiles in the layout depicted in Figure 13.4a; A contained eight single-step movements, following the principle compass directions; R yielded a reward of 100 on transitions to the goal state indicated with a G in Figure 13.4a, otherwise zero; and T was deterministic. All actions were available in every state, and actions yielded no change in state if a move into a wall was attempted. Our choice to use deterministic actions was for simplicity of exposition, and does not reflect a limitation of either the RL or HRL framework.

Architecture

The basic RL agent comprised actor and critic components. The actor maintained a set (matrix) of real-valued strengths (W) for each action in each state. The critic maintained a vector V of values, attaching a real number to each state.

Training

At the outset of training, action strengths and state values were initialised to zero; the state was initialised to the start location indicated in Figure 13.4a; and a time index t was initialised at zero. On each step of processing, t, an action was selected probabilistically according to the softmax equation:

$$P(a) = \frac{e^{W(s_t, a)/\tau}}{\sum_{a' \in A} e^{W(s_t, a')/\tau}} \tag{A.1}$$

where $P(a)$ is the probability of selecting action a at step t; $W(s_t, a)$ is the weight for action a in the current state; and τ is a temperature parameter controlling the tendency toward exploration in action selection (ten in our simulations). (The softmax equation is formally equivalent to one parameterisation of the drift-diffusion process (Bogacz *et al.*, 2006), closely related to the decision models discussed by Bogacz *et al.*, this volume.) The next state (s_{t+1}) was then determined based on the transition function T, and the reward for the transition (r_{t+1}) based on R. Using these, the temporal-difference (TD) prediction error (δ) was computed as

$$\delta = r_{t+1} + \gamma V(s_{s+1}) - V(s_t) \tag{A.2}$$

where γ is a discount factor (0.9 in our simulations). The TD prediction error was then used to update both the value function and the strength for the action just completed:

$$V(s_t) \leftarrow V(s_t) + \alpha_C \delta \tag{A.3}$$

$$W(s_t, a) \leftarrow W(s_t, a) + \alpha_A \delta. \tag{A.4}$$

The learning rate parameters α_C and α_A were set to 0.2 and 0.1, respectively. Following these updates, t was incremented and a new action was selected. The cycle was repeated until the goal state was reached, at which point the agent was returned to the start state, t was reinitialised, and another episode was run.

HRL Implementation

Our implementation of HRL was based on the options framework described by Sutton *et al.* (1999), but adapted to the actor–critic framework.

Task and representations
The set of available actions was expanded to include options in addition to primitive actions. Each option was associated with (1) an initiation set, indicating the states where the option could be selected; (2) a termination function, returning the probability of terminating the option in each state; and (3) a set of option-specific strengths W_o, containing one weight for each action (primitive or abstract) at each state.

For the four-rooms simulations, two options could be initiated in each room, each terminating deterministically at one of the room's two doors. Each option also had a pseudo-reward function, yielding a pseudo-reward of 100 at the option's termination state. For simplicity, each option was associated with strengths only for primitive actions (i.e., not for other options). That is, option policies were only permitted to select primitive actions. As indicated in the main text, options are ordinarily permitted to select other options. This more general arrangement is compatible with the implementation described here.

Architecture
In addition to the option-specific strengths just mentioned, the actor maintained a 'root' set of strengths, used for action selection when no option was currently active. The critic maintained a root-level value function plus a set of option-specific value functions V_o.

Training
Since primitive actions can be thought of as single-step options, we shall henceforth refer to primitive actions as 'primitive options' and temporally abstract actions as 'abstract options,' using the term 'option' to refer to both at once. The model was initialised as before, with all option strengths and state values initialised to zero. On each successive step, an option o was selected according to

$$P(o) = \frac{e^{W_{o_{ctrl}}(s_t, o)/\tau}}{\sum\limits_{o' \in O} e^{W_{o_{ctrl}}(s_t, o')/\tau}} \qquad (A.5)$$

where O is the set of available options, including primitive options; o_{ctrl} is the option currently in control of behaviour (if any); and $W_{o_{ctrl}}(s_t, o)$ is the option-specific – i.e., o_{ctrl}-specific – strength for option o (or the root strength for o in the case where no option is currently in control). Following identification of the next state and of the reward (including pseudo-reward) yielded by the transition, the prediction error was calculated for all *terminating* options, including primitive options, as

$$\delta = r_{cum} + \gamma^{t_{tot}} V_{o_{ctrl}}(s_{t+1}) - V_{o_{ctrl}}(s_{init}) \tag{A.6}$$

where t_{tot} is the number of timesteps elapsed since the relevant option was selected (one for primitive actions); $s_{t_{init}}$ is the state in which the option was selected; o_{ctrl} is the option whose policy selected the option that is now terminating (or the root value function if the terminating option was selected by the root policy); and r_{cum} is the cumulative discounted reward for the duration of the option:

$$r_{cum} = \sum_{i=1}^{t_{tot}} \gamma^{i-1} r_{t_{init}+i}. \tag{A.7}$$

Note that $r_{t_{init}+i}$ incorporated pseudo-reward only if $s_{t_{init}+i}$ was a subgoal state for o_{ctrl}. Thus, pseudo-reward was used to compute prediction errors 'within' an option, i.e., when updating the option's policy, but not 'outside' the option, at the next level up. It should also be remarked that, at the termination of non-primitive options, two TD prediction errors were computed, one for the last primitive action selected under the option and one for the option itself (see Figure 13.3).

Following calculation of each δ, value functions and option strengths were updated:

$$V_{o_{ctrl}}(s_{t_{init}}) \leftarrow V_{o_{ctrl}}(s_{t_{init}}) + \alpha_C \delta \tag{A.8}$$

$$W_{o_{ctrl}}(s_{t_{init}}, o) \leftarrow W_{o_{ctrl}}(s_{t_{init}}, o) + \alpha_A \delta. \tag{A.9}$$

The time index was then incremented and a new option/action selected, with the entire cycle continuing until the top-level goal was reached.

In our simulations, the model was first pre-trained for a total of 50 000 timesteps without termination or reward delivery at G. This allowed option-specific action strengths and values to develop, but did not lead to any change in strengths or values at the root level. Thus, action selection at the top level was random during this phase of training. In order to obtain the data displayed in Figure 13.4c, for clarity of illustration, training with pseudo-reward only was conducted with a small learning rate ($\alpha_A = 0.01$, $\alpha_C = 0.1$), reinitialising to a random state whenever the relevant option reached its subgoal.

Acknowledgements

The present work was completed with support from the National Institute of Mental Health, grant number P50 MH062196 (M.M.B.), the Human Frontiers Science Program (Y.N.), and from the National Science Foundation, grant number CCF-0432143 (A.C.B.). Any opinions, findings, and conclusions or recommendations expressed in this material are those of the authors and do not necessarily reflect the views of the funding agencies. The authors thank Carlos Brody, Jonathan Cohen, Scott Kuindersma, Ken Norman, Randy O'Reilly, Geoff Schoenbaum, Asvin Shah, Ozgur Simsek, Andrew Stout, Chris Vigorito, and Pippin Wolfe for useful comments on the work reported.

References

Agre, P. E. (1988). The dynamic structure of everyday life (Tech. Rep. No. 1085). Cambridge, MA: Massachusetts Institute of Technology, Artificial Intelligence Laboratory.

Aldridge, W. J. and K. C. Berridge (1998). Coding of serial order by neostriatal neurons: a 'natural action' approach to movement sequence. *J. Neurosci.* **18**: 2777–87.

Aldridge, J. W., K. C. Berridge, and A. R. Rosen (2004). Basal ganglia neural mechanisms of natural movement sequences. *Can. J. Physiol. Pharmacol.* **82**: 732–9.

Alexander, G. E., M. D. Crutcher, and M. R. DeLong (1990). Basal ganglia-thalamocortical circuits: parallel substrates for motor, oculomotor, 'prefrontal' and 'limbic' functions. *Prog. Brain Res.* **85**: 119–46.

Alexander, G. E., M. R. DeLong, and P. L. Strick (1986). Parallel organization of functionally segregated circuits linking basal ganglia and cortex. *Annu. Rev. Neurosci.* **9**: 357–81.

Allport, A. and Wylie, G. (2000). Task-switching, stimulus-response bindings and negative priming. In *Control of Cognitive Processes: Attention and Performance, XVIII*, ed. S. Monsell and J. Driver. Cambridge, MA: MIT Press, pp. 35–70.

Anderson, J. R. (2004). An integrated theory of mind. *Psychol. Rev.* 111: 1036–60.

Andre, D. and S. J. Russell (2001). Programmable reinforcement learning agents. *Adv. Neural Inf. Proc. Syst.* **13**: 1019–25.

Andre, D. and S. J. Russell (2002). State abstraction for programmable reinforcement learning agents. Paper presented at the Proceedings of the 18th National Conference on Artificial Intelligence.

Ansuini, C., M. Santello, S. Massaccesi, and U. Castiello (2006). Effects of end-goal on hand shaping. *J. Neurophysiol.* **95**: 2456–65.

Arbib, M. A. (1985). Schemas for the temporal organization of behaviour. *Hum. Neurobiol.* **4**: 63–72.

Asaad, W. F., G. Rainer, and E. K. Miller (2000). Task-specific neural activity in the primate prefrontal cortex. *J. Neurophysiol.* **84**: 451–9.

Averbeck, B. B. and D. Lee (2007). Prefrontal neural correlates of memory for sequences. *J. Neurosci.* **27**: 2204–11.

Badre, D. (2008). Cognitive control, hierarchy, and the rostro–caudal organization of the frontal lobes. *Trends Cogn. Sci.* **12**: 193–200.

Balleine, B. W. and A. Dickinson (1998). Goal-directed instrumental action: contingency and incentive learning and their cortical substrates. *Neuropharmacology* 37: 407–19.

Barto, A. G. (1995). Adaptive critics and the basal ganglia. In *Models of Information Processing in the Basal Ganglia*, ed. J. C. Houk and J. Davis and D. Beiser. Cambridge, MA: MIT Press, pp. 215–32.

Barto, A. G. and S. Mahadevan (2003). Recent advances in hierarchical reinforcement learning. *Discrete Event Dyn. S.* **13**: 343–79.

Barto, A. G., S. Singh, and N. Chentanez (2004). Intrinsically motivated learning of hierarchical collections of skills. *Proceedings of the 3rd International Conference on Development and Learning (ICDL 2004)*, pp. 112–19.

Barto, A. G. and Sutton, R. S. (1981). Toward a modern theory of adaptive networks: Expectation and prediction. *Psychol. Rev.* **88**: 135–70.

Barto, A. G., R. S. Sutton, and C. W. Anderson (1983). Neuronlike adaptive elements that can solve difficult learning control problems. *IEEE T. Syst. Man and Cyb.* **13**: 834–46.

Berlyne, D. E. (1960). *Conflict, Arousal and Curiosity*. New York: McGraw-Hill.

Bhatnagara, S. and J. R. Panigrahi (2006). Actor-critic algorithms for hierarchical Markov decision processes. *Automatica* **42**: 637–644.

Bogacz, R., E. Brown, J. Moehlis, P. Holmes, and J. D. Cohen (2006). The physics of optimal decision making: a formal analysis of models of performance in two-alternative forced-choice tasks. *Psychol. Rev.* **113**: 700–65.

Bor, D., J. Duncan, R. J. Wiseman, and A. M. Owen (2003). Encoding strategies dissociate prefrontal activity from working memory demand. *Neuron* **37**: 361–67.

Botvinick, M. and D. C. Plaut (2002). Representing task context: proposals based on a connectionist model of action. *Psychol. Res.* 66(4): 298–311.

Botvinick, M. and D. C. Plaut (2004). Doing without schema hierarchies: a recurrent connectionist approach to normal and impaired routine sequential action. *Psychol. Rev.* **111**(2): 395–429.

Botvinick, M. and D. C. Plaut (2006). Such stuff as habits are made on: a reply to Cooper and Shallice (2006). *Psychol. Rev.* **113**(4): 917–27.

Botvinick, M. M. (2007). Multilevel structure in behaviour and the brain: a model of Fuster's hierarchy. *Phil. Trans. Roy. Soc. B* **362**: 1615–26.

Botvinick, M. M. (2008). Hierarchical models of behavior and prefrontal function. *Trends Cogn. Sci.* **12**: 201–208.

Bruner, J. (1973). Organization of early skilled action. *Child Dev.* **44**: 1–11.

Bunge, S. A. (2004). How we use rules to select actions: a review of evidence from cognitive neuroscience. *Cogn. Affect. Behav. Ne.* **4**: 564–579.

Bunzeck, N. and E. Duzel (2006). Absolute coding of stimulus novelty in the human substantia nigra/VTA. *Neuron* **51**: 369–79.

Cohen, J. D., T. S. Braver, and R. C. O'Reilly (1996). A computational approach to prefrontal cortex, cognitive control and schizophrenia: recent developments and current challenges. *Phil. Trans. Roy. Soc. B* **351**: 1515–27.

Cohen, J. D., K. Dunbar, and J. L. McClelland (1990). On the control of automatic processes: a parallel distributed processing account of the Stroop effect. *Psychol. Rev.* **97**: 332–61.

Conway, C. M. and M. H. Christiansen (2001). Sequential learning in non-human primates. *Trends Cogn. Sci.* **5**: 539–46.

Cooper, R. and T. Shallice (2000). Contention scheduling and the control of routine activities. *Cogn. Neuropsychol.* **17**: 297–338.

Courtney, S. M., Roth, J. K., and Sala, J. B. (in press). A hierarchical biased-competition model of domain-dependent working memory maintenance and executive control. In N. Osaka and R. Logie and M. D'Esposito (Eds.), *Working Memory: Behavioural and Neural Correlates.* Oxford: Oxford University Press, pp. 369–384.

D'Esposito, M. (2007). From cognitive to neural models of working memory. *Phil. Trans. Roy. Soc. B* **362**: 761–72.

Daw, N. D., A. C. Courville, and D. S. Touretzky (2003). Timing and partial observability in the dopamine system. In *Advances in Neural Information Processing Systems*, 15. Cambridge, MA: MIT Press, pp. 99–106.

Daw, N. D., Y. Niv, and P. Dayan (2005). Uncertainty-based competition between prefrontal and striatal systems for behavioral control. *Nat. Neurosci.* **8**: 1704–11.

Daw, N. D., Y. Niv, and P. Dayan (2006). Actions, policies, values and the basal ganglia. In *Recent Breakthroughs in Basal Ganglia Research*, ed. E. Bezard. New York: Nova Science Publishers, pp. 369–84.

De Pisapia, N. and N. H. Goddard (2003). A neural model of frontostriatal interactions for behavioral planning and action chunking. *Neurocomputing* **52–54**: 489–95.

Dehaene, S. and J.-P. Changeux (1997). A hierarchical neuronal network for planning behavior. *Proc. Nat. Acad. Sci.* **94**: 13293–8.

Dell, G. S., Berger, L. K., and Svec, W. R. (1997). Language production and serial order. *Psychol. Rev.* **104**: 123–147.

Dietterich, T. G. (1998). The MAXQ method for hierarchical reinforcement learning. *Proceedings of the International Conference on Machine Learning*, pp. 118–26.

Dietterich, T. G. (2000). Hierarchical reinforcement learning with the maxq value function decomposition. *J. Artif. Intell. Res.* **13**: 227–303.

Elfwing, S., K. Uchibe, and H. I. Christensen (2007). Evolutionary development of hierarchical learning structures. *IEEE Trans. Evol. Comput.* **11**: 249–64.

Estes, W. K. (1972). An associative basis for coding and organization in memory. In *Coding Processes in Human Memory*, ed. A. W. Melton and E. Martin. Washington DC: V. H. Winston and Sons, pp. 161–90.

Ribas-Fernandes, J., A. Solway, C. Diuk, *et al.* (in press). A neural signature of hierarchical reinforcement learning. *Neuron*

Fischer, K. W. (1980). A theory of cognitive development: the control and construction of hierarchies of skills. *Psychol. Rev.* **87**: 477–531.

Fischer, K. W. and M. W. Connell (2003). Two motivational systems that shape development: epistemic and self-organizing. *B. J. Educ. Psychol.* **2**: 103–123.

Frank, M. J. and E. D. Claus (2006). Anatomy of a decision: striato-orbitofrontal interactions in reinforcement learning, decision making, and reversal. *Psychol. Rev.* **113**: 300–26.

Fujii, N. and A. M. Graybiel (2003). Representation of action sequence boundaries by macaque prefrontal cortical neurons. *Science* **301**: 1246–9.

Fuster, J. M. (1997). *The Prefrontal Cortex: Anatomy, Physiology, and Neuropsychology of the Frontal Lobe*. Philadelphia, PA: Lippincott-Raven.

Fuster, J. M. (2001). The prefrontal cortex – an update: time is of the essence. *Neuron* **30**: 319–33.

Fuster, J. M. (2004). Upper processing stages of the perception-action cycle. *Trends Cogn. Sci.* **8**: 143–5.

Gergely, G. and G. Csibra (2003). Teleological reasoning in infancy: the naive theory of rational action. *Trends Cogn. Sci.* **7**: 287–92.

Gopnik, A., C. Glymour, D. Sobel, *et al.* (2004). A theory of causal learning in children: causal maps and Bayes nets. *Psychol. Rev.* **111**: 1–31.

Gopnik, A. and L. Schulz (2004). Mechanisms of theory formation in young children. *Trends Cogn. Sci.* **8**: 371–7.

Grafman, J. (2002). The human prefrontal cortex has evolved to represent components of structured event complexes. In J. Grafman (ed.), *Handbook of Neuropsychology*. Amsterdam: Elsevier, pp. 157–74.

Graybiel, A. M. (1995). Building action repertoires: memory and learning functions of the basal ganglia. *Curr. Opin. Neurobiol.* **5**: 733–41.

Graybiel, A. M. (1998). The basal ganglia and chunking of action repertoires. *Neurobiol. Learn. Mem.* **70**: 119–36.

Greenfield, P. M. (1984). A theory of the teacher in the learning activities of everyday life. In *Everyday Cognition: Its Development in Social Context*, ed. B. Rogoff and J. Lave. Cambridge, MA: Harvard University Press, pp. 117–38.

Greenfield, P. M., K. Nelson, and E. Saltzman (1972). The development of rulebound strategies for manipulating seriated cups: a parallel between action and grammar. *Cogn. Psychol.* **3**: 291–310.

Greenfield, P. M. and L. Schneider (1977). Building a tree structure: the development of hierarchical complexity and interrupted strategies in children's construction activity. *Dev. Psychol.* **13**: 299–313.

Grossberg, S. (1986). The adaptive self-organization of serial order in behavior: speech, language, and motor control. In *Pattern Recognition by Humans and Machines, Volume 1: Speech, Perception*, ed. E. C. Schwab and H. C. Nusbaum. New York: Academic Press, pp. 187–294.

Hamilton, A. F. d. C. and S. T. Grafton (2008). Action outcomes are represented in human inferior frontoparietal cortex. *Cereb. Cortex* **18**: 1160–8.

Harlow, H. F., M. K. Harlow, and D. R. Meyer (1950). Learning motivated by a manipulation drive. *J. Exp. Psychol.* **40**: 228–34.

Haruno, M. and M. Kawato (2006). Heterarchical reinforcement-learning model for integration of multiple cortico-striatal loops: fMRI examination in stimulus-action-reward association learning. *Neural Networks* **19**: 1242–54.

Hayes-Roth, B. and F. Hayes-Roth (1979). A cognitive model of planning. *Cogn. Sci.* **3**: 275–310.

Hengst, B. (2002). Discovering hierarchy in reinforcement learning with HEXQ. *P. Int. C. Mach. Learn.* **19**: 243–50.

Holroyd, C. B. and M. G. H. Coles (2002). The neural basis of human error processing: Reinforcement learning, dopamine, and the error-related negativity. *Psychol. Rev.* **109**(4): 679–709.

Hoshi, E., K. Shima, and J. Tanji (1998). Task-dependent selectivity of movement-related neuronal activity in the primate prefrontal cortex. *J. Neurophysiol.* **80**: 3392–7.

Houk, J. C., C. M. Adams, and A. G. Barto (1995). A model of how the basal ganglia generate and use neural signals that predict reinforcement. In *Models of Information Processing in the Basal Ganglia*, ed. J. C. Houk and D. G. Davis. Cambridge, MA: MIT Press, pp. 249–70.

Joel, D., Y. Niv, and E. Ruppin (2002). Actor-critic models of the basal ganglia: new anatomical and computational perspectives. *Neural Networks* **15**: 535–47.

Johnston, K. and S. Everling (2006). Neural activity in monkey prefrontal cortex is modulated by task context and behavioral instruction during delayed-match-to-sample and conditional prosaccade–antisaccade tasks. *J. Cogn. Neurosci.* **18**: 749–65.

Jonsson, A. and A. Barto (2001). Automated state abstraction for options using the U-tree algorithm. In *Advances in Neural Information Processing Systems 13*. Cambridge, MA: MIT Press, pp. 1054–60.

Jonsson, A. and A. Barto (2005). A causal approach to hierarchical decomposition of factored MDPs. *Proceedings of the International Conference on Machine Learning 22*, pp. 401–408.

Kambhampati, S., A. D. Mali, and B. Srivastava (1998). Hybrid planning for partially hierarchical domains. In *Proceedings of the Fifteenth National Conference on Artificial Intelligence (AAAI-98)*. Madison, WI: AAAI Press, pp. 882–8.

Kaplan, F. and P.-Y. Oudeyer (2004). Maximizing learning progress: an internal reward system for development. In *Embodied Artificial Intelligence*, ed. F. Iida and R. Pfeifer and L. Steels. Berlin: Springer-Verlag, pp. 259–70.

Kearns, M. and S. Singh (2002). Near-optimal reinforcement learning in polynomial time. *Mach. Learn.* **49**: 209–32.

Koechlin, E., C. Ody, and F. Kouneiher (2003). The architecture of cognitive control in the human prefrontal cortex. *Science* **302**(5648): 1181–5.

Krueger, K. A. and P. Dayan (2008). Flexible Shaping. Presented at *Cosyne (Computational and Systems Neuroscience)*. Salt Lake City, Utah.

Laird, J. E., P. S. Rosenbloom, and A. Newell (1986). Chunking in soar: the anatomy of a general learning mechanism. *Mach. Learn.* **1**: 11–46.

Landrum, E. R. (2005). Production of negative transfer in a problem-solving task. *Psychol. Rep.* **97**: 861–6.

Lashley, K. S. (1951). The problem of serial order in behavior. In *Cerebral Mechanisms in Behavior: The Hixon Symposium*, ed. L. A. Jeffress. New York, NY: Wiley, pp. 112–36.

Lee, I. H., A. R. Seitz, and J. A. Assad (2006). Activity of tonically active neurons in the monkey putamen during initiation and withholding of movement. *J. Neurophysiol.* **95**: 2391–3403.

Lee, F. J. and N. A. Taatgen (2003). Production compilation: a simple mechanism to model complex skill acquisition. *Hum. Factors* 45: 61–76.

Lehman, J. F., J. Laird, and P. Rosenbloom (1996). A gentle introduction to Soar, an architecture for human cognition. In *Invitation to Cognitive Science*, Vol. 4, ed. S. Sternberg and D. Scarborough. Cambridge, MA: MIT Press, pp. 212–49.

Li, L. and T. J. Walsh (2006). Towards a unified theory of state abstraction for MDPs. Paper presented at the Ninth International Symposium on Artificial Intelligence and Mathematics.

Logan, G. D. (2003). Executive control of thought and action: in search of the wild homunculus. *Curr. Dir. Psychol. Sci.* **12**: 45–8.

Luchins, A. S. (1942). Mechanization in problem solving. *Psychol. Monogr.* **248**: 1–95.

MacDonald, A. W., III, J. D. Cohen, V. A. Stenger, and C. S. Carter (2000). Dissociating the role of the dorsolateral prefrontal and anterior cingulate cortex in cognitive control. *Science* **288**(5472): 1835–8.

MacKay, D. G. (1987). *The Organization of Perception and Action: A Theory for Language and Other Cognitive Skills*. New York: Springer-Verlag.

Mannor, S., I. Menache, A. Hoze, and U. Klein (2004). Dynamic abstraction in reinforcement learning via clustering. *Proceedings of the Twenty-First International Conference on Machine Learning*. New York: ACM Press, pp. 560–7.

Marthi, B., S. J. Russell, and J. Wolfe (2007). Angelic semantics for high-level actions. Paper presented at the Seventeenth International Conference on Automated Planning and Scheduling (ICAPS 2007), Providence, RI.

McGovern, A. (2002). Autonomous discovery of temporal abstractions from interaction with an environment. PhD thesis, University of Massachusetts.

Mehta, S., P. Ray, P. Tadepalli, and T. Dietterich (2008). Automatic discovery and transfer of MAXQ hierarchies. Paper presented at *International Conference on Machine Learning*, Helsinki, Finland.

Meltzoff, A. N. (1995). Understanding the intentions of others: re-enactment of intended acts by 18-month-old children. *Dev. Psychol.* **31**: 838–50.

Menache, I., S. Mannor, and N. Shimkin (2002). Dynamic discovery of sub-goals in reinforcement learning. *Proceedings of the Thirteenth European Conference on Machine Learning*, 295–306.

Middleton, F. A. and P. L. Strick (2002). Basal-ganglia 'projections' to the prefrontal cortex of the primate. *Cereb. Cortex* **12**: 926–35.

Miller, E. K. and J. D. Cohen (2001). An integrative theory of prefrontal cortex function. *Annu. Rev. Neurosci.* 24: 167–202.

Miller, G. A., E. Galanter, and K. H. Pribram (1960). *Plans and the Structure of Behavior*. New York: Holt, Rinehart and Winston.

Minton, S., P. J. Hayes, and J. Fain (1985). *Controlling Search in Flexible Parsing*. Paper presented at the Ninth International Joint Conference on Artificial Intelligence (IJCAI-85), Los Angeles.

Miyamoto, H., J. Morimoto, K. Doya, and M. Kawato (2004). Reinforcement learning with via-point representation. *Neural Networks* **17**: 299–305.

Monsell, S. (2003). Task switching. *Trends Cogn. Sci.* **7**(3): 134–40.

Monsell, S., N. Yeung, and R. Azuma (2000). Reconfiguration of task-set: is it easier to switch to the weaker task? *Psychol. Res.* **63**: 250–64.

Montague, P. R., P. Dayan, and T. J. Sejnowski (1996). A framework for mesencephalic dopamine based on predictive Hebbian learning. *J. Neurosci.* **16**: 1936–47.

Morris, G., D. Arkadir, A. Nevet, E. Vaadia, and H. Bergman (2004). Coincident but distinct messages of midbrain dopamine and striatal tonically active neurons. *Neuron* **43**: 133–43.

Muhammad, R., J. D. Wallis, and E. K. Miller (2006). A comparison of abstract rules in the prefrontal cortex, premotor cortex, inferior temporal cortex, and striatum. *J. Cogn. Neurosci.* **18**: 974–89.

Nason, S. and J. E. Laird (2005). Soar-RL: integrating reinforcement learning with Soar. *Cogn. Syst. Res.* **6**: 51–9.

Newell, A. and H. A. Simon (1963). GPS, a program that simulates human thought. In *Computers and Thought*, ed. E. A. Feigenbaum and J. Feldman. New York: McGraw-Hill, pp. 279–293.

Newtson, D. (1976). Foundations of attribution: the perception of ongoing behavior. In *New Directions in Attribution Research*, ed. J. H. Harvey, W. J. Ickes, and R. F. Kidd. Hillsdale, NJ: Erlbaum, pp. 223–48.

O'Doherty, J., H. Critchley, R. Deichmann, and R. J. Dolan (2003). Dissociating valence of outcome from behavioral control in human orbital and ventral prefrontal cortices. *J. Neurosci.* **79**: 31–9.

O'Doherty, J., P. Dayan, P. Schultz, *et al.* (2004). Dissociable roles of ventral and dorsal striatum in instrumental conditioning. *Science* **304**: 452–4.

O'Reilly, R. C. and M. J. Frank (2006). Making working memory work: a computational model of learning in prefrontal cortex and basal ganglia. *Neural Comput.* **18**: 283–328.

Oudeyer, P.-Y., F. Kaplan, and V. Hafner (2007). Intrinsic motivation systems for autonomous development. *IEE T. Evol. Comput.* **11**: 265–86.

Parent, A. and L. N. Hazrati (1995). Functional anatomy of the basal ganglia. I. The cortico-basal ganglia-thalamo-cortical loop. *Brain Res. Rev.* **20**: 91–127.

Parr, R. and S. Russell (1998). Reinforcement learning with hierarchies of machines. *Adv. Neural Inf. Proc. Syst.* **10**: 1043–9.

Pashler, H. (1994). Dual-task interference in simple tasks: data and theory. *Psychol. Bull.* **116**: 220–44.

Petrides, M. (1995). Impairments on nonspatial self-ordered and externally ordered working memory tasks after lesions to the mid-dorsal part of the lateral frontal cortex in the monkey. *J. Neurosci.* **15**: 359–75.

Piaget, J. (1936 [1952]). *The Origins of Intelligence in Children*. M. Cook, trans. New York: International Universities Press.

Pickett, M. and A. G. Barto (2002). PolicyBlocks: an algorithm for creating useful macro-actions in reinforcement learning. In *Machine Learning: Proceedings of the Nineteenth International Conference on Machine Learning*, ed. C. Sammut and A. Hoffmann. San Francisco: Morgan Kaufmann, pp. 506–13.

Postle, B. R. (2006). Working memory as an emergent property of the mind and brain. *Neurosci.* **139**: 23–8.

Ravel, S., P. Sardo, E. Legallet, and P. Apicella (2006). Influence of spatial information on responses of tonically active neurons in the monkey striatum. *J. Neurophysiol.* **95**: 2975–86.

Rayman, W. E. (1982). Negative transfer: a threat to flying safety. *Aviat. Space Envir. Md.* **53**: 1224–6.

Reason, J. T. (1992). *Human Error*. Cambridge: Cambridge University Press.

Redgrave, P. and K. Gurney (2006). The short-latency dopamine signal: a role in discovering novel actions? *Nat. Rev. Neurosci.* **7**: 967–75.

Roesch, M. R., A. R. Taylor, and G. Schoenbaum (2006). Encoding of time-discounted rewards in orbitofrontal cortex is independent of value. *Neuron* **51**: 509–20.

Rolls, E. T. (2004). The functions of the orbitofrontal cortex. *Brain Cogn.* **55**: 11–29.

Rougier, N. P., D. C. Noell, T. S. Braver, J. D. Cohen, and R. C. O'Reilly (2005). Prefrontal cortex and flexible cognitive control: rules without symbols. *Proc. Nat. Acad. Sci.* **102**: 7338–43.

Ruh, N. (2007). Acquisition and control of sequential routine activities: modelling and empirical studies. PhD thesis, University of London.

Rumelhart, D. and D. A. Norman (1982). Simulating a skilled typist: a study of skilled cognitive-motor performance. *Cogn. Sci.* **6**: 1–36.

Rushworth, M. F. S., M. E. Walton, S. W. Kennerley, and D. M. Bannerman (2004). Action sets and decisions in the medial frontal cortex. *Trends Cogn. Sci.* **8**: 410–17.

Ryan, R. M. and E. L. Deci (2000). Intrinsic and extrinsic motivation. *Contemp. Edu. Psychol.* **25**: 54–67.

Saffran, J. R., R. N. Aslin, and E. L. Newport (1996). Statistical learning by 8-month-old infants. *Science* **13**: 1926–8.

Saffran, J. R. and D. P. Wilson (2003). From syllables to syntax: multilevel statistical learning by 12-month-old infants. *Infancy* **4**: 273–84.

Salinas, E. (2004). Fast remapping of sensory stimuli onto motor actions on the basis of contextual modulation. *J. Neurosci.* **24**: 1113–18.

Schank, R. C. and R. P. Abelson (1977). *Scripts, Plans, Goals and Understanding.* Hillsdale, NJ: Erlbaum.

Schmidhuber, J. (1991). A possibility for implementing curiosity and boredom in model-building neural controllers. In *From Animals to Animats: Proceedings of the First International Conference on Simulation of Adaptive Behavior.* Cambridge: MIT Press, pp. 222–7.

Schneider, D. W. and G. D. Logan (2006). Hierarchical control of cognitive processes: switching tasks in sequences. *J. Exp. Psychol.* **135**: 623–40.

Schoenbaum, G., A. A. Chiba, and M. Gallagher (1999). Neural encoding in orbitofrontal cortex and basolateral amygdala during olfactory discrimination learning. *J. Neurosci.* **19**: 1876–84.

Schultz, W., P. Apicella, and T. Ljungberg (1993). Responses of monkey dopamine neurons to reward and conditioned stimuli during successive steps of learning a delayed response task. *J. Neurosci.* **13**: 900–913.

Schultz, W., P. Dayan, and P. R. Montague (1997). A neural substrate of prediction and reward. *Science* **275**: 1593–9.

Schultz, W., K. L. Tremblay, and J. R. Hollerman (2000). Reward processing in primate orbitofrontal cortex and basal ganglia. *Cereb. Cortex* **10**: 272–83.

Shallice, T. and P. W. Burgess (1991). Deficits in strategy application following frontal lobe damage in man. *Brain* **114**: 727–41.

Shima, K., M. Isoda, H. Mushiake, and J. Tanji (2007). Categorization of behavioural sequences in the prefrontal cortex. *Nature* **445**: 315–18.

Shima, K. and J. Tanji (2000). Neuronal activity in the supplementary and presupplementary motor areas for temporal organization of multiple movements. *J. Neurophysiol.* **84**: 2148–60.

Shimamura, A. P. (2000). The role of the prefrontal cortex in dynamic filtering. *Psychobiol.* **28**: 207–18.

Simsek, O., A. Wolfe, and A. Barto (2005). Identifying useful subgoals in reinforcement learning by local graph partitioning. *Proceedings of the Twenty-Second International Conference on Machine Learning (ICML 05)*. New York: ACM, pp. 816–23.

Singh, S., A. G. Barto, and N. Chentancz (2005). Intrinsically motivated reinforcement learning. In *Advances in Neural Information Processing Systems 17: Proceedings of the 2004 Conference*, ed. L. K. Saul, Y. Weiss, and L. Bottou. Cambridge, MA: MIT Press, pp. 1281–8.

Sirigu, A., T. Zalla, B. Pillon, *et al.* (1995). Selective impairments in managerial knowledge in patients with pre-frontal cortex lesions. *Cortex* **31**: 301–16.

Sommerville, J. and A. L. Woodward (2005a). Pulling out the intentional structure of action: the relation between action processing and action production in infancy. *Cognition* 95: 1–30.

Sommerville, J. A. and A. L. Woodward (2005b). Infants' sensitivity to the causal features of means–end support sequences in action and perception. *Infancy* **8**: 119–45.

Suri, R. E., J. Bargas, and M. A. Arbib (2001). Modeling functions of striatal dopamine modulation in learning and planning. *Neurosci.* **103**: 65–85.

Sutton, R. S. and A. G. Barto (1990). Time-derivative models of Pavlovian reinforcement. In *Learning and Computational Neuroscience: Foundations of Adaptive, Networks*, ed. M. Gabriel and J. Moore. Cambridge, MA: MIT Press, pp. 497–537.

Sutton, R. S. and A. G. Barto (1998). *Reinforcement Learning: An Introduction*. Cambridge, MA: MIT Press.

Sutton, R. S., D. Precup, and S. Singh (1999). Between MDPs and semi-MDPs: a framework for temporal abstraction in reinforcement learning. *Artif. Intell.* **112**: 181–211.

Tenenbaum, J. B. and R. R. Saxe, eds (2006). *Bayesian Models of Action Understanding*. Cambridge, MA: MIT Press.

Thrun, S. B. and A. Scwhartz (1995). Finding structure in reinforcement learning. In *Advances in Neural Information Processing Systems: Proceedings of the 1994 Conference*, ed. G. Tesauro, D. S. Touretzky, and T. Leen. Cambridge, MA: MIT Press, pp. 385–92.

Wallis, J. D., K. C. Anderson, and E. K. Miller (2001). Single neurons in prefrontal cortex encode abstract rules. *Nature* **411**: 953–6.

Wallis, J. D. and E. K. Miller (2003). From rule to response: neuronal processes in the premotor and prefrontal cortex. *J. Neurophysiol.* **90**: 1790–806.

Ward, G. and A. Allport (1997). Planning and problem-solving using the five-disc Tower of London task. *Q. J. Exp. Psychol.* **50**A: 59–78.

White, I. M. (1999). Rule-dependent neuronal activity in the prefrontal cortex. *Exp. Brain Res.* **126**: 315–35.

White, R. W. (1959). Motivation reconsidered: the concept of competence. *Psychol. Rev.* **66**: 297–333.

Wickens, J., R. Kotter, and J. C. Houk (1995). Cellular models of reinforcement. In *Models of Information Processing in the Basal Ganglia*, ed. J. L. Davis and D. G. Beiser. Cambridge, MA: MIT Press, pp. 187–214.

Wolpert, D. and J. Flanagan (2001). Motor prediction. *Curr. Biol.* **18**: R729–R732.

Wood, J. N. and J. Grafman (2003). Human prefrontal cortex: processing and representational perspectives. *Nature Rev. Neurosci.* **4**: 139–47.

Woodward, A. L., Sommerville, J. A., and Guajardo, J. J. (2001). How infants make sense of intentional action. In B. F. Malle and L. J. Moses and D. A. Baldwin (eds.), *Intentions and Intentionality: Foundations of Social Cognition*. Cambridge, MA: MIT Press, pp. 149–70.

Yamada, S. and S. Tsuji (1989). Selective learning of macro-operators with perfect causality. Paper presented at the IJCAI-89, Detroit, MI.

Yan, Z. and K. Fischer (2002). Always under construction: dynamic variations in adult cognitive microdevelopment. *Hum. Dev.* **45**: 141–60.

Zacks, J. M., T. S. Braver, M. A. Sheridan, *et al.* (2001). Human brain activity time-locked to perceptual event boundaries. *Nature Neurosci.* **4**: 651–5.

Zacks, J. M., N. K. Speer, K. M. Swallow, T. S. Braver, and J. R. Reynolds (2007). Event perception: a mind/brain perspective. *Psychol.Bull.* **133**: 273–93.

Zacks, J. M. and B. Tversky (2001). Event structure in perception and conception. *Psychol. Bull.* **127**: 3–21.

Zalla, T., P. Pradat-Diehl, and A. Sirigu (2003). Perception of action boundaries in patients with frontal lobe damage. *Neuropsychologia* **41**: 1619–27.

Zhou, W. and R. Coggins (2002). Computational models of the amygdala and the orbitofrontal cortex: a hierarchical reinforcement learning system for robotic control. In *Lecture Notes AI: LNAI 2557*, ed. R. I. McKay and J. Slaney. Berlin: Springer-Verlag, pp. 419–30.

Zhou, W. and R. Coggins (2004). Biologically inspired reinforcement learning: reward-based decomposition for multi-goal environments. In *Biologically Inspired Approaches to Advanced Information Technology*, ed. A. J. Ijspeert, M. Murata, and N. Wakamiya. Berlin: Springer-Verlag, pp. 80–94.

14 The medial reticular formation: a brainstem substrate for simple action selection?

Mark D. Humphries, Kevin N. Gurney, and Tony J. Prescott

Summary

The search for the neural substrate of vertebrate action selection has focused on structures in the fore- and mid-brain, particularly on the basal ganglia. Yet, the behavioural repertoire of decerebrate and neonatal animals suggests the existence of a relatively self-contained neural substrate for action selection in the brainstem. We propose that the medial reticular formation (mRF) is this substrate's main component, reviewing evidence that the mRF's inputs, outputs, and intrinsic organisation are consistent with the requirements of an action selection system. We argue that the internal architecture of the mRF is composed of interconnected neuron clusters; our quantitative model of this anatomy suggests the mRF's intrinsic circuitry constitutes a small-world network, and may have evolved to reduce axonal wiring. We use computational models to enumerate and illustrate potential configurations of action representation within the internal circuitry of the mRF. We show that each cluster's output could represent activation of an action component; thus, co-activation of a set of these clusters would lead to the coordinated behavioural response observed in the animal. New results are presented that provide evidence for an alternative scheme: inputs to the mRF are organised to contact clusters, but recruit a pattern of reticulo-spinal neurons from across clusters to generate an action. We propose that this reconciles the anatomical structure with behavioural data showing action sequencing is degraded, rather than individual actions lost, as the mRF is progressively lesioned. Finally, we consider the potential integration of the basal ganglia and mRF substrates for selection and suggest they may collectively form a layered/hierarchical control system.

14.1 Introduction

All animals must continuously sequence and coordinate behaviours appropriate to both their context and current internal state if they are to survive. It is natural to wonder what parts of the nervous system – the neural substrate – evolved to carry out this action selection process. For simpler animals, like the nematode worm *Caenorhabditis elegans*

Modelling Natural Action Selection, eds. Anil K. Seth, Tony J. Prescott and Joanna J. Bryson.
Published by Cambridge University Press. © Cambridge University Press 2012.

and the leech, a circumscribed behavioural repertoire is handled by specialist neurons that direct motor responses to specific stimuli (de Bono and Maricq, 2005; Kristan *et al.*, 2005; Stephens *et al.*, 2008).[1] The sensory apparatus and motor behaviours are largely a product of these animals' ecological niche, and hence so too is the neural network that handles the action selection process.

By contrast, vertebrates (particularly mammals) have a behavourial repertoire that is both extensible (by learning new action–outcome pairings) and flexible (by applying existing actions to new contexts). The evolution of this broader scope for behaviour seems related to the evolution of a central nervous system, the coalescing of all neural circuits into a single 'brain' and the appearance of many 'inter-neurons' between the primary sensory and motor neurons. Complexity of behaviour alone does not and cannot prove complexity of the underlying generating circuitry (Braitenberg, 1984), but flexibility and extensibility seem to require something interposed between sense and action.

The elaboration of the vertebrate nervous system has led to multiple, partially segregated neural systems that lie interposed between primary sensory and motor circuits. Each of the elaborated sensory, homeostatic, memory, planning, and emotion neural systems could in principle guide behaviour; yet each is essentially competing for access to a single final common motor pathway (Sperry, 1952) formed by the motor neurons of the spinal cord and cranial nerve nuclei. It has thus been proposed that the vertebrate brain has co-evolved (or co-opted) specialised and centralised neural systems for action selection (Prescott, 2007; Prescott *et al.*, 1999; Redgrave *et al.*, 1999), to handle both the competition between systems accessing the final motor pathway and the open-ended nature of a flexible, extensible behavioural repertoire.

The basal ganglia have been central to recent proposals for the neural substrate of the vertebrate action selection system (see, for example, Doya, 1999; Graybiel, 1995; Grillner *et al.*, 2005; Kropotov and Etlinger, 1999; Mink and Thach, 1993; Redgrave *et al.*, 1999; Rubchinsky *et al.*, 2003; and chapters in this volume). This collection of nuclei in the fore- and mid-brain are intimately involved in motor control: damage to the basal ganglia causes a wide variety of disorders with motor symptoms, such as Parkinson's disease (Zigmond and Burke, 2002). Moreover, in keeping with the hypothesis of evolved specialised action selection structures, they have been identified in all mammal species, homologous structures exist in the other amniotes (birds and reptiles), and the basic circuitry is conserved over all jawed vertebrates (Reiner *et al.*, 1998).

We have previously argued that, of all the structures of the vertebrate brain, the basal ganglia have the necessary inputs, outputs, and internal connectivity to function as the central switch of an action selection system (Prescott *et al.*, 1999; Redgrave *et al.*, 1999). Computational modelling of the intrinsic basal ganglia circuitry has demonstrated that

---

[1] That is not to say their behaviours are reducible to simple sensory-motor reflexes. The locomotive behaviour of *C. elegans* after the detection of food depends on how well fed they are (de Bono and Maricq, 2005): the internal milieu plays a role even with a brain of just 302 neurons. Even the idea of a stereotyped sensory-motor reflex in small-scale animals may be particularly misleading. They often display a stochastic motion response to repeated stimuli that stands in contrast to the highly repeatable movements of vertebrates.

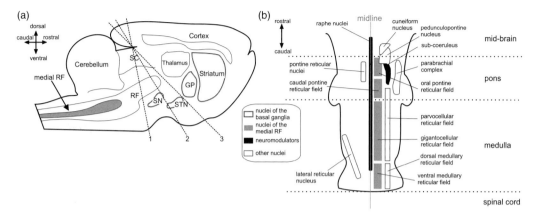

Figure 14.1 Anatomical locations of the putative action selection systems. (a) The relative locations of major nuclei and structures including the basal ganglia and the medial reticular formation (RF) shown on a cartoon sagittal section of rat brain. The dashed lines show the location of the three most-common decerebration lines – all the brain rostral to the line is removed, leaving hindbrain and spinal cord intact. GP: globus pallidus. SN: substantia nigra. STN: subthalamic nucleus. SC: superior colliculus. (b) Principal reticular formation fields, and associated nuclei in a schematic horizontal section from spinal cord to decerebration line 1 in (a). The raphe nuclei sit either side of the midline, and the other nuclei and fields are distributed symmetrically about the midline – the main fields and nuclei are illustrated to the right of the midline, those on the left are found beneath those on the right. The main components of the putative brainstem action selection system are in the medial RF. We retain names of major regions from Paxinos and Watson (1998) for consistency, but rename as 'fields' rather than 'nuclei' to reflect the lack of strong criteria for subdivisions (and extend the names to cover all cells in the medial RF at that anterior-posterior level).

it is capable of resolving competition between action-representing signals such that the basal ganglia output expresses the selection of the most appropriate action(s) and suppresses the others (Gurney *et al.*, 2001a, b; Humphries *et al.*, 2006b). At the same time, we readily acknowledge that the basal ganglia do not form the complete vertebrate action selection system (Prescott, 2007; Prescott *et al.*, 1999; Redgrave *et al.*, 1999).

The basal ganglia cannot be directly involved in all forms of action selection. Decerebrate animals and altricial (helpless at birth) neonates do not have fully intact basal ganglia, but are capable of expressing spontaneous behaviours and coordinated and appropriate responses to stimuli. During decerebration the entire brain anterior to the superior colliculus is removed, leaving only the hindbrain intact (Figure 14.1a). Yet the chronic decerebrate rat can, for example, spontaneously locomote, orient correctly to sounds, groom, perform coordinated feeding actions, and discriminate food types (Berntson and Micco, 1976; Berridge, 1989; Lovick, 1972; Woods, 1964). Such animals clearly have some form of intact system for simple action selection that both enables them to respond to stimuli with appropriate actions (more complex than simple spinal-level reflexes), and enables them to sequence behaviours – as demonstrated by the orienting, grasping (with jaw), and chewing initiated by placing food within their whiskers.

Even in intact animals, basal ganglia outputs do not directly control all the hindbrain and midbrain circuits that underpin these behaviours. Instead, these circuits may be controlled by parallel systems for action selection in other contexts (Swanson, 2000; Zahm, 2006). In particular, Holstege has championed the idea of the 'emotional motor system' that coordinates somatic and autonomic responses to valent stimuli, centred on the midbrain periacqueductal gray and the inputs it receives from the central amygdala and lateral hypothalamus (Holstege, 1995). It seems then that a neural circuit must both handle the coordination of simpler behaviours, and may arbitrate between multiple parallel brain systems by lying interposed between them and the final common motor pathway (Zahm, 2006).

Is there then a brainstem substrate for action selection? Such a substrate should have the necessary properties of a system specialised for action selection. We believe these to be the following (Redgrave et al., 1999). First, the system requires inputs that provide information about an animal's internal state and external context. Second, the system requires a method for computing the urgency (or salience) of each available action from the provided information, in some 'common currency' that allows comparison of their relative levels of support. Third, the system must have an internal configuration that allows for both the representation and the resolution of competition between actions. Fourth, the system must have outputs allowing the expression of the selected action. In addition, we may identify the substrate by the effect that manipulations of it have on the performance of actions.

Of the intact structures in the brainstem of both neonatal and decerebrate animals, we proposed that only the medial reticular formation (mRF) fulfils these criteria (Humphries et al., 2007), and is then the most likely substrate of a generalised simple action selection mechanism. This chapter fleshes out our argument that the mRF has the necessary properties of an action selection system. In particular we illustrate modelling of action selection in its numerous forms: conceptual models of brain function form the overarching theme; quantitative models of anatomy let us constrain the possible computations and representational forms supported by the neural system; quantitative models of dynamics let us explore the implications for action selection in the input–output relationships of the neural system.

Historically, we are not the first to note that the mRF may function as some form of selection device. Warren McCulloch and colleagues proposed the mRF was a 'mode selector', which set the global behavioural state of an animal – such as escape, feeding, and so on. To demonstrate the plausibility of their proposal, they created one of the first computational neuroscience models, and showed their interpretation of the mRF's structure could perform selection of signals (Kilmer et al., 1969). However, their emphasis was on the *ascending* projections of the RF, the connections to thalamus and cortex being responsible for setting the overall state of the animal. Our emphasis is on the dominant *descending* projections of the mRF, and the potential they have to directly control motor behaviour.

14.2   Where and what is the mRF?

The reticular formation (RF), broadly defined, is the main central mass of neurons that extend from the border with spinal cord, running through the medulla and pons, and terminating in the mesencephalon, underneath the superior colliculus (optic tectum in non-mammalian vertebrates) – see Figure 14.1. Clearly specifying the constituents of the 'reticular formation' is fraught with problems (Blessing, 1997). In the major reference work on the rat nervous system, Jones (1995) does not attempt a clean definition of the RF's extent or constituents. Rather, in common with other contemporary reviews (Holstege, 1995; Newman, 1995), Jones (1995) emphasises three major columns of cells on the long axis of the RF: a midline-hugging column of serotonergic cells, a large-celled medial column, and a smaller-celled lateral column (Figure 14.1b). The difficulties principally revolve around two problems: what constitutes a continuation of the lateral column, rather than a discretely identifiable nucleus; and the subdivisions of the medial column along all three axes of the brain.

Our interest here is with the medial column of larger neurons, and thus we may side-step the first problem to some extent. The second problem requires some resolution. The rat brain atlas of Paxinos and Watson (1998) labels subdivisions of the medial column as 'nuclei', and a rather large number of them. Jones (1995) softens this stance and calls them 'fields' to reflect the lack of strong criteria for demarcating the cell groups. Blessing (1997) takes this further: using the 'paragigantocellular' field as an example, he argues that on no grounds – cytoarchitecture, neurochemistry, or projections – can each 'field' or 'nucleus' be clearly dissociated from the tissue surrounding it. Indeed, Blessing (1997) is strongly critical of the whole concept of a 'reticular formation' and the loaded nature of that label: literally 'net-like', it conjures an impression of impenetrability and a mass of cells that respond as one – an impression embraced by earlier authorities on the RF (Scheibel and Scheibel, 1967).

We have sympathy with Blessing's position, and are not keen to add to the proliferation of names; at the same time we agree with Jones that, if we are to distinguish any subdivisions of the medial column, then the term 'field' is better than 'nucleus' to signify the continuity of the structures. We see no compelling reason to distinguish the multiple fields of the medial RF in the dorsal-ventral or medial-lateral axes. For our purposes the medial RF column is all the cells with bifurcating anterior–posterior axons that reach the spinal cord, and all the other cells interspersed among them. These run in parallel with the lateral RF column through the medulla and pons, up to the caudal/oral pons border. Along the anterior–posterior axis, there appear to be some minor distinctions within the medial column: the 'giant cells' appear part-way through the medulla, there is a cell-body light gap at the medulla–pons transition, and large cells disappear in the oral pons (Jones, 1995; Newman, 1985). Whether these distinctions correspond to anything other than anatomical variation is not clear.

Our choice is consistent with the RF of simpler vertebrates. In the lamprey, possibly the simplest extant vertebrate, four regions of the RF contain all spinally projecting neurons, and these form a medial column arranged along the anterior–posterior axis (Dubuc *et al.*, 2008). The lamprey is in many respects the epitome of our argument that the mRF forms a critical part of specialised action selection circuits. Like all vertebrates, the lamprey brain has the three primary divisions into hindbrain, midbrain, and forebrain, with homologues for many major regions of mammalian brains, including the basal ganglia. Yet, as the origin of around 90% of all axons reaching the spinal cord, the lamprey mRF is truly the final arbiter for access to the final common motor pathway.

14.3   Manipulations of mRF alter actions

An intact mRF is trivially necessary for action selection in the sense that lesions to specific parts of it cause coma and even death in humans (Parvizi and Damasio, 2003). Substantial cytoskeletal lesions have also been found in the mRF of Parkinson's disease patients (Braak *et al.*, 2000). Thus, like the basal ganglia, damage to the mRF may make a significant contribution to the symptomatic motor deficits of this disease.

Early studies showed that stimulation of the RF resulted in motor responses (Magoun and Rhines, 1946). Electrical stimulation of specific mRF regions can elicit locomotion in both mammals and lamprey (Deliagina *et al.*, 2002; Kinjo *et al.*, 1990; Whelan, 1996). Neurons within other regions of the mammalian mRF are critical for the maintenance of posture (Mori, 1987), the control of feeding behaviours (Lund *et al.*, 1998), and the generation of eye movements (Moschovakis *et al.*, 1996). In a comprehensive review, Siegel (1979) found multiple competencies were attributed to the mRF because its neural activity correlated with a wide range of responses to stimuli and with naturally occurring behaviours. He concluded that the only way to reconcile these conflicting data was to assume that mRF neuron activity controlled the specific muscle groups required to perform the behaviour or response being tested.

These studies are all consistent with Kuypers' classical concept of distinct lateral and medial descending motor control systems (Kuypers, 1964). Drawing together neuroanatomical and lesion studies, he proposed that the cortical-spinal and rubro-spinal tracts, terminating in the lateral spinal cord, were primarily responsible for skilled movements requiring the distal musculature, and that the reticulo-spinal tract, terminating in the medial spinal cord, was primarily responsible for gross movements requiring the proximal (or axial) musculature. Lesions of the medial system do not affect skilled movement, but do impair motor performance; conversely, lesions of the lateral system (or decortication) partially impair skilled movement, but do not impair overall motor performance (Iwaniuk and Whishaw, 2000). The behavioural repertoire of the decerebrate animal and the lamprey are thus both consistent with them only having Kuypers' medial system intact.

14.4   Inputs to the mRF

A substrate for action selection should have access to all the information necessary to compute an appropriate subsequent action. Numerous studies have demonstrated mRF neurons responding to a wide variety of stimuli, and many respond to multiple sensory modalities (Scheibel, 1984; Siegel, 1979). Classically, the small neurons in the lateral brainstem – the parvicellular area – were thought to relay sensory input to the medial brainstem (Scheibel and Scheibel, 1967). However, neurons in the parvicellular area receive input from a limited range of sensory sources (Shammah-Lagnado *et al.*, 1992), and many sensory systems provide primary or secondary afferents directly to the mRF.

The mRF receives input from each of the body's sensory, pain, vestibular (balance), visceral (organs), proprioceptive (muscle and joint), cardiovascular, and respiratory systems. Many of these have been demonstrated anatomically. Direct inputs have been traced from secondary nuclei in the whisker (Kleinfeld *et al.*, 1999), auditory (Cant and Benson, 2003), and vestibular systems (Yates and Stocker, 1998). The proprioceptive information carried by the ascending dorsal column is directly relayed to the mRF via collaterals from the gracile and cuneate nuclei (Salibi *et al.*, 1980). And the spino-reticular tract and collaterals from the spinothalamic tract, the primary routes for pain signals to the brain, are a major source of fibres reaching the mRF (Fields and Basbaum, 1978).

These anatomical inputs are consistent with the multi-modal responses recorded from mRF neurons. Individual neurons respond to somatic stimuli (Segundo *et al.*, 1967), and many respond to the stimulation of multiple body locations (Bowsher, 1970; Schulz *et al.*, 1983). A recent study of freely moving rats has shown that a single mRF cell can respond to visual, vestibular, olfactory, auditory, and tactile stimuli (Martin *et al.*, 2007). Remarkably, some presentations evoked sustained activity for seconds after the stimulus was withdrawn.

Such extensive activity may be a direct motor command elicited by the stimulus. Single lamprey reticulo-spinal neurons have a subthreshold response linearly related to the force of mechanical stimulation applied to the head, but supra-threshold stimulation evokes sustained spiking that lasts for several minutes (Prisco *et al.*, 2000). Sustained spiking by a set of responsive reticulo-spinal cells initiates locomotion by driving the spinal cord central pattern generators (Dubuc *et al.*, 2008). The somatic stimulation is directly relayed to the reticulo-spinal cells by the dorsal trigeminal nerve (Prisco *et al.*, 2000), showing that mRF cells can translate saliency of sensory information directly into motor activity.

Internal state changes also activate mRF neurons. Experimental manipulations of the cardiovascular (blood pressure and cardiac rhythm) and respiratory (rhythm, lung inflation and deflation) systems all activated mRF neurons (Langhorst *et al.*, 1983). Again, many of the recorded neurons showed responses to manipulations of both systems. Moreover, a combined study showed many mRF neurons respond to stimulation of multiple somatic regions and to manipulation of both cardiovascular and respiratory systems (Langhorst *et al.*, 1996). Thus, it seems the mRF has access to all information made available by an animal's external and internal sensory and monitoring systems. Moreover, because these inputs converge on single neurons, they are in a position to extract correlated input, providing a basis for the computation of an action's salience.

14.5   Outputs of the mRF

A substrate for action selection should also be able to express the outcome of the selection competition. The majority of neurons in the mRF project extensively to all levels of the spinal cord and to the cranial nerves (Eccles *et al.*, 1976; Jones, 1995; Torvik and Brodal, 1957). Axons of individual reticulo-spinal neurons can contact multiple spinal levels on both sides of the spinal cord (Peterson, 1979). Recent studies have shown the majority of reticulo-spinal neurons synapse on spinal inter-neurons (Matsuyama *et al.*, 2004). The anatomy of the mRF's output is thus consistent with the ability to control the axial musculature (trunk, limbs, neck) and the face.

Reticulo-spinal neurons have direct control over the activity of central pattern generators (CPGs) located in the spinal cord (Matsuyama *et al.*, 2004) and the brainstem (Lund *et al.*, 1998). The control of lamprey locomotion and posture is particularly well established. CPGs located in each spinal segment burst fire on alternate sides to contract the muscle fibres on each side of the body, with each CPG bursting in an overlapping sequence along the spinal cord, causing the undulating wave of motion that propels the lamprey (Grillner *et al.*, 1995). Swimming initiated by any stimulus is preceded by bilateral activity of reticulo-spinal cells, and total activity correlates with locomotion intensity (Deliagina *et al.*, 2000). (Similarly, though the details remain poorly worked out, Noga *et al.*, 2003, have provided evidence that mRF reticulo-spinal neurons directly drive the putative mammalian locomotion CPG). Asymmetry in the left–right mRF activity levels encodes turning towards the side with the greatest activity (Deliagina *et al.*, 2000).

Changes in lamprey posture occur either on its long axis (tilt) or around the long axis (roll). Rolling to one side causes activity in a group of mRF cells on the opposite side that returns the lamprey to dorsal side up, with the maximum number of active cells corresponding to the maximum displacement from vertical (90° of roll). Tilting is corrected by two bilateral groups of mRF cells, one firing to correct for upward tilt, the other to correct downward tilt; both have maximum activity at maximum displacement from horizontal (Deliagina *et al.*, 2002).

Individual lamprey reticulo-spinal cells, like their mammalian counterparts, project to different combinations of spinal neuron classes. This in turn correlates with the wide variety of spinal interneuron activity patterns elicited by stimulation of single reticulo-spinal cells (Dubuc *et al.*, 2008). Yet each reticulo-spinal cell has the same effect on each spinal segment it projects to (Deliagina *et al.*, 2002). Thus, there is evidence not only that individual mRF neurons contact structures able to directly express action, but also that their activity levels may encode the degree of behavioural activation, and that asymmetry in their activation encodes both movements and postural changes.

14.6 Internal circuitry of the mRF

The effects of manipulations of the mRF on behaviour and its external connectivity together make a compelling case for the involvement of the mRF in action selection. Demonstrating that it is able to represent and resolve action competitions is impeded by the lack of a clear picture of its internal anatomy. We describe here our recent work to solve this problem.

14.6.1   Known anatomy of the mRF

Classic Golgi staining work by the Schiebels (Scheibel and Scheibel, 1958, 1967) showed the existence of giant-bodied neurons with bifurcating axons and disc-like radial dendritic trees. They proposed that the giant neurons were arranged along the rostro-caudal axis like 'a stack of poker-chips'. Others have repeatedly described similar cells using a variety of staining techniques (see e.g., Bowsher and Westman, 1971; Newman, 1985; Ramon-Moliner and Nauta, 1966; Valverde, 1961). However, little work had been done to integrate more recent anatomical studies of the RF into a coherent picture of its internal structure. Therefore, we conducted an extensive literature review, leading us to propose the following structural organisation (Humphries *et al.*, 2006a).

We identified two main neuron classes. The *projection* neurons extend a bifurcating axon, predominantly sending the major branch caudally to the spinal cord and the minor branch rostrally toward the midbrain (the giant neuron of the Scheibels' Golgi studies belongs to this class). They make excitatory contacts on their targets, mostly via collaterals regularly branching from the main axon. Typically medium-to-giant in size, projection neurons have a characteristic radial dendritic field extending in the coronal (vertical, medio-lateral) plane but limited in the rostro-caudal axis. The dendrites thus seem positioned to sample from the multiple fibre tracts traversing the RF along the rostro-caudal axis, carrying the axons of many spinal, cortical, and sensory systems. Figure 14.2a shows the spatial relationships between these tracts, and the projection neurons' dendritic fields and axon trajectories. The *inter-neurons* project their axon almost entirely within the RF, predominantly along the medio-lateral axis, and make inhibitory contacts with their targets. There is good functional evidence for localised intra-mRF inhibition (Holmes *et al.*, 1994; Iwakiri *et al.*, 1995).

We proposed that mRF neurons are arranged into a series of stacked *clusters* (Figure 14.2b), each comprising a mix of projection and inter-neurons, and each delimited by the initial collateral from the projection neurons' axons – which occurs roughly 100 μm from the initial bifurcation. In other words, a cluster's rostral and caudal borders are defined by the first collateral in those directions from the projection neurons' axons. Thus, the inter-neurons project only within the cluster, and the projection neurons only contact neurons outside the cluster. This cluster structure is replicated on both sides of the midline (on both sides of the raphe nuclei in Figure 14.1b).

14.6.2   An anatomical model of the mRF

In Humphries *et al.* (2006a) we specified a *stochastic* model that generated a network with the proposed cluster organisation. Six parameters completely describe the network's structure. Two parameters determine the size of the network: each of the N_c clusters has n neurons (the total number of neurons is thus $T = N_c \times n$). One parameter determines the class of neuron: a certain proportion ρ of neurons in each cluster are deemed to be the projection neurons, the remainder are inter-neurons.

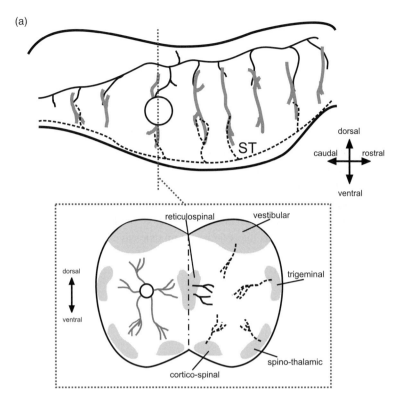

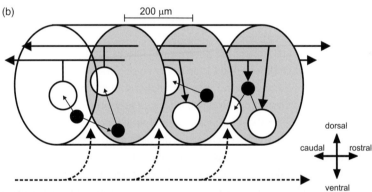

Figure 14.2 Anatomical organisation of the vertebrate medial reticular formation (mRF). (a) Organisation of the fibre tracts and orientations of the projection cells. The cartoon sagittal section of the brainstem shows the dendritic trees (thick grey lines) of the projection neurons (one neuron body shown, open circle) extending throughout the mRF along the dorso-ventral axis but extending little along the rostro-caudal axis. These dendritic trees contact axon collaterals of both passing fibre systems (black dashed line) and far-reaching axons of the projection neurons (the axon of the depicted neuron body is shown by the black solid line); the example fibre system is the spinothalamic tract (ST). A cartoon coronal section through the brainstem illustrates the radial dendritic tree of the projection neurons in this plane, with dendrite branches oriented towards axon collaterals emanating from the passing fibre tracts (grey regions). (b) The proposed mRF organisation: it comprises stacked clusters (three shown) containing medium-to-large projection neurons (open circles) and small-to-medium inter-neurons (filled circles); cluster limits (grey ovals) are defined by the initial collaterals from the projection neuron axons. The projection neurons' radial dendritic fields allow sampling of ascending and descending input from both other clusters (solid black lines) and passing fibre systems (dashed black line). The inter-neurons project within their parent cluster.

The other three parameters describe the connectivity and thus define the links between the neurons. The probability of each projection neuron contacting a given cluster is $P(c)$. This models the probability of the projection neuron's axon extending a collateral into that cluster. If a collateral is extended, then $P(p)$ is the probability of the projection neuron forming a connection with any given neuron in that cluster. Finally, $P(l)$ denotes the probability of an inter-neuron forming a connection with any other given neuron in its own cluster. We also proposed an alternative generating model for the cluster structure, based on the stochastic model, in which the neurons were wired together by a procedure analogous to the neural development process (Humphries *et al.*, 2006a); we refer to them collectively as the anatomical model.

14.6.3   Structural properties of the mRF

Quantifying anatomy in this way generates useful, and often surprising, insights of its own accord, as well as providing a sound basis for exploring dynamics of the neural system. First, just by specifying a set of parameters sufficient to describe its structure we can identify missing data. Estimates for the number of clusters N_c, number of neurons per cluster n, the proportion of projection neurons ρ, and the probability of contacting a cluster $P(c)$ could be determined from available anatomical data (Humphries *et al.*, 2006a). The synaptic connection parameters $P(p)$ and $P(l)$, on the other hand, do not have supporting values in the literature, and thus these were free parameters of the mRF anatomical model.

Studying the model across the parameters' ranges then informs us of the range of topologically distinct classes that the anatomy could fall in to. And having identified the possible classes, we can examine why the anatomy may have evolved to this state. We found that, to the extent it captures the mRF's organisation (and for all realistic values of the parameters given above), the anatomical model predicts the mRF is likely to be a *small-world*, but not *scale-free*, network at the individual neuron level (Humphries *et al.*, 2006a). A small-world network has two defining properties: its nodes are more clustered – more locally inter-connected – than would be expected if the same number of total links were made at random; its nodes are also linked by shorter paths than would be expected if the same number of total links were made uniformly. Small-worlds have been found in many real-world networks, including connections between airports, electricity grids, and food webs, suggesting that some general organisational principle is at work (see Albert and Barabasi, 2002, for review).

Why then is the mRF a small-world network? What functional advantages does it bestow? The structural properties of a small-world network imply certain dynamic properties – of rapid cross-network synchronisation, consistent stabilisation, and persistent activity – that may all be critical to the representation and resolution of competition between actions (briefly reviewed in Humphries *et al.*, 2006a). However, the presence of a small-world may also imply structural constraints. For example Mathias and Gopal (2001) demonstrated that, in a one-dimensional ring of nodes, small-world networks were formed when attempting to the find the optimal trade-off between total wire length and shortest path length.

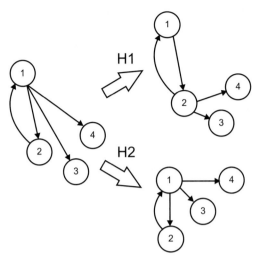

Figure 14.3 Two hypotheses of wiring efficiency. The total wiring length of a network (left) can be reduced in two ways. Hypothesis 1 (H1): if the node placement is crucial – due, say, to the position of the inputs to the network – then the wiring length may be minimised (for the same number of links) by moving the links while ensuring each node remains connected. Hypothesis 2 (H2): if the network configuration is crucial, then the wiring length may be minimised by moving the nodes while maintaining the links.

Could the cluster structure have thus evolved to optimise neural connectivity? Other neural structures appear to have optimised component placement to minimise total wiring length (Cherniak, 1994). This may be a priority of neural design, as it reduces energy usage during creation and maintenance of axons, and signal propagation along them (Laughlin and Sejnowski, 2003). We therefore asked if the cluster structure could reduce total axonal wire-length, testing the two hypotheses illustrated in Figure 14.3. First, the cluster structure could reduce the wiring connecting together neurons fixed in particular positions: that is, the neuron placement is critical, for example due to the position of input fibres, and the wiring is arbitrary to some extent. Second, the cluster structure could reduce the length of wiring required to achieve a particular network configuration: that is, the internal wiring is critical and the neuron position is arbitrary to some extent. The second hypothesis is akin to the problem of component placement optimisation (Cherniak, 1994).

A set of cluster model networks was generated by varying the synaptic connection probabilities over their plausible ranges. Each neuron was assigned a three-dimensional position within the estimated volume of its anatomical cluster. The total axonal wire length was then computed by calculating the Euclidean distance between each pair of connected neurons and summing over all pairs. For each generated cluster model network, two random networks were created to test each of the two hypotheses: first, a *randomly wired* network, to test if total wire length for the clustered neurons was less than for the randomly wired neurons; second, a *randomly positioned* network (ignoring cluster boundaries), to test if total wire length for the clustered neurons was less than for randomly positioned neurons.

We found that total wire length for the cluster structure was greater than that of the corresponding randomly wired network, but less than that of the corresponding randomly positioned network, for every generated cluster model network (Humphries *et al.*, 2007). Therefore, we concluded that the cluster structure of the mRF does not specifically reduce axonal wire length for a given neuron placement (first hypothesis), but wiring length is comparatively reduced for a given wiring configuration (second hypothesis), and thus may explain why the cluster structure has evolved.

14.7   Action representation in the mRF

Having examined both the structure of the mRF and possible reasons for the structure's existence, we turn now to the question of how that structure supports the representation and resolution of competition between actions. We begin by reviewing existing ideas on the functional organisation of the mRF.

14.7.1   Functional organisation of mRF

Many researchers have seen no functional organisation in the mRF. Early studies report stimulation of the RF resulting in either postural inhibition via descending projections to the spinal cord (Magoun and Rhines, 1946), or desynchronisation of the cortical EEG via ascending projections (Moruzzi and Magoun, 1949). This latter result famously gave rise to the concept of the ascending reticular activating system.[2] These results, along with the wide array of overlapping sensory inputs to the mRF that lack a demonstrable organisation (Segundo *et al.*, 1967), led some researchers to assert that mRF output was only a function of general sensory arousal (Hobson and Scheibel, 1980; Scheibel and Scheibel, 1967).

Though still widely discussed, the division of the RF into just two systems (ascending, facilitatory and descending, inhibitory) was refuted soon after by Sprague and Chambers (1954). By applying micro-stimulation at or near threshold to mRF neurons of awake animals, they were able to elicit a multitude of single and multiple limb movements. They saw little of the reported postural inhibition. More recent micro-stimulation studies of the mRF in the medulla have demonstrated both multiple movement and multiple muscle responses following the injection of short trains of low-amplitude current pulses (Drew and Rossignol, 1990). (The same micro-stimulation applied to the lateral medullary RF did not consistently result in movement, further evidence that the mRF is the substrate of action selection in the brainstem.) Neurons of the mRF thus have functionally specialised rather than general outputs.

How then might the mRF neurons be functionally organised? They are not topographically organised to match patterns of sensory input. No topographical projections to the mRF have ever been convincingly demonstrated, despite numerous attempts to

---

[2] As noted by Blessing (1997), this concept has been particularly difficult to remove from the EEG literature and neurobehavioural textbooks, despite its vagueness. The location and strength of stimulation applied by Moruzzi and Magoun (1949) would have activated a large range of disparate structures and fibres of passage, thus in no sense is there some identifiable 'activating system' located in the upper RF.

find them (Bowsher, 1970; Eccles *et al.*, 1976; Segundo *et al.*, 1967). Groves *et al.* (1973) reported that tactile stimuli were encoded in rough somatotopic form in the RF, but the methods used could not distinguish between recording from neuron bodies and from passing fibres, and their recording sites covered the whole coronal extent of the brainstem (Angel, 1977). On the output side, Peterson (1979) proposed a crude anterior–posterior topography of the reticulo-spinal projections, based on the combinations of elicited responses in motor neurons related to the neck, back, forelimb, and hindlimb. However, other studies of this system found no anatomical topography of the spinal projections (Eccles *et al.*, 1976; Torvik and Brodal, 1957), and neurons responding during movement of those body parts seem randomly inter-mingled (Siegel and Tomaszewski, 1983).

Beyond the work just detailed, there is little direct evidence on the functional organisation of the mRF. Rather, we can infer some potential forms of organisation from combining electrophysiology and anatomical data. We have thus explored the potential methods of representing and resolving action selection through simulation of new computational models. Given the paucity of guiding data, we cannot reach any firm conclusions here. Nonetheless, constructing and simulating computational models allows us to enumerate and illustrate the potential forms of action selection supported by the mRF.

14.7.2   Action selection at the cluster level

We could hypothesise that clusters in the mRF are functionally as well as anatomically distinct and are, therefore, the representational unit in the brainstem action selection system (Humphries *et al.*, 2007). Then the regions of cranial nerve nuclei and the spinal cord targeted by a cluster's projection neurons express the action selected by the mRF system. A variety of evidence supports this hypothesis.

Sensory input to the mRF may be arranged on a cluster basis. Neighbouring mRF neurons have overlapping somatic sensory fields, but distal pairs do not (Schulz *et al.*, 1983), and individual mRF neurons respond to multiple modalities (Martin *et al.*, 2007). Neighbouring pairs of mRF neurons have correlated activity in both awake (Siegel *et al.*, 1981) and anaesthetised (Schulz *et al.*, 1985) animals. In both studies, all neuron pairs separated by more than 200 μm showed no correlations. Many projection neurons have correlated activity with multiple movements, and the activity of near-neighbour projection neurons often does not correlate with the same movement or set of movements (Siegel and Tomaszewski, 1983). There is thus evidence for neighbouring neurons having common activity patterns, and that those shared patterns are on the scale of single anatomical clusters. The correlated activity between near-neighbour projection neurons in waking animals (Siegel *et al.*, 1981) would lead to the simultaneous recruitment of multiple muscle groups and movement types. We therefore proposed that sufficient activation of a cluster's projection neurons would lead to a coordinated behavioural response (Humphries *et al.*, 2007).

There is evidence for intra-mRF localisation of actions and competition between them. Stimulation of a medial pons region inhibits locomotion elicited from medial medulla (Iwakiri *et al.*, 1995). GABA antagonists injected into this medulla mRF region initiate locomotion (Kinjo *et al.*, 1990), suggesting a local inhibitory circuit is involved.

Separate groups of mRF cells seem to control motor neurons projecting to the trunk and hindlimb muscles (Szokol *et al.*, 2008). We thus used simulations of a population-level model to explore possible action representations and competition resolution, assuming that the cluster itself was the key representational element.

14.7.2.1   Single-action configuration

The output of each cluster could represent a complete action. The maximum number of representable actions is thus just N_c, and grows by 1 with each additional cluster. Action selection in such a circuit requires a winner-takes-all (WTA) competition, to reduce the set of potential actions to just the most appropriate one. To form a WTA-like circuit in a fully connected cluster structure (Figure 14.4b) the projection neuron population of each cluster must receive greater input (i.e., inhibition) from its corresponding inter-neuron population than from the combined input of its inter-cluster connections; otherwise the net effect of any sensory input to the network would be excitatory (in a symmetrical network).

One option for implementing such a WTA-like network is that the inhibitory *intra*-cluster connection from the cluster's inter-neuron population to its projection neuron population is very strong compared to any excitatory *inter*-cluster projections. Thus input from other clusters to both the inter-neuron and projection neuron populations will result in a net inhibitory effect on the projection neuron population. Indeed, synapse counts from projection neuron dendritic trees suggest this may be the case. Roughly 45% of the synapses on a projection neuron are GABAergic (Jones *et al.*, 1991) – and thus inhibitory – and inter-neurons are the primary (perhaps only) source of GABAergic input (Holmes *et al.*, 1994). Yet the proportion of inter-neurons to projection neurons is much smaller than this value. Thus, an inter-neuron input to a projection neuron would have a disproportionately larger effect than a projection neuron input, as it forms more synapses.

Simulation of a population-level model with such an architecture shows that the cluster structure can implement soft selection – that is, simultaneous selection of more than one action. Some thresholding of output would be required to implement hard selection – a true WTA competition – a threshold possibly set by the amount of cluster output required to sufficiently activate target neurons in the cranial nerve nuclei and spinal cord. However, the outputs for this simulation are, roughly, just the ratio of the corresponding inputs, which reduces the mRF architecture to a simple relay system.

Removing the excitatory inter-cluster connections to the projection neurons leaves only the inter-cluster projections to inter-neurons and thus would seem more able to implement a WTA circuit (Figure 14.4c). However, simulation of this altered model shows it does not implement a WTA circuit either: the output of the clusters are little different from their input values. The presence or absence of the long-range connections appears to have little impact on the mRF's ability to act as a selection mechanism if each cluster is assumed to represent a single action.

14.7.2.2   Subaction configuration

The existence of abundant long-range connections between projection neurons is not in doubt, and thus should be accounted for in a functional model of the mRF. It is possible that in the mRF some cluster-to-cluster projections preferentially target the inter-neuron populations, while others preferentially target the projection neuron populations. The output of a single cluster may then simultaneously inhibit some clusters and excite others. Excitation of a target cluster could correspond to recruitment of a compatible, perhaps essential, component of an action. Conversely, inhibition of a target cluster could correspond to the prevention of an incompatible, perhaps dangerous, component of an action. The output of each cluster thus activates a *subaction*, a component part of a coherent behaviour. This has a representational advantage over a single-action representation: the upper limit of potential unique subaction combinations is $2^{N_c} - 1$, and grows by 2^{N_c-1} with each additional cluster.

An example of a subaction configuration in the same three cluster model is shown in Figure 14.4d. In simulation, the outputs of both clusters 1 and 3 exceed the value of their inputs, and both have considerably greater output than cluster 2 (which has a much reduced output compared to its input). Thus, in this configuration, the output pattern is consistent with subactions 1 and 3 being activated, and subaction 2 being suppressed.

Even in this simple example we can see that, while reduced, activity in the 'losing' cluster(s) will rarely disappear completely. How then does this residual activity not affect the command encoded by the most active clusters? There is evidence that spinal cord circuits further clean-up the descending command signals, resulting in clean motor responses. Models have shown that the lamprey spinal locomotion CPG could band-pass filter its inputs from the mRF: the CPG oscillations – and hence swimming – are turned on within a range of mRF activity, but are off if the input is too low or too high (Jung *et al.*, 1996). Conversely, the spinal circuit can amplify small differences in the descending commands: the asymmetry in the bilateral mRF activity encoding turning is a small percentage of the total activity, but the spinal circuits turn this into muscle contraction on only one side of the body (Deliagina *et al.*, 2002). If all potential subaction combinations could be similarly cleaned up by the spinal cord circuit(s), then only the ordering and total activity of the outputs is important.

Having demonstrated that the subaction configuration works in principle, we did a preliminary assessment of its robustness over a range of inputs. The configuration depicted in Figure 14.4d supports just two actions, given that selection is based on the ordering of the output values: one action is clusters 1 and 3 both more active than cluster 2; the other action is cluster 2 more active than the others. We found that subaction selection is robust over a wide range of inputs, with the majority of input combinations to the three clusters resulting in correct selection of either clusters 1 and 3 together, or cluster 2 alone (Humphries *et al.*, 2007). The incorrect selections occurred for input combinations that were either all roughly equal, or when input to cluster 2 was roughly equal with either cluster 1 or 3 (and the other was low). Thus, this simple model of a configuration of the mRF's anatomy lacks a mechanism for resolving selection competitions between closely matched inputs.

14.7.3 Distributed action representation in the mRF

The proposed mapping of clusters to actions (or subactions) is not the only possibility: the anatomical organisation does not necessarily map directly onto a functional organisation. An alternative is suggested by a re-interpretation of the model of Kilmer *et al.* (1969).

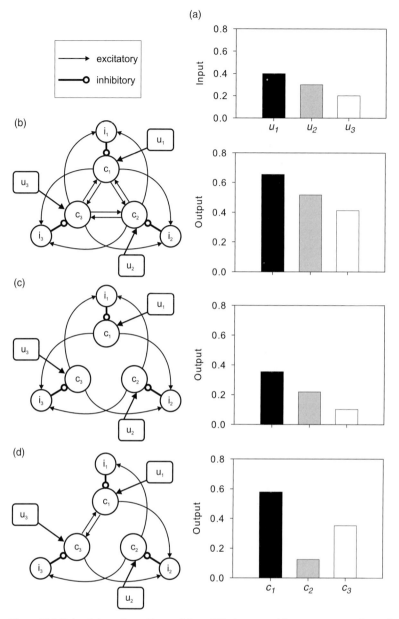

Figure 14.4 Potential configurations of the mRF cluster architecture as an action selection mechanism. (These illustrate connection schemes, not relative physical location.) Each configuration was instantiated as a population-level model and given the input values in (a). Cluster-specific total afferent input (u_n) targets only the cluster's projection neuron population (c_n), whose outputs drive some form of coherent behavioural response to that particular combination of input from sensory, pain, respiratory, and so forth, systems. A cluster's inter-neuron population (i_n) contacts only the projection neuron population. (b) Each cluster's projection neuron population represents a single action. Competition between actions is putatively resolved by a winner-takes-all (WTA) type circuit, formed by stronger relative weighting of the inhibitory within-cluster inter-neuron connections (open circles) than of the excitatory projection neurons connections to other clusters (arrows). However, the simulation outputs show that such a single-action configuration does not act as a winner-takes-all (WTA) circuit, but as an amplified relay of the inputs. (c) With all inter-cluster excitatory connections to projection neurons removed, a traditional WTA circuit seems to be created; yet the

What if the actions are represented by the parallel long axons of the projection neurons, rather than the clustered neuron bodies? That is, a few projection neurons from each (or many) of the clusters contribute their axons to a group which represents a single action (or subaction). The activity transmitted by that axon group to the spinal cord thus recruits the appropriate musculature for the action.

Remarkably, the general structure of the Kilmer *et al.* (1969) model is still consistent with the known organisation of the projection neurons in the mRF. We thus tested this model in embodied form (the original authors' long-held wish) as a controller for a robot in a survival task, to evaluate the possibility of it forming an action selection mechanism (Humphries *et al.*, 2005). We found the model as originally proposed could not sustain action selection, but, by evolving the model with a genetic algorithm, certain configurations could be found that did. Thus, the mRF may also be able to support action selection based on parallel representation of those actions. (However, inevitably, given its age, several aspects of the model were incorrect or implausible, or omitted features known from more modern studies of the mRF; this was in part the impetus for our work reviewed here.)

Some evidence for this scheme has been found in studies of grooming behaviour under progressive decerebration (Berridge, 1989). The brainstem alone is sufficient to generate and sequence all elements of a stereotypical chain of grooming actions. Decerebration cuts placed progressively lower in the brainstem did not delete whole elements of that syntax, as might be predicted by the subaction hypothesis. Rather, as more of the brainstem was lost, the sequencing of the whole chain became degraded, pointing to a widely distributed representation across the whole network.

14.7.4   Reconciling cluster-based and distributed action selection

A distributed representation of actions faces particular problems with generalisation and separation: similar patterns of sensory input should recall similar activity patterns (a loud noise to left should recruit motor commands for left-orienting irrespective of the exact amplitude) and different patterns of sensory input should recall substantially different activity patterns (corresponding to different motor commands).

We show this using a full dynamic version of the anatomical model, in which each neuron, rather than each population as above, is instantiated as a rate-coding unit (model details are given in Appendix A). Figure 14.5a shows that distributed input to the mRF

Figure 14.4 (cont.) simulation outputs show that this does not form a WTA circuit either. Moreover, it does not account for the existence of the long-range axons. (d) Each cluster's projection neuron population represents a subaction. Specific wiring configurations may create a circuit in which the sensory activation of a single cluster recruits other clusters representing compatible (or essential) subactions, via the inter-cluster connections between projection neurons. The combination of subactions then creates the coherent behavioural response observed in the animal. In simulation, the subaction configuration results in appropriate selection for the given inputs: activation of cluster 1 (c^1) results in concurrent recruitment of cluster 3, and inhibition of cluster 2.

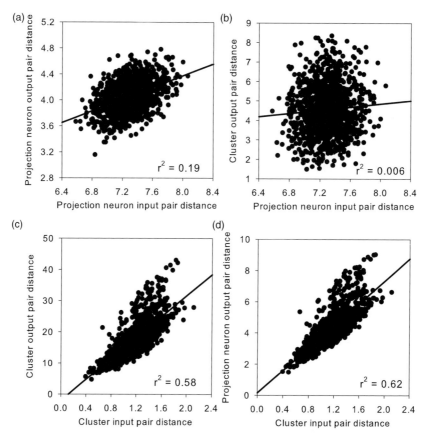

Figure 14.5 The cluster model of the mRF can encode similarity of its cluster inputs only. A full mRF anatomical model was built with eight clusters and 40 projection neurons per cluster, and instantiated as a dynamic model using rate-coding neurons (see Appendix A). We tested the model with randomly generated input vectors, each element taking a value in the interval [0,1]. We provided vectors of input to each projection neuron (panels a, b) or to each cluster (panels c, d) – in this case, all projection neurons in the same cluster received the same input; 50 input patterns were tested for each. At equilibrium, we read out the vector of projection neuron output (panels a, d) or total cluster output (panels b, c). We computed the Euclidean distance between each pair of input vectors and between the corresponding pair of output vectors: the closer the pair, the more similar the vectors. For each input–output combination, this gave $(50 \times 49)/2 = 1225$ unique pairs of input–output similarity, plotted in each panel. A perfect correlation across all pairs would show that relative input similarity was encoded perfectly by relative output similarity. We found that distributing input across all projection neurons resulted in weak correlation between input and output similarity for both (a) projection neuron and (b) total cluster output. Distributed input is thus unable to reliably generalise by recalling either similar cluster or projection neuron output. (c) Cluster input and output show a strong positive correlation of similarity: similar input vectors gave rise to similar output vectors, dissimilar input vectors gave rise to dissimilar output vectors. (d) Similarly, cluster input and projection neuron output show a strong positive correlation of similarity.

does indeed struggle to generalise similar inputs and separate dissimilar inputs, if we read-out neuron output across all the projection neurons. If instead we read-out total activity at the cluster level rather than at the projection neuron level (Figure 14.5b) then we see no correlation between input and output similarity. Restricting inputs to a per-cluster basis, we find total cluster output has strong correlation between input and output similarity (Figure 14.5c) – this, being equivalent to the population-level models explored above, shows that the cluster-level action representation schemes can successfully generalise and separate their input space. More interesting is that, for the same input, the projection neuron output from across the whole mRF shows equally strong correlation between input and output similarity (Figure 14.5d). The model thus suggests a reconciliation of the evidence for cluster-based and distributed representations: anatomically, the clusters are organised to receive common sensory inputs that then recall distributed action representations, and the synchrony of within-cluster cells in the mRF is caused by common sensory input.

Both of our conclusions here – cluster-based inputs increase similarity encoding, projection neuron read-out as good as cluster-based read-out – may not strike the reader as particularly surprising. Switching to a lower-dimensional input space, and driving many neurons with the same input, may inevitably improve the correlation between input and output similarity. But that misses two key insights: first, that input–output similarity is a problem at all; second, that only by studying the anatomical and dynamic models did we find a basis for reducing the input space. Future work will elaborate and further probe this reconciling hypothesis. For example, representational capacity is unknown, and depends on the threshold between 'similar' and 'dissimilar', potentially set by circuits in spinal cord.

14.8   Integration of the action selection systems

The mRF cluster model's inability to resolve competitions between (roughly) equally salient actions suggests the tantalising possibility that more complex action selection systems evolved partly to cope with ambiguous situations – complex systems which could, of course, encompass the basal ganglia. We sketch here how the proposed basal ganglia and mRF action selection mechanisms may interact.

There are three candidate control architectures that could encapsulate the combined action selection system, illustrated in Figure 14.6. First, a strict hierarchy of control, in which decisions made at higher levels limit those of lower levels. This is often taken to imply that lower levels encode more elementary actions than higher levels. The modelling work reported above supports this, and it is consistent with the decomposition of the control of grooming in rats: an intact basal ganglia is necessary to correctly sequence the components of the grooming routine (Berridge and Whishaw, 1992), but each component is encoded entirely within the brainstem (Berridge, 1989). The basal ganglia's primary route to the brainstem is via the pedunculopontine nucleus (PPN), which itself projects heavily into the mRF (Delwaide *et al.*, 2000; Jones, 1990). Some

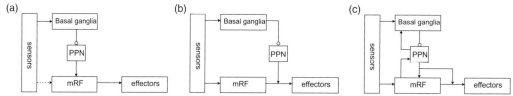

Figure 14.6 Alternative schemes for integrating the action selection substrates. (a) An hierarchical architecture: lower levels represent increasingly simple actions, selected by the higher layers. This is consistent with the output of the basal ganglia reaching the mRF via the pedunculopontine nucleus (PPN), and with the results of our modelling work. (b) A layered architecture: the mRF and basal ganglia form separate layers in a control system dealing with increasingly complex stimuli, the higher layers being able to veto the output of the lower layers. This design is consistent with the separate sensory input to the basal ganglia and mRF, and with the basal ganglia's access to the spinal cord via the PPN. (c) A combined architecture: the competences of each layer contribute to the whole system. This is consistent with the evidence for feedback pathways within the neural systems, particularly between the PPN and the basal ganglia. Arrows: excitatory pathways; open circles: inhibitory pathways.

functional and anatomical data, therefore, support a hierarchical architecture in which the basal ganglia dictates control of the mRF output (Figure 14.6a).

The second alternative is a layered architecture, such as Brooks' subsumption architecture (Brooks, 1991). Increasingly complex computations are supported by higher layers of this architecture and, while all layers compute in parallel, higher layers can veto the output of lower layers. There is considerable evidence that the sensorimotor mappings within the vertebrate brain are organised in this fashion (Prescott *et al.*, 1999). Do basal ganglia and mRF circuits thus run in parallel, with basal ganglia output able to veto mRF if necessary? (Figure 14.6b). The motor effects of Parkinson's disease (Zigmond and Burke, 2002), in which the basal ganglia are jammed in 'off' mode, suggests it is continually vetoing lower layers. In addition, the paradoxical results of Parkinson's disease interventions point to the existence of parallel systems. Following drug treatment with L-DOPA, Parkinsonian patients regain voluntary movement but continue to have problems controlling their axial musculature (Lakke, 1985), which is under the direct control of the mRF. Moreover, surgical interventions often destroy sections of the basal ganglia: the patients' recovery of voluntary movement after surgery (Marsden and Obeso, 1994) thus suggests destruction of the basal ganglia releases other action selection systems to work. Anatomically, this design has potential: the basal ganglia and mRF do receive separate inputs, and the basal ganglia can bypass the mRF and access the spinal cord via the PPN. However, this basal ganglia–PPN–spinal circuit may be limited to postural control only (Takakusaki *et al.*, 2004).

The third alternative is a combined hierarchical/layered system, given the data reviewed above that support each of those elements. In addition, a combined system incorporates some form of heterarchy in the control decomposition, in that lower levels can influence higher levels. Anatomically, the PPN projects extensively into the basal ganglia (Inglis and Winn, 1995), and the mRF may project to PPN (Jones, 1995) – see

Figure 14.6c. There is little research on what these ascending projections may be encoding, though the known properties of the PPN and mRF suggest, respectively, attentional arousal and motor feedback.

14.9   Further questions about the mRF

The current work is intended to move us closer to an understanding of the neural substrate of action selection in the vertebrate brain. Naturally it has opened up many questions, for which we can only hazard answers. Particularly difficult to understand is how the mRF is successfully wired up to turn patterns of sensory input into appropriate motor output. Questions about wiring have three distinct contributions from evolution, development, and plasticity. How did the mRF evolve through the vertebrate lineage? Does the lamprey embody the original locomotion-dominant solution, suitable for water, later adapted for land-based vertebrates and the greater elaboration of cortex? We know, for example, that mammalian mRF projection neurons receive input from the cortico-spinal pathway (Scheibel, 1984), not present in lamprey, and hence there is not a clean separation between the medial and lateral musculature controlling systems (Iwaniuk and Whishaw, 2000).

How does the mRF input and output reach the right targets during development? At birth, rat mRF already contains all the neurons present in the adult. Over the first two post-natal weeks the principal change is a massive growth then reduction in the number of dendritic spines (Hammer et al., 1981), suggesting a rapid phase of axonal wiring then massive pruning. We have already shown that a stochastic over-growth-then-pruning model can generate the proposed adult cluster structure (Humphries et al., 2006a), but this presupposed the presence of cues for axonal growth in the appropriate axes (anterior–posterior for projection neurons; medial–lateral for interneurons), and only addresses the internal structure, not the input–output wiring. A key example of correct wiring is the inputs to ventrolateral medulla, where many projection neurons controlling cardiac and respiratory system muscles are located (Blessing, 1997). Many, but not all, projection neurons from elsewhere in the mRF give off collaterals to this region, presumably to recruit cardio-respiratory changes in synchrony with changes in motor activity; aberrant wiring here would render an animal largely unable to function. Are mRF synapses plastic over the animal's lifetime, beyond initial development? It is often implicitly assumed that all excitatory synapses in the central nervous system are plastic. Plasticity has been indirectly (Breedlove et al., 1979) and directly (Alford et al., 1995) observed at synapses from afferent inputs to projection neurons. Yet, when we consider inputs to the ventrolateral medulla, we again must pause to consider that any such changes would have a direct effect on basic survival.

We looked at the difficulties of successfully wiring up both input–output and internal connectivity by attempting to evolve 'brainstem-only' subaction guided robots on a simple survival task, in which the robot had to gather food in one location and consume it in another (Humphries and Prescott, 2006). Each robot was controlled by a six-cluster population-level model, representing six subactions (four movement, two consumptive), with eight sensory inputs (four external, four internal). A genetic algorithm attempted to maximise the mean energy of the robot through successful coordination of all subactions in appropriate contexts, by evolving the wiring within the mRF model and between the sensory inputs and each cluster. We found that reliable wiring could not be evolved, despite trying many different search variants. The few successful evolved models were not robust, relying on a very high rate of energy return from consumed food, and their emergent behaviour was highly stereotyped. Hence this work nicely demonstrated the sheer complexity of the wiring task faced in the real mRF.

Beyond wiring, we have not touched here on the many potential roles for neuromodulators in the mRF. Receptors have been found for serotonin (Fay and Kubin, 2000; Stevens *et al.*, 1992), noradrenaline (Stevens *et al.*, 1994), and acetylcholine (Stevens *et al.*, 1993). Principal sources of these are, respectively, the brainstem raphe nuclei, subcoeruleus (Jones, 1995), and PPN and adjacent cholinergic cell bands (Jones *et al.*, 1991) – though local cholinergic cells within mRF are also numerous (Jones, 1990; Holmes *et al.*, 1994). Given the wide variety of roles ascribed to neuromodulators in the brain (Krichmar, 2008), any speculation here would be purely idle: serotonin, for example, is particularly strongly implicated in regulating activity of CPGs for whisking Hattox *et al.* (2003) and locomotion (Jordan *et al.*, 2008); acetylcholine plays a role in initiating locomotion from mRF of medulla (Kinjo *et al.*, 1990). What we do know is that neuromodulation in the mRF comes from both local and top-down sources.

Recent advances suggest we may soon get key information to address both these general questions and the specific hypotheses we have raised. Combined behavioural and neural recording in semi-intact preparations of suitable model species provides unparalleled data on functional organisation. Semi-intact lamprey work has featured heavily in our discussions here; ongoing work on the afferent control of locomotion from mesencephalic and higher structures promises to shed light on the integration of action selection systems (Dubuc *et al.*, 2008). Mesce *et al.* (2008) have produced compelling evidence that dedicated leech interneurons control components of whole behaviours, and each receive multi-modal sensory input; they drew attention to the strong analogy between this arrangement and the idea of 'subaction' coordinating clusters we proposed (Humphries *et al.*, 2007). Wiring of the mRF too is under new scrutiny. Recent work has established genetic markers for specific proteins that identify subpopulations of reticulo-spinal cells for characterisation of their inputs, outputs, and electrophysiology (Bretzner and Brownstone, 2008). Further, there are now mouse lines expressing selective neurotoxins for mRF cells (Kamal Sharma, personal communication), promising future studies relating specific cell loss to effects on behaviour. With this new data, and given the comparatively small numbers of neurons involved, we can test hypotheses of mRF wiring in full-scale models in the near future.

14.10   Final remarks

The reticular formation is a strange beast: where some see an undifferentiated neuron mass, responsive only to global sensory input, others see a conglomeration of functionally specific units. Both views contain an element of truth. The dense ascending input and intra-RF connectivity point to a system capable only of responding to stimulation with increased activation. Yet, stimulation of individual neurons within it elicits discrete, repeatable movements. We hope that by proposing the mRF as an action selection system we may unify these disparate views: the dense web of inputs provide the ability to extract correlated sensory information, the internal connectivity provides the substrate for the coordination of behavioural components, and the individual neurons drive the appropriate motor systems.

Our proposals partially rest on the structure of the mRF: if the cluster structure is an accurate depiction of the mRF's internal anatomy, then a likely method of representing and resolving action competitions is that the activity of a cluster's projection neuron population encodes the relative selection of an action component. This subaction configuration has the advantage of both providing a functional role for the collaterals of the long-range axons, and increasing the representational capacity of the system. It is possible that both clustered and parallel action representations co-exist: competing complex behaviours may be represented by parallel axon activity that recruits the necessary subactions for each behaviour by activating the appropriate clusters. Combining these representational schemes with the potential control decomposition across the basal ganglia and mRF makes for a fascinating, if daunting, proposition. At the very least, we hope our work inspires a re-evaluation of the mRF's functional significance.

Acknowledgements

This work was funded by the EPSRC (GR/R95722/01) and the European Union Framework 6 ICEA project.

Appendix A Basic form of the computational models

All computational models used leaky rate-coding units: the population-level models (section 14.7.2) to represent the average firing rate of that population; the full model (section 14.7.4) to represent the firing rate of a single neuron. The change in activity a is given by

$$\tau\dot{a} = -a + I, \tag{A.1}$$

where I is the summed, weighted, total of all unit outputs that reach this unit, and τ the time-constant. Output y of the unit is rectified to the interval $y \in [0, 1]$.

A single instantiation of a three-cluster anatomical model was used to derive the connection parameters of the population-level computational model. Each 100 neuron cluster had 80 projection neurons and 20 inter-neurons. The weights between neural populations were scalars proportional to the total number of connections between them. Details and the specific connection matrices used are given in (Humphries *et al.*, 2007).

A single instantiation of an eight-cluster model was used for the full dynamic model. Each cluster had 50 neurons, with 80% projection neurons. The connection probabilities were set as $P(p) = 0.1$, $P(c) = 0.25$ (the 'spatially-uniform' model from Humphries *et al.* (2006a)), and $P(l) = 0.25$. All excitatory connections had a weight of 0.1; all inhibitory connections had a weight of -0.924. This ensured that the total magnitude of inhibitory and excitatory weights was equal for the network. Unit time constant was set to $\tau = 2$ ms (Yen and Chan, 1993). The differential equations were solved using exponential Euler and a timestep of 0.1 ms. The simulations were run until either equilibrium was reached or 1000 timesteps elapsed. Equilibrium was defined as the total change in a over all units on consecutive timesteps being less than 10^{-6}. Every simulation reported here reached equilibrium before the timestep limit.

References

Albert., R. and A.-L. Barabasi (2002). Statistical mechanics of complex networks. *Rev. Mod. Phys.* **74**: 47–97.

Alford, S., I. Zompa, and R. Dubuc (1995). Long-term potentiation of glutamatergic pathways in the lamprey brainstem. *J Neurosci.* **15**: 7528–38.

Angel, A. (1977). Processing of sensory information. *Prog. Neurobiol.* **9**: 1–122.

Berntson, G. G. and D. J. Micco (1976). Organization of brainstem behavioral systems. *Brain Res. Bull.* **1**: 471–83.

Berridge, K. C. (1989). Progressive degradation of serial grooming chains by descending decerebration. *Behav. Brain Res.* **33**: 241–53.

Berridge, K. C. and I. Q. Whishaw (1992). Cortex, striatum and cerebellum: control of serial order in a grooming sequence. *Exp. Brain Res.* **90**: 275–90.

Blessing, W. W. (1997). *The Lower Brainstem and Bodily Homeostasis.* New York: Oxford University Press.

Bowsher, D. (1970). Place and modality analysis in caudal reticular formation. *J. Physiol.* **209**: 473–86.

Bowsher, D. and J. Westman (1971). Ultrastructural characteristics of the caudal and rostral brain stem reticular formation. *Brain Res.* **28**: 443–57.

Braak, H., U. Rub, D. Sandmann-Keil, *et al.* (2000). Parkinson's disease: affection of brain stem nuclei controlling premotor and motor neurons of the somatomotor system. *Acta Neuropathol. (Berl.)* **99**: 489–95.

Braitenberg, V. (1984). *Vehicles: Experiments in Synthetic Psychology.* Cambridge, MA: MIT Press.

Breedlove, S. M., D. J. McGinty, and J. M. Siegel (1979). Operant conditioning of pontine gigantocellular units. *Brain Res. Bull.* **4**: 663–7.

Bretzner, F. and R. M. Brownstone (2008). Characterization of genetically identified reticulospinal pathways. In *2008 Neuroscience Meeting Planner.* Washington, DC: Society for Neuroscience, Program No. 576.3.

Brooks, R. A. (1991). New approaches to robotics. *Science* **253**: 1227–32.

Cant, N. B. and C. G. Benson (2003). Parallel auditory pathways: projection patterns of the different neuronal populations in the dorsal and ventral cochlear nuclei. *Brain Res. Bull.* **60**: 457–74.

Cherniak, C. (1994). Component placement optimization in the brain. *J. Neurosci.* **14**: 2418–27.

de Bono, M. and A. V. Maricq (2005). Neuronal substrates of complex behaviors in C. elegans. *Annu. Rev. Neurosci.* **28**: 451–501.

Deliagina, T. G., P. V. Zelenin, P. Fagerstedt, S. Grillner, and G. N. Orlovsky (2000). Activity of reticulospinal neurons during locomotion in the freely behaving lamprey. *J. Neurophysiol.* **83**: 853–63.

Deliagina, T. G., P. V. Zelenin, and G. N. Orlovsky (2002). Encoding and decoding of reticulospinal commands. *Brain Res. Rev.* **40**: 166–77.

Delwaide, P. J., J. L. Pepin, V. De Pasqua, and A. M. de Noordhout (2000). Projections from basal ganglia to tegmentum: a subcortical route for explaining the pathophysiology of Parkinson's disease signs? *J. Neurol.* **247**(2): 75–81.

Doya, K. (1999). What are the computations of the cerebellum, the basal ganglia and the cerebral cortex? *Neural Networks* **12**: 961–74.

Drew, T. and S. Rossignol (1990). Functional organization within the medullary reticular formation of intact unanesthetized cat. I. Movements evoked by microstimulation. *J. Neurophysiol.* **64**: 767–81.

Dubuc, R., F. Brocard, M. Antri, *et al.* (2008). Initiation of locomotion in lampreys. *Brain Res. Rev.* **57**: 172–82.

Eccles, J. C., R. A. Nicoll, T. Rantucci, H. Taborikova, and T. J. Willey (1976). Topographic studies on medial reticular nucleus. *J. Neurophysiol.* **39**: 109–118.

Fay, R. and L. Kubin (2000). Pontomedullary distribution of 5-HT2A receptor-like protein in the rat. *J. Comp. Neurol.* **418**: 323–45.

Fields, H. L. and A. I. Basbaum (1978). Brainstem control of spinal pain-transmission neurons. *Annu. Rev. Physiol.* **40**: 217–48.

Graybiel, A. M. (1995). Building action repertoires: memory and learning functions of the basal ganglia. *Curr. Opin. Neurobiol.* **5**: 733–41.

Grillner, S., T. Deliagina, O. Ekeberg, *et al.* (1995). Neural networks that co-ordinate locomotion and body orientation in lamprey. *Trends Neurosci.* **18**: 270–79.

Grillner, S., J. Hellgren, A. Menard, K. Saitoh, and M. A. Wikstrom (2005). Mechanisms for selection of basic motor programs – roles for the striatum and pallidum. *Trends Neurosci.* **28**: 364–70.

Groves, P. M., S. W. Miller, M. V. Parker, and G. V. Rebec (1973). Organization by sensory modality in the reticular formation of the rat. *Brain Res.* **54**: 207–24.

Gurney, K., T. J. Prescott, and P. Redgrave (2001a). A computational model of action selection in the basal ganglia I: a new functional anatomy. *Biol. Cybern.* **85**: 401–10.

Gurney, K., T. J. Prescott, and P. Redgrave (2001b). A computational model of action selection in the basal ganglia II: analysis and simulation of behaviour. *Biol. Cybern.* **85**: 411–23.

Hammer, R. P.J., R. D. Lindsay, and A. B. Scheibel (1981). Development of the brain stem reticular core: an assessment of dendritic state and configuration in the perinatal rat. *Dev. Brain Res.* **1**: 179–90.

Hattox, A., Y. Li, and A. Keller (2003). Serotonin regulates rhythmic whisking. *Neuron* **39**: 343–52.

Hobson, J. A. and A. B. Scheibel (1980). The brainstem core: sensorimotor integration and behavioral state control. *Neurosci. Res. Program. Bull.* **18**: 1–173.

Holmes, C. J., L. S. Mainville, and B. E. Jones (1994). Distribution of cholinergic, GABAergic and serotonergic neurons in the medial medullary reticular formation and their projections studied by cytotoxic lesions in the cat. *Neuroscience* **62**: 1155–78.

Holstege, G. (1995). The basic, somatic, and emotional components of the motor system in mammals. In *The Rat Nervous System*, 2nd edn, ed. G. Paxinos. New York: Academic Press, pp. 137–54.

Humphries, M. D., K. Gurney, and T. J. Prescott (2005). Is there an integrative center in the vertebrate brainstem? A robotic evaluation of a model of the reticular formation viewed as an action selection device. *Adapt. Behav.* **13**: 97–113.

Humphries, M. D., K. Gurney, and T. J. Prescott (2006a). The brainstem reticular formation is a small-world, not scale-free, network. *Proc. Roy. Soc. B.* **273**: 503–11.

Humphries, M. D., K. Gurney, and T. J. Prescott (2007). Is there a brainstem substrate for action selection? *Phil. Trans. Roy. Soc. B* **362**: 1627–39.

Humphries, M. D. and T. J. Prescott (2006). Distributed action selection by a brainstem neural substrate: an embodied evaluation. In *From Animals to Animats 9: Proceedings of the Ninth International Conference on Simulation of Adaptive Behaviour*, Volume 4095., ed. S. Nolfi, G. Baldassarre, R. Calabretta, *et al.* Berlin, Germany: Springer Verlag, pp. 199–210.

Humphries, M. D., R. D. Stewart, and K. N. Gurney, (2006b). A physiologically plausible model of action selection and oscillatory activity in the basal ganglia. *J. Neurosci.* **26**: 12921–42.

Inglis, W. L. and P. Winn (1995). The pedunculopontine tegmental nucleus: where the striatum meets the reticular formation. *Prog. Neurobiol.* **47**: 1–29.

Iwakiri, H., T. Oka, K. Takakusaki and S. Mori (1995). Stimulus effects of the medial pontine reticular formation and the mesencephalic locomotor region upon medullary reticulospinal neurons in acute decerebrate cats. *Neurosci. Res.* **23**: 47–53.

Iwaniuk, A. N. and I. Q. Whishaw (2000). On the origin of skilled forelimb movements. *Trends Neurosci.* **23**: 372–6.

Jones, B. E. (1990). Immunohistochemical study of choline acetyltransferase-immunoreactive processes and cells innervating the pontomedullary reticular formation in the rat. *J. Comp. Neurol.* **295**: 485–514.

Jones, B. E. (1995). Reticular formation: cytoarchitecture, transmitters, and projections. In *The Rat Nervous System*, 2nd edn, ed. G. Paxinos. New York: Academic Press, pp. 155–71.

Jones, B. E., C. J. Holmes, E. Rodriguez-Veiga, and L. Mainville (1991). GABA-synthesizing neurons in the medulla: their relationship to serotonin-containing and spinally projecting neurons in the rat. *J. Comp. Neurol.* **313**: 349–67.

Jordan, L. M., J. Liu, P. B. Hedlund, T. Akay, and K. G. Pearson (2008). Descending command systems for the initiation of locomotion in mammals. *Brain Res. Rev.* **57**: 183–91.

Jung, R., T. Kiemel, and A. H. Cohen (1996). Dynamic behavior of a neural network model of locomotor control in the lamprey. *J. Neurophysiol.* **75**: 1074–86.

Kilmer, W. L., W. S. McCulloch, and J. Blum (1969). A model of the vertebrate central command system. *Int. J. Man. Mach. Stud.* **1**: 279–309.

Kinjo, N., Y. Atsuta, M. Webber, *et al.* (1990). Medioventral medulla-induced locomotion. *Brain Res. Bull.* **24**: 509–16.

Kleinfeld, D., R. W. Berg, and S. M. O'Connor (1999). Anatomical loops and their electrical dynamics in relation to whisking by rat. *Somatosens. Mot. Res.* **16**: 69–88.

Krichmar, J. L. (2008). The neuromodulatory system: a framework for survival and adaptive behavior in a challenging world. *Adapt. Behav.* **16**: 385–99.

Kristan, W. B., R. L. Calabrese, and W. O. Friesen (2005). Neuronal control of leech behavior. *Prog. Neurobiol.* **76**: 279–327.

Kropotov, J. D. and S. C. Etlinger (1999). Selection of actions in the basal ganglia thalamocortical circuits: review and model. *Int. J. Psychophysiol.* **31**: 197–217.

Kuypers, H. G. (1964). The descending pathways to the spinal cord, their anatomy and function. *Prog. Brain Res.* **11**: 178–202.

Lakke, J. P. (1985). Axial apraxia in Parkinson's disease. *J. Neurol. Sci.* **69**: 37–46.

Langhorst, P., B. Schulz, G. Schulz, and M. Lambertz (1983). Reticular formation of the lower brainstem. A common system for cardiorespiratory and somatomotor functions: discharge patterns of neighboring neurons influenced by cardiovascular and respiratory afferents. *J. Auton. Nerv. Syst.* **9**: 411–32.

Langhorst, P., B. G. Schulz, H. Seller, and H. P. Koepchen (1996). Convergence of visceral and somatic afferents on single neurones in the reticular formation of the lower brain stem in dogs. *J. Auton. Nerv. Syst.* **57**: 149–57.

Laughlin, S. B. and T. J. Sejnowski (2003). Communication in neuronal networks. *Science* **301**: 1870–4.

Lovick, T. A. (1972). The behavioural repertoire of precollicular decerebrate rats. *J. Physiol.* **226**: 4P–6P.

Lund, J. P., A. Kolta, K. G. Westberg, and G. Scott (1998). Brainstem mechanisms underlying feeding behaviors. *Curr. Opin. Neurobiol.* **8**: 718–24.

Magoun, H. W. and R. Rhines (1946). An inhibitory mechanism in the bulbar reticular formation. *J. Neurophysiol.* **9**: 165–71.

Marsden, C. D. and J. A. Obeso (1994). The functions of the basal ganglia and the paradox of stereotaxic surgery in Parkinson's disease. *Brain* **117**: 877–97.

Martin, E. M., C. Pavlides, and D. W. Pfaff (2007). Neurons in the medullary reticular formation with multimodal sensory response capacities. In *2007 Neuroscience Meeting Planner*. San Diego, CA: Society for Neuroscience, Program No. 403.11.

Mathias, N. and Gopal, V. (2001). Small worlds: how and why. *Phys. Rev. E.* **63**: 021117.

Matsuyama, K., F. Mori, K. Nakajima, *et al.* (2004). Locomotor role of the corticoreticular-reticulospinal-spinal interneuronal system. *Prog. Brain Res.* **143**: 239–49.

Mesce, K., T. Esch, and W. Kristan (2008). Cellular substrates of action selection: a cluster of higher-order descending neurons shapes body posture and locomotion. *J. Comp. Physiol. A Neuroethol. Sens. Neural Behav. Physiol.* **194**: 469–81.

Mink, J. W. and W. T. Thach (1993). Basal ganglia intrinsic circuits and their role in behavior. *Curr. Opin. Neurobiol.* **3**: 950–7.

Mori, S. (1987). Integration of posture and locomotion in acute decerebrate cats and in awake, freely moving cats. *Prog. Neurobiol.* **28**: 161–95.

Moruzzi, G. and H. W. Magoun (1949). Brain stem reticular formation and activation of the EEG. *Electroenceph. Clin. Neurophysiol.* **1**: 455–73.

Moschovakis, A. K., C. A. Scudder, and S. M. Highstein (1996). The microscopic anatomy and physiology of the mammalian saccadic system. *Prog. Neurobiol.* **50**: 133–254.

Newman, D. B. (1985). Distinguishing rat brainstem reticulospinal nuclei by their neuronal morphology. I. Medullary nuclei. *J. für Hirnforschung* **26**: 187–226.

Newman, D. B. (1995). Anatomy and neurotransmitters of brainstem motor systems. *Adv. Neurol.* **67**: 219–43.

Noga, B. R., D. J. Kriellaars, R. M. Brownstone, and L. M. Jordan (2003). Mechanism for activation of locomotor centers in the spinal cord by stimulation of the mesencephalic locomotor region. *J. Neurophysiol.* **90**: 1464–78.

Parvizi, J. and A. R. Damasio (2003). Neuroanatomical correlates of brainstem coma. *Brain* **126**: 1524–36.

Paxinos, G. and Watson, C. (1998). *The Rat Brain in Stereotaxic Coordinates*, 4th edn. San Diego, CA: Academic Press.

Peterson, B. W. (1979). Reticulospinal projections to spinal motor nuclei. *Annu. Rev. Physiol.* **41**: 127–40.

Prescott, T. J. (2007). Forced moves or good tricks in design space? landmarks in the evolution of neural mechanisms for action selection. *Adapt. Behav.* **15**: 9–31.

Prescott, T. J., P. Redgrave, and K. Gurney (1999). Layered control architectures in robots and vertebrates. *Adapt. Behav.* **7**: 99–127.

Prisco, G. V. D., E. Pearlstein, D. L. Ray, R. Robitaille, and R. Dubuc (2000). A cellular mechanism for the transformation of a sensory input into a motor command. *J. Neurosci.* **20**: 8169–76.

Ramon-Moliner, E. and W. J. Nauta (1966). The isodendritic core of the brain stem. *J. Comp. Neurol.* **126**: 311–35.

Redgrave, P., T. J. Prescott, and K. Gurney (1999). The basal ganglia: a vertebrate solution to the selection problem? *Neuroscience* **89**: 1009–23.

Reiner, A., L. Medina, and C. L. Veenman (1998). Structural and functional evolution of the basal ganglia in vertebrates. *Brain Res. Rev.* **28**: 235–85.

Rubchinsky, L. L., N. Kopell, and K. A. Sigvardt (2003). Modeling facilitation and inhibition of competing motor programs in basal ganglia subthalamic nucleus-pallidal circuits. *Proc. Natl. Acad. Sci. USA* **100**: 14427–32.

Salibi, N. A., N. E. Saade, N. R. Banna, and S. J. Jabbur (1980). Dorsal column input into the reticular formation. *Nature* **288**: 481–3.

Scheibel, A. B. (1984). The brainstem reticular core and sensory function. In *Handbook of Physiology. Section 1: The Nervous System*, ed. J. M. Brookhart, and V. B. Mountcastle. Bethesda, MD: American Physiological Society, pp. 213–56.

Scheibel, M. E. and A. B. Scheibel (1958). Structural substrates for integrative patterns in the brain stem reticular core. In *Reticular Formation of the Brain*, ed. H. H. E. A. Jasper. Boston, MA: Little and Brown.

Scheibel, M. E., and A. B. Scheibel (1967). Anatomical basis of attention mechanisms in vertebrate brains. In *The Neurosciences, A Study Program*, ed. G. C. Quarton, T. Melnechuk, and F. O. Schmitt. New York: The Rockefeller University Press, pp. 577–602.

Schulz, B., M. Lambertz, G. Schulz, and P. Langhorst (1983). Reticular formation of the lower brainstem. A common system for cardiorespiratory and somatomotor functions: discharge patterns of neighboring neurons influenced by somatosensory afferents. *J. Auton. Nerv. Syst.* **9**: 433–49.

Schulz, G., M. Lambertz, B. Schulz, P. Langhorst, and B. Krienke (1985). Reticular formation of the lower brainstem. A common system for cardio-respiratory and somatomotor functions. Cross-correlation analysis of discharge patterns of neighbouring neurones. *J. Auton. Nerv. Syst.* **12**: 35–62.

Segundo, J. P., T. Takenaka, and H. Encabo (1967). Somatic sensory properties of bulbar reticular neurons. *J. Neurophysiol.* **30**: 1221–38.

Shammah-Lagnado, S. J., M. S. Costa, and J. A. Ricardo (1992). Afferent connections of the parvocellular reticular formation: a horseradish peroxidase study in the rat. *Neuroscience* **50**: 403–25.

Siegel, J. M. (1979). Behavioral functions of the reticular formation. *Brain Res. Rev.* **1**: 69–105.

Siegel, J. M., R. Nienhuis, R. L. Wheeler, D. J. McGinty, and R. M. Harper (1981). Discharge pattern of reticular-formation unit pairs in waking and REM-sleep. *Exp. Neurol.* **74**: 875–91.

Siegel, J. M. and K. S. Tomaszewski (1983). Behavioral organization of reticular formation: studies in the unrestrained cat. I. Cells related to axial, limb, eye, and other movements. *J. Neurophysiol.* **50**: 696–716.

Sperry, R. W. (1952). Neurology and the mind-brain problem. *Amer. Sci.* **40**: 291–312.

Sprague, J. M. and W. W. Chambers (1954). Control of posture by reticular formation and cerebellum in the intact, anesthetized and unanesthetized, decerebrated cat. *Am. J. Physiol.* **176**: 52–64.

Stephens, G. J., B. Johnson-Kerner, W. Bialek, and W. S. Ryu (2008). Dimensionality and dynamics in the behavior of C. elegans. *PLoS Comput. Biol.* **4**: e1000028.

Stevens, D. R., S. Birnstiel, U. Gerber, R. W. McCarley, and R. W. Greene (1993). Nicotinic depolarizations of rat medial pontine reticular formation neurons studied in vitro. *Neuroscience* **57**: 419–24.

Stevens, D. R., R. W. McCarley, and R. W. Greene (1992). Serotonin1 and serotonin2 receptors hyperpolarize and depolarize separate populations of medial pontine reticular formation neurons in vitro. *Neuroscience.* **47**: 545–53.

Stevens, D. R., R. W. McCarley, and R. W. Greene (1994). The mechanism of noradrenergic alpha 1 excitatory modulation of pontine reticular formation neurons. *J. Neurosci.* **14**: 6481–87.

Swanson, L. W. (2000). Cerebral hemisphere regulation of motivated behavior. *Brain Res.* **886**: 113–64.

Szokol, K., J. C. Glover, and M.-C. Perreault (2008). Differential origin of reticulospinal drive to motorneurons innervating trunk and hindlimb muscles in the mouse revealed by optical recording. *J. Physiol.* **586**: 5259–76.

Takakusaki, K., K. Saitoh, H. Harada, and M. Kashiwayanagi (2004). Role of basal ganglia-brainstem pathways in the control of motor behaviors. *Neurosci. Res.* **50**: 137–51.

Torvik, A. and A. Brodal (1957). The origin of reticulospinal fibers in the cat; an experimental study. *Anat. Rec.* **128**: 113–37.

Valverde, F. (1961). Reticular formation of the pons and medulla oblongata: a Golgi study. *J. Comp. Neurol.* **116**: 71–99.

Whelan, P. J. (1996). Control of locomotion in the decerebrate cat. *Prog. Neurobiol.* **49**: 481–515.

Woods, J. W. (1964). Behavior of chronic decerebrate rats. *J. Neurophysiol.* **27**: 635–44.

Yates, B. J. and S. D. Stocker (1998). Integration of somatic and visceral inputs by the brainstem: functional considerations. *Exp. Brain Res.* **119**: 269–75.

Yen, J. C. and S. H. Chan (1993). Passive biophysical membrane properties of nucleus reticularis gigantocellularis neurons in brain slices from the rat. *Neurosci. Lett.* **159**: 5–8.

Zahm, D. S. (2006). The evolving theory of basal forebrain functional–anatomical 'macrosystems'. *Neurosci. Biobehav. Rev.* **30**: 148–72.

Zigmond, M. J. and R. E. Burke (2002). Pathophysiology of Parkinson's disease. In *Neuropsychopharmacology: The Fifth Generation of Progress*, ed. K. L. Davis, D. Charney, J. T. Coyle, and C. Nemeroff. Philadelphia: Lippincott Williams and Wilkins, pp. 1781–93.

15 Understanding decision-making deficits in neurological conditions: insights from models of natural action selection

Michael J. Frank, Anouk Scheres, and Scott J. Sherman

Summary

Models of natural action selection implicate fronto-striatal circuits in both motor and cognitive 'actions'. Dysfunction of these circuits leads to decision-making deficits in various populations. We review how computational models provide insights into the mechanistic basis for these deficits in Parkinson's patients and individuals with ventromedial frontal damage. We then consider implications of the models for understanding behaviour and cognition in attention deficit/hyperactivity disorder (ADHD). Incorporation of cortical norepinephrine function into the model improves action selection in noisy environments and accounts for response variability in ADHD. We close with more general clinical implications.

15.1 Introduction

Fronto-striatal dysfunction can lead to dramatic changes in cognition and action, as evidenced by various disorders with disturbances to this circuitry, including Parkinson's disease (PD), schizophrenia, attention deficit/hyperactivity disorder (ADHD), obsessive–compulsive disorder, Tourrette's syndrome, Huntington's disease and addiction (Nieoullon 2002). One might wonder how adaptive evolution of a brain system could lead to the complexity and diversity of behaviours associated with these disorders, especially since these behaviours generally do not occur spontaneously in animals. However, we could also turn this question on its ear and ask: how elegant must a neural system be to lead to more rational human behaviour? It may be an unfortunate but necessary corollary that the complexity required to produce adaptive thought and behaviour may be vulnerable to all manner of issues with the 'plumbing', which would have compounding effects on the overall system. Thus the trade-offs that come with adaptive human behaviour may be akin to those associated with a car that has electronic seat position control and GPS navigation – these luxurious amenities come with increased risk of something breaking in an unpredictable fashion.

Modelling Natural Action Selection, eds. Anil K. Seth, Tony J. Prescott and Joanna J. Bryson.
Published by Cambridge University Press. © Cambridge University Press 2012.

This chapter presents an attempt to understand decision-making deficits in various patients with neurological conditions, as informed by neurocomputational models of fronto-striatal circuitry. The prefrontal cortex (PFC) – often considered the seat of abstract thought and executive function – dynamically interacts with multiple subcortical and other cortical areas, and the whole system is dynamically modulated by dopamine and other neurotransmitters. It should be clear that even if our knowledge base for how each of these subsystems worked was perfect, it would nevertheless quickly become intractable to try to connect all the pieces together 'in your head' or on a figure. The use of computational models forces one to be explicit about each part of the system, and allows systematic exploration of how changes in a single parameter in one subsystem may propagate through the system and impact cognition and decision making. Of course, several computational approaches can be used at multiple levels of analysis – from the most biophysically detailed to highly abstract frameworks – each having its own merits, and none a panacea. The hallmark of a successful modelling endeavour should therefore be its ability to generate insights into the mechanisms needed to explain phenomena at a particular level of analysis (Dayan, 2001; O'Reilly and Munakata, 2000).

The computational models described below offer an integrative framework that attempts to link cellular and systems-level interactions with cognitive dysfunction in patients with dysfunction within the same neural circuitry, including PD, patients with ventromedial/orbital prefrontal damage, ADHD, and the effects of medications and surgical treatments of these conditions. The models do not attempt to provide precise quantitative fits to any particular data set, but rather to develop qualitative patterns of predictions that depend on key principles that drive the system. The development of these principles are constrained by data at both the neural and cognitive level, thereby minimising the number of plausible models consistent with the data. Moreover, the models have generated novel testable predictions at both the neural and behavioural levels. The details of the models and analyses are described elsewhere and in the appendices; here we focus on the higher level principles.

15.2   Neurocomputational framework

Building upon other theoretical/modelling work on the role of the basal ganglia (BG)–frontal cortical (FC) system in motor control (e.g., Beiser and Houk, 1998; Brown et al., 2004; Gurney et al., 2001; Houk and Wise, 1995; Mink, 1996), we have developed a series of neurocomputational models that explore the roles of this system in cognitive actions (Frank, Loughry, and O'Reilly, 2001; Frank, 2005; O'Reilly and Frank, 2006; Frank and Claus, 2006; Frank, 2006; see also Houk, 2005; Houk et al., 2007). All of the above models share the idea that BG–FC circuits play a key role in action selection.

Figure 15.1a shows the basic circuitry included in our models. Two main cell populations in the striatum have opposing effects on the selection of a given action, via divergent projections through BG nuclei, thalamus, and back to cortex. Activity in 'Go' neurons facilitates the execution of a response considered in cortex, whereas 'NoGo' activity suppresses (or prevents the facilitation of) competing responses. Dopamine (DA)

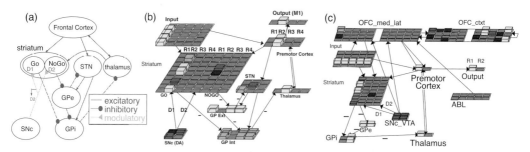

Figure 15.1 (a)The striato-cortical loops, including the direct ('Go') and indirect ('NoGo') pathways of the basal ganglia. The Go cells disinhibit the thalamus via GPi, facilitating the execution of an action represented in cortex. The NoGo cells have an opposing effect by increasing inhibition of the thalamus, and suppressing action execution. Dopamine from the SNc excites synaptically driven Go activity via D1 receptors, and inhibits NoGo activity via D2 receptors. GPi: internal segment of globus pallidus; GPe: external segment of globus pallidus; SNc: substantia nigra pars compacta; STN: subthalamic nucleus. (b) Neural network model of this circuit Frank (2005, 2006). Squares represent units, with height reflecting neural activity. The premotor cortex selects one of four responses (R1–R4) via direct projections from the sensory input, and is modulated by BG projections from thalamus. Go units are in the left half of the striatum layer; NoGo in the right half, with separate columns for the four responses). In the case shown, striatum Go is stronger than NoGo for R2, inhibiting GPi, disinhibiting the thalamus, and facilitating R2 execution in cortex. A tonic level of dopamine is shown in SNc; a burst or dip ensues in a subsequent error feedback phase (not shown), driving Go/NoGo learning. The STN exerts a dynamic 'Global NoGo' function on response execution, and adaptively modulates the threshold at which actions are selected depending on the degree of cortical response conflict (Frank, 2006). (c) Modelling BG interactions with orbitofrontal cortex in decision making (Frank and Claus, 2006). The BG model is as in (b). In addition, medial and lateral OFC areas receive graded information about reward/punishment magnitude information from the ABL (amygdala), which have a top-down effect on responding within the striatum, and directly on premotor cortex, allowing more flexible behaviour. *OFC-ctxt* is a context layer that maintains recent reinforcement information in working memory and biases activity in *OFC-med-lat* for use in behavioural decisions.

modulates the relative balance of these pathways, exciting synaptically driven Go activity via D1 receptors, while inhibiting NoGo activity via D2 receptors (Aubert *et al.*, 2000; Gerfen, 1992; Hernandez-Lopez *et al.*, 1997; Hernandez-Lopez *et al.*, 2000). Further, via diffuse projections to BG output nuclei (Parent and Hazrati, 1995), the subthalamic nucleus (STN) may exert a Global NoGo signal on the execution of all responses, which can prevent premature responding when multiple competing responses are being evaluated (Frank, 2006). Simulated DA depletion in the model results in emergent oscillatory activity in BG nuclei; these oscillations are characteristic of Parkinson's tremor (e.g., Bergman *et al.*, 1994; Terman *et al.*, 2002), and are eliminated with both real and simulated STN lesions (Frank, 2006; Ni *et al.*, 2000). Thus, although the models are intended to address decision-making functions of BG–FC circuitry, they are also constrained by data at the lower neural level of analysis. Furthermore, by virtue of interactions with different areas of the FC (Alexander *et al.*, 1986; Houk, 2005), the models show how the BG can participate in a wide range of cognitive functions, from relatively 'low-level' tasks such as procedural learning (Frank, 2005), up to 'higher-level' tasks such as working memory (Frank *et al.*, 2001; O'Reilly and Frank, 2006) and decision making (Frank and Claus, 2006).

Given that the BG participate in selecting among various competing low-level motor responses, it is natural to extend this functionality to include higher-level decisions. A key question is, how do the BG *know* which decision has the highest value? Insight comes from various experiments showing that when monkeys are rewarded following a correct choice, transient increases in dopamine firing are observed (Schultz, 2002). Conversely, choices that do not lead to reward are associated with DA dips (pauses in DA firing) that drop below baseline (e.g., Satoh *et al.*, 2003; Schultz, 2002), with longer duration pauses when rewards are highly expected (Bayer *et al.*, 2007). Similar DA-dependent processes have been inferred to occur in humans during positive and negative reinforcement using neuroimaging techniques (Delgado *et al.*, 2000; Frank *et al.*, 2005; Holroyd and Coles, 2002). In our models, these DA bursts and dips modify learning in Go and NoGo striatal units. Via D1 receptors, phasic DA bursts during rewards enhance neural activity and synaptic plasticity in those Go units that are activated by the stimulus–response conjunction, while having opposite effects via D2 receptors in the NoGo pathway; this functionality is supported by various lines of neurobiological evidence (e.g., Centonze *et al.*, 2001; Frank, 2005; Mahon *et al.*, 2003; for reviews, see Cohen and Frank, 2009; Frank and O'Reilly, 2006). Striatal units not activated by the particular input stimulus do not learn. The net result is that DA bursts support 'Go' learning to reinforce the good choice in response to a particular stimulus, while DA dips support 'NoGo' learning to avoid bad choices (Brown *et al.*, 2004; Frank, 2005). That is, a lack of DA releases NoGo cells from their tonic D2 inhibition, allowing them to become more excited than their Go counterparts, and driving 'Hebbian' learning in the opposite direction to DA bursts. Supporting this account, D2 receptor blockade (simulating the lack of D2 stimulation during dips) is associated with enhanced NoGo activity in the indirect pathway and associated increases in corticostriatal plasticity (Centonze *et al.*, 2004; Robertson *et al.*, 1992). Recent plasticity studies also support this model, whereby a lack of D2 stimulation in striatopallidal NoGo cells is required for LTP (Shen *et al.*, 2008).

As DA bursts and dips reinforce Go and NoGo representations in the BG, our model showed that the most adaptive (i.e., rewarding) responses are facilitated while less adaptive ones are suppressed. Further, as the BG learns to facilitate adaptive responses, the associated adaptive representations become enhanced directly in premotor cortical areas (via modification of input to premotor synaptic strengths). In this way, DA reward processes within the BG may ingrain prepotent motor 'habits' in cortical areas (Frank, 2005). Once these behaviours are ingrained, there is less need for selective facilitation by the BG. This is consistent with observations that dopaminergic integrity within the BG is critical for the acquisition but not execution of instrumental responses (Choi *et al.*, 2005; Smith-Roe and Kelley, 2000), and with recent observations that learning-related activity is initially seen in the BG and only later in frontal cortex (Delgado *et al.*, 2005; Pasupathy and Miller, 2005; Seger and Cincotta, 2006).

Next, we review how models of this circuitry can account for decision-making deficits in clinical populations.

15.3   Applying the models to clinical populations

15.3.1   Parkinson's disease and dopamine manipulations

PD is a progressive neurodegenerative disease that selectively damages dopaminergic cells targeting the BG. The most obvious behavioural changes associated with PD are muscular rigidity, slowness of movements, and tremor. However, motor neurons themselves are not damaged, and patients can perform movements quite smoothly under some circumstances. Instead, these patients may have difficulty selecting among various competing motor actions and executing the most appropriate one. A long standing hypothesis is that depleted DA in PD leads to an imbalance of the direct and indirect pathways (Albin *et al.*, 1989). In effect, the threshold for facilitating a motor programme is raised (Mink, 1996; Wichmann and DeLong, 2003). The observation that treatment with DA agonists and L-Dopa sometimes leads to jerking movements, or *dyskinesia* (McAuley, 2003) is consistent with this hypothesis by shifting the balance the other way and making the threshold for motor execution too low (Gerfen, 2003).

A number of cognitive changes also exist in PD, and these are often complex and seemingly unrelated, ranging from deficits in *reinforcement learning and decision making* (i.e., choosing among multiple menu items at a restaurant and learning from the outcome of this decision) to *working memory* (holding and manipulating information in the mind, as in mental arithmetic) and *attentional control* (directing attention to task-relevant versus distracting information). Rather than proposing separate mechanisms for the various cognitive and motor impairments in PD, our approach unifies the diverse pattern of results by adopting a mechanistic approach that attempts to decipher the underlying roles of the BG/DA system. In fact, the various deficits can all be accounted for by a reduced dynamic range of DA signals within the BG of the models (Frank, 2005). Indeed, although executive dysfunction is sometimes assumed to be due to prefrontal deficits, frontal-like cognitive dysfunction in early stage PD is correlated with striatal, and not prefrontal, DA measures (Kaasinen *et al.*, 2000a; Müller *et al.*, 2000; Remy *et al.*, 2000). Our models suggest that low striatal DA leads to diminished Go signals and difficulty in the *updating* of prefrontal representations, leading to frontal-like deficits (Frank, 2005; Frank and O'Reilly, 2006; Moustafa *et al.*, 2008b; O'Reilly and Frank, 2006; see also Hazy *et al.*, this volume).

We have tested various aspects of the hypothesised roles of the BG/DA system in action selection. First, we demonstrated support for a central prediction of our model regarding dopamine involvement in 'Go' and 'NoGo' cognitive reinforcement learning (Frank *et al.*, 2004). We tested PD patients on and off DA medication. We predicted that decreased DA levels in PD would enable patients to avoid selecting options that had been associated with negative reinforcement, due to spared NoGo learning, but that these patients would have more difficulty making choices that had high reward value (which depends on DA bursts). We further predicted that DA medications used to treat PD (L-Dopa and D2 receptor agonists) should alleviate the Go learning deficit, but would block the effects of DA dips needed to support NoGo learning, as was simulated to account for other medication-induced cognitive deficits in PD (Frank, 2005). To test

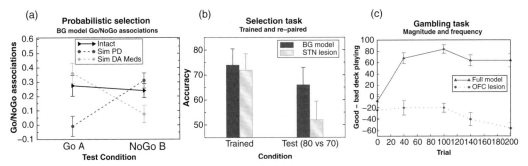

Figure 15.2 (a) BG model Go and NoGo associations recorded from the striatum after learning that choosing stimulus A is rewarding in 80% of trials and choosing Stimulus B is rewarding only in 20%. Parkinson's disease was simulated (Sim PD) by reducing DA input to the striatum, and medication was simulated (Sim DA Meds) by increasing tonic DA levels and reducing phasic DA dips. These qualitative patterns predicted learning biases in PD patients on and off medication (Frank *et al.*, 2004). (b) The contributions of the subthalamic nucleus to decision making were explored (Frank, 2006). STN lesions improved PD-like symptoms in the model (not shown) but induced premature and inappropriate responding when having to choose among two positively reinforced responses (80% versus 70%). (c) The orbitofrontal cortex (OFC) is critical in the model for adaptive decision making when the magnitudes of decision outcomes (rewards and losses) are more relevant than their probability of occurrence (Frank and Claus, 2006), providing a mechanistic explanation for decision making deficits in patients with OFC damage.

this idea, we developed a paradigm to dissociate the ability to select good actions versus avoiding bad ones. Indeed, patients who had abstained from taking medication were better at avoiding the selection of negative stimuli (NoGo choices) than they were at Go choices. In contrast, patients taking their regular dose of medication were better at Go learning and selection, but were relatively impaired at NoGo learning (Frank *et al.*, 2004). These same learning biases were observed in the model (Figure 15.2a), and have since been replicated by our and other labs in a number of paradigms (Bodi *et al.*, 2009; Cools *et al.*, 2006; Frank *et al.*, 2007b; Moustafa *et al.*, 2008a).

According to the model, L-Dopa medication enhanced Go choices via increases in spike-dependent DA release (Harden and Grace, 1995; Pothos *et al.*, 1998), consistent with beneficial L-Dopa effects on other tasks thought to depend on DA bursts (Shohamy *et al.*, 2004). Moreover, the tendency for medication to *impair* NoGo learning was similarly predicted by the model, as DA medications (especially D2 agonists) would tonically stimulate D2 receptors and may effectively block the effects of DA dips needed to learn NoGo (Frank, 2005). This effect was previously simulated in the model to explicitly account for medication-induced reversal learning deficits in PD, in which patients are impaired at learning to reverse stimulus–reward contingencies (Cools *et al.*, 2001; Swainson *et al.*, 2000). Cools *et al.* (2006) independently confirmed more specific model predictions, showing that reversal learning deficits are selectively observed for NoGo learning to a previously rewarded stimulus. Others have confirmed this medication-induced NoGo learning deficit in categorisation tasks that require learning from negative outcomes (Bodi *et al.*, 2009). Finally, the preserved NoGo learning in non-medicated patients, or *de novo* never-medicated patients (Bodi *et al.*, 2009), is readily explained by the notion that this learning depends on DA dips that remove DA from the synapse (so as to disinhibit NoGo neurons expressing D2 receptors). While low tonic DA levels in PD may still be sufficient to inhibit highly sensitive D2 receptors (e.g., Creese *et al.*, 1983; Goto and Grace, 2005), these may also make it more likely that all DA is removed from the synapse during DA dips. Further, the D2 receptor supersensitivity observed in PD (Kaasinen *et al.*, 2000b; Rinne *et al.*, 1990) would make NoGo neurons particularly sensitive to DA dips. Indeed, striatopallidal NoGo cells are more excitable in conditions of reduced DA (Surmeier *et al.*, 2007).

15.3.1.1   Dopamine manipulation in healthy participants

We have also tested predictions for a more general role for BG/DA in cognitive function by administering low doses of dopamine agonists/antagonists to young, healthy participants (Frank and O'Reilly, 2006). The drugs used (cabergoline and haloperidol) were selective for D2 receptors, which are by far most prevalent in the BG. By acting on presynaptic D2 receptors, low doses of these drugs modulate the amount of phasic DA released in the BG (e.g., Wu *et al.*, 2002). Again, results were consistent with our model: increases in DA were associated with better Go choices, whereas decreases in DA were associated with better NoGo performance. These same effects extended to higher level cognitive actions. As reviewed by Hazy *et al.* (this volume), our models show that these same Go/NoGo mechanisms can also drive the updating of working memory representations in PFC (Frank *et al.*, 2001; O'Reilly and Frank, 2006). In support of this consistent account, drug-induced BG/DA increases selectively enhanced working memory updating of task-relevant (i.e., 'positively-valenced'), but not distracting ('negatively-valenced') information; DA decreases had the opposite effect (Frank and O'Reilly, 2006). Functional imaging studies reveal that individual differences in the ability to screen out distractors from working memory are associated with BG activity, likely in the indirect pathway (McNab and Klingberg, 2007). Overall, these results show that the BG/DA system modulation of learning and action selection is not restricted to the relatively extreme case of PD.

15.3.1.2   Deep brain stimulation in Parkinson's disease

In addition to DA medications, PD patients are increasingly often treated with deep brain stimulation (DBS), a surgical treatment that places electrodes in the subthalamic nucleus. This type of therapy generally improves motor symptoms and activities of daily living, but its effects on cognition are not well understood, with both enhancements and impairments reported (e.g., Witt *et al.*, 2004). Our models may be useful in this regard, in that they can simulate when decision-making abilities are enhanced, and when they might be hindered, from increases or decreases in subthalamic activity (Frank, 2006). Our model suggests that the STN provides a dynamic 'Global NoGo' or 'Hold your horses' signal that prevents premature responding when faced with multiple good decision options (Figure 15.2b). This signal allows the system to take a longer time to integrate over all possibilities before selecting the best choice, and is suggestive of a key role of the STN in classical speed–accuracy trade-offs. This account is also consistent with effects of STN lesions on premature responding in choice paradigms in rats (Baunez and Robbins, 1998; Baunez *et al.*, 2001).

Moreover, our model predicts that the STN 'hold your horses' signal is dynamically modulated by the degree of decision conflict, as represented in premotor cortical areas, potentially extending into the dorsal anterior cingulate (ACC). This region is consistently activated under conflict conditions (Yeung *et al.*, 2004) and has direct projections to the STN (Orieux *et al.*, 2002). Thus, when choosing among two responses that have had similar positive reinforcement histories ('win–win' decisions), the associated conflicting cortical representations lead to a larger intensity and longer duration STN signal (Frank, 2006). We have previously observed modulation of cortical conflict signals in healthy participants using electrophysiological measures thought to reflect ACC activity (Frank *et al.*, 2005). Notably, these conflict signals depended on the kinds of decisions that should elicit conflict in the particular individual. Those biased to learn more from the positive outcomes of their decisions showed conflict signals when making win–win decisions, whereas those who learned more from their errors showed greater conflict during lose–lose decisions (i.e., when having to choose among two responses that were both likely to be incorrect). Our model predicts that the effect of these conflict signals in modulating choice behaviour may in part be mediated via the STN. Recent studies with patients on and off DBS provide initial confirmatory support for this notion: whereas patients off DBS showed intact ability to slow down during high conflict decisions, when their stimulators were turned on – thereby disrupting STN function – they no longer slowed down, and even showed impulsive speeded responding under high conflict conditions (Frank *et al.*, 2007b). Such impulsivity as a function of DBS has recently been shown to exist in patients' day-to-day lives (Hlbig *et al.*, 2009). Ultimately, we believe that a combined modelling/empirical approach can be used to constrain stimulation parameters to minimise the potential negative impact of DBS on decision making.

Finally, the model suggests that a different mechanism is responsible for observations that PD patients taking D2 agonists can develop spontaneous onset of pathological gambling (e.g., Dodd *et al.*, 2005). Although this behaviour is also characterised as impulsive, our models suggest it may be due to an inability to learn from losses, rather than an inability to take more time to make high-conflict decisions as in DBS. Specifically, medications continually stimulate DA receptors and effectively block the effects of DA dips during the experience of losses, thereby preventing NoGo learning in the BG, while preserving Go learning from rewards; this undue biasing of decision outcomes would further ingrain the behaviour as a habitual response. Our recent study reported such a dissociation, whereby medications impaired avoidance learning but not high-conflict slowing, and DBS produced the opposite pattern of results (Frank *et al.*, 2007b). However, the 'basic' BG model may not be sufficient to fully account for the data. As described next, frontal reward regions may play a key role in incorporating the inherent graded differences in the *magnitudes* of gains and losses associated with gambling experiences.

15.3.2   Decision–making deficits in ventromedial/orbitofrontal patients

Despite preliminary support for its predictions, the BG model as described above is not adequate to account for more complex, 'real-world' decisions. In particular, it is not well equipped to pay appropriate weight either to relative differences in the magnitudes of gains and losses, or to the recency of reinforcement contingencies. For such functions, the more advanced and adaptive orbitofrontal cortex (OFC) may be necessary to complement the functions of the more primitive BG/DA system (Frank and Claus, 2006). Indeed, patients with OFC damage (but intact BG/DA system) make dramatic decision–making errors in their everyday lives, as well as the laboratory (e.g., Bechara *et al.*, 1998). In our explorations of the unique OFC contributions to decision making (Figure 15.1c), the OFC maintains recently experienced rewards and punishments and their relative magnitudes in an active state (via persistent neural firing), and has a top-down effect on the BG and premotor regions to guide behaviour (Frank and Claus, 2006). This model is based on a substantial body of evidence for OFC representation of reward and punishment magnitude information, which it receives from the amygdala, and for the persistent maintenance of this activity in working memory (e.g., Hikosaka and Watanabe, 2000; Holland and Gallagher, 2004; Schoenbaum and Roesch, 2005). These representations can bias behaviour (Wallis and Miller, 2003), via efferent projections to the striatum and motor cortical areas.

Our combined BG/OFC model offers a mechanistic explanation of impaired decision-making processes and reversal learning deficits in OFC patients (Bechara *et al.*, 1998; Fellows and Farah, 2003; Rolls, 1996), and further accounts for irrational patterns of decisions in healthy populations (e.g., Kahneman and Tversky, 1979; Frank and Claus, 2006). We showed that the more primitive BG/DA system is sufficient for (relatively slow) learning to make choices based on their frequencies of positive versus negative reinforcement (not shown; see Frank and Claus, 2006). But OFC integrity is necessary for faster learning of more recent contingencies, and for making choices that lead to less probable but larger rewards over those that are more certain but yield smaller expected values (Figure 15.2c), consistent with patterns of data observed in rats with and without OFC damage (Mobini *et al.*, 2002). These authors further showed that OFC is necessary for making choices that lead to larger but delayed rewards instead of smaller, immediate rewards. The implication of our model is that choosing based on delayed rewards depends on working memory for action–outcome contingencies, and requires suppression of responses that would lead to immediate rewards (which the BG would be able to learn itself). Recent neuroimaging results in humans support this account, showing striatal activity during the selection of immediate rewards, and OFC activity when participants suppressed this choice in favour of a later delayed reward (McClure *et al.*, 2004).

Thus our model suggests that the core decision-making deficit in OFC patients is in assigning reinforcement value to decisions based on the magnitude and recent temporal context of expected outcomes. In tasks involving only probability learning (i.e., reward magnitudes are the same for all choice), the Frank and Claus (2006) model predicts that the OFC is helpful for rapid initial acquisition of reinforcement contingencies, but that the BG system is sufficient after further training (Frank and Claus, 2006). Such a pattern was recently confirmed in a study in which OFC patients showed deficits relative to controls only in the early acquisition phase of a probabilistic classification task (Chase *et al.*, 2008). In healthy participants, individual differences in rapid acquisition of stimulus–reinforcement contingencies and trial-to-trial behavioural adjustments as a function of decision outcomes were predicted by the *COMT* gene (Frank *et al.*, 2007a), a marker of prefrontal (and especially orbitofrontal) cortical dopamine levels (Slifstein *et al.*, 2008). Conversely, individual differences in the ability to integrate reinforcement probabilities over many trials, and to discriminate between subtly different probabilities, were predicted by genes controlling striatal (but not prefrontal) dopamine function (Frank *et al.*, 2007a; Frank *et al.*, 2009; Klein *et al.*, 2007).

In contrast to OFC patients, the models predict that non-medicated PD patients should show intact working memory maintenance of reward value information in OFC, given that this frontal area interacts with ventral striatal areas that are spared in mild to moderate PD. However, medication is thought to 'overdose' the ventral striatal-OFC circuit with DA (e.g., Cools *et al.*, 2001). In addition to blocking DA dips in the BG, this could prevent the encoding of large losses in OFC, while sparing or even enhancing the magnitudes of gain representations (Frank and Claus, 2006). Taken together, this combination could present an attractive account for the documented effects of medication on gambling behaviour in PD (Dodd *et al.*, 2005).

15.3.3 Attention deficit/hyperactivity as a disorder of action selection

ADHD is a common childhood-onset psychiatric condition, characterised by age-inappropriate levels of inattention and/or hyperactivity–impulsivity. In order to qualify for either of the three subtypes of ADHD (inattentive subtype, hyperactive/impulsive subtype, or combined subtype), symptoms need to be present in more than one situation (for example, at home and in school), and need to cause impairment. Prevalence estimates of ADHD in childhood range from 3–7% (APA, 1994). Although overall ADHD symptoms decline with age, about 15% of individuals who had ADHD in childhood meet full criteria for ADHD in adulthood, and 65% meet partial criteria (see Faraone *et al.*, 2006, for a meta-analysis). ADHD is a highly heritable psychiatric condition, with a mean heritability estimate of 76% (Faraone *et al.*, 2005). In candidate-gene studies, a number of dopaminergic and serotonergic genes are implicated in ADHD, each with a small effect size (Faraone *et al.*, 2005). The majority of children respond well to psychostimulant drugs, with at least 62% showing significant and clinically relevant reduction of ADHD symptoms (Swanson *et al.*, 2001). Neuropsychological studies have mainly focused on the domain of executive function. Deficits in response inhibition, although modest in effect size, are reliably associated with ADHD (Willcutt *et al.*, 2005). Recent research has shown that motivational processes may, independent of response inhibition deficits, account for a large proportion of ADHD symptoms (Solanto *et al.*, 2001).

Here we consider the possibility that ADHD can be thought of as a disorder in action selection. A dysfunction in the circuitry that selects among multiple possible actions and inappropriately facilitates one of them is conceptually attractive for capturing the core deficits in both motor and cognitive domains. The complexity of behavioural phenotypes and associated neurobiological underpinnings motivates the need for solid theoretical foundations (Pennington, 2005) that ultimately may help determine when and when not to medicate a symptomatic child. Below we review evidence for dysfunctional BG-frontal circuits in ADHD, before elaborating potential implications of action selection models. We then show how incorporation of norepinephrine function into the model can account for additional effects of the disorder.

15.3.3.1 Structural, functional, and dopamine effects in attention deficit/hyperactivity disorder

A recent review of the literature on structural brain imaging in ADHD clearly demonstrates reduced volumes in frontal and striatal areas (Krain and Castellanos, 2006), despite earlier reported inconsistent effects in smaller sample studies (Baumeister and Hawkins, 2001). A longitudinal study with a large sample has clearly demonstrated reductions in brain volumes in ADHD (Castellanos et al., 2002), including volumes of total cerebrum, cerebellum, gray and white matter of the frontal lobes, and caudate nucleus compared to healthy controls. These findings remained unchanged after controlling for differences in estimated IQ, height, weight, and handedness, and were not due to the use of psychostimulant drugs. Reduced brain volumes remained stable over time, suggesting that they result from early genetic or environmental influences. Interestingly, by age 16 caudate volumes in ADHD were no longer smaller than those in healthy controls, potentially related to the reduction in ADHD motor symptoms with increasing age.

Functional MRI studies in children and adolescents with ADHD have mainly focused on studying the neural basis of executive control, and response inhibition, in particular. Generally, fMRI studies have found reduced activation in striatal and frontal regions in ADHD during executive control and response inhibition, using tasks such as the Go/No-Go task, stop task, and Stroop colour–word test (Booth et al., 2005; Durston et al., 2003; Rubia et al., 1999; Vaidya et al., 2005; Zang et al., 2005). Often, reduced frontostriatal activation in ADHD is accompanied by increased activation in other brain areas (Bush et al., 2005). Studies with medication-naive subjects demonstrate that frontostriatal abnormalities during executive control are not due to the use of psychostimulant drugs (e.g., Vaidya et al., 2005).

While a complex disorder such as ADHD is unlikely to be a function of any single neurotransmitter, DA dysfunction of some sort – whether genetic, environmental, or a combination – is relatively undisputed. In a comprehensive review of the behavioural and biological bases of ADHD, the authors concluded that hypodopaminergic function in three striato-cortical loops are responsible for core deficits in DA-mediated reinforcement and extinction (Sagvolden et al., 2005). This is supported by observations that both children and adults with ADHD have abnormally high densities of dopamine transporters (DATs) which remove too much DA from the synapse (Dougherty et al., 1999; Krause et al., 2000). Some have suggested that low levels of tonic DA are accompanied by *heightened* phasic DA signals in ADHD, due to reduced DA stimulation onto inhibitory autoreceptors that regulate phasic release (Grace, 2001; Solanto, 2002). However, other data suggest that stimulants do not have preferential action on autoreceptors (Ruskin et al., 2001). Further, Sagvolden and colleagues (2005) propose that the tight regulation between tonic and phasic DA is dysregulated in ADHD, resulting in stunted phasic DA responses, despite low tonic DA. The latter position fits with findings showing that methylphenidate (Ritalin) increases extracellular striatal DA (Volkow *et al.*, 2001), and enhances synaptic DA associated with phasic responses (Schiffer *et al.*, 2006).

Given the above changes in fronto-striatal and DA systems, it is natural to consider ADHD as a disorder of action selection. Although it is premature to develop a computational model for all the sources of brain dysfunction in ADHD, we can nevertheless consider the implications of the models with respect to the hypodopaminergic hypothesis, which has gained increasing support. We then consider symptoms that are more readily explained by noradrenergic mechanisms, as informed by other computational models.

By virtue of interactions with multiple frontal circuits, it is possible that a single 'low-level' mechanism may be responsible for diverse behavioural effects at the systems level. Thus reduced BG/DA signals would decrease Go signals for reinforcing appropriate motor behaviours and raise the threshold for when to update information to be robustly maintained in the PFC. In the BG/PFC models, cortico-cortical projections allow a stimulus present in the environment to reach and activate PFC, independent of BG signals. BG Go signals are particularly important for selectively updating task-relevant information to be maintained once a stimulus is no longer present, and in the face of ongoing distractors (Frank *et al.*, 2001; Hazy *et al.*, this volume; McNab and Klingberg, 2007; Moustafa *et al.*, 2008b; O'Reilly and Frank, 2006). Reduced BG Go signals would therefore lead to apparent hypofrontality due to reductions in selective maintenance of task-relevant information, and increased distractibility. Further, we think the same functions may apply with respect to ventral striatum and the updating of orbitofrontal representations of reward value (see Frank and Claus, 2006). In this case, DA reductions would lead to impairments in the updating and subsequent maintenance of large magnitude, long term reward values to bias behaviour and motivational processes.

15.3.3.2 Reward anticipation and temporal discounting in attention deficit/hyperactivity disorder

The hypo-DA hypothesis suggests that ADHD may be associated with a core deficit in motivational/reward processes. In a recent fMRI study, adolescents with ADHD had reduced activation in the ventral striatum when they anticipated receiving monetary gains (Scheres *et al.*, 2007). This reduction in activation may potentially reflect reduced DA levels in ventral striatum in ADHD, and was selectively associated with symptoms of impulsivity/hyperactivity (and not inattention), suggesting distinct neural mechanisms for the subtypes. In certain contexts, ADHD is associated with unusually strong preferences for small immediate rewards over larger delayed rewards (e.g., Sonuga-Barke, 2005), consistent with reduced striatal Go signals for updating long-term motivational information in OFC. However, we note that reduced phasic DA and ventral striatal activity should also be associated with reduced sensitivity to immediate rewards (e.g., McClure *et al.*, 2004). Given the above-mentioned reduction in ventral striatum during reward anticipation in ADHD (Scheres *et al.*, 2007), one might expect relative impairments in sensitivity to immediate rewards. Indeed, evidence for this position was found in a study on temporal reward discounting in children and adolescents with ADHD

(Scheres *et al.*, 2006). In this case, controls were actually more susceptible to immediate rewards: whereas 73% of ADHD subjects maximised their gains by waiting for the large delayed reward, only 58% of the control group did so. We are currently testing the contexts in which preferences are seen for immediate versus delayed rewards in ADHD, and the role of ventral striatum.

A clear model prediction is that reduced BG phasic DA should lead to Go learning deficits, which should be ameliorated by DA medications, in the probabilistic learning task described above. The BG/PFC models suggest that BG/DA reductions should also lead to impaired Go signals for updating task-relevant information into prefrontal working memory representations (Frank and O'Reilly, 2006). We found consistent evidence for this account in adult ADHD subjects tested on and off their regular dose of stimulant medications (Frank *et al.*, 2007c).

15.3.3.3   Norepinephrine in attention deficit/hyperactivity disorder and action selection

One problem with this hypodopaminergic hypothesis usually unaddressed is why low DA levels in ADHD are not associated with Parkinson-like symptoms? First, it is likely that DA levels are much lower in PD patients, given that PD symptoms do not arise until DA is depleted by approximately 75–80%. Second, whereas PD patients simply do not have DA available, DA synthesis and availability is intact in ADHD. Thus patients may try to self-regulate their DA levels, as seen in rats who self administer more amphetamine when DA receptors are partially blocked pharmacologically (Robbins and Everitt, 1999). Intriguingly, patients may achieve these DA increases by their own hyperactive movements: matrix neurons of the striatum that are involved in motor selection can disinhibit DA release via striatonigral projections (e.g., Joel and Weiner, 2000).

Moreover, while DA depletion is the core biological deficit in PD, norepinephrine (NE) regulation is also thought to be disturbed in ADHD (e.g., Biederman and Spencer, 1999). The NE hypothesis is particularly well supported by the beneficial effects of the specific NE transporter blocker atomoxetine (e.g., Swanson *et al.*, 2006). In this regard, it is instructive to consider effects of NE in physiological recordings, behaviour, and computational models of action selection. While a complete review of this topic is outside the scope of this chapter, we present a brief summary (see Aston-Jones and Cohen, 2005 for a full review).

Like DA cells, firing states of NE-releasing neurons in the locus coeruleus (LC) come in both tonic and phasic modes. In both electrophysiological recordings and computational simulations, LC cells release phasic NE bursts during periods of focused attention, infrequent target detection, and good task performance. This phasic NE burst is thought to reflect the outcome of the response selection process and serves to facilitate response execution. In contrast, poor performance is accompanied by a high tonic, but low phasic, state of LC firing. The authors simulated the effects of these LC modes on action selection such that NE modulated the gain of the activation function in cortical response units (Usher *et al.*, 1999). They showed that phasic NE release leads to 'sharper' cortical representations and a tighter distribution of reaction times, whereas the high tonic state was associated with more RT variability. They further hypothesised that increases in tonic NE during poor performance may be adaptive, in that it may enable the representation of alternate competing cortical actions during exploration of new behaviours.

This model has clear implications for ADHD. It is possible that ADHD participants are stuck with an intermediate high tonic, low phasic level of NE, leading to a preponderance of multiple cortical representations. This would result in variability in reaction times and distractibility of prefrontal representations. Indeed, studies that report within-subject RT variability consistently show that children with ADHD are more variable in their responses (Castellanos *et al.*, 2005; Leth-Steensen *et al.*, 2000). Notably, a recent study showed that this variability correlated with NE, but not dopamine function, as measured in urinary metabolites (Llorente *et al.*, 2006).

15.3.3.4   Simulating norepinephrine function in action selection and attention deficit/hyperactivity disorder

Given the purported role of the BG circuitry in action selection, one might question whether these cortical NE selection effects would apply within the context of a BG–cortical model. To explore potential interactions between the systems, here we added a simulated LC layer to the standard BG model. In particular, we explored the effects of LC modulation of premotor cortical units, which reciprocally project back to the LC (Figure 15.3a). Following Usher *et al.* (1999), the gain (i.e., slope) of the activation function (see Appendix A) of premotor units was dynamically modulated in proportion to the LC unit response. This effectively makes cortical units more responsive and can increase the network signal to noise ratio, as hypothesised for NE (Servan-Schreiber *et al.*, 1990). Thus, whereas the default gain parameter of cortical units in our modelling framework is statically set to 600 (O'Reilly and Munakata, 2000), we applied a dynamic function to the gain γ of the premotor units:

$$\gamma = 20 + 600 * (LC_{act})^2 \tag{15.1}$$

where LC_{act} ranges from 0 to 1 and is the mean ratecoded activation of LC units. The resulting gain is relatively low when LC activity is low, and increases monotonically with increasing LC/NE activation. Low LC firing, and hence premotor gain, is associated with low-level noisy activation of multiple noisy premotor unit responses (some noise is essential for initial exploration of possible actions; Frank, 2005). However, sufficient premotor activity can elicit a phasic burst in LC unit activity via top-down premotor-LC excitatory projections. Critically, this LC burst does not occur unless premotor activity is sufficiently high, such that it is preferentially elicited by stimulus-evoked activity (due to prior stimulus-response learning from the input layer to the desired cortical response). This depiction is consistent with (1) the idea that LC phasic responses reflect the outcome of a task-related decisional process (Aston-Jones and Cohen, 2005), (2) observations that frontal cortical stimulation produces excitatory LC phasic responses (Jodo *et al.*, 1998), and (3) electrophysiological recordings showing that frontal activity precedes LC phasic activity (Jodo *et al.*, 2000).

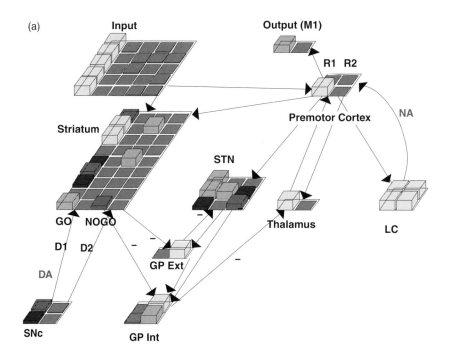

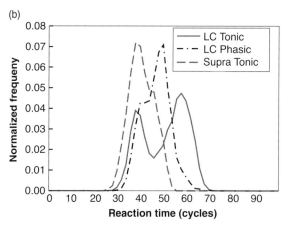

Figure 15.3 (a) Standard BG model with additional simulated cortical norepinephrine (NE) effects. The locus coeruleus (LC) fires phasically upon sufficient activation of premotor units, and reciprocally modulates the gain of these units via simulated NE. (b) Normalised distributions for model reaction times (number of processing cycles before the BG facilitates a response). The LC phasic mode is associated with a narrow distribution of reaction times, peaking at 50 cycles. In the tonic mode (LC units tonically 50% activated), noisy activation of both competing responses leads to a bimodal distribution and overall more RT variability, potentially explaining the variability seen in ADHD. In the 'supra-tonic' mode, LC activity was tonically set to maximal firing rates, leading to faster RTs. (c) Percent accuracy in the same simple choice discrimination simulated to generate (b). High accuracy is seen in the phasic LC mode, as premotor responsiveness is boosted only in the presence of a task-relevant stimulus-response association. The tonic and supra-tonic modes lead to activation of alternative noisy responses, which can get inappropriately executed if not dynamically modulated by the LC.

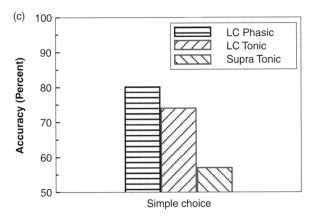

Figure 15.3 (*cont.*)

Moreover, the cortically driven phasic LC/NE burst reciprocally enhances the gain γ of cortical units, which facilitates the execution of the most active cortical representation by allowing it to dominate over alternative noisy units. This conceptualisation is very similar to (and indeed was motivated by) that of Aston-Jones and Cohen (2005), but applies even in our model of BG–cortical interactions. Although the BG circuitry enables the facilitation of a desired response together with suppression of alternative responses, the LC/NE effects modulate the strength of inputs to the BG system. As previously noted, the BG cannot select a desired response itself – this response has to first be sufficiently activated (or 'considered') in cortex before the BG can gate its execution (Frank, 2005). As we shall see, the LC/NE modulation affects both *when* the target response is facilitated and in some cases, *which* response is ultimately executed.

To demonstrate the effect of LC modulation, we trained our BG model to select between two alternative choices in response to two separate input stimuli A and B (each represented by a column of input units). Response 1 ($R1$) was positively reinforced (DA burst) on 80% of stimulus A trials, whereas $R2$ was reinforced on 80% of stimulus B trials. Networks were trained for 50 trials and easily learned this simple discrimination via standard BG/DA modulation of Go and NoGo learning. Note that as $R1$ is increasingly facilitated by the BG in response to stimulus A, Hebbian learning principles drive learning directly between the stimulus A input and $R1$ premotor cortical units (see above). In this manner, premotor cortex comes to eventually preferentially activate $R1$ ($R2$) in response to stimulus A (B), even prior to BG facilitation; this premotor action selection is subsequently facilitated by LC cortical modulation, BG Go signals, and associated thalamic activation.

To assess the effects of NE on reaction times, we generated an RT distribution across 5000 trials of response selection after the initial training (with no further learning). The stimulus onset was delayed by approximately 30 cycles on each trial, so that during initial network processing, premotor activity only reflected intrinsic noise to a similar degree in $R1$ and $R2$ units. In the intact simulations, baseline tonic LC firing was low ($LC_{act} = 0.05$), and the resulting low gain of premotor units prevented noisy responses from being amplified. Once the stimulus (e.g., A) was presented, the appropriate response ($R1$) became preferentially active as a function of direct cortico-cortical weights. The resulting LC burst further facilitated the active $R1$ representation, which was then swiftly accompanied by a BG Go signal. This scenario leads to a narrow distribution of model reaction times across trials (Figure 15.3b).

To simulate dysfunctional NE processes (as hypothesised for ADHD), baseline tonic LC firing was set high (50% maximal firing rate), and premotor to LC connections were severed so that no phasic burst was elicited. In this case, the intermediate gain of premotor units led to enhanced noisy activity in the absence of a task-relevant stimulus. Thus in stimulus A trials, if $R1$ happened to be more active than $R2$ when the A was presented, $R1$ was immediately facilitated. However, if $R2$ was more active due to noise, then the stimulus-evoked $R1$ activity led to increased response conflict in the premotor cortex, due to simultaneous $R1/R2$ representations. This cortical conflict in turn led to longer decision times (see above discussion on the STN and Frank, 2006). The overall pattern across trials led to a bimodal RT distribution for the LC tonic mode, with more variable and somewhat overall slower RTs, as is observed in ADHD. This bimodal distribution demonstrates that the same mechanisms responsible for simultaneous activation of responses (and associated exploratory behaviour) can lead to reaction time variability. Supporting this conjecture, in our recent study with adult ADHD participants, we found a very strong correlation between greater RT variability and erratic trial-to-trial switching when participants were off their stimulant medications (Frank *et al.*, 2007c). Both of these measures were captured by increased tonic NE in the model.

Finally, to demonstrate the need for a phasic (dynamic) LC signal, and to control for overall differences in premotor unit gain, we ran a 'supra-tonic' condition in which the LC units were tonically active at maximal firing rates (to the same degree as maximal phasic activity). The tonically high gain led to overall more excitable premotor units and facilitated response execution, as evidenced by faster RTs. However, the lack of an adaptive LC signal for modulating premotor gain caused networks to be more likely to choose the incorrect response (in this case, $R2$) when stimulus A arrives (Figure 15.3c). This is because if noise happens to favour $R2$ the high cortical gain can cause inappropriate execution.

Figure 15.4 shows RT variability and accuracy as a continuous function of LC tonic firing rate, in addition to the simple tonic (0.5) and supra-tonic (1.0) levels. Overall, intermediate tonic levels are associated with high RT variability, due to noisy activation of competing responses. As tonic levels increase, noisy activity is likely to be facilitated, and RT variability decreases at the cost of increased error rates. This trade-off demonstrates the need for an adaptive LC modulated gain.

Overall these simulations (and recent empirical studies) show that a dynamic LC signal is adaptive in modulating motor responsiveness. Simulated LC/NE dysfunction leads to more variable reaction times and simultaneous activation of multiple responses, which could lead to exploratory behaviour. This may provide a framework by which to formally investigate NE-related deficits in ADHD.

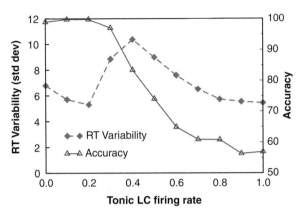

Figure 15.4 RT variability (standard deviation of processing cycles) and accuracy as a function of tonic LC firing rate (with no phasic response). Intermediate tonic LC levels are associated with high RT variability, while high tonic (supratonic) levels are associated with narrower distributions, with a cost in accuracy.

The NE account may also help explain response inhibition deficits in ADHD. Phasic LC responses would be expected to occur during the infrequent 'stop-signals' in inhibition tasks, and these may transiently enhance processing in frontal and BG regions that support response inhibition. Supporting this account, increases in NE by atomoxetine leads to enhanced response inhibition in both healthy participants and those with ADHD (Chamberlain *et al.*, 2006; Overtoom *et al.*, 2003). In the BG, NE may enhance Global NoGo signals via excitatory effects in the STN (Arcos *et al.*, 2003), and/or in inferior frontal regions which in turn activate STN (Aron and Poldrack, 2006).

In sum, both DA and NE effects can account for various deficits in action selection in ADHD. It is plausible that NE effects are primarily involved in response inhibition and variability, while DA effects are involved in motivational/reward processes, supporting the independence of these symptoms (Solanto *et al.*, 2001). We are hopeful that further investigation of the interactions between BG/DA and cortical NE effects in our models will provide increasingly refined predictions that can be tested empirically

15.4   Clinical implications of basal ganglia modelling

The classical model of BG connections as described by Gerfen (1992) and others has had great heuristic value in explaining the effects of DA replacement therapy and surgical intervention in PD. This model was also of importance in the development of deep brain stimulation utilising the subthalamic nucleus as the target (Benabid, 2003). The evolution of this static anatomical model to a network-based model which encompasses phasic changes in DA release, multiple feedback loops with variable delays, and plastic changes based on Hebbian principles, will be important in further refining our clinical approaches to BG disorders, including the associated deficits in decision making. The effect of chronic D2 stimulation by D2 agonists to selectively diminish the impact of negative consequences while leaving positive rewards intact can easily be extrapolated to predict gambling addictions in patients treated with D2 selective agonists. Indeed such effects have been reported in patients with PD and must be considered during the initiation of DA replacement therapy. As these drugs are now finding widespread use in the treatment of restless leg syndrome (which affects more than 5% of the general population), the effect on decision making has important public health ramifications. Patients with ADHD have increased risk of developing substance abuse later in life (e.g., Disney et al., 1999). Modelling of BG circuitry will be helpful in the development of specific psychological tests to screen for potentially adverse effects of new dopaminergic drugs on behaviour. Deep brain stimulation of BG structures has become the treatment of choice for advanced PD and is increasingly being applied to other neurological conditions including experimental trials in Tourette's syndrome and obsessive–compulsive disorder (Dell'Osso et al., 2005). Despite the increasingly common use of this technique, basic questions remain regarding the optimum clinical application. For example, treatment of PD can be accomplished by deep brain stimulation in either the internal segment of globus pallidus (GPi) or the STN with nearly equal improvement in motor function (Anderson et al., 2005). Modelling suggests that there may be important non-motor, cognitive effects of deep brain stimulation that differ between these two anatomical targets. Interference of STN function, which is thought to provide a Global NoGo signal in the face of multiple competing incipient motor plans, could lead to impulsive behaviour. At a low-level, this could lead to an 'impulsive gait' that has been observed in some patients where improvement in motor function leads to increased falls if the patient fails to account for residual difficulties with balance. At a higher level, there may be impairment of fronto-striatal circuitry that leads to more global behavioural impulsivity. Clinical trials that test the predictions of BG modelling on decision making will be critical for selecting the proper therapeutic option.

Selective modulation of BG pathways using advanced neurobiological techniques hold great potential for psychiatric treatment. One important challenge that remains is the separation of effects on motor and cognitive circuits. DA receptor blocking drugs that are useful in the treatment of schizophrenia and mania have a crossover effect in the motor portion of the striatum where serious side-effects such as Parkinsonism and tardive dyskinesia occur. Similarly, DA replacement therapy and deep brain stimulation for movement disorders leads to neuropsychiatric side-effects due to action in the cognitive and emotional circuits of the caudate and ventral striatum. One approach to this problem would be to capitalise on the wide anatomic separation of motor, cognitive, and emotional circuits in the striatum. A viral gene transfer vector that selectively modulates the indirect or direct pathway could be constructed based on cell type specific promoters coupled to ion channel-modifying sequences which shape the electrical output response of the neuron. When injected into the relevant area of the striatum, this agent would selectively control the Go or NoGo pathway in a limited sector of basal ganglia loops. This scenario may not be too far in the future since viral gene transfer vectors that modify synaptic transmission in the indirect pathway are currently in Phase 1 trials (see Luo et al., 2002).

Having a robust computational model will be critical for exploring how these effects interact at the dynamic systems level, and in response to changing task demands. For example, while the described effect of DA on striatal D1 receptors is excitatory, this is only true for spiny neurons that are in the 'up-state' (i.e., high membrane potential driven by synaptic activity); in contrast, D1 activation is inhibitory on those in the 'down-state' (Hernandez-Lopez et al., 1997). Because this state-dependent modulation is inherently dynamic in nature, simulation of tonic D1 modulation effects (as in viral gene transfers) will be critical for assessing their potential benefit. It is acknowledged that therapies that operate at the ion channel level will require more detailed biophysical models than those presented here (e.g., Wolf et al., 2005). Nevertheless, abstractions of these functions may still be useful in the systems level of analysis. In our BG model, the D1 membrane potential modulation is simulated by a contrast enhancement function on the gain of Go neuron activation, such that the most active units are strengthened while less active units are suppressed. In this manner, Go learning during DA bursts is restricted to the most active synapses, and is prevented in more weakly active synapses (Frank, 2005) – allowing the model to learn Go to a response only in an appropriate stimulus context. See Cohen et al. (2002) for a similar discussion on the theoretical benefits of interplay between abstract and biophysically detailed models of D1 receptor effects in prefrontal cortex.

Appendix A   Basic basal ganglia model

This appendix outlines the implementational details for the 'basic' BG model described in the main text (i.e., without the orbitofrontal cortex). For details of the OFC model, please see Frank and Claus (2006). The model code, written in PDP[++], can be obtained by emailing the corresponding author at mfrank@u.arizona.edu. For animated video captures of model dynamics during response selection and learning, please see www.u.arizona.edu/~mfrank/BGmodel_movies.html.

Implementational details

The model is implemented using the Leabra framework (O'Reilly, 2001; O'Reilly and Munakata, 2000). Leabra uses point neurons with excitatory, inhibitory, and leak conductances contributing to an integrated membrane potential, which is then thresholded and transformed via an $x/(x + 1)$ sigmoidal function to produce a rate code output communicated to other units (discrete spiking can also be used, but produces noisier results). Each layer uses a k-winners-take-all (kWTA) function that computes an inhibitory conductance that keeps roughly the k-most active units above firing threshold and keeps the rest below threshold.

The membrane potential V_m is updated as a function of ionic conductances g with reversal (driving) potentials E as follows:

$$\Delta V_m(t) = \tau \sum_c gc(t)\overline{gc}(E_c - V_m(t)) \tag{A.1}$$

with three channels c corresponding to: e excitatory input; l leak current; and i inhibitory input. Following electrophysiological convention, the overall conductance is decomposed into a time-varying component $g_c(t)$ computed as a function of the dynamic state of the network, and a constant $\overline{gc}$ that controls the relative influence of the different conductances. The equilibrium potential can be written in a simplified form by setting the excitatory driving potential (E_e) to 1 and the leak and inhibitory driving potentials (E_l and E_i) of 0:

$$V_m^\infty = \frac{g_e \overline{g_e}}{g_e \overline{g_e} + g_l \overline{g_l} + g_i \overline{g_i}} \qquad (A.2)$$

which shows that the neuron is computing a balance between excitation and the opposing forces of leak and inhibition.

This equilibrium form of the equation can be understood in terms of a Bayesian decision making framework (O'Reilly and Munakata, 2000). The excitatory net input/conductance $g_e(t)$ or η_j is computed as the proportion of open excitatory channels as a function of sending activations times the weight values:

$$\eta_j = g_e(t) = \langle x_i w_{ij}\rangle = \frac{1}{n}\sum_i x_i w_{ij}. \qquad (A.3)$$

The inhibitory conductance is computed via the kWTA function described in the next section, and leak is a constant.

Activation communicated to other cells (y_j) is a thresholded (Θ) sigmoidal function of the membrane potential with gain parameter γ:

$$y_j(t) = \frac{1}{\left(1 + \dfrac{1}{\gamma[V_m(t) - \Theta]_+}\right)} \qquad (A.4)$$

where $[x]+$ is a threshold function that returns 0 if $x < 0$ and x if $x > 0$. Note that if it returns 0, we assume $y_j(t) = 0$, to avoid dividing by 0. As it is, this function has a very sharp threshold, which interferes with graded learning mechanisms (e.g., gradient descent). To produce a less discontinuous deterministic function with a softer threshold, the function is convolved with a Gaussian noise kernel ($\mu = 0$, $\sigma = 0.005$), which reflects the intrinsic processing noise of biological neurons:

$$y_j^*(x) = \int_{-\infty}^{\infty} \frac{1}{\sqrt{2\pi}\sigma} e^{-z^2/(2\sigma^2)} y_j(z - x)dz \qquad (A.5)$$

where x represents the $[V_m(t) - \Theta]+$ value, and $y_j^*(x)$ is the noise-convolved activation for that value.

Connectivity and mechanics of the basal ganglia model

The network's job is to select one of four responses (R1–R4), depending on the task and the sensory input. At the beginning of each trial, incoming stimuli directly activate a response in premotor cortex (PMC). However, these direct connections are not strong enough to elicit a robust response in and of themselves; they also require bottom-up support from the thalamus. The job of the BG is to integrate stimulus input with the dominant response selected by PMC, and based on what it has learned in past experience, either facilitate (Go) or suppress (NoGo) that response.

Within the overall thalamocortical circuit, there are multiple parallel subloops that are isolated from each other, separately modulating the different responses. This allows for the BG to *selectively* gate one response, while continuing to suppress the other(s). The striatum is divided into two distributed subpopulations. The columns on the left are 'Go' units for each of the potential responses, and have simulated D1 receptors. The columns on the right are 'NoGo' units, and have simulated D2 receptors. The Go columns project only to the corresponding column in the GPi (direct pathway), and the NoGo columns to the external segment of globus pallidus (GPe; indirect pathway). Both GPe columns inhibit the associated column in GPi, so that striatal Go and NoGo activity have opposing effects on GPi. Finally, each column in GPi tonically inhibits the associated column of the thalamus, which is reciprocally connected to premotor cortex. Thus, if Go activity is stronger than NoGo activity for R1, the left column of GPi will be inhibited, removing tonic inhibition (i.e., disinhibiting) of the corresponding thalamus unit, and facilitating its execution in premotor cortex.

The above parallel and convergent connectivity is supported by anatomical evidence discussed in Frank (2005). The network architecture simply supports the existence of connections, but how these ultimately influence behaviour depends on their relative strengths. The network starts off with random weights and representations in both the BG and cortical layers are learned. Input to striatal units are initialised with random synaptic weights with a Gaussian distribution, with $\mu = 0.5$, $\sigma = 0.25$. Distributed activity within each striatal column enables different Go and NoGo representations to develop for various stimulus configurations during the course of training. Therefore whereas the different columns in the striatum represent Go and NoGo units for different responses, the different rows enable units with different initial random synaptic connectivity to become specialised to respond to particular stimulus–response conjunctions.

Subthalamic nucleus connectivity with other basal ganglia and cortical structures

The STN was included in the model in accordance with known constraints on its connectivity in BG circuitry (Frank, 2006). First, the STN forms part of the 'hyperdirect' pathway, so-named because cortical activity targets the STN, which directly excites GPi, bypassing the striatum altogether (Nambu *et al.*, 2000). Thus initial activation of the STN by cortex leads to an initial excitatory drive on the already tonically active GPi, effectively making the latter structure more inhibitory on the thalamus, and therefore less likely to facilitate a response. Further, the STN gets increasingly excited with increasing cortical activity. Thus, if several competing responses are activated, the STN sends a stronger 'Global NoGo' signal which allows the BG system to fully consider all possible options before sending a Go signal to facilitate the most adaptive one.

Second, the STN and GPe are reciprocally connected in a negative feedback loop, with the STN exciting the GPe and the GPe inhibiting the STN (Parent and Hazrati, 1995). The connections from STN to GPe are diffuse, and therefore are not likely to be

Table 15.1 BG model parameters for model described in Frank (2006), which selects among four responses and includes the STN. First two rows indicate standard default parameters used in hundreds of simulations with Leabra software; these parameters are used in the model except where noted with an * for specialised functions of the BG layers. Striatal units have a higher firing threshold θ and higher gain γ during DA bursts ('+DA'), and lower γ during DA dips, to simulate contrast enhancement and reduction (Frank, 2005). GP and STN units have higher than normal E_l, $\overline{g_i}$ and V_{rest}, leading to tonic baseline activity in the absence of synaptic input. Thal units have high $\overline{g_i}$ and low $\overline{g_e}$ enabling a default strong inhibition from BG output and only allowing top-down excitatory activity if disinhibited, thereby serving a gating function. Premotor units have Gaussian noise added to the membrane potential, learn with a slow learning rate via purely Hebbian learning. k (kWTA) parameters are shown for striatum and premotor areas, which have within-layer lateral inhibition.

Param	Value	Param	Value	Param	Value	Param	Value	Param	Value	Param	Value
E_l	0.15	$\overline{g_l}$	0.10	E_i	0.15	$\overline{g_i}$	1.0	E_e	1.00	$\overline{g_e}$ 1.0	1.0
V_{rest}	0.15	Θ	0.25	γ	600	k_{hebb}	.01	ε	.001		
Striatum	(k = 4)	$\overline{g_l}$	1.0*	Θ, +DA	0.32*	γ	2500*	γ, +DA	10000*	γ, –DA	300*
GPi		E_l	0.28*	$\overline{g_l}$	3.0*	V_{rest}	0.26*				
GPe		E_l	0.26*	$\overline{g_l}$	1.0*	V_{rest}	0.26*				
STN		E_l	0.2*	$\overline{g_l}$	1.0*	V_{rest}	0.25*				
Thal		$\overline{g_l}$	1.7*	$\overline{g_e}$	0.5*						
Premotor	(k = 3)	ε	1e-5*	k_{hebb}	1*	V_m noise	μ = .0015	V_m noise	σ = .0015		

involved in suppressing a specific response. Of the STN neurons that project to GPe, the vast majority also project to GPi (Sato *et al.*, 2000). In the model, each STN neuron receives projections from two randomly selected GPe neurons. This was motivated by data showing that multiple GPe neurons converge on a single STN neuron (Karachi *et al.*, 2005). In contrast, each GPe neuron receives diffuse projections from all STN neurons (but with randomly different synaptic weights).

Inhibition within and between layers

Inhibition *between* layers (i.e., for GABAergic projections between BG layers) is achieved via simple unit inhibition, where the inhibitory current g_i for the unit is determined from the net input of the sending unit.

For *within* layer lateral inhibition (used in the striatum and premotor cortex), Leabra uses a kWTA function to achieve inhibitory competition among units within each layer (area). The kWTA function computes a uniform level of inhibitory current for all units in the layer, such that the $k + 1$th most excited unit within a layer is generally below its firing threshold, while the kth is typically above threshold. Activation dynamics similar to those produced by the kWTA function have been shown to result from simulated inhibitory interneurons that project both feedforward and feedback inhibition (O'Reilly and Munakata, 2000). Thus, although the kWTA function is somewhat biologically implausible in its implementation (e.g., requiring global information about activation states and using sorting mechanisms), it provides a computationally effective approximation to biologically plausible inhibitory dynamics. Table 15.1 gives BG model parameters for the model described in Frank (2006).

kWTA is computed via a uniform level of inhibitory current for all units in the layer as follows:

$$g_i = g_{k+1}^{\Theta} + q(g_k^{\Theta} - g_{k+1}^{\Theta})$$

(A.6)

where $0 < q < 1$ (0.25 default used here) is a parameter for setting the inhibition between the upper bound of $g_k{}^{\Theta}$ and the lower bound of g_{k+1}^{Θ}. These boundary inhibition values are computed as a function of the level of inhibition necessary to keep a unit right at threshold:

$$g_i^{\Theta} = \frac{g_e^* \bar{g}_e (E_e - \Theta) + g_i \bar{g}_l (E_l - \Theta)}{\Theta - E_i}$$

(A.7)

where g_e^* is the excitatory net input

Two versions of kWTA functions are typically used in Leabra. In the kWTA function used in the Striatum, g_k^{Θ} and g_{k+1}^{Θ} are set to the threshold inhibition value for the kth and $k + 1$ th most excited units, respectively. Thus, the inhibition is placed to allow k units to be above threshold, and the remainder below threshold.

The premotor cortex uses the *average-based* kWTA version, g_k^{Θ} is the average g_i^{Θ} value for the top k most excited units, and g_{k+1}^{Θ} is the average of g_i^{Θ} for the remaining $n - k$ units. This version allows for more flexibility in the actual number of units active depending on the nature of the activation distribution in the layer and the value of the q parameter (which is set to default value of 0.6). This flexibility is necessary for the premotor units to have differential levels of activity during settling (depending on whether or not a single response has been facilitated), and also allows greater activity in high-conflict trials.

Learning

Synaptic connection weights were trained using a reinforcement learning version of Leabra. The learning algorithm involves two phases, and is more biologically plausible than standard error backpropagation. In the *minus phase*, the network settles into activity states based on input stimuli and its synaptic weights, ultimately 'choosing' a response. In the *plus phase*, the network resettles in the same manner, with the only difference being a change in simulated dopamine: an increase of substantia nigra pars compacta (SNc) unit firing from 0.5 to 1.0 for correct responses, and a decrease to zero SNc firing for incorrect responses (Frank, 2005).

For learning, Leabra uses a combination of error-driven and Hebbian learning. The error-driven component is the symmetric midpoint version of the GeneRec algorithm (O'Reilly, 1996), which is functionally equivalent to the deterministic Boltzmann machine and contrastive Hebbian learning (CHL), computing a simple difference of a pre and postsynaptic activation product across these two phases. For Hebbian learning, Leabra uses essentially the same learning rule used in competitive learning or mixtures-of-Gaussians which can be seen as a variant of the Oja normalisation (Oja, 1983). The error-driven and Hebbian learning components are combined additively at each connection to produce a net weight change.

The equation for the Hebbian weight change is:

$$\Delta_{hebb} w_{ij} = x_i^+ y_j^+ - y_j^+ w_{ij} = y_j^+ (x_i^+ - w_{ij}) \tag{A.8}$$

and for error-driven learning using CHL:

$$\Delta_{err} w_{ij} = \left(x_i^+ y_j^+\right) - \left(x_i^- y_j^-\right) \tag{A.9}$$

which is subject to a soft-weight bounding to keep within the 0–1 range:

$$\Delta_{sberr} w_{ij} = [\Delta_{err}] + (1 - w_{ij}) + [\Delta_{err}] - w_{ij}. \tag{A.10}$$

The two terms are then combined additively with a normalised mixing constant k_{hebb}:

$$\Delta w_{ij} = \varepsilon[k_{hebb}(\Delta_{hebb}) + (1 - k_{hebb})(\Delta_{sberr})]. \tag{A.11}$$

Appendix B   Additional details for locus coeruleus/norepinephrine simulations

The model used for these simulations was a standard BG model selecting among two responses, with additional LC modulation. In the standard model, there are 25 input units of which a subset represent particular stimulus cues. For example, in the LC simulations stimulus A was represented by the first column of input units, whereas stimulus B was represented by the fourth column of units. The Striatum and premotor cortex have to learn to facilitate the appropriate response associated with the combination of input features. Each response in premotor cortex is represented by a column of two units. This allows for a more distributed representation of motor activity, because activation of $R1$ involves high unit activity in both motor units of the same column.

As specified in the main text, the effect of LC activation was to dynamically modulate the gain γ of the activation function of premotor units according to the following function.

$$\gamma = 20 + 600 * (LC_{act})^2 \tag{B.1}$$

where LC_{act} ranges from 0 to 1 and is the mean rate-coded activation of LC units, and γ affects the activation function in Equation (A.3). To demonstrate the effects of tonic/phasic activation on noise in premotor units, the Gaussian distribution for noise in the membrane potential of these units was increased to $\mu = .0035$ $\sigma = 0.005$. The stimulus input was also delayed at the beginning of each trial by approximately 30 cycles. This was accomplished by 'soft-clamping' the input layer, so that input units did not activate immediately upon trial onset but instead needed to integrate activity with a slow membrane potential time constant $\tau = 0.1$ and input gain $= 0.05$. These effects combine to produce more noisy activity in premotor units prior to stimulus processing, which is more realistic than standard conditions in which each trial is initiated with no activation in the network and input stimuli can then directly activate appropriate units in the rest of the network without having to compete with ongoing noise. The effects show that phasic

LC activity can therefore make the model more robust to noise, while tonic activity is associated with more sensitivity to noise.

Reaction times were calculated by determining when a particular response was facilitated by the BG. This amounts to recording from thalamic neurons, which facilitate the execution of responses upon being disinhibited by BG Go signals. RTs were calculated as the number of network processing cycles until one of the thalamic unit activity reaches 0.9 (90% maximal value). The actual value does not much matter because thalamic neurons are completely silent until disinhibited, at which point they increase sharply in activity. Similar patterns were observed when recording from M1, but in that case it is less clear how to define when a response is actually executed, because M1 units become somewhat active from initial premotor activity prior to BG facilitation, so the thalamic units provide a more discrete RT readout.

References

Albin, R. L., A. B. Young, and J. B. Penney (1989). The functional anatomy of basal ganglia disorders. *Trends Neurosci.* **12**: 366–75.

Alexander, G. E., M. R. DeLong, and P. L. Strick (1986). Parallel organization of functionally segregated circuits linking basal ganglia and cortex. *Annu. Rev. Neurosci.* **9**: 357–81.

Anderson, V. C., K. J. Burchiel, P. Hogarth, J. Favre, and J. P. Hammerstad (2005). Pallidal vs. subthalamic nucleus deep brain stimulation in Parkinson disease. *Archiv. Neurol.* **62**(4): 554–60.

APA (ed.) (1994). *Diagnostic and Statistical Manual of Mental Disorders*, 4th edn. Washington DC: American Psychiatric Press.

Arcos, D., A. Sierra, A. Nuez, *et al.* (2003). Noradrenaline increases the firing rate of a subpopulation of rat subthalamic neurones through the activation of alpha 1-adrenoceptors. *Neuropharmacol.* **45**(8): 1070–9.

Aron, A. R. and R. A. Poldrack (2006). Cortical and subcortical contributions to stop signal response inhibition: role of the subthalamic nucleus. *J. Neurosci.* **26**: 2424–33.

Aston-Jones, G. and J. D. Cohen (2005). An integrative theory of locus coeruleus-norepinephrine function: adaptive gain and optimal performance. *Annu. Rev. Neurosci.* **28**: 403–50.

Aubert, I., I. Ghorayeb, E. Normand, and B. Bloch (2000). Phenotypical characterization of the neurons expressing the D1 and D2 dopamine receptors in the monkey striatum. *J. Comp. Neurol.* **418**: 22–32.

Baumeister, A. A. and M. F. Hawkins (2001). Incoherence of neuroimaging studies of attention deficit/hyperactivity disorder. *Clin. Neuropharmacol.* **24**(1): 2–10.

Baunez, C., T. Humby, D. M. Eagle, *et al.* (2001). Effects of STN lesions on simple versus choice reaction time tasks in the rat: preserved motor readiness, but impaired response selection. *Eur. J. Neurosci.* **13**: 1609–16.

Baunez, C. and T. W. Robbins (1998). Bilateral lesions of the subthalamic nucleus induce multiple deficits in an attentional task in rats. *Eur. J. Neurosci.* **9**(10): 2086–99.

Bayer, H. M., B. Lau, and P. W. Glimcher (2007). Statistics of midbrain dopamine neuron spike trains in the awake primate. *J. Neurophysiol.* **98**(3): 1428–39.

Bechara, A., H. Damasio, D. Tranel, and S. W. Anderson (1998). Dissociation of working memory from decision making within the human prefrontal cortex. *J. Neurosci.* **18**, 428–37.

Beiser, D. G. and J. C. Houk (1998). Model of cortical-basal ganglionic processing: encoding the serial order of sensory events. *J. Neurophysiol.* **79**: 3168–88.

Benabid, A. L. (2003). Deep brain stimulation for Parkinson's disease. *Curr. Opin. Neurobiol.* **13**(6): 696–706.

Bergman, H., T. Wichmann, B. Karmon, and M. R. DeLong (1994). The primate subthalamic nucleus. II. Neuronal activity in the MPTP model of Parkinsonism. *J. Neurophysiol.* **72**: 507–20.

Biederman, J. and T. Spencer (1999). Attention-deficit/hyperactivity disorder (ADHD) as a noradrenergic disorder. *Biol. Psychiatry* **46**(9): 1234–42.

Bodi, N., S. Keri, H. Nagy, *et al.* (2009). Reward-learning and the novelty-seeking personality: a between- and within-subjects study of the effects of dopamine agonists on young Parkinson's patients. *Brain*, **132**(9), 2385–95.

Booth, J. R., D. D. Burman, J. R. Meyer, *et al.* (2005). Larger deficits in brain networks for response inhibition than for visual selective attention in attention deficit/hyperactivity disorder (ADHD). *J. Psychol. Psyc.* **46**(1): 94–111.

Brown, J., D. Bullock, and S. Grossberg (2004). How laminar frontal cortex and basal ganglia circuits interact to control planned and reactive saccades. *Neural Networks* **17**: 471–510.

Bush, G., E. M. Valera, and L. J. Seidman (2005). Functional neuroimaging of attention-deficit/hyperactivity disorder: a review and suggested future directions. *Biol. Psychiat.* **57**(11): 1273–84.

Castellanos, F. X., P. P. Lee, W. Sharp, *et al.* (2002). Developmental trajectories of brain volume abnormalities in children and adolescents with attention-deficit/hyperactivity disorder. *JAMA* **288**: 1740–8.

Castellanos, F. X., E. J. S. Sonuga-Barke, A. Scheres, *et al.* (2005). Varieties of attention-deficit/hyperactivity disorder-related intra-individual variability. *Biol. Psychiat.* **57**: 1416–23.

Centonze, D., Picconi, B., Gubellini, P., Bernardi, G., and Calabresi, P. (2001). Dopaminergic control of synaptic plasticity in the dorsal striatum. *Eur. J. Neurosci.* **13**: 1071–7.

Centonze, D., A. Usiello, C. Costa, *et al.* (2004). Chronic haloperidol promotes corticostriatal long-term potentiation by targeting dopamine d2l receptors. *J. Neurosci.* **24**: 8214–22.

Chamberlain, S. R., U. Müller, A. D. Blackwell, *et al.* (2006). Neurochemical modulation of response inhibition and probabilistic learning in humans. *Science* **311**(5762): 861–3.

Chase, H. W., L. Clark, C. E. Myers, *et al.* (2008). The role of the orbitofrontal cortex in human discrimination learning. *Neuropsychologia* **46**(5): 1326–37.

Choi, W. Y., P. D. Balsam, and J. C. Horvitz (2005). Extended habit training reduces dopamine mediation of appetitive response expression. *J. Neurosci.* **25**(29): 6729–33.

Cohen, J. D., T. S. Braver, and J. W. Brown (2002). Computational perspectives on dopamine function in prefrontal cortex. *Curr. Opin. Neurobiol.* **12**: 223–9.

Cohen, M. X. and M. J. Frank (2009). Neurocomputational models of basal ganglia function in learning, memory and choice. *Behav. Brain Res.* **199**(1): 141–56.

Cools, R., L. Altamirano, and M. D'Esposito (2006). Reversal learning in Parkinson's disease depends on medication status and outcome valence. *Neuropsychologia* **44**: 1663–73.

Cools, R., R. A., Barker, B. J. Sahakian, and T. W. Robbins (2001). Enhanced or impaired cognitive function in Parkinson's disease as a function of dopaminergic medication and task demands. *Cereb. Cortex* **11**: 1136–43.

Creese, I., D. R. Sibley, M. W. Hamblin, and S. E. Leff (1983). The classification of dopamine receptors: relationship to radioligand binding. *Annu. Rev. Neurosci.* **6**: 43–71.

Dayan, P. (2001). Levels of analysis in neural modeling. In *Encyclopedia of Cognitive Science*. London: MacMillan Press.

Delgado, M. R., M. M. Miller, S. Inati, and E. A. Phelps (2005). An fMRI study of reward-related probability learning. *NeuroImage* **24**: 862–73.

Delgado, M. R., L. E. Nystrom, C. Fissell, D. C. Noll, and J. A. Fiez (2000). Tracking the hemodynamic responses to reward and punishment in the striatum. *J. Neurophysiol.* **84**: 3072.

Dell'Osso, B., A. C. Altamura, A. Allen, and E. Hollander (2005). Brain stimulation techniques in the treatment of obsessive-compulsive disorder: current and future directions. *CNS Spectr.* **10**(12): 966–79, 983.

Disney, E. R., I. J. Elkins, M. McGue, and W. G. Iacono (1999). Effects of ADHD, conduct disorder, and gender on substance use and abuse in adolescence. *Am. J. Psychiat.* **156**(10): 1515–21.

Dodd, M. L., K. J. Klos, J. H. Bower, *et al.* (2005). Pathological gambling caused by drugs used to treat Parkinson disease. *Archiv. Neurol.* **62**(9): 1377–81.

Dougherty, D. D., Bonab, A. A., Spencer, T. J., Rauch, S. L., Madras, B. K., and Fischman, A. J. (1999). Dopamine transporter density in patients with attention deficit hyperactivity disorder. *Lancet* **354**: 2132–3.

Durston, S., N. T. Tottenham, K. M. Thomas, *et al.* (2003). Differential patterns of striatal activation in young children with and without ADHD. *Biol. Psychiat.* **53**: 871–8.

Faraone, S. V., J. Biederman, and E. Mick (2006). The age-dependent decline of attention deficit hyperactivity disorder: a meta-analysis of follow-up studies. *Psychol. Med.* **36**(2): 159–65.

Faraone, S. V., R. H. Perlis, A. E. Doyle, *et al.* (2005). Molecular genetics of attention-deficit/hyperactivity disorder. *Biol. Psychiat.* **57**(11): 1313–23.

Fellows, L. K. and Farah, M. J. (2003). Ventromedial frontal cortex mediates affective shifting in humans: evidence from a reversal learning paradigm. *Brain* **126**: 1830–7.

Frank, M. J. (2005). Dynamic dopamine modulation in the basal ganglia: a neurocomputational account of cognitive deficits in medicated and non-medicated parkinsonism. *J. Cogn. Neurosci.* **17**: 51–72.

Frank, M. J. (2006). Hold your horses: a dynamic computational role for the subthalamic nucleus in decision making. *Neural Networks* **19**: 1120–36.

Frank, M. J. and E. D. Claus (2006). Anatomy of a decision: striato-orbitofrontal interactions in reinforcement learning, decision making, and reversal. *Psychol. Rev.* **113**(2): 300–326.

Frank, M. J., B. Doll, J. Oas-Terpstra, and F. Moreno (2009). Prefrontal and striatal dopaminergic genes predict individual differences in exploration and exploitation. *Nature Neurosci.* **12**: 1062–8.

Frank, M. J., B. Loughry, and R. C. O'Reilly (2001). Interactions between the frontal cortex and basal ganglia in working memory: a computational model. *Cogn. Affect. Behav. Neurosci.* **1**: 137–60.

Frank, M. J., A. A. Moustafa, H. M. Haughey, T. Curran, and K. E. Hutchison (2007a). Genetic triple dissociation reveals multiple roles for dopamine in reinforcement learning. *Proc. Nat. Acad. Sci. USA* **104**: 16311–6.

Frank, M. J. and R. C. O'Reilly (2006). A mechanistic account of striatal dopamine function in human cognition: psychopharmacological studies with cabergoline and haloperidol. *Behav. Neurosci.* **120**: 497–517.

Frank, M. J., J. Samanta, A. A. Moustafa, and S. J. Sherman (2007b). Hold your horses: impulsivity, deep brain stimulation, and medication in Parkinsonism. *Science* **318**: 1309–12.

Frank, M. J., A. Santamaria, R. C. O'Reilly, and E. Willcutt (2007c). Testing computational models of dopamine and noradrenaline dysfunction in attention deficit/hyperactivity disorder. *Neuropsychopharmacol.* **32**: 1583–99.

Frank, M. J., L. C. Seeberger, and R. C. O'Reilly, (2004). By carrot or by stick: cognitive reinforcement learning in Parkinsonism. *Science* **306**: 1940–3.

Frank, M. J., B. S. Woroch, and T. Curran (2005). Error-related negativity predicts reinforcement learning and conflict biases. *Neuron* **47**: 495–501.

Gerfen, C. R. (1992). The neostriatal mosaic: multiple levels of compartmental organization in the basal ganglia. *Annu. Rev. Neurosci.* **15**: 285–320.

Gerfen, C. R. (2003). D1 dopamine receptor supersensitivity in the dopamine-depleted striatum animal model of Parkinson's disease. *Neuroscientist* **9**: 455–62.

Goto, Y. and A. A. Grace (2005). Dopaminergic modulation of limbic and cortical drive of nucleus accumbens in goal-directed behavior. *Nature Neurosci.* **8**: 805–12.

Grace, A. A. (2001). Psychostimulant actions on dopamine and limbic system function: relevance to the pathophysiology and treatment of ADHD. In *Stimulant Drugs and ADHD: Basic and Clinical Neuroscience*, ed. M. V. Solanto and A. F. T. Arnsten. New York: Oxford University Press, pp. 134–55.

Gurney, K., T. J. Prescott, and P. Redgrave (2001). A computational model of action selection in the basal ganglia. I. A new functional anatomy. *Biol. Cybern.* **84**: 401–10.

Harden, D. G. and A. A. Grace (1995). Activation of dopamine cell firing by repeated L-Dopa administration to dopamine-depleted rats: its potential role in mediating the therapeutic response to L-Dopa treatment. *J Neurosci.* **15**(9): 6157–6166.

Hernandez-Lopez, S., J. Bargas, D. J. Surmeier, A. Reyes, and E. Galarraga (1997). D1 receptor activation enhances evoked discharge in neostriatal medium spiny neurons by modulating an l-type Ca2 + conductance. *J. Neurosci.* **17**: 3334–42.

Hernandez-Lopez, S., T. Tkatch, E. Perez-Garci, *et al.* (2000). D2 dopamine receptors in striatal medium spiny neurons reduce L-type Ca^{2+} currents and excitability via a novel Plc[beta]1-IP3-calcineurin-signaling cascade. *J. Neurosci.* **20**(24): 8987–95.

Hikosaka, K. and M. Watanabe (2000). Delay activity of orbital and lateral prefrontal neurons of the monkey varying with different rewards. *Cereb. Cortex* **10**: 263–71.

Hlbig, T. D., W. Tse, P. G. Frisina, *et al.* (2009). Subthalamic deep brain stimulation and impulse control in Parkinson's disease. *Eur. J. Neurol.* **16**(4), 493–7.

Holland, P. C. and M. Gallagher (2004). Amygdala-frontal interactions and reward expectancy. *Curr. Opin. Neurobiol.* **14**(2): 148–55.

Holroyd, C. B. and M. G. H. Coles (2002). The neural basis of human error processing: reinforcement learning, dopamine, and the error-related negativity. *Psychol. Rev.* **109**: 679–709.

Houk, J. C. (2005). Agents of the mind. *Biol. Cybern.* **92**(6): 427–37.

Houk, J. C., C. Bastianen, D. Fansler, *et al.* (2007). Action selection and refinement in subcortical loops through basal ganglia and cerebellum. *Phil. Trans. Roy. Soc. B, Biol. Sci.* **362**(1485), 1573–83.

Houk, J. C. and S. P. Wise (1995). Distributed modular architectures linking basal ganglia, cerebellum, and cerebral cortex: their role in planning and controlling action. *Cereb. Cortex* **5**: 95–110.

Jodo, E., C. Chiang, and G. Aston-Jones (1998). Potent excitatory influence of prefrontal cortex activity on noradrenergic locus coeruleus neurons. *Neuroscience* **83**: 63.

Jodo, E., Y. Suzuki, and Y. Kayama (2000). Selective responsiveness of medial prefrontal cortex neurons to the meaningful stimulus with a low probability of occurrence in rats. *Brain Res.* **856**(1–2): 68–74.

Joel, D. and I. Weiner (2000). The connections of the dopaminergic system with the striatum in rats and primates: an analysis with respect to the functional and compartmental organization of the striatum. *Neuroscience* **96**: 451.

Kaasinen, V., K. Nagren, J. Hietala, *et al.* (2000a). Extrastriatal dopamine D2 and D3 receptors in early and advanced in Parkinson's disease. *Neurology* **54**: 1482–7.

Kaasinen, V., H. Ruottinen, K. Nagren, *et al.* (2000b). Upregulation of putaminal dopamine D2 receptors in early Parkinson's disease: a comparative PET study with [11C]raclopride and [11C]N-methylspiperone. *J. Nucl. Med.* **41**(1): 65–70.

Kahneman, D. and A. Tversky (1979). Prospect theory: an analysis of decision under risk. *Econometrica* **47**: 263–91.

Karachi, C., J. Yelnik, D. Tand, *et al.* (2005). The pallidosubthalamic projection: an anatomical substrate for nonmotor functions of the subthalamic nucleus in primates. *Movement Disord.* **20**: 172–80.

Klein, T. A., J. Neumann, M. Reuter, *et al.* (2007). Genetically determined differences in learning from errors. *Science* **318**(5856): 1642–45.

Krain, A. L. and F. X. Castellanos (2006). Brain development and ADHD. *Clin. Psychol. Rev.* **26**(4): 433–44.

Krause, K., S. H. Dresel, J. Krause, H. F. Kung, and K. Tatsch (2000). Increased striatal dopamine transporter in adult patients with attention deficit hyperactivity disorder: effects of methylphenidate as measured by single photon emission computed tomography. *Neurosci. Lett.* **285**: 107–110.

Leth-Steensen, C., Z. K. Elbaz, and V. I. Douglas (2000). Mean response times, variability, and skew in the responding of ADHD children: a response time distributional approach. *Acta Psychol.* **104**: 167–90.

Llorente, A. M., R. G. Voigt, C. L. Jensen, *et al.* (2006). Performance on a visual sustained attention and discrimination task is associated with urinary excretion of norepineprhine metabolite in children with attention-deficit/hyperactivity disorder (AD/HD). *Clinical Neuropsychol.* **20**(1): 133–44.

Luo, J., M. G. Kaplitt, H. L. Fitzsimons, *et al.* (2002). Subthalamic gad gene therapy in a Parkinson's disease rat model. *Science* **298**(5592): 425–9.

Mahon, S., G. Casassus, C. Mulle, and S. Charpier (2003). Spike-dependent intrinsic plasticity increases firing probability in rat striatal neurons in vivo. *J. Physiol.* **550**(Pt 3): 947–59.

McAuley, J. H. (2003). The physiological basis of clinical deficits in Parkinson's disease. *Prog. Neurobiol.* **69**: 27–48.

McClure, S. M., D. I. Laibson, G. Loewenstein, and J. D. Cohen (2004). Separate neural systems value immediate and delayed rewards. *Science* **306**: 503–507.

McNab, F. and Klingberg, T. (2007). Prefrontal cortex and basal ganglia control access to working memory. *Nature Neurosci.* **11**(1): 103–107.

Mink, J. W. (1996). The basal ganglia: focused selection and inhibition of competing motor programs. *Prog. Neurobiol.* **50**: 381–425.

Mobini, S., S. Body, M.-Y. Ho, *et al.* (2002). Effects of lesions of the orbitofrontal cortex on sensitivity to delayed and probabilistic reinforcement. *Psychopharmacol.* **160**: 290–8.

Moustafa, A. A., M. X. Cohen, S. J. Sherman, and M. J. Frank (2008a). A role for dopamine in temporal decision making and reward maximization in Parkinsonism. *J. Neurosci.* **28**(47): 12294–304.

Moustafa, A. A., S. J. Sherman, and M. J. Frank (2008b). A dopaminergic basis for working memory, learning, and attentional shifting in Parkinson's disease. *Neuropsychologia* **46**: 3144–56.

Müller, U., T. Wächter, H. Barthel, M. Reuter, and D. Y. von Cramon (2000). Striatal [123i]beta-CIT SPECT and prefrontal cognitive functions in Parkinson's disease. *J. Neural Transm.* **107**: 303–19.

Nambu, A., H. Tokuno, I. Hamada, *et al.* (2000). Excitatory cortical inputs to pallidal neurons via the subthalamic nucleus in the monkey. *J. Neurophysiol.* **84**: 289–300.

Ni, Z., R. Bouali-Benazzouz, D. Gao, A. Benabid, and A. Benazzouz (2000). Changes in the firing pattern of globus pallidus neurons after the degeneration of nigrostriatal pathway are mediated by the subthalamic nucleus in rat. *Eur. J. Neurosci.* **12**: 4338–44.

Nieoullon, A. (2002). Dopamine and the regulation of cognition and attention. *Prog. Neurobiol.* **67**: 53–83.

Oja, E. (1983). A simplified neuron model as a principal component analyzer. *J. Math. Biol.* **15**: 267–73.

O'Reilly, R. C. (1996). Biologically plausible error-driven learning using local activation differences: the generalized recirculation algorithm. *Neural Comput.* **8**(5): 895–938.

O'Reilly, R. C. (2001). Generalization in interactive networks: the benefits of inhibitory competition and Hebbian learning. *Neural Comput.* **13**: 1199–242.

O'Reilly, R. C. and M. J. Frank (2006). Making working memory work: a computational model of learning in the prefrontal cortex and basal ganglia. *Neural Comput.* **18**: 283–328.

O'Reilly, R. C. and Y. Munakata (2000). *Computational Explorations in Cognitive Neuroscience: Understanding the Mind by Simulating the Brain.* Cambridge, MA: MIT Press.

Orieux, G., C. Franois, J. Féger, and E. C. Hirsch (2002). Consequences of dopaminergic denervation on the metabolic activity of the cortical neurons projecting to the subthalamic nucleus in the rat. *J. Neurosci.* **22**: 8762–70.

Overtoom, C. C. E., M. N. Verbaten, C. Kemner, *et al.* (2003). Effects of methylphenidate, desipramine, and l-dopa on attention and inhibition in children with attention deficit hyperactivity disorder. *Behav. Brain Res.* **145**: 7–15.

Parent, A. and L. N. Hazrati (1995). Functional anatomy of the basal ganglia. II. the place of subthalamic nucleus and external pallidum in basal ganglia circuitry. *Brain Res. Rev.* **20**: 128–54.

Pasupathy, A. and E. K. Miller (2005). Different time courses for learning-related activity in the prefrontal cortex and striatum. *Nature* **433**: 873–6.

Pennington, B. F. (2005). Toward a new neuropsychological model of attention-deficit/hyperactivity disorder: subtypes and multiple deficits. *Biol. Psychiat.* **57**(11): 1221–3.

Pothos, E. N., V. Davila, and D. Sulzer (1998). Presynaptic recording of quanta from midbrain dopamine neurons and modulation of the quantal size. *J. Neurosci.* **18**(11): 4106–18.

Remy, P., P. L. Jackson, and M. J. Ribeiro (2000). Relationships between cognitive deficits and dopaminergic function in the striatum of Parkinson's disease patients: a pet study. *Neurology* **54**: A372.

Rinne, U. K., A. Laihinen, J. O. Rinne, *et al.* (1990). Positron emission tomography demonstrates dopamine D2 receptor supersensitivity in the striatum of patients with early Parkinson's disease. *Move. Disord.* **5**(1): 55–9.

Robbins, T. W. and B. J. Everitt (1999). Drug addiction: bad habits add up. *Nature* **398**(6728): 567–70.

Robertson, G. S., S. R. Vincent, and H. C. Fibiger (1992). D1 and d2 dopamine receptors differentially regulate c-fos expression in striatonigral and striatopallidal neurons. *Neuroscience* **49**: 285–96.

Rolls, E. T. (1996). The orbitofrontal cortex. *Phil. Trans. Roy. Soc. B Biol. Sci.* **351**: 1433–44.

Rubia, K., S. Overmeyer, E. Taylor, *et al.* (1999). Hypofrontality in attention deficit/hyperactivity disorder during higher-order motor control: a study with functional MRI. *Amer. J. Psychiat.* **156**: 891–6.

Ruskin, D. N., D. A. Bergstrom, A. Shenker, *et al.* (2001). Drugs used in the treatment of attention-deficit/hyperactivity disorder affect postsynaptic firing rate and oscillation without preferential dopamine autoreceptor action. *Biol. Psychiat.* **49**(4): 340–50.

Sagvolden, T., E. B. Johansen, H. Aase, and V. A. Russell (2005). A dynamic developmental theory of attention-deficit/hyperactivity disorder (ADHD) predominantly hyperactive/impulsive and combined subtypes. *Behav. Brain Sci.* **28**(3): 397–419; Discussion: 419–68.

Sato, F., M. Parent, M. Levesque, and A. Parent (2000). Axonal branching pattern of neurons of the subthalamic nucleus in primates. *J. Comp. Neurol.* **424**: 142–52.

Satoh, T., S. Nakai, T. Sato, and M. Kimura (2003). Correlated coding of motivation and outcome of decision by dopamine neurons. *J. Neurosci.* **23**: 9913–23.

Scheres, A., M. Dijkstra, E. Ainslie, *et al.* (2006). Temporal and probabilistic discounting of rewards in children and adolescents: effects of age and ADHD symptoms. *Neuropsychologia* **44**: 2092–103.

Scheres, A., M. P. Milham, B. Knutson, and F. X. Castellanos (2007). Ventral striatal hyporesponsiveness during reward anticipation in attention-deficit/hyperactivity disorder. *Biol. Psychiat.* **61**(5): 720–4.

Schiffer, W. K., N. D. Volkow, J. S. Fowler, *et al.* (2006). Therapeutic doses of amphetamine or methylphenidate differentially increase synaptic and extracellular dopamine. *Synapse* **59**(4): 243–51.

Schoenbaum, G. and M. Roesch (2005). Orbitofrontal cortex, associative learning, and expectancies. *Neuron* **47**(5): 633–6.

Schultz, W. (2002). Getting formal with dopamine and reward. *Neuron* **36**: 241–263.

Seger, C. A. and C. M. Cincotta (2006). Dynamics of frontal, striatal, and hippocampal systems during rule learning. *Cereb. Cortex* **16**(11): 1546–5.

Servan-Schreiber, D., H. Printz, and J. D. Cohen (1990). A network model of catecholamine effects: gain, signal-to-noise ratio, and behavior. *Science* **249**: 892–5.

Shen, W., M. Flajolet, P. Greengard, and D. J. Surmeier (2008). Dichotomous dopaminergic control of striatal synaptic plasticity. *Science* **321**(5890): 848–51.

Shohamy, D., C. E. Myers, S. Grossman, J. Sage, and M. A. Gluck (2004). The role of dopamine in cognitive sequence learning: evidence from Parkinson's disease. *Behav. Brain Res.* **156**(2): 191–9.

Slifstein, M., B. Kolachana, E. H. Simpson, *et al.* (2008). COMT genotype predicts cortical-limbic D1 receptor availability measured with [11C]NNC112 and PET. *Molec. Psychiat.* **13**(8): 821–7.

Smith-Roe, S. L. and A. E. Kelley (2000). Coincident activation of NMDA and dopamine D1 receptors within the nucleus accumbens core is required for appetitive instrumental learning. *J. Neurosci.* **20**: 7737–42.

Solanto, M. V. (2002). Dopamine dysfunction in AD/HD: integrating clinical and basic neuroscience research. *Behav. Brain Res.* **130**: 65–71.

Solanto, M. V., H. Abikoff, E. Sonuga-Barke, *et al.* (2001). The ecological validity of delay aversion and response inhibition as measures of impulsivity in AD/HD: a supplement to the NIMH multimodal treatment study of AD/HD. *J. Abnorm. Child Psych.* **29**(3): 215–28.

Sonuga-Barke, E. J. S. (2005). Causal models of attention-deficit/hyperactivity disorder: from common simple deficits to multiple developmental pathways. *Biol. Psychiat.* **57**(11): 1231–8.

Surmeier, D. J., J. Ding, M. Day, Z. Wang, and W. Shen (2007). D1 and D2 dopamine-receptor modulation of striatal glutamatergic signaling in striatal medium spiny neurons. *Trends Neurosci.* **30**(5): 228–35.

Swainson, R., R. D. Rogers, B. J. Sahakian, *et al.* (2000). Probabilistic learning and reversal deficits in patients with Parkinson's disease or frontal or temporal lobe lesions: possible adverse effects of dopaminergic medication. *Neuropsychologia* **38**: 596–612.

Swanson, C. J., K. W. Perry, S. Koch-Krueger, *et al.* (2006). Effect of the attention deficit/hyperactivity disorder drug atomoxetine on extracellular concentrations of norepinephrine and dopamine in several brain regions of the rat. *Neuropharmacology* **50**: 755–60.

Swanson, J. M., H. C. Kraemer, S. P. Hinshaw, *et al.* (2001). Clinical relevance of the primary findings of the MTA: success rates based on severity of ADHD and odd symptoms at the end of treatment. *J. Am. Acad. Child Psy.* **40**(2): 168–79.

Terman, D., J. E. Rubin, A. C. Yew, and C. J. Wilson (2002). Activity patterns in a model for the subthalamopallidal network of the basal ganglia. *J. Neurosci.* **22**: 2963–76.

Usher, M., J. D. Cohen, D. Servan-Schreiber, J. Rajkowski, and G. Aston-Jones (1999). The role of locus coeruleus in the regulation of cognitive performance. *Science* **283**: 549–54.

Vaidya, C. J., S. A. Bunge, N. M. Dudukovic, *et al.* (2005). Altered neural substrates of cognitive control in childhood ADHD: evidence from functional magnetic resonance imaging. *Am. J. Psychiat.* **162**(9): 1605–13.

Volkow, N. D., G. J. Wang, J. S. Fowler, *et al.* (2001). Therapeutic doses of methylphenidate significantly increase extracellular dopamine in the human brain. *J. Neurosci.* **21**: RC121.

Wallis, J. D. and E. K. Miller (2003). From rule to response: neuronal processes in the premotor and prefrontal cortex. *J. Neurophysiol.* **90**: 1790–806.

Wichmann, T. and M. R. DeLong (2003). Pathophysiology of Parkinson's disease: the MPTP primate model of the human disorder. *Ann. NY Acad. Sci.* **991**: 199–213.

Willcutt, E. G., A. E. Doyle, J. T. Nigg, S. V. Faraone, and B. F. Pennington (2005). Validity of the executive function theory of attention-deficit/hyperactivity disorder: a meta-analytic review. *Biol. Psychiat.* **57**: 1336–46.

Witt, K., U. Pulkowski, J. Herzog, *et al.* (2004). Deep brain stimulation of the subthalamic nucleus improves cognitive flexibility but impairs response inhibition in Parkinson disease. *Arch. Neurol.* **61**: 697–700.

Wolf, J. A., J. T. Moyer, M. T. Lazarewicz, *et al.* (2005). NMDA/AMPA ratio impacts state transitions and entrainment to oscillations in a computational model of the nucleus accumbens medium spiny projection neuron. *J. Neurosci.* **25**(40): 9080–95.

Wu, Q., M. E. A. Reith, Q. D. Walker, *et al.* (2002). Concurrent autoreceptor-mediated control of dopamine release and uptake during neurotransmission: an in vivo voltammetric study. *J. Neurosci.* **22**: 6272–81.

Yeung, N., M. M. Botvinick, and J. D. Cohen (2004). The neural basis of error detection: conflict monitoring and the error-related negativity. *Psychol. Rev.* **111**(4): 931–59.

Zang, Y.-F., Z. Jin, X.-C. Weng, *et al.* (2005). Functional MRI in attention-deficit hyperactivity disorder: evidence for hypofrontality. *Brain Dev.* **27**(8): 544–50.

16 Biologically constrained action selection improves cognitive control in a model of the Stroop task

Tom Stafford and Kevin N. Gurney

Summary

The Stroop task is a paradigmatic psychological task for investigating stimulus conflict and the effect this has on response selection. The model of Cohen *et al.* (1990) has hitherto provided the best account of performance in the Stroop task, but there remains certain key data that it fails to match. We show that this failure is due to the mechanism used to perform final response selection – one based on the diffusion model of choice behaviour (Ratcliff, 1978). We adapt the model to use a selection mechanism which is based on the putative human locus of final response selection, the basal ganglia/thalamo-cortical complex (Redgrave *et al.*, 1999). This improves the match to the core human data and, additionally, makes it possible for the model to accommodate, in a principled way, additional mechanisms of cognitive control that enable better fits to the data. This work prompts a critique of the diffusion model as a mechanism of response selection, and the features that any response mechanism must possess to provide adaptive action selection. We conclude that the consideration of biologically constrained solutions to the action selection problem is vital to the understanding and improvement of cognitive models of response selection.

16.1 Introduction

The Stroop task provides a thoroughly explored experimental framework for investigating cognitive aspects of selection. In this task, subjects have to name the ink colour of word-strings which can themselves spell out the name of a colour. When the ink-colour and the word-name contradict each other response selection is slowed and is more prone to error (compared to conditions where the word-name is neutral or is congruent with respect to the ink-colour). This is 'the Stroop Effect'. A simple reversal of the task, that of reading the word-name and ignoring the ink-colour, does not produce an opposite effect (a 'reverse Stroop' effect).

The asymmetrical interaction of the colour-naming and word-naming processes can be interpreted within an automaticity framework (MacLeod, 1991; Posner and Snyder,

Modelling Natural Action Selection, eds. Anil K. Seth, Tony J. Prescott and Joanna J. Bryson.
Published by Cambridge University Press. © Cambridge University Press 2012.

1975). Here, word-reading is an 'automatic' or 'overlearnt', response which is triggered on stimulus presentation and difficult to interrupt, and colour-naming is a controlled process which is not automatic and is liable to interference from word-reading. Variations on the basic Stroop task have been successful in clarifying the nature of automatic processing (Besner and Stolz, 1999; Besner, Stolz, and Boutilier, 1997; Blais and Besner, 2007; Dishon-Berkovits and Algom, 2000; Durgin, 2000).

Here, however, we wish to focus on the Stroop task as defining a process of selection. The Stroop task has a long history of use in the investigation of aspects of response selection at a cognitive level (Macleod, 1991) and, more recently, at the neural level (MacLeod and MacDonald, 2000). In particular, while early processing of stimulus information is clearly important to an understanding of the Stroop task, the final response uttered on each trial is subject to the constraints imposed by a response or decision mechanism, which must translate internal cognitive states into motor action.

Much progress has been made in investigating decision mechanisms in simple two-alternative choice tasks. Mathematical models of such simple decisions are able to accurately predict the patterns of reaction times (RTs) and errors across task variations, and there is a considerable history in psychology of their development and refinement (Luce, 1986; Ratcliff and Smith, 2004). More recently it has been possible to connect these models with neurophysiological data (Ratcliff et al., 2003; Reddi et al., 2003) and with an information theoretic foundation for optimal decision making (Bogacz et al., 2006; Bogacz et al., this volume). These developments promise an exciting period of cross-fertilisation between neurobiological and psychological perspectives on simple decisions (Gold and Shadlen, 2007; Opris and Bruce, 2005; Platt, 2002; Smith and Ratcliff, 2004). The current work investigates how one instance of this class of model serves selection in a model of the more complex Stroop task.

An additional perspective on decision making is supplied by workers in neuroscience, animal behaviour, ethology, and robotics who have defined, and explored solutions to, the problem of *action selection*: the resolution of conflicts between competing requests for behavioural expression through a final common motor path (Redgrave et al., 1999).

The aim of the present work was to determine whether a biologically plausible model of the putative locus of action selection in humans (the basal ganglia) could work as the response mechanism in a model of a cognitive task (the Stroop task). This is therefore a first step in making links between possible neural substrates for action selection, neural correlates of decision making, and cognitive processes of selection.

16.2   Modelling the Stroop task

In a seminal paper, Cohen et al. (1990) described a model of processing in the Stroop task and variants.

This simple connectionist model (hereafter 'the Cohen model') involves the translation of a localist input representation into a response representation, via a feed-forward two-layer network trained with standard backpropagation. The architecture is shown in Figure 16.1. The main features of this network are:

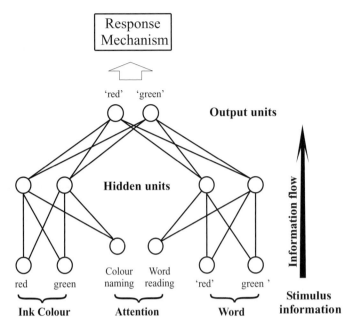

Figure 16.1 Architecture of the Cohen model.

1. Differential training of the network: word inputs are presented at ten times the frequency of colour inputs during training. This results in a stronger weighting of signals representing this aspect of the stimulus.
2. Attentional sensitisation: the network implements attention as an additional input which offsets a bias (in effect a default inhibition) on all hidden units. This interacts with the sigmoidal output function of the units so that moderately sized colour or word input signals do not result in a commensurate increase in output, unless presented in combination with attentional input. Signals in the word-processing pathway are, however, large enough to partially overcome the default inhibition without the aid of attentional input.
3. RTs are generated by the dynamics of a response mechanism that works with evidence accumulation: the two output units of the network are taken to indicate, at each time step, the evidence favouring each response. This evidence is compared and the difference accumulated, until the total crosses a threshold, when a response is said to have been made.

The current work focuses on the third element above: the response mechanism and its role in determining overall model behaviour.

The Cohen model matches the basic Stroop data very well (see Figure 16.2). Not only does the model capture the quantitative difference that word-reading is faster than colour-naming, and unaffected by the word information, but it also matches the asymmetry between the size of the interference effect (the slowing of colour-naming due to contradictory word-information) and the facilitation effect (the speeding of colour-naming due to compatibility with the word-information). All the stimulations presented,

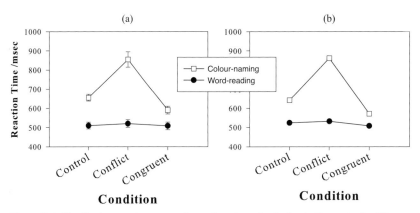

Figure 16.2 The fundamental pattern of reaction times in the basic Stroop tasks. There are two tasks: word-reading (filled circles) and colour-naming (unfilled squares). Within each task there are three possible conditions; in the congruent condition the word and the colour agree, in the conflict condition the word and the colour disagree, in the control condition the irrelevant element is neutral with respect to the target. Empirical data, (a) from Dunbar and MacLeod (1984) for which standard error bars are shown, and (b) simulation data from replication of model of Cohen *et al.* (1990).

both our model and our replication of Cohen's model, are shown run without added noise, since this does not affect the mean results.

In addition to matching the fundamental data, the model gives an implementational definition of automaticity: automaticity arises from greater strength of processing. In a connectionist framework this means stronger weightings between stimulus and response (as in the Cohen model), or additional connections between modules involved in stimulus response translation (as in other connectionist models of Stroop processing, Herd *et al.*, 2006; Phaf *et al.*, 1990; Zhang *et al.*, 1999). Either way the implication is that there is no sharp dichotomy between 'automatic' processes and 'controlled' processes, and, additionally, that other quantitative differences, such as response time differences, arise out of this single fundamental mechanistic difference.

A plausible alternative theory of Stroop processing – and of automatic processing in general – is that more automatic processes are those in which pre-response processing is faster. This theory suggests that Stroop interference is due to the response evoked by the (contradictory) word element of the stimulus arriving at some response bottleneck earlier, creating slower selection of the opposite (and correct) response when it arrives there (we can posit that in a connectionist network this would be reflected by faster transference times between stimulus input and the model response mechanism which arbitrates action selection). This theory may be tested in so-called stimulus-onset asynchrony (SOA) experiments. These involve the two elements of the conventional Stroop stimulus, the word and colour, being presented asynchronously. This manipulation allows either element to appear before the other and thus, it is assumed, to be given a 'headstart' in perceptual processing.

The experimental data are shown in Figure 16.3a. By convention SOAs which involve the to-be-ignored element being presented first are labelled negative. Clearly no amount

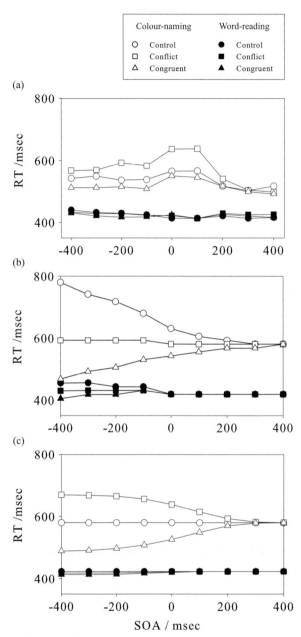

Figure 16.3 Empirical data, (a) for the Stroop tasks with stimulus-onset asynchrony (SOA) (from Glaser and Glaser, 1982). Simulation data, (b) replication of Cohen *et al*. (1990), (c) using the basal ganglia response mechanism. Negative SOAs represent the irrelevant element of the stimulus appearing before the target element, positive SOAs represent the target element appearing before the irrelevant element.

of headstart for colour-information (i.e., at negative SOAs) allows it to interfere with word-reading (Glaser and Glaser, 1982), demonstrating that the automaticity of word-reading is not a consequence of enhanced speed of processing. For colour-naming, the word element causes interference if it appears at any point before colour processing is finished (up to 300 ms after the appearance of the colour element – close to the asymptotic limit for RTs). Additionally, the appearance of the word before the colour always causes interference, however long the subject is given to accommodate to the presence of the word. This, and other results which contradict the automaticity as speed-of-processing account (Dunbar and MacLeod, 1984), leave the automaticity as strength-of-processing account more preferable (this is not to say that strength-of-processing accounts do not imply that automatic processes will be faster than controlled processes – they do – rather they merely assert that speed of processing is a byproduct of a more fundamental distinction between the two types of processes rather than being causative in itself).

The original simulation data for the SOA manipulation within the Cohen model are shown in Figure 16.3b. The Cohen model simulates the correct relative ordering of the RTs in all conditions with respect to the empirical data. Cohen *et al.* (1990) note some discrepancy between their simulation and the model – first, that in the simulations colour information does interfere with word reading, albeit marginally, and that, second, the influence of word information on colour reading is not reduced but increases for SOAs before -200 ms. These discrepancies would not contradict the empirical data, and hence a strength of processing account, if the size of these effects was limited to that shown over the range originally tested by Cohen *et al.* (1990). The size of the interference and facilitation effects are not, however – as Cohen *et al.* (1990) suggest – asymptotic with increasingly negative SOA (as shown in Figure 16.4). Given this, it is of concern that the primary model of the automaticity-based account of Stroop processing, the Cohen model, is not able to simulate the primary data which falsifies the speed-of-processing account but instead produces a pattern of RTs which would, if true, appear to validate a speed-of-processing account.

16.2.1 Limitations of the Cohen model with stimulus-onset asynchrony are failures of response selection

Our replication of Cohen *et al.*'s (1990) model shows that, beyond the range of data of SOA values they originally present, the trends visible in the original data continue so that the model behaves inconsistently with the strength-of-processing account and consistently with the experimentally disproved speed-of-processing account of automaticity in the Stroop task (see Figure 16.4).

Consider the change in the simulated RTs as SOA gets more negative – as the to-be-ignored element of the stimulus appears increasingly before the to-be-responded-to element. For the colour-naming task in the conflict condition the model RT increases as the word element slows selection based on the colour. Eventually, beyond –1300 ms, the word is presented early enough to prompt a response on its own. This response will be an incorrect one, since in the conflict condition the word is opposite to the colour. RTs now start to decrease with increasingly negative SOAs because the RT is defined as the

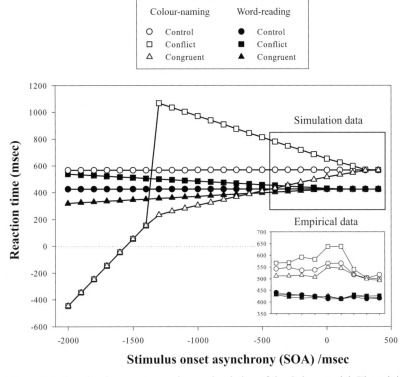

Figure 16.4 The stimulus-onset asynchrony simulation of the Cohen model. The original range of data shown by Cohen *et al.* (1990) is demarcated by the box. The simulation data corresponds roughly to the empirical data over this range (−400 to +400 ms) but beyond that diverges.

time between the onset of the to-be-responded-to stimulus element and the occurrence of selection. So RT eventually falls below zero because selection occurs *before* the onset of the colour (this is highlighted in Figure 16.4 by the point at which the RT lines cross the dotted line representing zero on the RT axis). If the word is congruent to the colour information then there is comparable interference, but this reveals itself as a speeding of the correct response (which likewise falls below zero RT beyond –1500 ms). Note that from here the time between the onset of the irrelevant element and selection is constant, so that beyond this point the rate of the decrease in RT becomes a function of the decrease in SOA, not of changes in model output.

For the same fundamental reasons, in the word-naming task the conflict and congruent conditions diverge in the same way (albeit over a longer time span, the point at which word-reading times fall below zero SOA is not shown here). Thus, the model behaves in accordance with the experimentally disproved speed-of-processing account: presenting colour information ahead of word information creates a reverse Stroop effect – colour information interferes with word-reading. This is surprising, not least because the stated purpose of the model was to validate a strength of processing account.

Here we trace this flaw to the response mechanism used in the model. Cohen's model of Stroop processing explicitly draws on the choice behaviour literature (Luce, 1986) and adopts an exact analogue of the diffusion model (Ratcliff, 1978; Ratcliff and McKoon, 2008; Ratcliff and Smith, 2004) to resolve the response selection problem presented by the Stroop task. In the diffusion model the balance of evidence regarding the two possible responses at each point in time is used to adjust a running total. The momentary balance of evidence is defined by the strength of evidence in favour of one response minus the strength of evidence in favour of the other. At each time step the change in the running total is drawn from a normal distribution with a mean defined by the balance of evidence (in this case, this is the difference between the output units of the connectionist front end). When this total, which reflects the accumulated evidence, crosses either a positive threshold (indicating selection of one response) or a negative threshold (indicating selection of the other response) selection occurs. The diffusion model has been shown to be an analytically tractable form of several connectionist models of decision making, and an optimal decision algorithm for a two-choice decision situation (Bogacz *et al.*, 2006), where either desired accuracy or time-to-decision is specified (obviously these two mutually constrain each other). Further, potential neurobiological correspondences to the evidence accumulation processes of the diffusion model have been identified (Bogacz and Gurney, 2007; Gold and Shadlen, 2000; Ratcliff *et al.*, 2003; Reddi *et al.*, 2003).

The diffusion model response mechanism takes the outputs of the connectionist 'front-end' of the Cohen model as inputs. Because the model, like all connectionist models, works on graded signals there is always some input due to the to-be-ignored stimulus, even if this is very small due to the attentional inhibition. In the case of the colour-naming task, it is integral to the model's function that some influence of the word-element of the stimulus survives attentional selection and comes to influence the response stage. Without this feature the basic effect of Stroop interference would not be present. However, in SOA conditions, this influence of the to-be-ignored element may accumulate indefinitely. This affects selection time to an extent proportional to the time it is presented multiplied by the strength of evidence conveyed. So arbitrarily small amounts of evidence can provoke erroneous selection if presented for long enough, or they can massively slow correct selection (because accumulated evidence for the opposite response must be overcome).

The fact that Cohen *et al.*'s (1990) model involves a response mechanism is ignored in textbook treatments of the model (Ellis and Humphreys, 1999; O'Reilly and Munakata, 2000; Sharkey and Sharkey, 1995) and even overlooked in Cohen *et al.*'s own analysis of the function of the model (Cohen *et al.*, 1990). This reflects, we argue, a regrettable, but not untypical, neglect of the action selection problem in psychology. Reinforcing this view, we have recently shown how, contrary to the original account of Cohen *et al.* (1990), it is the response mechanism, not the neuronal transfer function, which generates the important differences in RTs between conditions (Stafford and Gurney, 2004), and it is the response mechanism which explains the asymmetry in the magnitudes of the interference and facilitation effects in the Cohen model (a matter about which there has been some debate, MacLeod and MacDonald, 2000).

In summary, our investigation of evidence accumulation as a mechanism of selection in the Cohen model of the Stroop task will have general implications for theories of selection. The core element in this investigation is to show how a more biologically realistic response mechanism – a model of action selection in the basal ganglia – overcomes the deficiencies noted here.

16.3   The basal ganglia and thalamic complex as a response mechanism in a cognitive task

The basal ganglia are a set of subcortical nuclei that have been implicated in a range of motor and cognitive functions (Balleine *et al.*, 2009; Brown *et al.*, 1997). Recently we have provided a unified account of basal ganglia function by hypothesising that they are a key element in resolving the action selection problem by serving as a central 'switch' or arbiter between action requests (Redgrave *et al.*, 1999). Recent neuropsychological evidence supporting this idea has been reported by Yehene and colleagues (Yehene *et al.*, 2008). Anatomically this hypothesis is plausible because the basal ganglia receive widespread input from all over the brain, including many areas of the cortex (Parent and Hazrati, 1993) and subcortex (McHaffie *et al.*, 2005). Outputs from the basal ganglia project back, directly or indirectly, to their input targets, forming closed anatomical loops (Alexander and Crutcher, 1990; McHaffie *et al.*, 2005). For loops including cortex, this occurs indirectly via the thalamus. We focus, first, on those aspects of our decision circuitry that make use of the basal ganglia alone.

16.3.1   The basal ganglia and action selection

Our model of the circuitry intrinsic to the basal ganglia is drawn directly from our earlier work (Gurney *et al.*, 2001a). This, in turn, is based on the known anatomy and physiology of the vertebrate basal ganglia, shown in Figure 16.5a and described in detail in several recent reviews (e.g., Mink, 1996; Smith *et al.*, 1998). The main input nuclei of the basal ganglia are the striatum and the subthalamic nucleus (STN). The STN is the only source of excitation within the basal ganglia. In primates, the major output nuclei are the internal segment of the globus pallidus (GPi), and substantia nigra pars reticulata (SNr). These nuclei provide extensively branched GABAergic efferents to functionally related zones of the ventral thalamus (which in turn projects back to the cerebral cortex), the midbrain and hind-brain areas critical for movement (e.g., Kha *et al.*, 2001). The external segment of the globus pallidus (GPe) is an internal source of inhibition within the basal ganglia. Two separate striatal populations have been identified (Gerfen and Young, 1988): (1) a population that contains the neuropeptides substance P and dynorphin, and preferentially expresses the D1 subtype of dopamine receptors; and (2) a population that contains enkephalin and preferentially expresses the D2 subtype of dopamine receptors. In most accounts of basal ganglia anatomy, the D1-preferential population is usually associated with projections to SNr and GPi alone, while its D2 counterpart is associated with projections to GPe (Gerfen *et al.*, 1990).

The basic assumption underlying our model was that the brain is processing, in parallel, a large number of sensory, cognitive, and motivational streams or 'channels',

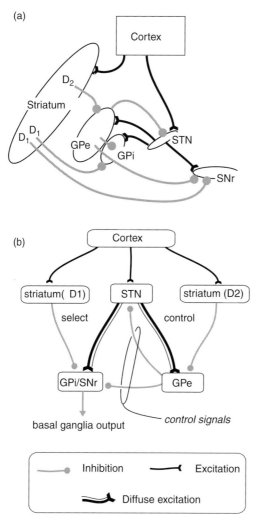

(a)

(b)

Inhibition   Excitation

Diffuse excitation

Figure 16.5 Basal ganglia anatomy and functional architecture. (a) Basal ganglia anatomy used as the basis for the model. (b) New functional architecture for basal ganglia (Gurney *et al.*, 2001a) used in the current work. See text for details.

each of which may be requesting/promoting different actions to be taken. For effective use of limited motor resources, it is necessary to suppress the majority of these requests while allowing the expression of only a small number (in some cases just one). This channel-based scheme is consonant with the view that the basal ganglia comprise a series of afferent and efferent parallel processing streams or loops (Alexander *et al.*, 1986; Hoover and Strick, 1993; Middleton and Strick, 2002). At the systems level, the smallest neuronal population we needed to consider was, therefore, the set of neurons responsible for a single channel within each of the basal ganglia nuclei.

A further assumption was that, implicit in the representation of each action, there is an encoding of its *salience* or propensity to be selected for execution. In our model, we assumed that channel salience had already been extracted from phasic excitatory input by processes in the basal ganglia input nuclei. The input to the model, therefore, was simply the scalar-valued salience of each channel. The basal ganglia output is inhibitory and tonically active. Selection then occurs via selective disinhibition of target structures (Chevalier and Deniau, 1990) which include (as well as thalamus) premotor areas of the brainstem. Once inhibition has been released in this way, the corresponding behaviour is enacted. In summary then, large salience signal inputs at the striatum and STN select for low signal outputs at SNr/GPi.

We used the computational premise of selection to guide our interpretation of basal ganglia anatomy in functional terms. One architectural feature that may be invoked in this respect is the diffuse excitation from STN to its targets – GPe and SNr/GPi (Parent and Hazrati, 1993, 1995) – in combination with more focused inhibition from striatum to the same nuclei. This constitutes an off-centre, on-surround network that can perform a selection function, as noted by Mink and Thach (1993). However, it is not clear a priori what function GPe serves in this scheme, since it is not an output nucleus of the basal ganglia able to implement selection directly. We resolved this problem by observing that, while selection could be performed in principle by the complex of striatum (D1), STN, and SNr/GPi alone, the relative levels of excitation and inhibition required to achieve this function were only obtained (and indeed guaranteed) by the inhibition supplied by GPe. We therefore hypothesised that the GPe acts within a control pathway (comprising striatum (D2), STN and GPe) as a source of control signals for the selection pathway (striatum (D1), STN, SNr/GPi). The new functional architecture described above (Gurney et al., 2001a) is shown in Figure 16.5b. Note that it is quite different from the prevailing 'direct/indirect' pathway scheme of Albin et al (1989), and hypothesises a different role for GPe from that posited by Hazy et al. (this volume) and Frank et al. (this volume).

The resulting model (Gurney et al., 2001b) was able to successfully select and switch between channels based on their input salience. In addition, the model allowed dopaminergic modulation of basal ganglia function in ways compatible with disorders of dopamine function (e.g., Parkinson's disease). While, the role of dopamine is not discussed here, we note that the model is rich enough, in principle, to account for data derived from studies with relevant clinical populations.

16.3.2   Including the thalamic complex

As noted above, the basal ganglia sits in a wider anatomical context comprising closed loops of cortex–basal ganglia–thalamus–cortex. In previous work, we modelled such loops by embedding the basal ganglia model (described above) into a loop incorporating motor and somatosensory cortex (Humphries and Gurney, 2002). In that instance, there are well-understood anatomical relations between these cortical areas, basal ganglia, and specific nuclei within the thalamus. In the current work, the specific areas of cortex associated with word reading and colour processing are not well understood. We therefore adopt a simplified version of the model in Humphries and Gurney (2002) by using only a single cortical area (Figure 16.6).

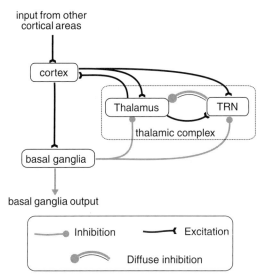

input from other
cortical areas

cortex

Thalamus   TRN

thalamic complex

basal ganglia

basal ganglia output

——• Inhibition   ——◀ Excitation

—— Diffuse inhibition

Figure 16.6 The model of cortico-basal ganglia-thalamo-cortical loops. Adapted from Humphries and Gurney (2002).

Further, whereas in the somatosensory/motor loop the thalamic nucleus is identified as the ventrolateral (VL) thalamus (Price, 1995), here it is left non-specific and is labelled 'Thalamus' in Figure 16.6. A component common to both the original and simplified scheme is the thalamic reticular nucleus (TRN) which sends diffuse inhibition to Thalamus. The extended thalamo-cortical model retains the channel-based scheme of the basal ganglia model and reciprocal connections between thalamus and TRN imply the latter acts as a distal lateral inhibition mechanism for the former. Input to the model comes from other cortical areas and constitutes an initial representation of salience.

The original somatosensory/motor loop model displays enhanced selection capabilities in several respects when compared with the model of the basal ganglia alone (Humphries and Gurney, 2002). Further, using these models in robot controllers has shown that their selection behaviour is of sufficient efficiency and sophistication to be behaviourally adequate in realistic environments (Girard *et al.*, 2003; Prescott *et al.*, 2006). Details of these models can be found in Gurney *et al.* (2001a) and Humphries and Gurney (2002), and also in the annotated code which is provided in the electronic supplementary material which accompanies Stafford and Gurney (2007).

16.3.3 Combining the Cohen model with the basal ganglia response mechanism

It is natural to ask if the extended thalamo-cortical-basal ganglia model, viewed as a decision mechanism, can perform appropriate selection in a cognitive task. The model was developed with a view to accounting for action selection in the domain of systems neuroscience with no intention, originally, of being used to generate RT data. The model's ability to account for such data would therefore serve to validate it further, and open up further possibilities for investigating biologically plausible response mechanisms in the study of cognition.

The rationales for the connectionist Cohen model and our systems neuroscience model are quite different. The Cohen model is a minimal connectionist model designed to test a high-level hypothesis about automatic and controlled processing. On the other hand, our basal ganglia models are biologically constrained, respecting the known anatomy of the target circuits, and were designed to test the hypothesis that those specific circuits could support action selection. Further, whereas learning is a key component of the Cohen model, it does not figure in our models of basal ganglia and thalamus.

There are, however, sufficient points of contact between the two models to allow them to be joined in a unified scheme. Thus, the model in Figure 16.6 is built out of standard leaky integrator neurons (Arbib, 1995) – a feature that it shares with the Cohen model – so that they both utilise a common signal representation denoting neuronal population responses.

The reaction-time behaviour of the model is read from the output units of basal ganglia. Recall that these represent neuron populations providing tonic (continuous background) inhibition to motor targets, and that selection occurs on those channels whose inhibitory output is sufficiently reduced. Reaction time is then interpreted as the time to selection, which is the time from stimulus onset to reduction of basal ganglia output on the selected channel to some threshold value. Moreover, we suppose that this selection threshold may be greater than zero. Although a zero output would demonstrate unequivocal selection, it is unrealistic to suppose that a population of neurons have to be held in a completely silent state for a behaviourally meaningful period of time to allow selection.

Given these observations, a combined model was constructed using the connectionist 'front-end' of the Cohen model (see Figure 16.7). This performed initial stimulus processing to provide initial salience input to the thalamo-cortical-basal ganglia model which constituted the response mechanism. The latter uses two channels mimicking the possible outcomes in the Stroop task.

The neural network component of Cohen *et al.*'s model performs what is normally thought of as the cognitive elements of the task: stimulus–response translation, attentional control and learning. Only one minor change is required to this 'front-end' to make it compatible with the basal ganglia model response mechanism. The output units of the original Cohen model have resting values of 0.5, the midpoint of their output range which lies in the interval [0, 1]. This is inconsistent with our new interpretation of these signals as salience values, since it indicates that all possible responses have moderately strong saliences at rest. In the combined model, the resting values of the front-end are set to 0.1, indicating a weakly salient input to the basal ganglia (small changes in weight initialisation are also required as a consequence of this manipulation; for details see Stafford (2003).

In all other respects the combined model is exactly as published by Cohen *et al.* (1990), except with the basal ganglia model replacing evidence accumulation as the method of final response selection. The basal ganglia thalamo-cortical model used is exactly as published elsewhere (Gurney *et al.*, 2001b; Humphries and Gurney, 2002).

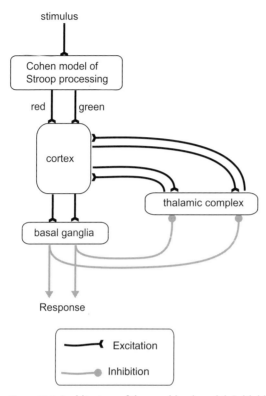

Figure 16.7 Architecture of the combined model. Initial inputs are processed by the connectionist 'front-end' of the Cohen model as described in Cohen *et al*. (1990). Outputs representing the evidence in favour of the two possible responses are interpreted as initial salience inputs to the cortical component of the thalamo-cortical-basal ganglia model in Figure 16.6. The basal ganglia outputs determine which response occurs (the output channel which first passes a selection threshold) and the reaction time (the time required to reach that threshold).

16.3.4   Simulations I: matching basic empirical data

The combined model successfully replicates the basic (colour-naming) Stroop task, and the word-reading variation (see Figure 16.8). This shows that the model is capable of performing basic selection in a cognitive task, and of producing realistic RT values.

The ability to realistically model learning phenomena is a key benefit of connectionist models. The combined model mimics the power-law function of learning (Figure 16.9), just as the original Cohen model does (note that no learning takes place in the response mechanism component in either model). This demonstrates that the learning dynamic captured by the connectionist front-end is not interfered with by the use of the basal ganglia response mechanism; graded changes in the signals from the front end are converted into appropriately graded changes in RTs.

The SOA task reveals that using the basal ganglia as a response mechanism provides a superior fit to the data than when using the original response mechanism (Figure 16.3c). Within the original range of the SOA values the simulation data more closely matches

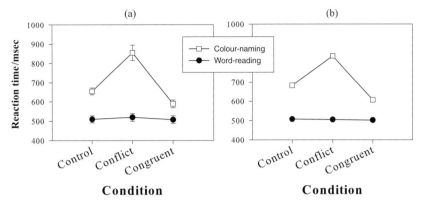

Figure 16.8 Comparing (a) empirical and (b) simulation reaction times when using the basal ganglia model as the response mechanism for the basic Stroop task. Empirical data is from Dunbar and MacLeod (1984), for which standard error bars are shown.

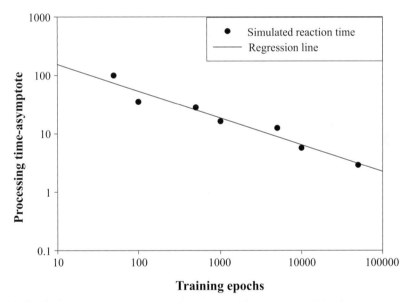

Figure 16.9 The model conforms to the power law of practice (Logan, 1988). Both axes use a log scale. Simulation results are shown as dots. The simple regression for the data is shown as a straight line and follows the form log_{10}(Processing time) $= 2.65 - 0.46 \times log_{10}$(epochs). $R^2 = 0.948$.

the empirical data. Running the model at extended SOA values (Figure 16.10) confirms that RTs using the basal ganglia response mechanism are stable. At negative SOAs, the salience output caused by the to-be-ignored element of the stimulus is not sufficient to cause selection. Thus, using the basal ganglia response mechanism, the model makes the correct selection at all SOA values. In addition, the amount of interference and facilitation it causes is limited. This is reflected in the stabilisation of RTs at SOAs below -400 ms.

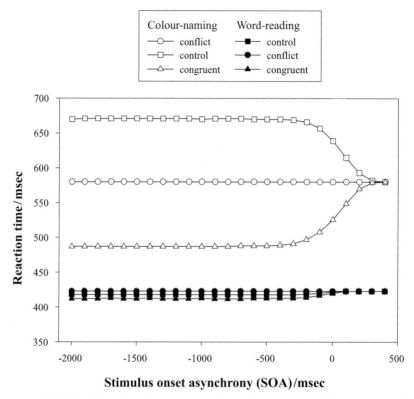

Figure 16.10 Simulation stimulus-onset asynchrony data at an extended range when using the basal ganglia model as the response mechanism.

16.3.5   Simulations II: dynamic attentional inhibition

Providing the model with stability under SOA conditions makes further manipulations possible which bring the model up to date, in a principled way, with developments in our understanding of automatic processing and cognitive control. It has been suggested that selection in the Stroop task is dynamically controlled by a process that monitors for conflicts (located in the anterior cingulate cortex) and increases attentional control in response (Botvinick, 2007; Botvinick, *et al.*, 2001; Botvinick *et al.*, 2004). Two additional simulations presented here demonstrate that using the basal ganglia model as the response mechanism allows the use of dynamic-attentional modulation to enhance the match to the empirical data.

Here, we do not propose an account of conflict monitoring, nor tie it to any specific anatomical location. Instead we implement solely the essential feature that the appearance of the to-be-ignored element provokes, after some delay, an increase in the attentional inhibition acting on it. The length of the delay used here is 100 ms which accords well with the timescale of phenomena such as negative priming, (see May *et al.*, 1995, for a review) and neurophysiological recordings of activity suppression due to

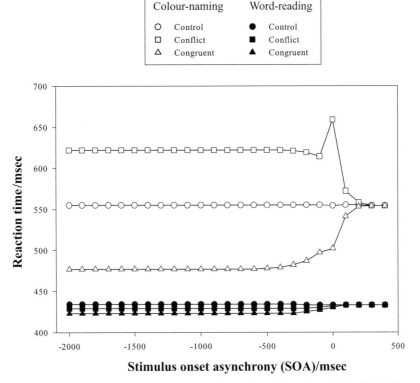

Figure 16.11 Simulation stimulus-onset asynchrony data when using the basal ganglia model as the response mechanism and with the addition of 'dynamic attentional modulation'.

attentional processes (Chelazzi *et al.*, 1998). See Usher and McClelland (2001) for a discussion of the time-course of activity during choice selection.

The implementation of attentional modulation in our model is achieved in the following way. After 100 ms (simulated) the inhibition on the relevant hidden units of the Cohen model is increased in magnitude from the default value of -4 to -4.9, the value used by Cohen *et al.* (1990) in their simulations of the SOA task (at all values of the SOA). Thus dynamic attentional modulation is a modification of the mechanism that already exists in the model for implementing attentional selection, using parameters that have already been established. The parameterisation of the attentional modulation could have been finessed, but we sought to test the validity of the idea without such ad-hoc modifications.

Figure 16.11 shows the simulation results for the model with this dynamic attentional modulation. Reaction times in the colour-naming conflict condition now peak around the 0 ms SOA point, and flatten-off at a lower level, as occurs in the empirical results (Figure 16.3a) – this is an improvement over both the Cohen model and the combined model without dynamic attentional modulation. This simulation both solves the stability problem and matches the peak and decline in RTs that the empirical data shows.

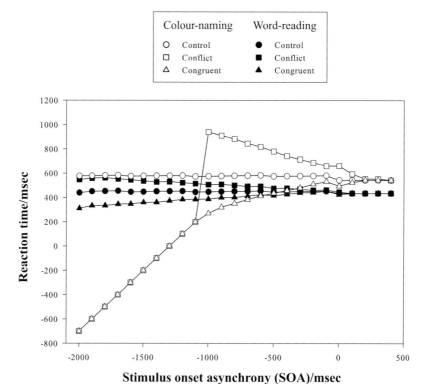

Figure 16.12 Simulation stimulus-onset asynchrony data when using the original Cohen *et al.* (1990) model with the diffusion model as the response mechanisms with the addition of 'dynamic attentional modulation'.

In contrast, with dynamic attentional modulation the original Cohen model does not successfully match the empirical data (see Figure 16.12). Because the stability problem is not resolved, the to-be-ignored stimulus element still provokes erroneous selection at long enough SOAs, and causes unrealistic amounts of response-time interference before that.

16.4   Discussion

Our primary result is that a neurobiologically plausible model of action selection allows the successful simulation of reaction times in the Stroop task, despite the fact that the model construction was structurally and functionally guided by quite different principles. Although the front-end of the model was explicitly designed to do Stroop processing it is the response mechanism which is responsible for converting signal outputs into RTs. Structurally, the model was constrained by the known functional neuroanatomy of the basal ganglia; functionally, it was a quantitative interpretation of our action

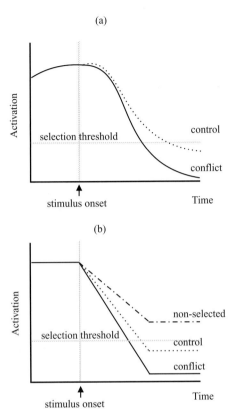

Figure 16.13 Selection in the basal ganglia. (a) Output signals from example runs of the model in the conflict (solid line) and control (dotted line) conditions. (b) Schematic illustration of the way in which final equilibrium output governs selection and reaction time (RT). A selected signal with fast RT (solid line), a selected signal with larger RT (dotted line) and a non-selected signal (dot-dash line) are shown.

selection hypothesis (Redgrave *et al.*, 1999). The basal ganglia model was not explicitly designed to simulate RTs, nor was it constrained by human cognitive performance, yet when processing outputs from the front-end of the Cohen *et al.* (1990) model it has advantages over the diffusion model, which was explicitly designed to simulate RTs, in simulating RTs.

16.4.1   Why the basal ganglia model successfully simulates reaction times

The model captures the basic Stroop (Figure 16.8) and learning (Figure 16.9) phenomena because, for moderately sized saliences, selection time is based on the relative difference between the to-be-selected salience and the competing salience (if any). To understand the emergence of RT differences in the basal ganglia model, consider Figure 16.13. Panel (a) shows traces (directly from the simulation) of the output signals corresponding to the correct response, in a control and a conflict condition; these signals cross the selection threshold and therefore produce a behavioural response. Note that the output signal in the conflict condition falls to a lower level than in the control condition. It is this final level to which the signal drops which defines the rate at which the signal drops and hence the time to selection. The final signal level is, in turn, dependent on the relative difference between the to-be-selected salience and the competing salience (if any).

The schematic diagram of signal time courses (Figure 16.13b) clarifies the way in which final equilibrium output governs selection and RT. The rate of decrease of the output signal has the same relation to time-to-selection as the drift rate (strength-of-evidence) does to mean RT in the diffusion model. However, because the rate of decrease in the basal ganglia model is ultimately determined by the final output signal resting level, selection does not always occur. In particular small saliences – which might result from a to-be-ignored stimulus – do not drive the output down beyond the selection threshold.

It is because the basal ganglia model is designed to operate continuously that it has equilibrium final states. Thus, in the idealised situation of unchanging inputs, all patterns of input eventually produce unchanging output states. In particular, for some patterns of input the final output state indicates that no action is selected. In more realistic situations, with noisy input, the basal ganglia-thalamo-cortical model is stable to small transient fluctuations in salience (Humphries and Gurney, 2002). It is with small saliences, and when dealing with successive rather than simultaneous inputs, that the advantages of using a selection mechanism that has non-selection equilibrium states is revealed. Both of these cases are revealed by comparison of the SOA simulations (Figures 16.4 and 16.10).

16.4.2   Weaknesses of the diffusion model

Our simulations illustrate a situation in which simple evidence accumulation is a non-adaptive choice process. The failure of the Cohen model on the SOA simulations is due to a model feature which is neither trivial nor irrelevant. The empirical existence of the basic Stroop interference effect demonstrates that response activation from the to-be-ignored word element of the stimulus must, at least to some extent, 'break through' any initial attentional inhibition. This activity, arriving at the response mechanism before the response activation of the colour element, is enough, in the Cohen model, to cause selection. The erroneous selection produced at long SOAs shows that a response mechanism must not make selections based on inconsequentially low inputs.

The Cohen model evidence accumulation mechanism has no minimal threshold on inputs, and no decay of accumulated evidence. This means that there are no equilibrium states and it is constantly being driven to enforce selection, no matter how long this takes. By extension, the diffusion model, the general form of the evidence accumulation mechanism used, contains no capacity for not making a selection. This is a serious flaw. At a minimum, it indicates that the context within which the diffusion model of selection is used cannot be ignored or assumed.

16.4.3   Alternative solutions

We have considered how the choice of response mechanism affects performance in simulation of the Stroop task. Other mechanisms for matching the core empirical data could be envisaged. Cohen and Huston (1994) adapt the model of Cohen *et al.* (1990) to provide a better match to the SOA data. They do this by removing the diffusion model response mechanism entirely and having selection triggered by activation on the output units crossing a fixed threshold. This solves the problem of selection by arbitrarily small activations, since they do not reach the selection threshold.

    This approach allows a fit to the data, but the removal of an explicit response mechanism raises some additional questions. Cohen and Huston's (1994) model, in this respect, bears some similarity to the Usher and McClelland (2001) model of perceptual choice. Both models use a single network for processing stimuli and for selecting responses using a simple threshold. Bogacz *et al.* (this volume) have provided extensions and discussions of the optimality of the Usher and McClelland model. This model considers mechanisms of choice comprised of neuron-like elements but removed from a realistic cognitive or biological architecture. Although models without explicit response mechanisms can fit behavioural data (Cohen and Huston, 1994) or be shown to make optimal decisions (Bogacz *et al.*, this volume; Usher and McClelland, 2001) two issues remain unaddressed. First, which neural structures implement the model? Second, how is the optimal decision making provided by the model adaptively controlled?

    Our approach has been to consider action representation and response selection separately, as in the original Cohen model, and to provide an account of response selection based upon the basal ganglia, as the proposed vertebrate solution to the selection problem. The benefits of using a centralised rather than distributed selection mechanism are discussed in Prescott *et al.* (1999). Amongst these benefits is the greater theoretical ease of coordinating between multiple competing neural loci – both in terms of lower wiring cost and in the ability to centrally mediate the equivalent of thresholds.

16.4.4   Benefits of the basal ganglia model

The simulation of the SOA paradigm highlights two properties which the basal ganglia as a selection mechanism brings to the combined model to improve the possible account of the data. The first, as already discussed, is the lack of incorrect selection for arbitrarily small saliences. The second is the limit on the maximum possible influence of concurrently or consecutively active inputs. Priming of RTs, whether positive or negative, occurs because activity on other channels alters the basal ganglia output signals, at a subselection level, thereby affecting the time it takes for outputs to drop below the selection threshold. A similar process occurs in the diffusion model, but accumulated evidence is not limited – and can ultimately lead to incorrect selection (as discussed above). Figure 16.14 shows the geometry of selection interference in both response mechanisms. In the diffusion model (Figure 16.14a) the increase in RT due to a preceding to-be-ignored stimulus is a function of the size of that signal multiplied by time – the longer the to-be-ignored stimulus is presented, the greater the size of the interference effect. If

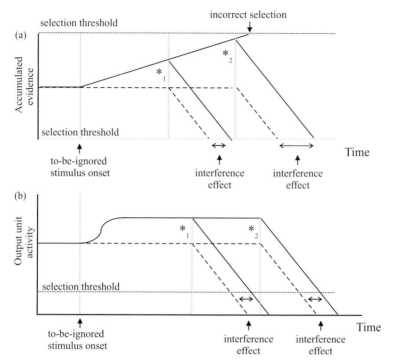

Figure 16.14 Interference in (a) the diffusion model and (b) the basal ganglia model response mechanisms. Signals in the diffusion model represent the accumulated evidence in favour of two possible responses, selection is indicated by crossing either the positive or negative evidence thresholds. Signals in the basal ganglia represent the activity on the to-be-selected action channel, selection is indicated by activity on that channel dropping below the selection threshold. Solid lines show signals subject to interference from a preceding input, dashed lines show signals without this competition. The signal courses for the early or later appearance of the to-be-responded-to stimulus are shown (indicated by points $*_1$ and $*_2$ respectively), and the corresponding size of the interference effects is indicated.

the to-be-ignored stimulus is presented for long enough and the accumulated evidence reaches the selection threshold then an incorrect response is made. In the basal ganglia model (Figure 16.14b) the amount of increase in RT due to a to-be-ignored stimulus is solely a function of the magnitude of the salience that the to-be-ignored stimulus provokes. Because, as discussed above, the basal ganglia model has equilibrium final states, some of which do not indicate selection, the rise in the output signal associated with the correct response is limited and does not increase with time after a certain point. The increase in RT result is commensurately limited, and thus the correct response is selected efficiently.

This is an example of the general 'clean switching' property which has been identified as a desirable feature of any selection mechanism (Redgrave et al., 1999). A response mechanism needs to work in real-time, continuously, dealing with the successive selection of actions and interruption of old actions by new. The SOA paradigm illustrates just one situation where human action selection demonstrates clean switching. The benefits the basal ganglia model brings to modelling the Stroop task demonstrate the value of considering the constraints of natural action selection within cognitive models.

16.4.5   The diffusion model in the context of action selection

That the evidence accumulation response mechanism, on the other hand, has only one type of final state (that of selecting an action) and it continuously moves towards this state, has implications for the diffusion model as a model of response selection. The diffusion model embodies the inevitable progression towards selection because all inputs are integrated into a running total of activity, without any decay of that activity. This 'perfect integration' is actually a requirement of the proof that the diffusion model performs optimally (Bogacz *et al.*, 2006; Smith and Ratcliff, 2004), at least for a restricted class of choices. The simulation of the SOA experiments reveals that selection by perfect integration can be unadaptive in at least some circumstances. This particular case of the general problem of clean-switching illustrates that adaptive action selection involves criteria beyond those which have been used to define decision-optimality (i.e., criteria beyond those pertaining to the kind of simple choices which have hitherto been the main focus of analysis of choice behaviour). This is not to say that the diffusion model, or diffusion-like processes, are inappropriate for selection. Indeed, it has recently been proposed that the basal ganglia architecture is able to perform optimal decision making in a manner akin to the diffusion model, but between multiple alternatives (see Bogacz and Gurney, 2007). The diffusion model reflects an optimal way of integrating information if the possible choices are defined, the sources of evidence static and if the point at which the choice process begins is a given. Our claim is only that evidence accumulation and the diffusion model alone cannot provide a full account of adaptive action selection. For this wider problem mechanisms are required which signal the appropriate initialisation of the accumulation process, and which reset it or effectively overcome previous accumulation of evidence. The basal ganglia-thalamo-cortical model provides a first step towards the integration of the decision-optimal diffusion model into the wider context of adaptive action selection.

16.4.6   Conclusions and future work

This work validates our model against the basic Stroop phenomena. Use of the basal ganglia model as the response mechanism improves the fit that can be made to the empirical data and highlights necessary features response mechanisms should contain, the lack of which was overlooked in the previous account by Cohen *et al.* (1990). Utilising an adaptive, action selection-based response mechanism in the model of Stroop task, allows the principled addition to the model of dynamic attentional modulation (Botvinick *et al.*, 2001, 2004). Use of the basal ganglia model also extends the account of Stroop processing to connect with the neurobiology of selection.

From a wider perspective, there is a 'theoretical purity' to testing models outside of the domain that they were developed in. First, the basal ganglia model, while not designed to account for RTs, successfully managed to do so. Second, the biologically grounded model of the basal ganglia also deals appropriately with signals provided by a more abstract connectionist model of a cognitive task. This depended on a common signal interpretation at the interface between the two model components in terms of population rate codes. We therefore suggest that this offers a useful tactic in any high level cognitive modelling that would enable the gradual replacement of abstract model components with more biologically realistic counterparts. Note, however, that this approach does not undermine the principled use of connectionist modelling in quantitative testing of cognitive hypotheses. Thus, in our present context, the model proposed by Cohen *et al*. (1990) was a test of the hypothesis that the Stroop effect could be accounted for in a framework in which the 'strength of processing' devoted to a perceptual or cognitive process determined its status as more or less automatic (or controlled) in relation to other processes. Our work does not challenge the validation of this particular hypothesis since the 'front-end' of the model still tests it perfectly adequately.

Finally, the ability of the model to deal with an arbitrary number of inputs will provide opportunities for future modelling investigations of additional selection paradigms. Making connections to the underlying neurobiology enriches the account possible of Stroop processing. In particular, we anticipate that the existing provision for dopaminergic modulation of signal processing in our model will allow future tests of the model against various pathologies, such as schizophrenia. Our model will also need to be broadened to account for learning within the basal ganglia. Developing a full account of the interaction of plasticity with decision making will be an important test of all existing models of action selection.

Acknowledgements

We thank Mark Humphries and two anonymous reviewers for their comments on an earlier version of this chapter.

References

Albin, R. L., A. B. Young, and J. B. Penney (1989). The functional anatomy of basal ganglia disorders. *Trends Neurosci*. **12**: 366–75.

Alexander, G. E. and M. D. Crutcher (1990). Functional architecture of basal ganglia circuits: neural substrates of parallel processing. *Trends Neurosci*. **13**: 266–72.

Alexander, G. E., M. R. Delong, and P. L. Strick (1986). Parallel organization of functionally segregated circuits linking basal ganglia and cortex. *Annu. Rev. Neurosci*. **9**: 357–81.

Arbib, M. (1995). Introducing the neuron. In *The Handbook of Brain Theory and Neural Networks*, ed. M. Arbib. Cambridge, MA: MIT Press, pp. 266–72.

Balleine, B. W., M. Lijeholm, and S. B. Ostlund (2009). The integrative function of the basal ganglia in instrumental conditioning. *Behav. Brain Res*. **199**(1): 43–52.

Besner, D. and J. Stolz (1999). Context dependency in Stroop's paradigm: when are words treated as nonlinguistic objects? *Can. J. Exp. Psychol*. **53**(4): 374–80.

Besner, D., J. A. Stolz, and C. Boutilier (1997). The Stroop effect and the myth of automaticity. *Psychon. Bull. Rev.* **4**(2): 221–5.

Blais, C. and D. Besner (2007). A reverse Stroop effect without translation or reading difficulty. *Psychon. Bull. Rev.* **14**(3): 466–9.

Bogacz, R., E. Brown, J. Moehlis, P. Holmes, and J. D. Cohen (2006). The physics of optimal decision making: a formal analysis of models of performance in two-alternative forced-choice tasks. *Psychol. Rev.* **113**(4): 700–765.

Bogacz, R. and K. Gurney (2007). The basal ganglia and cortex implement optimal decision making between alternative actions. *Neural Comput.* **19**(2): 442–77.

Botvinick, M. M. (2007). Conflict monitoring and decision making: reconciling two perspectives on anterior cingulate function. *Cogn. Aff. Behav. Neurosci.* **7**(4): 356–66.

Botvinick, M. M., T. S. Braver, D. M. Barch, C. S. Carter, and J. D. Cohen (2001). Conflict monitoring and cognitive control. *Psychol. Rev.* **108**(3): 624–52.

Botvinick, M. M., J. D. Cohen, and C. S. Carter (2004). Conflict monitoring and anterior cingulate cortex: an update. *Trends Cogn. Sci.* **8**(12): 539–46.

Brown, L. L., J. S. Schneider, and T. I. Lidsky (1997). Sensory and cognitive functions of the basal ganglia. *Curr. Opin. Neurobiol.* **7**(2): 157–63.

Chelazzi, L., Duncan, J., Miller, E. K., and Desimone, R. (1998). Responses of neurons in inferior temporal cortex during memory-guided visual search. *J. Neurophysiol.* **80**(6): 2918–40.

Chevalier, G. and J. Deniau (1990). Disinhibition as a basic process in the expression of striatal functions. *Trends Neurosci.* **13**: 277–81.

Cohen, J. D., K. Dunbar, and J. L. McClelland (1990). On the control of automatic processes: a parallel distributed-processing account of the Stroop effect. *Psychol. Rev.* **97**(3): 332–61.

Cohen, J. D. and T. A. Huston (1994). Progress in the use of interactive models for understanding attention and performance. *Attention and Performance* **15**: 453–76.

Dishon-Berkovits, M. and D. Algom (2000). The Stroop effect: it is not the robust phenomenon that you have thought it to be. *Mem. Cogn.* **28**(8): 1437–49.

Dunbar, K. and C. M. MacLeod (1984). A horse race of a different color: Stroop interference patterns with transformed words. *J. Exp. Psychol. Human* **10**(5): 623–39.

Durgin, F. H. (2000). The reverse Stroop effect. *Psychon. Bull. Rev.* **7**(1): 121–5.

Ellis, R. and G. Humphreys (1999). *Connectionist Psychology: A Text with Readings*. Hove, UK: Psychology Press Ltd.

Gerfen, C. R., T. M. Engber, L. C. Mahan, *et al.* (1990). D1 and D2 dopamine receptor regulated gene expression of striatonigral and striatopallidal neurons. *Science* **250**: 1429–31.

Gerfen, C. R. and Young, W. S. III (1988). Distribution of striatonigral and striatopallidal peptidergic neurons in both patch and matrix compartments: an in situ hybridization histochemistry and fluorescent retrograde tracing study. *Brain Res.* **460**: 161–7.

Girard, B., V. Cuzin, A. Guillot, K. N. Gurney, and T. J. Prescott (2003). A basal ganglia inspired model of action selection evaluated in a robotic survival task. *J. Integr. Neurosci.* **2**(2): 179–200.

Glaser, M. O. and W. R. Glaser (1982). Time course analysis of the Stroop phenomenon. *J. Exp. Psychol. Human* **8**(6): 875–94.

Gold, J. I. and M. N. Shadlen (2000). Representation of a perceptual decision in developing oculomotor commands. *Nature* **404**(6776): 390–4.

Gold, J. I. and M. N. Shadlen (2007). The neural basis of decision making. *Annu. Rev. Neurosci.* **30**: 535.

Gurney, K., T. J. Prescott, and P. Redgrave (2001a). A computational model of action selection in the basal ganglia I: a new functional anatomy. *Biol. Cybern.* **85**(6): 401–10.

Gurney, K., T. J. Prescott, and P. Redgrave (2001b). A computational model of action selection in the basal ganglia: II: analysis and simulation of behaviour. *Biol. Cybern.* **85**(6): 411–23.

Herd, S. A., M. T. Banich, and R. C. O'Reilly (2006). Neural mechanisms of cognitive control: an integrative model of Stroop task performance and fMRI data. *J. Cogn. Neurosci.* **18**(1): 22–32.

Hoover, J. E. and P. L. Strick (1993). Multiple output channels in the basal ganglia. *Science* **259**: 819–21.

Humphries, M. D. and K. N. Gurney (2002). The role of intra-thalamic and thalamocortical circuits in action selection. *Network-Comp. Neural* **13**(1): 131–56.

Kha, H. T., D. I. Finkelstein, D. Tomas, *et al.* (2001). Projections from the substantia nigra pars reticulata to the motor thalamus of the rat: single axon reconstructions and immunohistochemical study. *J. Comp. Neurol.* **440**(1): 20–30.

Logan, G. (1988). Toward an instance theory of automatization. *Psychol. Rev.* **95**(4): 492–527.

Luce, R. (1986). *Response Times: Their Role in Inferring Elementary Mental Organisation*. New York: Clarendon Press.

MacLeod, C. (1991). Half a century of research on the Stroop effect: an integrative review. *Psychol. Bull.* **109**(2): 163–203.

MacLeod, C. and P. MacDonald (2000). Interdimensional interference in the Stroop effect: uncovering the cognitive and neural anatomy of attention. *Trends Cogn. Sci.* **4**(10): 383–91.

May, C. P., M. J. Kane, and L. Hasher (1995). Determinants of negative priming. *Psychol. Bull.* **118**(1): 35–54.

McHaffie, J. G., T. R. Stanford, B. E. Stein, V. Coizet, and P. Redgrave (2005). Subcortical loops through the basal ganglia. *Trends Neurosci.* **28**: 401–407.

Middleton, F. A. and P. L. Strick (2002). Basal-ganglia 'projections' to the prefrontal cortex of the primate. *Cereb. Cortex* **12**: 926–35.

Mink, J. W. (1996). The basal ganglia: focused selection and inhibition of competing motor programs. *Prog. Neurobiol.* **50**: 381–425.

Mink, J. W. and W. T. Thach (1993). Basal ganglia intrinsic circuits and their role in behavior. *Curr. Opin. Neurobiol.* **3**: 950–7.

Opris, I. and C. J. Bruce (2005). Neural circuitry of judgment and decision mechanisms. *Brain Res. Rev.* **48**(3): 509–526.

O'Reilly, R. C. and Y. Munakata (2000). *Computational Explorations in Cognitive Neuroscience: Understanding the Mind by Simulating the Brain*. Cambridge, MA: MIT Press.

Parent, A. and L. N. Hazrati (1993). Anatomical aspects of information processing in primate basal ganglia. *Trends Neurosci.* **16**: 111–116.

Parent, A. and Hazrati, L. N. (1995). Functional anatomy of the basal ganglia. 1. the cortico-basal ganglia-thalamo-cortical loop. *Brain Res. Rev.* **20**: 91–127.

Phaf, R. H., A. H. C. Vanderheijden, and P. T. W. Hudson (1990). Slam: a connectionist model for attention in visual selection tasks. *Cogn. Psychol.* **22**(3): 273–341.

Platt, M. (2002). Neural correlates of decisions. *Curr. Opin. Neurobiol.* **12**(2): 141–8.

Posner, M. and C. Snyder (1975). Attention and cognitive control. In *Information Processing and Cognition*, ed. R. Solso. Hillsdale, NJ: Erlbaum, pp. 55–85.

Prescott, T. J., F. M. Montes Gonzalez, K. Gurney, M. D. Humphries, and P. Redgrave (2006). A robot model of the basal ganglia: behavior and intrinsic processing. *Neural Networks* **19**(1): 31–61.

Prescott, T. J., P. Redgrave, and K. Gurney (1999). Layered control architectures in robots and vertebrates. *Adapt. Behav.* **7**(1): 99–127.

Price, J. (1995). Thalamus. In *The Rat Nervous System* Vol. 2, ed. G. Paxinos. New York: Academic, pp. 629–48.

Ratcliff, R. (1978). A theory of memory retrieval. *Psychol. Rev.* **85**: 59–108.

Ratcliff, R., A. Cherian, and M. Segraves (2003). A comparison of macaque behavior and superior colliculus neuronal activity to predictions from models of two-choice decisions. *J. Neurophysiol.* **90**(3): 1392–407.

Ratcliff, R. and G. McKoon (2008). The diffusion decision model: theory and data for two-choice decision tasks. *Neural Comput.* **20**(4): 873–922.

Ratcliff, R. and P. Smith (2004). A comparison of sequential sampling models for two-choice reaction time. *Psychol. Rev.* **111**(2): 333–67.

Reddi, B., K. Asrress, and R. Carpenter (2003). Accuracy, information, and response time in a saccadic decision task. *J. Neurophysiol.* **90**(5): 3538–46.

Redgrave, P., T. J. Prescott, and K. Gurney (1999). The basal ganglia: a vertebrate solution to the selection problem? *Neuroscience* **89**(4): 1009–23.

Sharkey, A. and N. Sharkey (1995). Cognitive modeling: psychology and connectionism. In *The Handbook of Brain Theory and Neural Networks*, ed. M. Arbib. Cambridge, MA: MIT Press, pp. 200–203.

Smith, Y., M. D. Bevan, E. Shink, and J. P. Bolam (1998). Microcircuitry of the direct and indirect pathways of the basal ganglia. *Neuroscience* **86**: 353–87.

Smith, P. and R. Ratcliff (2004). Psychology and neurobiology of simple decisions. *Trends Neurosci.* **27**(3): 161–8.

Stafford, T. (2003). Integrating psychological and neuroscientific constraints in models of Stroop processing and action selection. PhD thesis, University of Sheffield. Available at http://www.abrg.group.shef.ac.uk/.

Stafford, T. and K. Gurney (2004). The role of response mechanisms in determining reaction time performance: Piéron's law revisited. *Psychon. Bull. Rev.* **11**(6): 975–87.

Stafford, T. and K. Gurney (2007). Biologically constrained action selection improves cognitive control in a model of the Stroop task. *Phil. Trans. Roy. Soc. B.* **362**: 1671–84.

Usher, M. and J. L. McClelland (2001). The time course of perceptual choice: the leaky, competing accumulator model. *Psychol. Rev.* **108**(3): 550–92.

Yehene, E., N. Meiran, and N. Soroker (2008). Basal ganglia play a unique role in task switching within the frontal-subcortical circuits: evidence from patients with focal lesions. *J. Cogn. Neurosci.* **20**(6): 1079–93.

Zhang, H. Z. H., J. Zhang, and S. Kornblum (1999). A parallel distributed processing model of stimulus–stimulus and stimulus–response compatibility. *Cogn. Psychol.* **38**(3): 386–432.

17 Mechanisms of choice in the primate brain: a quick look at positive feedback

Jonathan M. Chambers, Kevin N. Gurney, Mark D. Humphries, and Tony J. Prescott

Summary

The mammalian brain's decision mechanism may utilise a distributed network of positive feedback loops to integrate, over time, noisy sensory evidence for and against a particular choice. Such loops would mitigate the effects of noise and have the benefit of decoupling response size from the strength of evidence, which could assist animals in acting early at the first signs of opportunity or danger. This hypothesis is explored in the context of the sensorimotor control circuitry underlying eye movements, and in relation to the hypothesis that the basal ganglia serve as a central switch acting to control the competitive accumulation of sensory evidence in positive feedback loops representing alternative actions. Results, in support of these proposals, are presented from a systems-level computational model of the primate oculomotor control. This model is able to reproduce behavioural data relating strength of sensory evidence to response time and accuracy, while also demonstrating how the basal ganglia and related oculomotor circuitry might work together to manage the initiation, control, and termination of the decision process over time.

17.1 Introduction

Whether it is a cheetah deciding whether its prey is veering left or right, a rabbit deciding whether that movement in the bushes is friend or foe, or a poker player wondering if his opponent has a stronger hand, infinitesimally small variations in sensory input can give rise to vastly different behavioural outcomes: the cheetah veers left and not right, the rabbit flees or continues grazing, the card player bets a month's salary or folds. The outcome of such decisions can be critical, even a matter of life or death, which is why there will have been tremendous evolutionary pressure to develop decision-making mechanisms that can extract maximal utility from limited sensory information. In this chapter, using the oculomotor system as an exemplar, we argue that the vertebrate basal ganglia (BG) are one of the results of that evolutionary pressure and explore how these

Modelling Natural Action Selection, eds. Anil K. Seth, Tony J. Prescott and Joanna J. Bryson.
Published by Cambridge University Press. © Cambridge University Press 2012.

structures tame and exploit positive feedback loops (henceforth PFBLs) within the brain in order to make the most of limited information.

In humans, the usual behavioural outcome arising from a change in our visual environment is that we reorient our gaze in order to investigate that change. Indeed, we typically make rapid, ballistic eye movements, termed saccades, two or three times per second. As one of the most frequent actions we perform, deciding where to look next is therefore one of the most common decisions we make.

We are all familiar with the idea of 'taking our time' in order to make the right decision, but how long is long enough? Amid the convoluted anatomy of the primate oculomotor system one can discern a relatively short pathway from the retina to the superior colliculus (SC) and back to the extraocular muscles. The SC responds to visual stimulation in approximately 40 ms and electrical stimulation of its deeper layers can trigger a saccade within 20 ms (Wurtz and Goldberg, 1989). Consequently, this pathway could, in principle, initiate a saccade in response to a visual stimulus in 60 ms. However, in humans, visually triggered saccades are typically elicited with a response time (RT) of 200 ms or more. It would seem then that the brain 'takes its time' even when making this most common of decisions.

Curiously, the amount of time an individual takes to decide where to look next is highly variable. When a subject is asked to repeatedly saccade to a light appearing unpredictably in their peripheral vision, the distribution of their RTs is heavily skewed with the majority of responses beginning a few hundred milliseconds after stimulus onset but with a long tail of responses with some taking a second or more (Carpenter and Williams, 1995). Furthermore, the instructions given to a participant in such a study can dramatically affect this distribution. For instance, an emphasis on accuracy tends to shift the distribution towards longer response times, while an emphasis on speed has the opposite effect (Reddi and Carpenter, 2000). Not only are we able to adjust the length of time we take to react to externally cued events, we are, of course, also able to voluntarily move our eyes in order to achieve arbitrary goals, such as reading the words of this article. It would seem, therefore, that deciding where to look next is a non-trivial problem.

The diffusion model (Ratcliff, 1978) is an influential psychological model of decision making that can account for the brain's variable procrastination in reaching decisions. The model assumes that sensory evidence in favour of alternative responses is fundamentally noisy, whether due to the environment (e.g., tall grass obscuring a cheetah's prey), or due to random neural activity in the brain. Key to the model is the idea that the brain accumulates, or integrates, evidence over time in order to mitigate the effects of this noise, only making a decision when the difference in evidence for and against an action reaches a threshold level. The model is able to account for the skewed distribution of RTs obtained in saccadic studies and also provides insight into how the trade-off between speed and accuracy can be controlled by modifying the decision threshold. With a low threshold the model is able to make fast selections but is more likely to make errors due to noise. With a high threshold, the model integrates the evidence for longer and makes fewer errors since there is more time to average out the noise contribution.

Remarkably, under laboratory conditions the integration of evidence has indeed been observed in the brain. The stochastic motion discrimination task (Britten *et al.*, 1993), presents a monkey with a situation not wholly dissimilar to that faced by the hypothetical cheetah described above. The animal is presented with a display containing moving dots, a proportion of which are moving left on some trials and right on others, while the remaining dots move randomly (thus providing environmental noise). The difficulty of the task can be varied by adjusting the motion strength i.e., by changing the relative number of dots moving coherently. The monkey is given a reward for correctly indicating in which direction the majority of dots are moving by making a saccade, in the same direction, to one of two targets flanking the dot display.

The medial temporal (MT) area of visual cortex is stimulated by this task as neurons in this area are highly sensitive to motion. More specifically, each MT neuron is responsive to motion in a particular direction so that their firing rate indicates the extent to which their preferred motion is present in the current visual scene. Consequently, on a trial in which the net flow of dots is to the left, MT neurons that are sensitive to leftward motion have an average firing rate that is higher than that of neurons sensitive to rightward motion (Britten *et al.*, 1993). For the motion discrimination task, therefore, the noisy neural activity in area MT can be thought of as the evidence that the brain has available in order to decide where to look next.

The integration of area MT's evidence appears to occur in downstream oculomotor structures that are implicated in the planning and execution of saccades (Ditterich *et al.*, 2003; Gold and Shadlen, 2007; Schall, 2001). For instance, in the lateral intra-parietal (LIP) area neurons that are able to trigger saccades to the left or right target exhibit a ramp-like build-up of activity as the animal observes the moving dots (Roitman and Shadlen, 2002; Shadlen and Newsome, 2001). Allowing the animal to respond at its own pace, Roitman and Shadlen (2002) demonstrated that both the accuracy and speed of decisions increase with motion strength and that this corresponds with a steeper rise of activity in those LIP neurons with motor fields centred on the target that the animal ultimately saccades to. LIP neurons corresponding to the alternative target also demonstrate an initial increase in firing rate but this is suppressed below baseline rates prior to saccade generation. Taken together, these findings support the idea that LIP neurons represent the accumulation of evidence for and against a particular saccade. This, and the finding that the decision process is completed when LIP neurons reach a threshold firing rate, suggests that the brain utilises a decision algorithm similar to the diffusion model.

17.1.1   The oculomotor system

In order to explore how the circuitry of the brain implements a diffusion-model-like decision mechanism we now consider the anatomy of the oculomotor system of which a simplified circuit diagram is illustrated in Figure 17.1. In particular, we focus on those areas that are known to be involved in the production of visually guided saccades, as the model of the oculomotor system we present later is restricted to these areas.

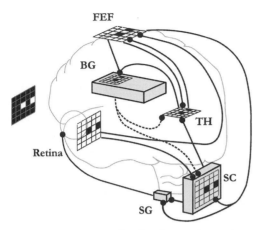

Figure 17.1 Brain areas forming the reactive oculomotor system. SC: superior colliculus; SG: saccadic generator; TH: thalamus; FEF: frontal eye fields; BG: basal ganglia. Solid and dashed lines denote excitatory and inhibitory projections, respectively.

17.1.1.1 The superior colliculus

Retinal ganglion cells project directly to the SC (Schiller and Malpeli, 1977), a multi-layered, midbrain structure, that preserves the spatial organisation of its retinal input. Figure 17.2 shows the basic connectivity of the SC as implemented in the model of Arai *et al.* (1994) (hereafter referred to as the Arai model) which we have incorporated into our own large-scale model (discussed in the methods section). The superficial layer of the SC relays its phasic retinal input to deeper motor layers, which in turn, send excitatory projections to a set of brainstem nuclei, collectively known as the saccadic generator (SG) circuit, which provide closed-loop control of the eye muscles (Sparks, 2002). The deeper layers of the SC also receive excitatory input from several frontal, visual, auditory, and somatosensory areas of cortex, so that saccades can be triggered voluntarily, or in response to processed visual features, localised noises, or physical contact with the body (Stein and Meredith, 1993).

17.1.1.2 The frontal eye field

Another important source of input to the SC comes from the frontal eye fields (FEF), an area of the frontal lobes implicated in saccade generation. In addition to projecting to the SC, the FEF also project directly to the SG so that a person or monkey with an SC lesion is still able to generate saccades. The FEF has reciprocal connections with both prefrontal and posterior cortices constituting the 'where pathway' of visual processing (Ungerleider and Mishkin, 1982). The input it receives from the dorsolateral prefrontal cortex (DLPFC) is implicated in the generation of voluntary saccades, while that from posterior cortices, including LIP, relays information concerning the location of salient visual targets. The nature of the processing that takes place in the 'where pathway' is not important for our purposes (indeed, in our depiction of this circuit in Figure 17.1 we have greatly simplified it by showing a direct connection between the retina and the FEF), other than to say that it preserves a retinotopic organisation throughout. The reciprocal

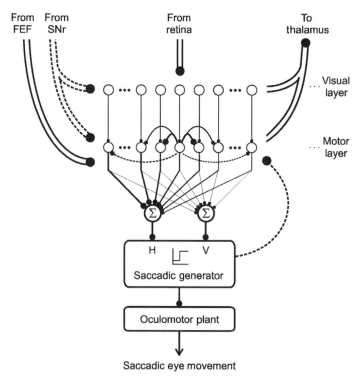

Figure 17.2 A model of the superior colliculus based on Arai *et al.* (1994). Solid and dashed lines denote excitatory and inhibitory projections, respectively. Double-lines denote topographic projections. See text for description.

connectivity between FEF and the posterior cortices suggests that FEF is both activated by the sensory information fed forward, and able to feed back the results of any frontal processing to those areas supplying the sensory information (see Cisek, this volume, for a similar proposal relating to the reach system). The evolution of build-up activity in LIP observed during the motion discrimination task could, therefore, be partially driven by the FEF.

17.1.1.3   The saccadic generator

The inner workings of the SG are beyond the scope of this chapter, however, one important detail of its operation is key to understanding later discussions. Models of the SG invariably incorporate a population of neurons found in the nucleus raphe interpositus known as the omni-pause-neurons (OPNs) (Langer and Kaneko, 1990). These neurons derive their name from the fact that they exhibit a pause in baseline firing just prior to saccade generation. They are thought to actively inhibit the brainstem neurons that drive changes in eye position and as such OPNs represent the oculomotor system's final gateway, blocking saccades until they themselves are silenced. OPNs are indirectly inhibited by those areas of the SC and FEF which represent potential saccade targets, while they are excited by the foveal regions of these structures (Buttner-Ennever *et al.*,

1999; Gandhi and Keller, 1997, 1999; Segraves, 1992; Stanton *et al.*, 1988). The fixation and saccade regions of the SC and FEF therefore provide the SG with conflicting commands, these being 'maintain fixation' and 'saccade to a new location', respectively. It is likely then that the relative level of activity in the fixation and saccade regions of the SC determines which of these two behaviours is expressed. Correspondingly, Munoz and Istvan (1998) have demonstrated that a decline in fixation activity is concomitant with the build up of target-related activity in the SC. This finding suggests that competitive dynamics within the oculomotor system must suppress ongoing fixation activity before a saccade can be generated.

17.1.1.4   The visuo-motor response

The visually guided saccade task is one of the most common paradigms used to probe activity within the oculomotor system. For this task the animal is trained to maintain active fixation of a central stimulus and to then saccade to a suddenly appearing target stimulus in peripheral vision. Electrophysiological studies with primates have revealed that neurons in the SC, FEF, and LIP display remarkably similar patterns of activity during this task (Ferraina *et al.*, 2002). First, neurons that represent the fovea show a tonic activation while the animal is maintaining fixation, and this appears to be largely endogenous in origin as it is not reliant on a fixation stimulus being present (Munoz and Wurtz, 1993). Second, neurons representing target coordinates display increases in activity that are time-locked to target stimulus onset, saccade onset or both – response classes that are respectively referred to as visual, motor, or visuo-motor (Figure 17.3; Munoz and Wurtz, 1995).

When animals produce saccades with a short RT it is often hard to discern separate visual and motor peaks, although careful analysis of the data reveals them to be present (Sparks *et al.*, 2000). Experiments in which the animal must delay its saccade make distinct peaks much more apparent. Under the delay paradigm the motor component displays a steady build-up of activity not dissimilar to that observed in the motion discrimination task described earlier (Wurtz *et al.*, 2001). Hanes and Schall (1996) demonstrated that the onset of the saccade is time-locked to the instant at which the motor activity in FEF reaches a threshold level, and similar thresholds have been found for LIP (Roitman and Shadlen, 2002) and SC (Pare and Hanes, 2003). Interestingly, as the build-up of motor activity continues towards threshold, there is a concomitant decrease in fixation activity. Recall that under the motion discrimination task it appears that decisions are only completed when there is sufficient difference between the elevated activity of the LIP neurons representing the chosen target and the suppressed activity of those representing the alternative target (Roitman and Shadlen, 2002). Similarly, under the visually guided saccade paradigm where the animal is making a choice between maintaining fixation and saccading to the target stimulus it would seem that, just as for the motion discrimination task, there is a requirement for a sufficiently large difference in the activity representing the competing alternatives, i.e., between fixation- and saccade-related activity. The oculomotor model we present later in this article incorporates the idea that OPNs are responsible for delaying action until this condition is met or, in other

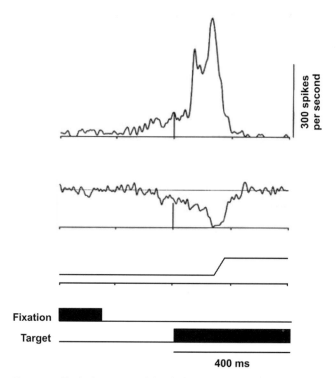

300 spikes per second

Fixation

Target

400 ms

Figure 17.3 Typical target- and fixation-related activity in the intermediate layers of monkey superior colliculus (SC) recorded during a visually guided saccade. Top trace shows a clear bimodal visuo-motor response in SC motor layer. Middle trace shows fixation-related activity reducing as target-related activity builds up. Bottom trace shows approximation of eye position for the same period. Data adapted from Munoz and Wurtz (1995).

words, that the OPNs implement thresholding in the brain's evidence accumulation mechanism for saccadic eye movements.

17.1.2   Accumulation by positive feedback

Given that the motor component of the visuo-motor response appears to represent the active process of decision making and that it is observed throughout the oculomotor system, it is interesting to consider what neural circuitry underlies it. Models seeking to address this question have largely concentrated on the cortical microcircuitry (Ditterich *et al.*, 2003; Usher and McClelland, 2001; Wang, 2002). Of these, the model proposed by Wang (2002) provides the most biologically plausible account of how populations of cortical neurons might accurately integrate sensory evidence by exploiting recurrent excitatory connections between neighbouring neurons. Arai *et al.* (1994) also offered local recurrent excitation as the most likely explanation for the build-up of motor activity observed in SC prior to a saccade. However, inspection of Figure 17.1 reveals that the oculomotor system contains at least two additional positive feedback loops: SC–TH–FEF–SC, and FEF–TH–FEF (TH = thalamus) (Haber and McFarland, 2001; Sommer and Wurtz, 2004) formed *between* oculomotor areas. Given this interconnectivity, it seems likely that the build-up of motor activity observed throughout the oculomotor system arises through the combination of PFBLs formed between neighbouring neurons within each oculomotor area, and by PFBLs formed by the long-range projections between these areas.

To understand the way in which positive feedback can be used to perform integration, consider the block diagram shown in Figure 17.4a which shows a simple rise-to-threshold mechanism with blocks f, b, and m, representing neural populations, which for the purpose of this discussion can be thought of as leaky integrators (Arbib, 2003), with an output limited to a minimum firing rate of zero, and a maximum of y_{max}. A salience signal c representing the sensory and/or motivational 'evidence' supporting an action, is fed into a closed loop formed by blocks f and b, the output of which is passed to block m, which provides the motor signal y^m, that drives the action. Block m also receives an inhibitory signal θ (assumed constant), which acts as a threshold to ensure that no action is produced until the output of the closed loop y^f exceeds a critical value. This architecture is loosely based on the oculomotor system (as shown in Figure 17.1), with the single loop formed by f and b representing the combined effect of SC–SC, SC–TH–FEF–SC, and FEF–FEF loops, and θ representing the threshold effect of the omni-pause neurons in the saccadic generator circuit. Accordingly, the signal β represents the inhibitory influence of the BG on these loops, the effect of which we shall consider shortly. We first consider the effect of the gains w^{fb}, and w^{bf}, which represent the synaptic weights of the projection from f to b and from b to f respectively. The closed loop gain G, of the subsystem formed by f and b is given by

$$G = w^{fb}w^{bf}. \tag{17.1}$$

Figure 17.4b shows the response of the system in Figure 17.4a, to a step change in salience of Δc, for different values of G. For $G > 1$, y^f is unstable and grows exponentially before saturating at y_{max}, so that action is guaranteed provided the selection threshold θ is less than y_{max}. In this situation, activity in the loop is self-sustaining, so that even when the salience signal returns to zero, the output of f remains saturated. For $G < 1$, y^f is stable and has an equivalent open-loop gain of $1/(1 - G)$, so that the final value of y^m is not guaranteed to reach saturation, but instead depends on the size of the salience signal c. Under this condition, the output of f tracks the salience signal, returning to zero when the salience signal does so.

With $G = 1$ the model exhibits the interesting behaviour of marginal stability, for which y^f increases linearly (after fast transients related to the neural time constant have settled) before reaching saturation. Recall that the diffusion model requires the temporal integration of evidence. With $G = 1$ this system approximates an ideal integrator and, as such, represents a way in which a pair of neurons, whose membrane voltages decay on a millisecond timescale, might accurately integrate information over the hundreds of milliseconds typically taken to make decisions. The circuit also makes clear another potential benefit that positive feedback can add to a selection system, namely the ability to raise weak sensory (and motivational) salience signals to the level required to elicit

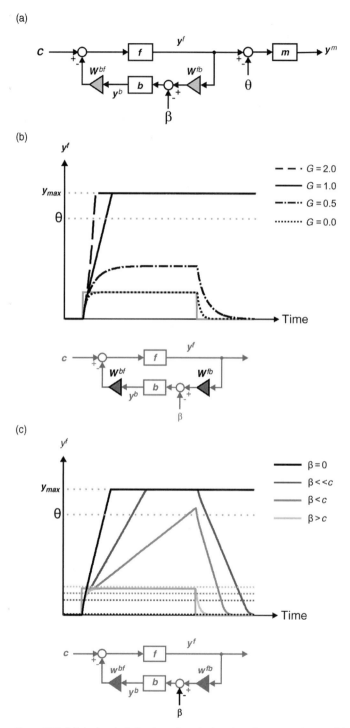

Figure 17.4 (a) A simple behavioural control system incorporating positive feedback. (b) The effect of varying the closed loop gain G; dashed line: $G = 2$; solid line: $G = 1$; dash-dot line: $G = 0.5$; dotted line: $G = 0$. (c) The effect of varying the level of loop inhibition β; dashed line: $\beta = 0$; solid line: $\beta \ll \Delta c$; dash-dot line: $\beta < \Delta c$; dotted line: $\beta \geq \Delta c$. See text for details.

action. Unchecked, this amplification will cause even the weakest of salience signals to trigger its corresponding behaviour, so that a system like this will seldom be at rest. This may upon first consideration sound rather inefficient, however, ethological models suggest such a scheme underlies animal behaviour. As Roeder (1975) points out: 'animals are usually "doing something" during most of their waking hours, especially when in good health and under optimal conditions'.

One potential benefit that arises from this tendency to act, is that problems are dealt with before they become unmanageable. For instance, in the absence of any other deficits, a mildly hungry animal will set about finding, and consuming food, thus ensuring that its hunger is sated before its energy levels become dangerously low. Accordingly, McFarland (1971) has shown that a hypothetical model of action selection incorporating positive feedback is able to account for animal feeding patterns. The oculomotor system could also be described as being unnecessarily active, however, orienting towards even weakly salient objects might provide an animal with an unexpected opportunity, or give it sufficient forewarning to avoid impending danger. By guaranteeing that motor signals reach saturation, positive feedback also acts to decouple the magnitude of a response from the magnitude of the salience signal driving it so that, for instance, a saccade's metrics (e.g., speed, duration) are largely independent from the properties of the stimulus that triggered it.

17.1.3   Competition in the oculomotor system

Much of the research into the neurobiology of decision making has focussed on LIP and recent models of decision making are consistent with the idea that this area is responsible for decision making. Under these proposals populations of neurons representing alternative actions compete with each other through mutual- (Usher and McClelland, 2001), feed-forward- (Ditterich *et al.*, 2003), or pooled-inhibition (Wang, 2002). Despite these architectural differences it has been demonstrated empirically (Ratcliff and Smith, 2004) and analytically (Bogacz *et al.*, 2006) that all three architectures can implement the diffusion process if appropriate parameters are selected.

Despite this, there is reason to suspect that LIP is not the sole seat of oculomotor decision making. As described in our review of the oculomotor system above, the ramp-like rise to threshold of motor activity observed in LIP is also observed within the FEF and SC, two areas that, like LIP, receive input from areas of extrastriate cortex (including area MT), and are able to elicit saccades. Lesion studies have revealed considerable redundancy amongst these structures. LIP lesions having relatively little effect on oculomotor function (Li *et al.*, 1999). Lesions to either FEF or SC produce more profound deficits (Dias and Segraves, 1999; Schiller and Chou, 1998), but only dual lesions of both FEF and SC can cause a permeant loss of function (Schiller *et al.*, 1980).

One possible interpretation of this apparent redundancy is that each of the oculomotor areas has some intrinsic capacity for action selection. More specifically, it may be the case that, as has been suggested for LIP, both FEF and SC have a local micro-circuit capable of independently implementing the diffusion process. If oculomotor decisions are computed in this distributed fashion then it would suggest that participating structures must coordinate with each other in order to ensure that conflicting motor commands are not issued to the brainstem.

An alternative interpretation of the oculomotor system's redundancy is that decisions are not computed in a distributed fashion but, rather, centrally by a dedicated selection mechanism. Redgrave *et al.* (1999) have argued that a centralised architecture is superior to a distributed architecture in terms of connectivity and metabolic efficiency.

To understand why this is the case consider, for instance, the mutual inhibition model of Usher and McClelland (2001). In this model, neurons representing saccades to alternative locations compete with each other via reciprocal inhibitory connections. While there is certainly evidence of reciprocal inhibition within cortex (Windhorst, 1996), if neurons representing saccades to all visual coordinates are to compete with each other, then neurons in every part of the retinotopic map in LIP would have to be connected to those in every other part. Evidence for sufficiently long-range inhibitory connectivity is lacking, and this is perhaps unsurprising given that such many-to-many connectivity would be a costly method of facilitating competition in terms of developmental overheads and metabolic consumption. This cost is compounded if similar connectivity is also necessary within FEF and SC, as it would presumably have to be under a distributed selection architecture. For these reasons we feel it is unlikely that the brain implements selection in this distributed fashion.

Redgrave *et al.* (1999) suggested that BG might constitute a centralised selection mechanism that offers a more efficient method of selecting between alternative actions. Under this proposal, structures which generate potentially conflicting motor commands send 'bids for action' to a central arbitrator, which chooses amongst them and signals this choice back to the bidding structures. The idea that the BG are involved in action selection is a recurring theme in the literature (Kropotov and Etlinger, 1999; Mink, 1996) and forms the basis of a unifying hypothesis of BG function that incorporates known anatomy and physiology (Prescott *et al.*, 1999; Redgrave *et al.*, 1999). Recent work by Bogacz and Gurney has lent further weight to this proposed role for the BG by demonstrating that their intrinsic connectivity can be interpreted as a minimal neural implementation of an optimal hypothesis testing algorithm (Bogacz and Gurney, 2007; Bogacz *et al.*, this volume).

Anatomical and functional evidence also support this role for the BG within the oculomotor system. FEF and TH both project to the input nuclei of the BG with retinotopic projections (Harting *et al.*, 2001; Hikosaka *et al.*, 2000), so that the SC–SC, SC–TH–FEF–SC, and FEF–TH–FEF positive feedback loops identified earlier can each provide either direct or indirect bids to the BG. Also, the substantia nigra pars reticulata (SNr) – one of the output nuclei of the BG – provides strong tonic inhibition to the TH and SC so that the BG can impose choices upon the same positive feedback loops. Indeed, this inhibitory output is known to pause prior to saccade initiation (Hikosaka *et al.*, 2000) suggesting that the BG are acting to gate the build-up of saccade-related activity within the oculomotor system.

Having established that connectivity between the BG and oculomotor structures conforms to the expectations of a centralised selection scheme, we now consider the computation performed by the BG. Gurney *et al.* (2001) suggest that the intrinsic connectivity of the BG implements a form of feed-forward selection network. Figure 17.5 shows their computational model (hereafter referred to as the Gurney model), and provides a description of how intrinsic BG processing achieves signal selection. A key assumption is that the topography of BG inputs is preserved throughout the BG nuclei so that competing actions are represented by activity in distinct channels. The extent to which a channel is selected is determined by the difference between its input salience and the sum of all other input saliences. The calculation takes place in SNr, where diffuse excitatory input from the subthalamic nucleus (STN) effectively provides the sum of channel activity, and focused inhibitory input from D1 striatal cells provides a measure of individual channel activity. The diffuse STN projection allows inter-channel communication, so that input to a given BG channel acts to raise the level of inhibition outputted from all other channels. Thus, the growth rate of motor activity in a BG controlled PFBL, will depend not only on the sensory input driving it, but also on the activity in other BG controlled loops. So, for instance, in the visually guided saccade paradigm, activity in a loop corresponding to the fixation coordinate will affect activity in a loop corresponding to the target coordinate.

Returning to the simple model shown in Figure 17.4a, we now consider the effect of the inhibitory input β, which represents the effect of SNr inhibition upon oculomotor PFBLs. Figure 17.4c shows the response of the system to a step change in salience of Δc, for different values of β and with the loop weights set to give ideal integration ($G = 1$). When the inhibitory input to the loop is greater or equal to the salience signal i.e., $\beta \geq \Delta c$, the positive feedback is effectively disabled because the input to b is zero or less. Consequently, the system behaves like a first order system, with its output settling at the level of its input. Under these circumstances, action is not guaranteed and will depend upon the magnitude of the salience signal c. For $\beta < \Delta c$ the feedback becomes active as soon as y^f exceeds β, causing a linear increase in y^f with a rate determined by the difference $\Delta c - \beta$, thus guaranteeing that y^m reaches y_{max}, and overcomes the selection threshold. The inhibitory input also provides a means of overcoming the self-sustaining property of the loop, causing activity to decay linearly at a rate, again determined by $\Delta c - \beta$, when the salience signal returns to zero. From this it is clear that β acts as both a threshold for activation of the PFBL, and a rate controller for the evolution of activity in the loop. Or, in other words, β determines whether 'evidence accumulation' is initiated, is able to scale the rate of accumulation, and can help passively terminate the accumulation process by removing accumulated evidence.

Having explored the properties of a single PFBL under inhibitory control, the remainder of this chapter examines the behaviour of multiple PFBLs in the context of a computational model of the primate oculomotor system. As pictured in Figure 17.1, this system can be thought of as a set of parallel loops, like those in Figure 17.4, each one corresponding to a different spatial coordinate. A key difference, according to the approach taken here, is that each loop's β input is determined by the competitive dynamics of the BG. The model described below is a revised version of the oculomotor system model

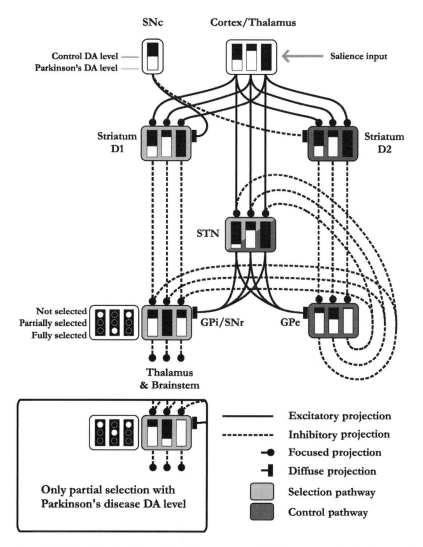

Figure 17.5 The intrinsic BG model of Gurney *et al.* (2001), assumes that duplicate salience input is sent to the subthalamic nucleus (STN) and striatum, which is further subdivided in two groups of cells classified by the type of dopamine (DA) receptor they express (D1 and D2). The globus pallidus internal segment (GPi) and substantia nigra pars reticulata (SNr) – which together form the output nuclei of the basal ganglia (BG) – send inhibitory projections back to the thalamus and to the motor nuclei in the brainstem (e.g., the superior colliculus). Spontaneous, tonic activity in the STN guarantees that this output is active by default, so that all motor systems are blocked. Gurney *et al.* (2001) identify two separate functional pathways within the BG. The selection pathway is responsible for disinhibiting salient actions: salience input to a channel activates D1, which then inhibits GPi/SNr thus silencing inhibitory output in the channel. The diffuse projection from STN to GPi/SNr means that all channels receive an increased excitatory drive. This is offset in the most active channel by the inhibitory input from D1, but goes unchecked in less active channels thus acting to block unwanted actions. The control pathway defined by Gurney *et al.* (2001) incorporates the globus pallidus external segment (GPe), and provides capacity-scaling by ensuring that STN activity does not become excessively high when multiple channels have non-zero salience, thus assuring full disinhibition of the winning channel irrespective of the number of competing channels. Because the striatal input to the control and selection pathways utilise different DA receptors, changes in tonic DA levels affect them differentially. Consequently, when DA is reduced to Parkinson's disease-like levels, the balance between the two pathways is disturbed resulting in residual inhibition on the selected channel (inset).

proposed by Chambers (2007), and hereafter referred to as the Chambers model. This model was previously shown to be able to reproduce data from several visually guided experimental paradigms. Here, we will demonstrate that a simplified version of the model can also reproduce data from a 'noisy' two-alternative, forced-choice task similar to the motion discrimination task reviewed earlier. Specifically, we will demonstrate that the model is able to reproduce appropriate RT distributions and error rates, and demonstrate a relationship between RT and the strength of sensory evidence relative to noise levels. We will also show that plasticity within the BG could provide a means of adaptively controlling the accumulation process. Before presenting these results, we provide a brief overview of the original model (see Chambers, 2007, for a full description) together with details of the modifications made for the purposes of the current study.

17.2   Methods

The Chambers model simulates, from perception to action, the full sensorimotor competency of visually guided saccade generation. More specifically, the model simulates an experimental display, the retina, the SC (based on the model of Arai et al., 1994) (Figure 17.2), FEF, TH, the BG (based on the model of Gurney et al., 2001) (Figure 17.5), the SG (based on the model of Gancarz and Grossberg 1998), and the eyeball and its musculature.

    The model explicitly tests the 'central switch' hypothesis of Redgrave et al. (1999) as the BG is the only structure in the model able to inhibit the build-up of motor activity i.e., reciprocal inhibition within cortex and the SC is not modelled. The BG is modelled using a two-dimensional version of the Gurney et al. model (described in the preceding section), which receives one-to-one excitatory projections from FEF and TH and sends a one-to-one inhibitory projection to SC and back to TH.

    The model also tests the hypothesis that a distributed network of PFBLs acts in concert to integrate evidence for and against specific saccades. Local positive feedback is modelled within SC via reciprocal excitatory connectivity between neighbouring neurons (with weights reducing with distance as modelled by Arai and Keller, 2005; Arai et al., 1994), long-range positive feedback loops are modelled by one-to-one projections between SC, TH, and FEF.

    The Chambers model also tests the idea that the SG is involved in managing the accumulation process. The model incorporates the biologically plausible model of the SG proposed by Gancarz and Grossberg (1998), which converts the spatially distributed representation of a saccade target, as found in SC and FEF, into the appropriate temporal signals necessary to drive the extra-ocular musculature. In the Chambers model the activity of the OPNs is determined by activity in the FEF and SC: foveal activity acts to increase OPN output, thus preventing saccades, while activity in the periphery inhibits the OPNs thus facilitating saccade generation. Under this interpretation of the anatomy, the OPNs are therefore ultimately responsible for setting the threshold for action within the oculomotor system.

    Finally, the Chambers model also incorporates evidence suggesting that the SG provides negative feedback to the SC as a saccade is generated (Goossens and Van Opstal,

2000; Soetedjo *et al.*, 2002). It is suggested that this inhibitory signal provides a means of actively resetting the decision mechanism by removing previously accumulated evidence.

For the current study, several changes were made to the Chambers model in order to simplify its interpretation and speed its execution time. First, the original model reproduced the log-polar representation of visual space found throughout the oculomotor system. Here we have removed this and simply represent visual space linearly in order to simplify the interpretation of results. Second, the Gancarz and Grossberg (1998) model of the SG was not included. Instead, we approximate the behaviour of this model by taking the centroid of combined SC and FEF activity just prior to saccade generation. Furthermore, we assume that saccades are made instantaneously, thus removing the need to simulate the dynamics of the eyeball. One aspect of the Gancarz model that is retained, however, is the inclusion of OPNs. These are modelled as a single leaky integrator excited and inhibited respectively by the foveal, and peripheral representations of FEF and SC. The centroid of saccade-related activity is sampled, and a saccade generated, when OPN activity reaches zero, and is not sampled again for a simulated refractory period of 100 ms (this prevents the eye from being continually repositioned despite the OPN remaining at zero for a short duration). At the same time that the centroid is taken, an inhibitory signal is injected into the build-up layer of the SC, simulating the feedback from the SG to the SC.

It has previously been demonstrated that the Chambers model can reproduce behavioural data from several visually guided experimental paradigms (Chambers, 2007). In this chapter, we seek to demonstrate that the model can also reproduce data from a 'noisy' two-alternative, forced-choice task similar to the motion discrimination task reviewed earlier. It was not possible to test the oculomotor model with the motion discrimination task as it lacks a representation of area MT and is, as a consequence, unable to simulate tasks that require the subject to make a discrimination based on stimulus motion.

We instead simulate an alternative paradigm which requires the subject to make a discrimination based on stimulus luminance. Under this paradigm, which has been utilised by Ludwig *et al.* (2005), the subject is first presented with a central fixation stimulus, which is abruptly extinguished and replaced with two spatially separated target stimuli. The subject is required to saccade to the brighter of the two targets. The luminance of the targets varies randomly over the course of the trial, with values being drawn from a normal distribution. The distributions used for each target have the same variance but different means. Task difficulty can be adjusted by altering the difference in mean luminance relative to the power of the noise or, in other words, by adjusting the signal to noise ratio.

In order to explore the selection capabilities of this system and its similarity to the diffusion model, we investigate its behaviour under four conditions:

- The control condition: the dimmer target has a mean luminance that is 95% that of the brighter target.
- A high luminance condition: the luminance of both targets is increased from the control value by 10%.

- A high contrast condition: the luminance of the brighter target is increased from the control value so that the dimmer target has a luminance that is 90% that of the brighter target.
- A low weight condition: the targets have the same mean luminance as the control condition, but the model's cortico- and thalamo-striatal weights are reduced to 90% of their control value.

We simulate the luminance discrimination task by generating a two-dimensional array that represents the world, a subregion of which is inputted into a retinal model. The subregion that is sampled depends on the current simulated eye position, which is initially set to be at the centre of the world-array where the fixation stimulus is also located. The retinal model is a two-layer network, with one layer that responds phasically to luminance increases and one which produces a tonic output proportional to luminance level. Both retinal layers project to the FEF layer, while only the phasic layer projects to the superficial layer of SC (which in turn relays that input to the deep layer of SC). These projections both introduce a 50 ms delay to simulate delays introduced by retinal processing and axonal propagation.

A random number generator provides input into the FEF layer of the model in order to simulate the combined effects of environmental and neural noise. This noise source is temporally filtered using a low pass Butterworth filter in order to decouple the power spectrum of the noise from the simulation frequency of the model.

Each experimental condition is simulated for 400 trials with a sampling frequency of 400 Hz. A trial consists of 2 s of simulated activity. The fixation stimulus is presented from 50 ms to 600 ms, and is then exchanged for the target stimuli which remains on for the remainder of the trial (Figure 17.6a).

In each trial, if the endpoint of a generated saccade is within $\pm$ 2° of the target with the higher mean luminance it is considered to be a correct response. Trials producing saccades that land elsewhere, or that fail to produce a saccade at all, are considered to have produced incorrect responses. Response accuracy was evaluated with the binomial test (one-sided) of the null hypothesis that the accuracy of a given test condition was the same as that for the control condition. The effect of test condition and response outcome (correct or incorrect) upon response time were assessed by two-factor ANOVA with Tukey post-hoc analyses. For all tests a level of $p < 0.05$ was considered significant.

17.3   Results

17.3.1   Accumulation dynamics in the oculomotor model

We first review the operation of the model during a single trial of the luminance discrimination task in order to highlight what each part of the modelled anatomy contributes to the decision process. Figure 17.6 shows typical model activity during a trial conducted under the control condition. This trial highlights the effect of noise on the decision process as the model erroneously selects the target with the lower mean luminance.

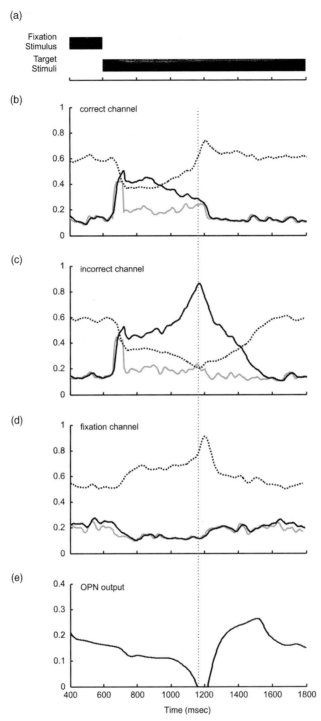

Figure 17.6 Model activity for a trial resulting in the selection of the incorrect target under the control condition. (a) Experimental timing; fixation onset occurred 350 ms prior to the period shown; fixation offset and dual target onset was simultaneous. (b) Output of neurons within the channel corresponding to the correct target, i.e., neurons with a receptive field centred on the correct target; for this and (c) and (d), the solid and broken black lines correspond to output from FEF and SNr, respectively; the grey line corresponds to sensory input supplied to FEF, i.e., the combination of retinal input and the noise source. (c) Neural output from the incorrect target channel. (d) Neural output from fixation channel. (e) Output from the omni-pause-neurons (OPNs). The vertical dropline denotes the instant at which a saccade to the incorrect target was initiated.

17.3.1.1   Initiation

Figure 17.6 shows activity in a subset of model layers from 200 ms prior to target onset. There are a number of things to note about this period, and that immediately following target onset. First, as can be seen from Figures 17.6b and c, noise in the target channels prior to target onset is not integrated thus ensuring that the system does not make spontaneous saccades in response to noise. This resistance to noise is due to the inhibitory output from SNr acting upon TH and SC, which ensures that the net input to these structures is negative thus preventing positive feedback dynamics from being initiated by the SC–SC, FEF–TH–FEF, and SC–TH–FEF–SC PFBLs upon which the model's accumulation dynamics rely.

Recall that the Gurney *et al.* (2001) BG model generates a baseline inhibitory output in the absence of salient input so that, in effect, downstream structures have a brake applied by default. Also recall that, when the BG model does have salient input, the level of SNr output is increased in losing channels (Figure 17.5). Prior to the target onset the BG selects the fixation channel (as this is the only channel with external input) and, as a consequence, all other channels, including the target channels, receive above baseline inhibition. This selection is evident from the slight reduction in SNr activity in the fixation channel (Figure 17.6d) relative to that in the target channels (Figures 17.6b and c). The reduction in fixation channel SNr activity is relatively small owing to a manipulation we made to simulate the influence of prefrontal cortex (PFC) upon the oculomotor BG. We explain this in the following section.

At 650 ms into the trial, retinal input corresponding to target onset reaches the FEF layer (Figures 17.6b and c) injecting a 'pulse-step' waveform of input into FEF and thus the model's system of PFBLs. The initial phasic burst is sufficiently large to overcome the effect of SNr inhibition on TH and SC, thus allowing the accumulation dynamic to be initiated. The 'pulse' also acts to rapidly establish a 'beach-head' of accumulated evidence in the system's PFBLs which subsequently feeds into the BG and causes a corresponding reduction in SNr activity thus enabling the integration of the 'step' over time.

One interpretation of this scheme, is that the burst of activity generated by stimulus onset is a form of interrupt signal, signalling that there is a stimulus that may warrant breaking from ongoing fixation. With this interpretation in mind, it is interesting to note that when a predictable stimulus onset acts to distract an animal from obtaining reward on a saccadic task, the corresponding phasic burst of activity (as observed in superficial SC) becomes attenuated over the course of several trials (Goldberg and Wurtz, 1972). It is likely that this attenuation prevents the accumulation of sensory evidence corresponding to the distracter, thus diminishing its ability to trigger a saccade. Later we will propose that the BG, in conjunction with PFC, may be involved in this pre-attentive habituation.

17.3.1.2   Competitive accumulation

Under the control condition, the contrast between targets is low compared to the level of noise. As a result of this the accumulated activity in each target's channel is very similar post target onset (Figures 17.6b and c). Correspondingly, the level of SNr activity applied to each channel is also similar, so that the BG grant neither channel a significant advantage over the other. Initially then, the rate of accumulation is mainly dependent on the strength of evidence for each target, as provided by tonic retinal input. However, as a result of the noise in the system, accumulated evidence in favour of the incorrect target takes an early lead in the particular trial shown in the figure. The BG circuitry responds to this increase in the incorrect target's channel activity by reducing SNr activity further for this channel, while increasing that to all other channels.

As a result of the change in relative SNr activity the BG imposes a bias on the accumulation process that favours evidence in the leading channel over that of losing channels. In other words, the system shows a primacy effect, favouring early evidence over that which comes later. In the trial shown, the accumulated evidence in the correct target's channel, despite having the higher mean input, is not able to overtake that in the incorrect target's channel which leads to an increase in this BG mediated bias. At approximately 950 ms the SNr input to the correct target's channel increases to such a level that the net input to that channel's accumulator circuit is negative, thus causing activity therein to decline. Conversely, SNr input to the incorrect target's channel continues to decrease, accelerating the rate of evidence accumulation in favour of making an erroneous saccade. This separation of signals is consistent with the findings of Roitman and Shadlen (2002) using the motion discrimination task. In the following sections we suggest that the increase in decision signal contrast that results from this separation is key to both the correct programming of saccadic movements and to facilitating rapid learning within the BG.

The BG-mediated competition between channels is also able to account for the mutual exclusivity between target and fixation activity reported by Munoz and Istvan (1998). Prior to target onset, the fixation channel is the most active channel although, as Figure 17.6d shows, the accumulation dynamic has not significantly amplified the input signal in this channel. The model was manipulated in order to prevent accumulation in the fixation channel, as early experiments, in which build-up was permitted, produced unrealistically prolonged RTs because residual fixation activity competed strongly with burgeoning target activity. Accumulation was prevented by providing additional drive to the fixation channel's D2 pathway in the BG, which has the effect of increasing SNr output for that channel. This is consistent with earlier work (Chambers and Gurney, 2008), which demonstrated a mechanism via which associative areas of the PFC might manipulate the behaviour of motor systems by top-down inputs to motor striatum. Our manipulation therefore represents the effect of frontal associative systems having learnt to restrict the effective salience of fixation stimuli relative to novel peripheral onsets.

17.3.1.3 Selection, enaction, and accumulator reset

In our interpretation of the oculomotor anatomy, the OPNs represent the final barrier to action and, thus, indirectly determine when the decision process is over. Figure 17.6e shows the activity in the OPNs over the course of the trial. Recall that fixation activity in FEF and SC excites the OPNs while target-related activity inhibits them. At 1150 ms the sum of target-related activity is sufficiently large compared to fixation activity that the OPNs are silenced and the saccade generation process is commenced.

The SG model generates a saccade to the centroid of summated FEF and SC activity (approximating the behaviour of the more biologically plausible Gancarz model) and so it is critical to accurate target acquisition that the BG competitive dynamics produce a clear peak of accumulator activity centred on the chosen target, while suppressing activity elsewhere as seen in Figures 17.6b and c. We model saccades as an instantaneous shift in eye position. The visual consequence of this shift is that the target stimuli move to different locations on the retina. For the trial shown, the saccade was accurate and so the incorrect target is now at the centre of the retina.

Post-selection it is critical that accumulated evidence is removed otherwise the system will continue to generate a staircase of saccades with the same relative displacement as the first (an effect that is observed when SC is driven continuously by micro-stimulation; Breznen et al., 1996). As Figure 17.6c shows, activity in the selected channel does indeed begin to decay after saccade generation. The model discards accumulated evidence both passively and actively. As the simple system shown in Figure 17.4c shows, removal of excitatory input can lead to passive decay of activity. An eye movement moves the target stimuli to a different part of the retina which, owing to the zero-luminance background used in the featured experiment, causes the target channels to lose their excitatory input. This reduction can be seen in the input trace in Figures 17.6b and c, and the increase in fixation channel activity resulting from target acquisition can be seen in Figures 17.6d.

In a natural scene there is every possibility that during, and immediately after, a saccade there *will* be salient input at the retinal coordinate the saccade target previously occupied. Consequently, *active* suppression of accumulated evidence is required in order to guarantee that accumulated evidence will be removed. One approach the oculomotor system appears to utilise is the active blocking of visual input whilst the eye is moving, a phenomenon known as 'saccadic suppression' (Thiele et al., 2002). Another active method is the robust negative feedback from the SG to the SC which effectively eliminates the SC–TH–FEF–SC and SC–SC feedback loops. The current model is tuned so that the combined effect of its distributed positive feedback loops approximates a single loop with a closed loop gain of unity (as shown in Figure 17.4c). Consequently, active suppression of two of these loops reduces the effective gain below unity so that the system loses its ideal integrator properties. We modelled both forms of active suppression as a brief burst of inhibition applied to the retina and the SC at the instant that a saccade is triggered.

17.4   Conclusions

The preceding sections have shown that the model is able to cleanly select between multiple options (albeit incorrectly in the given example) when provided with physiologically plausible inputs. Furthermore, the model illustrates that the accumulation dynamic observed throughout the oculomotor system can be reproduced through the inhibitory control of a distributed positive feedback network. Also, although not modelled, feedback to LIP, from FEF, could in principle induce a similar pattern of activity in that area, consistent with observations. Key control issues not addressed by abstract

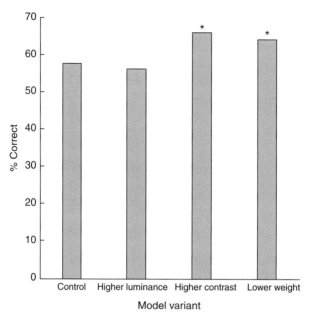

Figure 17.7 Percentage of trials that produced a saccade to the correct target for each of the experimental conditions. Asterisks indicate that the test condition produced a significant increase in accuracy compared to control condition.

mathematical models such as initiation thresholds, and reset mechanisms, have been shown to have physiological correlates in the guise of baseline SNr output and brainstem feedback respectively. We now consider the affect of sensory evidence and internal processing on the decision process.

17.4.1   Accuracy, response time, and the effect of learning

Figure 17.7 shows how successful the model was in selecting the brightest target under the four experimental conditions. These results demonstrate that an increase in absolute target luminance does not produce a significant change in accuracy ($p < 0.05$), while increasing stimulus contrast between stimuli does ($p < 0.05$). This is consistent with findings from the motion discrimination task in which increased motion contrast gives rise to increased response accuracy (Roitman and Shadlen, 2002). That increased stimulus contrast improves accuracy is perhaps unsurprising as this arises as a natural consequence of competitive dynamics. A less intuitive finding is that lowering cortico- and thalamo-striatal weights also produces a significant increase in accuracy ($p < 0.05$) similar in magnitude to that produced by increased contrast. This manipulation reduces the efficacy with which accumulated evidence within a given channel is able to request a reduction in the SNr activity applied to it. Because SNr levels are higher for a given level of accumulated evidence, under this condition, the accumulation dynamic progresses more slowly (as illustrated in Figure 17.4c). By being forced to 'take its time' in this way, the accumulation process is better able to average out the effects of noise and in so doing

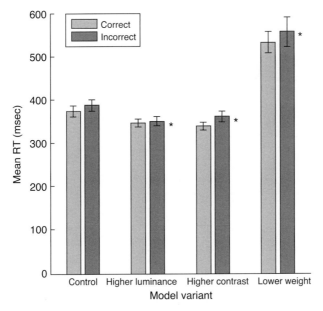

Figure 17.8 Median response time (RT) for correct and incorrect trials for each of the experimental conditions. Asterisks indicate that the test condition produced a significantly different mean RT compared to the control condition.

reduces the error rate. This result highlights the potential role that striatal plasticity may play in modulating the dynamics of decision making.

Figure 17.8 shows how the mean RT of correct and incorrect trials varies between experimental conditions. Both test condition and outcome (correct or incorrect) had a significant effect on RT ($p < 0.05$), while the interaction did not. Post-hoc tests revealed that both the high luminance and high contrast condition produced significant reductions in RT ($p < 0.05$), while the lower weight condition produced a significant increase in RT ($p < 0.05$). These results highlight that, while lowering cortico- and thalamo-striatal weights produced a similar increase in accuracy to increased target contrast, it comes at the cost of prolonged RT, the same trade-off observed when subjects voluntarily elect to increase their response accuracy in a saccadic task. The finding that the RT of incorrect trials is significantly longer than that of correct trials is consistent with findings from the motion discrimination task (Roitman and Shadlen, 2002). This property of the model arises from the fact that on error trials (such as that shown in Figure 17.6) the losing channel actually has the higher mean input. This means that, despite having a greater SNr input, the accumulated evidence in the losing channel can grow at a similar rate to that in the lead channel. This increased level of competition prolongs the selection process as it restricts the ability of the BG to further increase the contrast in SNr output.

Figure 17.9 shows the distribution of RTs achieved under each experimental condition for correct trials only. Figure 17.9a represents the RT data as histograms and clearly shows that the distributions of RT under each condition each exhibit a rightward skew

(a)

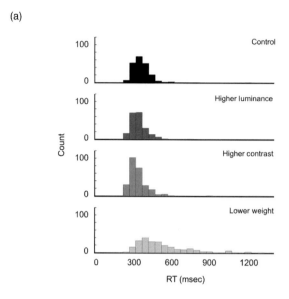

(b)

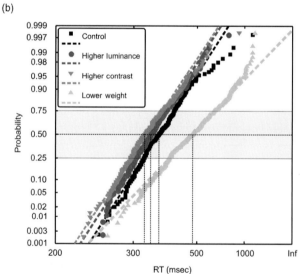

Figure 17.9 Response time (RT) distributions for correct trials under each experimental condition. (a) Histograms of RT distribution for each condition. (b) Reciprobit plots of RT distribution for each condition. See text for explanation.

as discussed in Section 17.1. It is also clear that the distribution for the lower weight condition is significantly more skewed than that of any other condition.

Although intuitive to understand, it is hard to compare distributions represented as histograms. In Figure 17.9b we therefore show the RT distributions as a reciprobit plot. This type of plot is most commonly used to compare RT data with the assumptions of the LATER model of Carpenter (1981), which models decision making as a race to threshold between evidence accumulators that do not inhibit each other. Although our model differs considerably from the LATER model, it is useful to try and characterise the RT distribution produced by our model using the relatively simple LATER framework.

First, the fact that each condition's plotted results form straight lines (for the inner quartiles at least) indicates that the reciprocal of RT has a normal distribution, indicating that the RT skew exhibited under each condition is consistent with a linear rise to threshold. Second, the distributions for the higher luminance and higher contrast conditions appear to be leftwards shifted versions of that for the control condition indicating that the mean rate of evidence accumulation is increased under these conditions. Finally, the fact that the distribution for the lower weight condition is both rightwards shifted and of reduced gradient, indicates that the mean rate of evidence accumulation is lower under this condition, but also that the total amount of evidence to be accumulated is increased, i.e., the distance between the initial evidence level and the threshold for action is increased.

17.5   Discussion

In this chapter we have demonstrated that the oculomotor anatomy, when viewed as a parallel array of, largely independent, BG-controlled PFBLs, appears to implement a decision mechanism with properties similar to the diffusion model. Further, we have shown that the BG (as conceptualised by Gurney et al., 2001) are able to arbitrate between alternative actions represented by accumulated sensory evidence, whilst also providing a threshold for the initiation of the accumulation process and a means of resetting accumulated evidence once an action has been initiated. We have demonstrated that this system, in the process of arbitrating between competing signals, also acts as to amplify its inputs so that cortical motor commands are of a standardised magnitude irrespective of stimulus strength. Finally, we have demonstrated that changes in synaptic weights within the striatum (the BG input nucleus) are able to adjust the system's RT/accuracy trade-off.

As described in Section 17.1 there are several computational models that ascribe observed accumulation dynamics to the cortical micro-circuitry (Ditterich et al., 2003; Usher and McClelland, 2001; Wang, 2002). The evidence we have presented in this chapter does not rule out the possibility that cortical circuitry fulfils an arbitration role, but does serve to highlight the possibility that this function might be performed centrally, by the BG. This view is consistent with other models that highlight the role of BG in controlling the build-up of motor activity in PFBLs (Arai et al., 1994; Grossberg and Pilly, 2008). We now seek to highlight two key advantages that the BG may offer as a centralised selection architecture.

17.5.1   Potential advantages of centralised selection by the basal ganglia

17.5.1.1   Algorithm refinement
As described above, the oculomotor model presented in this chapter has properties in common with the diffusion model. It can be demonstrated that, for two-alternative forced-choice tasks, the diffusion model is mathematically equivalent to an optimal statistical

test known as the sequential probability ratio test (SPRT) (Wald, 1947). The equivalent optimal statistical test for decisions involving more than two alternatives is called the *multihypothesis* sequential probability ratio test (MSPRT) (Baum and Veeravalli, 1994). Bogacz and Gurney have demonstrated that the intrinsic connections of the BG can be interpreted as a minimal neural implementation of the MSPRT algorithm (Bogacz and Gurney, 2007; Bogacz *et al.*, this volume). Thus, while it may, in principle, be possible to optimally select between two alternatives using the cortical micro-circuit, there is evidence that the specialised architecture of the BG may be best suited to resolving such competitions where there are more than two alternatives. One advantage of separating out this specialised selection function from cortex, may be that cortical specialisations are able to evolve without affecting the optimality of decision making while, at the same time, all modalities requiring decision making, benefit from evolutionary improvements to the BG.

In their model of BG, Bogacz and Gurney (2007) made the simplifying assumption that evidence accumulation occurred independently from the BG, i.e., accumulators feed integrated evidence into the BG but are not, in turn, affected by it. The model we present here therefore differs from that of Bogacz and Gurney, in that the output of the BG inhibits the PFBLs that feed into it. This change affects the relative importance of sensory evidence supplied over the course of the decision making process.

The diffusion model (and MSPRT) treats all evidence equally throughout the decision process so that evidence arriving just prior to action selection has the same influence on the decision process as the earliest evidence. Our model, in contrast, does not treat all evidence equally because losing accumulators are inhibited (by BG output) to a greater extent than the lead channel, so that as evidence accumulation in the lead channel approaches the selection threshold, losing channels must supply evidence at an ever increasing rate if they are to reverse the decision. In other words, whereas the diffusion model (and MSPRT) chooses between actions based on the quantity of evidence alone, the oculomotor system, as we have interpreted it, chooses based upon evidence and ongoing commitment to an action, i.e., as accumulated evidence increases, commitment to the leading decision starts to dominate with evidence from losing channels having a reduced influence. The policy implemented by the model therefore values conviction over accuracy.

It may be that our model has more in common with a variant of the diffusion process proposed by Busemeyer and Townsend (1993), which includes a term that is related to the current value of accumulated evidence. Support for an evidence inequality in decision making comes from the work of Ludwig *et al.* (2005) who tested human subjects using the same luminance discrimination paradigm described here. These authors found that the initial 100 ms of stimulus presentation had the greatest influence upon the participant's ultimate decision with later information having little or no effect.

17.5.1.2   Adaptive learning

In addition to their candidate role as the vertebrate brain's 'central switch' (Redgrave *et al.*, 1999), there is good evidence to suggest that the BG play a critical role in reward-based learning (Hollerman *et al.*, 2000) so that they are perhaps better thought of as an '*adaptive* central switch'. In this chapter, we have demonstrated that striatal efficacy can affect accumulation dynamics and hence the RT/accuracy trade-off implemented. Consistent with this role is the fact that striatum receives convergent input from both sensory cortex and most areas of the pre-frontal cortex (PFC), suggesting that the 'context-aware' PFC is able to directly influence action selection. This begs the question: what constitutes evidence? In the oculomotor system, for instance, DLPFC provides excitatory input to FEF and oculomotor BG (see Johnston and Everling, 2008, for review), suggesting that 'endogenous evidence' in DLPFC could augment, or even act as a substitute for 'exogenous evidence' from sensory cortices. This might lead to faster selection times for visible targets or the generation of purely voluntary eye movements to locations for which there is no sensory evidence.

In addition to being involved in decisions to act, it may be that PFC, through its influence on BG, is able to control decisions not to act. Certain tasks require that the subject withhold a response that they would ordinarily elicit, and it would appear that the BG provide a means of blocking habitual behaviour when necessary. Using a model derived from the architecture presented in this chapter, we have recently explored the role of the 'indirect pathway' (involving D2-type medium spiny neurons) in *inaction* selection (Chambers and Gurney, 2008). This work sought to demonstrate how PFC can, via a cortico-striatal projection, learn to either selectively facilitate or block the accumulation of sensory evidence by exploiting PFC neurons that have an asymmetrical influence on the D1- and D2-type neurons present in a given channel. The model is able to successfully reproduce results from the non-match to sample task used by Hasegawa *et al.* (2004) for which success relies on the participant overriding the 'habitual' tendency to attend to a primed location.

Acknowledgements

This research was supported by the EPSRC Doctoral Training Award scheme and by the EPSRC-funded REVERB project (EP/C516303/1). The authors are grateful to members of the Adaptive Behaviour Research Group at the University of Sheffield for their advice and comments.

References

Arai, K. and E. L. Keller (2005). A model of the saccade-generating system that accounts for trajectory variations produced by competing visual stimuli. *Biol. Cybern.* **92**(1): 21–37.

Arai, K., E. L. Keller, and J. Edelman (1994). Two-dimensional neural network model of the primate saccadic system. *Neural Networks* **7**(6/7): 1115–35.

Arbib, M. (2003). *The Handbook of Brain Theory and Neural Networks*. Cambridge, MA: MIT Press.

Baum, C. W. and V. V. Veeravalli (1994). A sequential procedure for multihypothesis testing. *IEEE T. Inform. Theory* **40**(6): 1994–2007.

Bogacz, R., E. Brown, J. Moehlis, P. Holmes, and J. D. Cohen (2006). The physics of optimal decision making: a formal analysis of models of performance in two-alternative forced-choice tasks. *Psychol. Rev.* **113**(4): 700–65.

Bogacz, R. and K. Gurney (2007). The basal ganglia and cortex implement optimal decision making between alternative actions. *Neural Comput.* **19**(2): 442–77.

Breznen, B., S. M. Lu, and J. W. Gnadt (1996). Analysis of the step response of the saccadic feedback: system behavior. *Exp. Brain Res.* **111**(3): 337–44.

Britten, K. H., M. N. Shadlen, W. T. Newsome, and J. A. Movshon (1993). Responses of neurons in macaque MT to stochastic motion signals. *Vis. Neurosci.* **10**(6): 1157–69.

Busemeyer, J. R. and J. T. Townsend (1993). Decision field theory: a dynamic-cognitive approach to decision making in an uncertain environment. *Psychol. Rev.* **100**(3): 432–59.

Buttner-Ennever, J. A., A. K. Horn, V. Henn, and B. Cohen (1999). Projections from the superior colliculus motor map to omnipause neurons in monkey. *J. Comp. Neurol.* **413**(1): 55–67.

Carpenter, R. H. and M. L. Williams (1995). Neural computation of log likelihood in control of saccadic eye movements. *Nature* **377**(6544): 59–62.

Carpenter, R. H. S. (1981). Oculomotor procrastination. In *Eye Movements: Cognition and Visual Perception*, ed. D. F. Fisher, R. A. Monty, and J. W. Senders. Hillsdale, NJ: Lawrence Erlbaum Associates, pp. 237–46.

Chambers, J. M. (2007). *Deciding where to look: a study of action selection in the oculomotor system*. PhD thesis, University of Sheffield.

Chambers, J. M. and K. Gurney (2008). A computational model of inaction-selection in multiple domains of basal ganglia. *SFN Abst.* **472**.7.

Dias, E. C. and M. A. Segraves (1999). Muscimol-induced inactivation of monkey frontal eye field: effects on visually and memory-guided saccades. *J. Neurophysiol.* **81**(5): 2191–214.

Ditterich, J., M. E. Mazurek, and M. N. Shadlen (2003). Microstimulation of visual cortex affects the speed of perceptual decisions. *Nat. Neurosci.* **6**(8): 891–8.

Ferraina, S., M. Pare, and R. H. Wurtz (2002). Comparison of cortico-cortical and cortico-collicular signals for the generation of saccadic eye movements. *J. Neurophysiol.* **87**(2): 845–58.

Gancarz, G. and S. Grossberg (1998). A neural model of the saccade generator in the reticular formation. *Neural Networks* **11**(7–8): 1159–74.

Gandhi, N. J. and E. L. Keller (1997). Spatial distribution and discharge characteristics of superior colliculus neurons antidromically activated from the omnipause region in monkey. *J. Neurophysiol.* **78**(4): 2221–5.

Gandhi, N. J. and E. L. Keller (1999). Activity of the brain stem omnipause neurons during saccades perturbed by stimulation of the primate superior colliculus. *J. Neurophysiol.* **82**(6): 3254–67.

Gold, J. I. and M. N. Shadlen (2007). The neural basis of decision making. *Annu. Rev. Neurosci.* **30**: 535–74.

Goldberg, M. E. and R. H. Wurtz (1972). Activity of superior colliculus in behaving monkey. I. Visual receptive fields of single neurons. *J. Neurophysiol.* **35**(4): 542–59.

Goossens, H. H. and A. J. Van Opstal (2000). Blink-perturbed saccades in monkey. II. Superior colliculus activity. *J. Neurophysiol.* **83**(6): 3430–52.

Grossberg, S. and P. K. Pilly (2008). Temporal dynamics of decision-making during motion perception in the visual cortex. *Vision Res.* **48**(12): 1345–73.

Gurney, K., T. J. Prescott, and P. Redgrave (2001). A computational model of action selection in the basal ganglia. II. Analysis and simulation of behaviour. *Biol. Cybern.* **84**(6): 411–23.

Haber, S. and N. R. McFarland (2001). The place of the thalamus in frontal cortical-basal ganglia circuits. *Neuroscientist* **7**(4): 315–24.

Hanes, D. P. and J. D. Schall (1996). Neural control of voluntary movement initiation. *Science* **274**(5286): 427–30.

Harting, J. K., B. V. Updyke, and D. P. Van Lieshout (2001). Striatal projections from the cat visual thalamus. *Eur. J. Neurosci.* **14**(5): 893–6.

Hasegawa, R. P., B. W. Peterson, and M. E. Goldberg (2004). Prefrontal neurons coding suppression of specific saccades. *Neuron* **43**(3): 415–25.

Hikosaka, O., Y. Takikawa, and R. Kawagoe (2000). Role of the basal ganglia in the control of purposive saccadic eye movements. *Physiol. Rev.* **80**(3): 953–78.

Hollerman, J. R., L. Tremblay, and W. Schultz (2000). Involvement of basal ganglia and orbitofrontal cortex in goal-directed behavior. *Prog. Brain Res.* **126**: 193–215.

Johnston, K. and S. Everling (2008). Neurophysiology and neuroanatomy of reflexive and voluntary saccades in non-human primates. *Brain Cogn.* **68**(3): 271–83.

Kropotov, J. D. and S. C. Etlinger (1999). Selection of actions in the basal ganglia-thalamocortical circuits: review and model. *Int. J. Psychophysiol.* **31**(3): 197–217.

Langer, T. P. and C. R. Kaneko (1990). Brainstem afferents to the oculomotor omnipause neurons in monkey. *J. Comp. Neurol.* **295**(3): 413–27.

Li, C. S., P. Mazzoni, and R. A. Andersen (1999). Effect of reversible inactivation of macaque lateral intraparietal area on visual and memory saccades. *J. Neurophysiol.* **81**(4): 1827–38.

Ludwig, C. J., I. D. Gilchrist, E. McSorley, and R. J. Baddeley (2005). The temporal impulse response underlying saccadic decisions. *J. Neurosci.* **25**(43): 9907–12.

McFarland, D. (1971). *Feedback mechanisms in animal behavior*. New York: Academic Press.

Mink, J. W. (1996). The basal ganglia: focused selection and inhibition of competing motor programs. *Prog. Neurobiol.* **50**(4): 381–425.

Munoz, D. P. and P. J. Istvan (1998). Lateral inhibitory interactions in the intermediate layers of the monkey superior colliculus. *J. Neurophysiol.* **79**(3): 1193–209.

Munoz, D. P. and R. H. Wurtz (1993). Fixation cells in monkey superior colliculus. I. Characteristics of cell discharge. *J. Neurophysiol.* **70**(2): 559–75.

Munoz, D. P. and R. H. Wurtz (1995). Saccade-related activity in monkey superior colliculus. I. Characteristics of burst and buildup cells. *J. Neurophysiol.* **73**(6): 2313– 33.

Pare, M. and D. P. Hanes (2003). Controlled movement processing: superior colliculus activity associated with countermanded saccades. *J. Neurosci.* **23**: 6480–9.

Prescott, T. J., P. Redgrave, and K. Gurney (1999). Layered control architectures in robots and vertebrates. *Adapt. Behav.* **7**: 99.

Ratcliff, R. (1978). A theory of memory retrieval. *Psychol. Rev.* **85**: 59–108.

Ratcliff, R. and P. L. Smith (2004). A comparison of sequential sampling models for two-choice reaction time. *Psychol. Rev.* **111**(2): 333–67.

Reddi, B. A. and R. H. Carpenter (2000). The influence of urgency on decision time. *Nat. Neurosci.* **3**(8): 827–30.

Redgrave, P., T. J. Prescott, and K. Gurney (1999). The basal ganglia: a vertebrate solution to the selection problem? *Neurosci.* **89**(4): 1009–1023.

Roeder, K. (1975). Feedback, spontaneous activity, and behaviour. In Baerends, G., Beer, C., and Manning, A. (eds), *Function and Evolution in Behaviour. Essays in Honour of Professor Niko Tinbergen, F.R.S.* Oxford: Clarendon Press, pp. 55–70.

Roitman, J. D. and M. N. Shadlen (2002). Response of neurons in the lateral intraparietal area during a combined visual discrimination reaction time task. *J. Neurosci.* **22**(21): 9475–89.

Schall, J. D. (2001). Neural basis of deciding, choosing and acting. *Nat. Rev. Neurosci.* **2**(1): 33–42.

Schiller, P. H. and I. H. Chou (1998). The effects of frontal eye field and dorsomedial frontal cortex lesions on visually guided eye movements. *Nat. Neurosci.* **1**(3): 248–53.

Schiller, P. H. and J. G. Malpeli (1977). Properties and tectal projections of monkey retinal ganglion cells. *J. Neurophysiol.* **40**(2): 428–445.

Schiller, P. H., S. D. True, and J. L. Conway (1980). Deficits in eye movements following frontal eye-field and superior colliculus ablations. *J. Neurophysiol.* **44**(6): 1175–89.

Segraves, M.A. (1992). Activity of monkey frontal eye field neurons projecting to oculomotor regions of the pons. *J. Neurophysiol.* **68**(6): 1967–85.

Shadlen, M. N. and W. T. Newsome (2001). Neural basis of a perceptual decision in the parietal cortex (area LIP) of the rhesus monkey. *J. Neurophysiol.* **86**(4): 1916–36.

Soetedjo, R., C. R. Kaneko, and A. F. Fuchs (2002). Evidence that the superior colliculus participates in the feedback control of saccadic eye movements. *J. Neurophysiol.* **87**(2): 679–95.

Sommer, M. A. and R. H. Wurtz (2004). What the brain stem tells the frontal cortex. I. Oculomotor signals sent from superior colliculus to frontal eye field via mediodorsal thalamus. *J. Neurophysiol.* **91**(3): 1381–402.

Sparks, D., W. H. Rohrer, and Y. Zhang (2000). The role of the superior colliculus in saccade initiation: a study of express saccades and the gap effect. *Vision Res.* **40**(20): 2763–77.

Sparks, D. L. (2002). The brainstem control of saccadic eye movements. *Nat. Rev. Neurosci.* **3**(12): 952–64.

Stanton, G. B., M. E. Goldberg, and C. J. Bruce (1988). Frontal eye field efferents in the macaque monkey: I. Subcortical pathways and topography of striatal and thalamic terminal fields. *J. Comp. Neurol.* **271**(4): 473–92.

Stein, B. E. and M. A. Meredith (1993). *The Merging of the Senses*. Cambridge, MA: MIT Press.

Thiele, A., P. Henning, M. Kubischik, and K. P. Hoffmann (2002). Neural mechanisms of saccadic suppression. *Science* **295**(5564): 2460–2.

Ungerleider, L. G. and Mishkin, M. (1982). Two cortical visual systems. In *Analysis of Visual Behavior*, ed. D. J. Ingle, M. A. Goodale, and R. J. W. Mansfield. Cambridge, MA: MIT Press, pp. 549–86.

Usher, M. and J. L. McClelland (2001). The time course of perceptual choice: the leaky, competing accumulator model. *Psychol. Rev.* **108**(3): 550–92.

Wald, A. (1947). *Sequential Analysis*. New York: Wiley.

Wang, X. J. (2002). Probabilistic decision making by slow reverberation in cortical circuits. *Neuron* **36**(5): 955–68.

Windhorst, U. (1996). On the role of recurrent inhibitory feedback in motor control. *Prog. Neurobiol.* **49**(6): 517–87.

Wurtz, R. H. and M. E. Goldberg, eds (1989). *The Neurobiology of Saccadic Eye Movements*. Amsterdam: Elsevier.

Wurtz, R. H., M. A. Sommer, M. Pare, and S. Ferraina (2001). Signal transformations from cerebral cortex to superior colliculus for the generation of saccades. *Vision Res.* **41**(25–26): 3399–412.

Part III

Action selection in social contexts

18   Introduction to Part III: action selection in social contexts

Joanna J. Bryson, Tony J. Prescott, and Anil K. Seth

In nature, action selection is rarely purely an individual matter; rather, adaptive action selection usually involves a social context. As Seth demonstrates in Part I, the apparently irrational behaviour of an individual viewed in isolation can, in fact, be optimal when considered in a semi-social context that includes competing conspecifics. Importantly, the agents in Seth's model express no explicitly social behaviour – there are no direct costs or benefits associated with social interactions. Rather, agents in the model interact indirectly via their effects on resource distribution in the environment. This demonstrates the ubiquity of social phenomena in nature, which of course will, in general, lead to selective pressure for social adaptations.

The final section of our volume is dedicated to studies of action selection in an explicitly social context. All of the models here *do* include social actions for individuals to select among. Once we begin to consider societies, however, it also becomes apparent that we can study action selection at the level of the society itself, and how such selection emerges from individual behaviour. In this introduction, we discuss the evolutionary and theoretical background underlying social action selection whilst briefly highlighting some of the contributions of subsequent chapters regarding current controversies in this field.

18.1   Simulations as explanations of pro-social behaviour

Just as it can be a mistake to model an individual without its social environment, it can also be a mistake to model a society without taking sufficient care to model the perception, memory, and action selection of the individual. The most egregious error along these lines leads to the still-pervasive misconception that costly pro-social behaviour – altruism – is difficult to evolve (e.g., Watson *et al.*, 2009; Boesch *et al.*, 2010). This misconception fundamentally hampers the understanding of social behaviour, and therefore of human and animal behaviour more generally.

The problem of altruism is that on the simplest level, paying a penalty to help another reduces your own probability of reproduction relative to that other. Thus a naïve view of the 'survival of the fittest' leads to the expectation that altruism is maladaptive – yet

Modelling Natural Action Selection, eds. Anil K. Seth, Tony J. Prescott and Joanna J. Bryson.
Published by Cambridge University Press. © Cambridge University Press 2012.

pro-social behaviour is pervasive in nature. Hamilton (1964) provides a simple explanation. First, altruistic actions can be adaptive if their benefit to others, multiplied by the relatedness of these others to the actor paying the cost, outweighs the cost to the actor. Second, because individuals move at a finite rate, have a finite lifespan, and start life at the same location as their mothers, physical proximity will correlate with relatedness for individuals of the same species. This property, known as *viscosity* facilitates altruism by removing the need for more complex kin-recognition systems.

Unfortunately, some theoretical biologists overlooked the fact that individuals are not identical, or that variation is not evenly distributed in space and time, leading to a history of contradictory theoretical results concerning altruism (Sober and Wilson, 1998). Artificial intelligence (AI) simulations that include time and continuous (real-valued) spatial location have, for example, demonstrated that altruistic acts can be adaptive, provided that they increase the carrying capacity of the environment local to the altruistic actors (Mitteldorf and Wilson, 2000; Čače and Bryson, 2007). Similarly, some authors argued that altruism could not invade a selfish population because altruism in isolation is a maladaptive trait. Simulation clarifies that in the real world, fluctuations due to predator–prey dynamics mean that population levels are not always at carrying capacity for the environment. This allows maladaptive traits to survive and reproduce for long enough that collective advantages can be realised (Čače and Bryson, 2007; Alizon and Taylor, 2008).

Although the chapters in this book do not explicitly deal with altruism, this issue serves to illustrate the value of simulation in exploring the impact of complex real-world dynamics on social behaviour. Further, it serves to provide a biological context for some of the social behaviours described below.

18.2   Levels of selection: ultimate goals and action-selection mechanisms

Darwin (1859) described natural selection in the context of individual organisms, but more recent evolutionary theory has focussed on the most basic and purest level of replication. A sexually reproducing animal never truly duplicates itself, but rather mixes its genes with those of another individual. Dawkins (1982) clarifies the relationship between individual animals and natural selection by referring to genes (the theoretical entities hypothesised to replicate themselves in biological evolution) as *replicators*, and the organisms that contain these genes as *vehicles*. From the perspective of the genes, there is little difference between an animal and a society (Sober and Wilson, 1998; West *et al.*, 2007). Both are a form of vehicle, and each level of abstraction can be seen as creating or affecting selective pressures. For example, a primate species that lives collectively reduces threat, and therefore pressure from predation, by increasing the probability that some animal will see an approaching predator and alert the whole troop (McNamara and Houston, 1992). On the other hand, group living brings its own pressures. For example, animals require time and skills for affiliative behaviour which increase the probability that an animal stays healthy, wins or avoids fights, and has reproductive opportunities.

Recently, some have argued that in eusocial species such as bees and termites, the colony should be viewed as a sort of 'super-organism' (Gardner and Grafen, 2009; Hölldobler and Wilson, 2008). Whether or not this hypothesis is true, the selective pressures of accuracy and speed are similar for the action selection of a group as for an individual. As Marshall, Bogacz, Dornhaus, Kovacs, and Franks (this volume) describe, there are striking parallels between decision making in primate brains and the collective decision making in social insect colonies. In both systems, separate populations (the first of neurons, the second of individual insects) accumulate evidence, each for one alternative among a number of possible choices. In both systems, when one population reaches a threshold level of certainty, the collective as a whole acts as if it has made a decision favouring that population's alternative. Further, for both systems, the threshold at which action occurs can be varied according to local pressures for speed (which lowers the threshold of accumulated information) and accuracy of decision making (which raises it). Marshall *et al.* also indicate that social insect colonies may be able to achieve statistically optimal collective decision making with respect to minimising decision time for any given error rate. In providing this general theoretical framework for decision making, Marshall *et al.* also make testable predictions which will allow further work in social insect research to examine whether real-world decision making follows these principles.

18.3   Levels of selection, emergence, and cognition in social behaviour

The introduction of the social level of action selection leads to new ways to consider the cognitive capacities of individuals. Having established that selection can result in similar mechanisms at a variety of levels (Marshall *et al.*, this volume), and that actions may be evolved and selected that serve a variety of selective pressures or individual goals (Crabbe, this volume), we open the question of how much intellectual work is done by individuals. Does apparently clever behaviour indicate that another species possesses a rich mental life, perhaps similar to our own? How and to what extent does the mental life that we experience really affect our own behaviour?

Whilst, at the level of folk psychology, there is a general preference for complex cognitive explanations of primate and human behaviour, modelling studies tend to favour Occam's principle that the simplest explanation is also the most probable. Many simulations have found that surprisingly complex behaviour can be explained through relatively simple cognitive mechanisms. This approach has become known as 'cognitive minimalism'. An example of this is the well-known and widely published Hemelrijk (1999) DomWorld agent-based model of primate social structure. In many primate species, dominant males grant access to resources to females when they are sexually receptive and capable of reproduction. Hemelrijk has used DomWorld as evidence that this apparent exchange of favours occurs simply because males are attracted to females during that period, and that females also tend to become more dominant themselves when they engage in more social interactions. Bryson, Ando, and Lehmann (this volume) re-analyse the DomWorld model and some of the data it seeks to explain. Bryson *et al.* argue that

DomWorld cannot fully account for observed dominance patterns, raising the possibility that a more cognitive explanation of this behaviour may be required after all. On a methodological level, this chapter demonstrates that agent-based models are – like any other scientific hypothesis – open to analysis, extension, refutation, and confirmation.

Cognitive minimalism remains, nevertheless, an impressively successful strategy for modelling natural action selection in social contexts. Rands, Pettifor, Rowcliffe, and Cowlishaw (this volume) use optimised agent-based modelling to consider optimal foraging behaviour not only in terms of calories consumed, but also in terms of avoiding predation. They consider a variety of parameters for a model of how animals might combine these two concerns. By default their agents have a desire to stay within a safe distance of other conspecifics, but if sufficiently hungry they will prioritise good foraging over safety. Since currently there is no suitable biological database for Rands *et al.* to attempt to match, their model is presented in a more general form as a series of predictions concerning how grouping behaviour will vary with cognitive abilities such as perception. Their model also demonstrates an emergent propensity for animals to cohere with others with similar current physical state. This is a known property of some social species, such as fish (Blakeslee *et al.*, 2009).

18.4   Precise matches to quantitative data: voting mechanisms in animals and humans

To show how social simulation can be used to account for detailed quantitative data and behaviour, we close this volume with two accounts of voting mechanisms for collective action selection – one in apes, the other in humans.

Hill, Logan, Sellers, and Zappala (this volume) look to account for group action selection for navigation and resource consumption as it varies per season for a specific species in a specific African field site in the De Hoop Nature Reserve of South Africa. These authors present a spatial simulation which precisely models the 200×200 study grid used by field researchers studying a particular troop of chacma baboons (*Papio hamadryas ursinus*). The baboons themselves are modelled in a metabolically accurate way based on established knowledge of baboon physiology. From here Hill *et al.* attempt to account for observed individual action selection between the high-level goals of foraging, drinking, socialising, and resting, and also the collective selection of the next range area that the troop will move to. Here Hill *et al.* assume a voting model, where the troop moves when a simple majority of animals agree a direction. Whilst their initial model matches the general behaviour of the baboon troop, Hill *et al.* acknowledge that accounting for the exact patterns of habitat exploitation as they vary over the year is much more difficult. A more accurate match is achieved in a refined model that also includes a measure of resource depletion.

Our final chapter completes Part III's bridge from the biological into the social sciences, by addressing social decision making in the human realm. Laver, Sergenti, and Schilperoord (this volume) model action selection by political parties as an explicit, rather than emergent, consequence of the desires of their electorate. Laver *et al.* also use a spatial agent-based model, but here 'space' represents beliefs or desires across axes of political positions, such as conservative versus liberal. These authors build on an existing model of Laver (2005) of political parties, which included a typology of strategies, e.g., STICKER ideological parties that maintain a single position, AGGREGATOR democratic parties which take the mean position of their voters, and HUNTER opportunistic parties that wander ideological space looking to maximise votes. The original model was able to match and categorise the strategies of real national parties in the Republic of Ireland. In their chapter, Laver *et al.* extend the original model to include party birth and death. They find that this revised model accounts for a range of interesting political phenomena, such as the fact that new parties tend to begin in very peripheral parts of the policy space. Further, they identify a set of rules that can be used to easily recognise whether a party is using the democratic or opportunistic strategy based on its location in policy space. Finally, they also present results concerning the representativeness of a political system consisting of particular mixes of types of parties and the political life-span of various strategies.

18.5   Modelling, action selection, and science

Our goal with this volume is not only to present examples of good science being conducted through the application of artificial models, but also to provide a survey of techniques for modelling natural action selection. The chapters of this final part of our volume make a significant contribution here as several of the authors explicitly attend to methodological questions. For instance, Marshall *et al.* unify two fields of research – neuroscience and entomology – using a generalisable framework that is potentially extensible to other biological domains. At a more meta-theoretic level, Bryson *et al.* discuss the position of AI models in ordinary science. While some have argued that agent-based modelling is a 'third way' to do science, Bryson *et al.* argue that a model is just a scientific hypothesis, to be tested, extended, supported, refuted, and adapted like any other. In particular, theories-as-models can be perfectly shared when the source code for the model is openly released, thus improving and accelerating scientific communication. In this final section Laver *et al.*, Hill *et al.*, and Bryson *et al.* demonstrate how such extension and critique can work, whilst Rands *et al.* and Marshall *et al.* provide useful discussions of methodology and extend the investigation of optimality that has been a recurring theme of this volume.

References

Alizon, S. and P. Taylor (2008). Empty sites can promote altruistic behaviour. *Evolution* **62**(6): 1335–44.

Blakeslee, C., N. Ruhl, W. Currie, and S. McRobert (2009). Shoaling preferences of two common killifish (*Fundulus heteroclitus* and *F. diaphanus*) in the laboratory and in the field: a new analysis of heterospecific shoaling. *Behav. Proc.* **81**(1): 119–125.

Boesch, C., C. Bolé, N. Eckhardt, and H. Boesch (2010). Altruism in forest chimpanzees: the case of adoption. *PLoS One* **5**(1): e8901, doi:10.1371/journal.pone.0008901.

Čače, I. and J. J. Bryson (2007). Agent based modelling of communication costs: why information can be free. In *Emergence and Evolution of Linguistic Communication*, ed. C. Lyon, C. L. Nehaniv, and A. Cangelosi. London: Springer, pp. 305–322.

Darwin, C. (1859). *On the Origin of Species by Means of Natural Selection*. London: John Murray.

Dawkins, R. (1982). *The Extended Phenotype: The Gene As the Unit of Selection*. London: W.H. Freeman and Company.

Gardner, A. and A. Grafen (2009). Capturing the superorganism: a formal theory of group adaptation. *J. Evol. Biol.* **22**(4): 659–671.

Hamilton, W. D. (1964). The genetical evolution of social behaviour. *J. Theor. Biol.* **7**: 1–52.

Hemelrijk, C. K. (1999). An individual-oriented model on the emergence of despotic and egalitarian societies. *Proc. Roy. Soc. B Biol. Sci.* **266**: 361–9.

Hölldobler, B. and E. O. Wilson (2008). *The Superorganism*. Norton, London.

Laver, M. J. (2005). Policy and the dynamics of political competition. *Amer. Pol. Sci. Rev.* **99**(2): 263–81.

McNamara, J. M. and A. I. Houston (1992). Evolutionarily stable levels of vigilance as a function of group size. *Anim. Behav.* **43**(4): 641–58.

Mitteldorf, J. and D. S. Wilson (2000). Population viscosity and the evolution of altruism. *J. Theor. Biol.* **204**(4): 481–96.

Sober, E. and D. S. Wilson (1998). *Unto Others: The Evolution and Psychology of Unselfish Behavior*. Cambridge, MA: Harvard University Press.

Watson, K. K., J. H. Ghodasra, and M. L. Platt (2009). Serotonin transporter genotype modulates social reward and punishment in rhesus macaques. *PLoS ONE* **4**(1): e4156.

West, S. A., A. S. Griffin, and A. Gardner (2007). Evolutionary explanations for cooperation. *Curr. Biol.* **17**: R661–R672.

19 Agent-based models as scientific methodology: a case study analysing the DomWorld theory of primate social structure and female dominance

Joanna J. Bryson, Yasushi Ando, and Hagen Lehmann

Summary

A scientific methodology must provide two things: first a means of explanation, and second, a mechanism for improving that explanation. It is also advantageous if a methodology facilitates communication between scientists. Agent-based modelling (ABM) is a method for exploring the collective effects of individual action selection. The explanatory force of the model is the extent to which an observed meta-level phenomena can be accounted for by the behaviour of its micro-level actors. But to demonstrate ABM is truly a scientific method, we must demonstrate that the theory it embodies can be verified, falsified, extended, and corrected. This chapter contains a case study demonstrating ABM as biological science. We show that agent-based models like any scientific hypotheses can be tested, critiqued, generalised, or specified. After first reviewing the state of the art for ABM as a methodology, we present our case: an analysis of Hemelrijk's DomWorld, a widely published model of primate social behaviour. Our analysis shows some significant discrepancies between the model and the behaviour of the genus we compare it to, the macaques. We then demonstrate that the explanation embodied in the DomWorld model is not fragile: its other results are still valid and can be extended to compensate for the problems identified. This robustness is a significant advantage of experiment-based artificial intelligence modelling techniques over purely analytic modelling.

19.1   Introduction

Agent-based modelling (ABM) is a method for testing the collective effects of individual action selection. More generally, ABM allows the examination of macro-level effects from micro-level behaviour. Science requires understanding how an observed characteristic of a system (e.g., a solid) can be accounted for by its components (e.g., molecules). In ABM we build models of both the components and the environment in which they

Modelling Natural Action Selection, eds. Anil K. Seth, Tony J. Prescott and Joanna J. Bryson.
Published by Cambridge University Press. © Cambridge University Press 2012.

exist, and then observe whether the overall system-level behaviour of the model matches that of the target (or *subject*) system.

ABM is a sufficiently new technique that there is still some controversy in its use, and still some unevenness in its application and description in scientific papers. Most critically, there is not enough established methodological practice for incorporating modelling results into true scientific discourse. In this chapter, we discuss ABM and the techniques for its analysis. We also present a case study where we analyse, critique, and extend one of the most extensively published ABMs in biology, Hemelrijk's DomWorld (Hemelrijk, 1999, 2000, 2002, 2004; Hemelrijk *et al.*, 2003, 2005, 2008). DomWorld provides an explanation of systematic differences in social organisation observed in closely related primate species.

Section 19.2 reviews the recent literature on analysing ABM, and assesses how this applies to the specific case of modelling in the biological sciences. We then provide the background information necessary for understanding DomWorld: the literature describing the target system we test the model against (macaque social behaviour) and a thorough description of the model and its results. In Section 19.4 we analyse DomWorld. Finally, we conclude by illustrating our earlier discussion of ABM as a scientific methodology in light of our analysis of DomWorld. We show that ABM produces not fragile analytic models, but rather robust scientific hypotheses, open to critique, extension, and circumscription.

19.2   Analysing agent-based modelling

In order for a methodology to be useful to science, it must provide two things: first a means of explanation, and second, a mechanism for improving that explanation. The explanatory force of the model is the extent to which an observed meta-level phenomena can be accounted for by the behaviour of its micro-level actors. Where models are running programs, they are tested by sampling their behaviour both over time and over a number of runs. Different experimental runs may use either the same parameters, in order to discover the range of possible results due only to the effects of random variation; or use systematically varying parameter values to test the significance of each parameter set or *condition*. The behaviour of the model system is then compared with the behaviour of the target system.

Axelrod (1985) is credited with founding ABM with his evolutionary simulations of cooperative behaviour (Axelrod and Hamilton 1981; though see Hogeweg and Hesper, 1979). He is still one of the area's main advocates. In the appendix of a recent text on the topic, Axelrod and Tesfatsion (2006) describe four research goals for the ABM field:

1. *Empirical*: 'Why have large-scale regularities evolved and persisted, even when there is little top-down control?'
2. *Normative understanding*: 'How can agent-based models be used as laboratories for the discovery of good designs?'

3. *Heuristic*: 'How can greater insight be attained about the fundamental causal mechanisms in social systems?'
4. *Methodological advancement*: 'How [can we] best provide ABM researchers with the methods and tools they need to undertake the rigorous study of social systems . . . and to examine the compatibility of experimentally-generated theories with real-world data?'

The bulk of the present chapter focuses on the fourth, methodological question as applied to biology. In the present volume, science in general subsumes Axelrod's third heuristic question – we achieve greater understanding by doing science. The type of models we examine focus primarily on empirical rather than normative problems, as best suits biology. In the present section we focus primarily on the methodological issue of 'compatibility' between theory and data, which in the ABM literature is often called the problem of *validation*.

19.2.1 Validation and analytic solutions

As ABM has become more prevalent in the social sciences and, particularly, in business and public policy, there has been an increasing emphasis on developing methods of verification and validation (Balci, 1998; Kennedy *et al.*, 2006). *Verification* is the process of making certain a model runs as designed. In science, this is roughly equivalent to ensuring that good experimental practice has been followed. *Validation* is the process of making certain the model actually models the target system. Our main thesis for this chapter is this: when ABMs are used for biology, validation is equivalent to hypothesis testing. We will begin by discussing validation, then return to verification shortly.

There is a common perception that ABMs are so complex (that is, have so many parameters) that they can be made to easily match any data or predict any outcome, but that having done so the system will have no capacity for generalisation, and therefore no predictive power. In practice, however, building and debugging an ABM is a difficult skill, and matching datasets is not easy. While it is true that ultimately most datasets can be matched, the principle value of the model is expressing what aspects need to be changed in order to generate these various outcomes. Where the data is behavioural, the model aspects that determine it are the model's theory of action selection.

If a model is built first to a set of justified assumptions, and *subsequently* matches a dataset with minimal adjustment, then it is generally considered to be at least partially validated. Of course, the more datasets it matches, the better-validated the model becomes. As this notion of *better*-validated implies, validation is not simply a state that either holds or does not hold for a model. Rather a model, like any scientific hypothesis, becomes more *probable* (given the data) the more it is validated. But a model never becomes perfectly certain (Box, 1979). The only exception is if a model becomes understood to such an extent that it can be *proven* correct in a logical or formal analytic sense.

Many people see formal analytic models as preferable to ABM for this reason, but there are several reasons to use ABM. First, even formally correct models can be wrong if their premises or assumptions are incorrect (Bundy *et al.*, 2005) – thus ABM with its more experimental approach can actually help *verify* a model by proving it *valid*. Second, ABM is sometimes more accessible or intuitive. Such models can consequently play an important role in scientific understanding, including *developing* a formal analytic understanding of a system by helping explore the space of possible solutions (Axtell, 2000). And finally, there are large classes of dynamic systems which are not amenable to closed analytic solutions (Axelrod, 1997, Axtell, 2000). Particularly interesting to biologists are those involving the open-ended co-evolution of multiple interdependent species.

Returning to the matter of verification, this issue is most nefarious in purely formal systems, where validation is not grounded in real-world data. Formal systems are used in mathematics and similar disciplines as a mechanism of knowledge *discovery*, and therefore verification is both more critical and more difficult. When validation is performed via hypothesis testing against real-world data, validation itself serves as a form of verification. To the extent a computational model reliably matches and predicts a target system's performance, then it *is* a model, in the formal sense of the word.

Verification in this sort of scientific process becomes a process of *model understanding*. Part of this process can be simplifying or generalising the model, or better determining the biological correlates of its components. This verification-like process is useful not only for AI modelling, but for all sorts of formal theories in biology. For example, Wynne (1998) provides a neat history of the development of ever-simpler models of transitive inference learning (see also Delius and Siemann, 1998).

19.2.2   Agent-based models as scientific hypotheses

For biology, there are only two important criteria for validating an ABM. These are the same as for validating any behavioural model:

1. Does the behaviour of the ABM match the behaviour of the target system within the standard metrics of hypothesis evaluation?
2. Do all the attributes of the agents and their environment have plausible biological correlates in the target system?

Regarding the 'standard metrics', these depend largely on the success of previous explanatory efforts. If the literature contains no prior explanation or model, then it may be sufficient to show a qualitative similarity between the model and the target system. The model is now a theory explaining the data, and as the first one it is necessarily the best. However, if there is another competing model, then we need to use standard statistical hypothesis testing to decide which will be the better match.

For the second criterion, the issue is whether the modeller has given the artificial agents any capacities that real subjects could not or arguably would not possess. For example, if we tried to explain the origins of theory of mind by using artificial agents that actually had perfect access to each other's internal state, then we might have simply modelled the presumed end state of the system while providing no explanation for how that capacity came into existence. Note, however, that such a model might be useful if the true end-state of the system was in doubt. For example, we might show that our 'perfect knowledge' theory-of-mind agents were actually less socially capable than agents with imperfect knowledge. This might lead us to change some of our assumptions, e.g., from believing more-social agents must be more perceptive, to some other explanation, such as more-social agents require a higher capacity for propagating social norms.

We recommend that the analysis of an ABM should be a three phase process. The first phase is a *replication* of the ABM. This may not seem (or even be) strictly necessary in the case where the model is publicly available – the results in that case can be checked just by rerunning the original model on another computer. However, reimplementing the model from its description in the literature can be a valuable exercise. Reimplementation may uncover important aspects of the model that the model's original authors either took for granted, overlooked, or even forgot about during the course of their research (King, 1995; Axtell *et al.*, 1996). As we mentioned earlier, an ABM may be valid without actually having been fully verified or understood. This is true of any scientific hypothesis; part of the scientific method is improving this understanding of a theory as a community.

Once the critical attributes of the model are well-understood, we can enter the second phase of ABM analysis, *model understanding*. Here, we carefully consider what the implied or the explicit correlates of those attributes are. Again, just as in any science, we go through a process of finding testable predictions and implications that result from our hypothesis. The third and final phase is *testing* these predictions and implications, looking first into the extant literature, and then (if necessary) to proposing and executing new experiments.

19.3   Primate societies and the DomWorld model

We now present a case study. We analyse DomWorld, a model which provides an explanation for the variety of social structures we see in different species of primates. We begin this study by providing background information on the target biological systems and features that DomWorld is intended to model.

19.3.1   Primate social structure

Most primate species are highly social. They live in structured societies. The structure of these societies is often characterised along a single axis based primarily on social tolerance and conciliatory tendency. *Tolerance* is expressed when a dominant animal allows a subordinate to take advantage of a resource in its presence. *Reconciliation* is when animals that were involved in an aggressive interaction participate in affiliative behaviour (e.g., grooming or clasping) shortly after the incident. This appears to happen most frequently between animals which have strong affiliative relationships, such as kin.

Tolerance is considered technically as one of the most basic forms of conflict resolution for a social species (de Waal and Luttrell, 1989), though, of course, it 'resolves' the conflict by avoiding it in the first place. It might be difficult to see tolerance as an action to be selected, since tolerance may seem more like a form of *inaction*. However, if an agent is inclined to preserve resources (including its own social rank), then expressing tolerance can require considerable inhibition of strong inclinations. In some species, this is achieved by the apparently deliberate averting of gaze in order to avoid witnessing a desired event. For example, a mother who desires to allow a tantrum-throwing juvenile to feed may look away from a particular morsel (de Waal, 2000). This shift in visual attention is necessary if witnessing such an event would automatically trigger an emotional/species-typical response that would lead to conflict and prevent the desired result (the juvenile feeding).

For species at the low end of the tolerant/conciliatory axis, the vast majority of conflicts are unidirectional – that is, a subordinate makes no effort to retaliate against an attack by a dominant, and would almost never initiate an attack on a dominant. Conflicts tend to be infrequent but, when they occur, high-intensity (e.g., biting). Conciliatory behaviour after the conflict is rare. At the high end of the spectrum, conflicts are both more frequent and bidirectional, the majority being met with protests or counter-attacks, but their aggressive intensity is typically low (e.g., vocalisations, slapping). In the most extremely conciliatory species even unrelated participants reconcile after around 50% of conflicts (Thierry, 2006). Van Schaik (1989) refers to these two extremes as *despotic* for the low end and *egalitarian* for the high. Though these terms are obviously anthropomorphic, they are well-established and have strong mnemonic value.

Thierry *et al.* (2004) propose that the macaques are a particularly good model genus for studying primate social organisation (see also Thierry, 1985; de Waal and Luttrell, 1989; Preuschoft and van Schaik, 2000). There are approximately 21 macaque species (the exact number depends on taxonomic dispute, Thierry *et al.*, 2004), all fairly closely genetically related. Thierry (2006) divides these species into four clusters on the tolerant/conciliatory axis. Rhesus (*Macaca mulatta*, familiar from zoos and laboratories) and Japanese (*M. fuscata*) macaques fall into the most despotic category. The stump-tailed macaques (*M. arctoides*) used by de Waal and Johanowicz (1993) in their seminal cross-rearing studies with rhesus are in the second-most egalitarian cluster, while the Tonkean (*M. tonkeana*) and crested (*M. nigra*) are in the most egalitarian cluster.

19.3.2   The DomWorld model

The DomWorld model was originally derived from another seminal ABM, the Hogeweg and Hesper (1983) MIRROR model (Hogeweg, 1988; Hemelrijk, 1999). MIRROR is an ABM which, among other things, was used to model the emergence of party composition of chimpanzees and fission–fusion dynamics in primate societies in general (te Boekhorst and Hogeweg, 1994). The results of these older simulations were based on variables not seen in basic DomWorld, such as food availability and the number of agents.

Hemelrijk was already a well-established primatologist when she published her first DomWorld paper in 1999 (Hemelrijk *et al.*, 1992; Kummer *et al.*, 1996). DomWorld follows good methodological practice by reducing the complexity of the MIRROR model to its most essential components. Later work reintroduces attributes such as food into the now better-understood system (Hemelrijk *et al.*, 2003).

The only addition to DomWorld made between 1999 and the 2002 model this analysis focuses on is the 'attraction procedure' added to the motion rules to simulate sexual attraction (Hemelrijk, 2002). We describe this in §19.3.3.3, which is on tumescence, not here as part of the basic model.

Describing the technical aspects of an ABM requires describing three things: the environment, the agents' state, and the agents' behaviour.

19.3.2.1   The DomWorld environment

The DomWorld environment is flat and undifferentiated. On a computer screen it looks like a square, however the top and bottom edges of the screen are contiguous. That is, if an agent goes off the top of the environment it will reappear at the bottom. Similarly the left and right edges are connected. Consequently, the world is said to be a *torus* since building such a world in reality would require a doughnut shape. This is a standard simplifying assumption for abstract behaviour models (e.g., Laver *et al.*, this volume), though models concerned with realistic environmental behaviour such as Hill *et al.* (this volume) work with more realistic maps.

The DomWorld environment is typically populated by eight agents – four males and four females. The world is large enough (given the agents' visual range) that agents could in theory become 'lost' out of view of the troop. One task for their intelligence is to ensure this does not happen. Agents in DomWorld do not eat, die, or reproduce. They only wait, move around, and occasionally perform dominance interactions.

19.3.2.2   DomWorld agents

Agents have a set of characteristics or *parameters* that describe their individual differences. Some of these parameters are fully *dynamic*, that is they change during an individual's 'lifetime' during an experimental run. The dynamic parameters for each agent in DomWorld are:

- Their x, y position on the 2D surface.
- Their **Dom** value. This determines the agent's dominance rank. Its initial value is determined by the sex of the agent, but it changes as a result of dominance interactions.
- A **waiting period**. When an agent stops moving, it will 'resolve' to sit still for a brief random amount of time. This models foraging or resting in the wild. This period is shortened if there is a nearby dominance interaction (cf. Galef, 1988).

Some parameters are determined per run of the experiment and therefore remain fixed over the course of that run. In DomWorld these *run-dependent parameters* are:

- The **sex** of each agent.
- Each agent's **StepDom**, which describes the level or intensity of aggression. This is species and sex specific: values are much higher for despotic than egalitarian conditions, and slightly higher for males than females.

Some parameters of an ABM are set by the experimenter in the course of developing the system into a reasonable model of the target system. Once determined by the modeller, these values are not changed at all over the course of the experiment. In DomWorld these *static parameters* are:

- The **field of view**, an angle that determines how much an agent sees around its direction of motion (the agents always look straight ahead).
- The **max view**, the furthest they can see.
- **Near view**, a distance within which the agents feel comfortably in the troop.
- **Personal space**, the minimum distance two agents can have between each other without engaging in a dominance interaction.

19.3.2.3   DomWorld agent behaviour

The basic motion dynamics of DomWorld are very like those described by Reynolds (1987) as necessary for flocking. The attractive force that provides coherence for the groups is the fact that as an agent moves towards the nearest other agent it sees if that agent is more than **near view** away. If an agent cannot see any other agent, it will rotate until it does. Separation (or *repulsion* as Reynolds terms it) is maintained by the fact that whenever two agents come within **personal space** of each other, they tend to engage in a dominance interaction (see below). The result of the interaction is that one agent will chase the other away from their joint location. There is no correlate in DomWorld of Reynolds' *alignment*; consequently the troop as a whole does not move quickly or in any persistent direction. DomWorld troops mill around rather than truly flocking.

When one agent sees another within its **personal space** it engages in an agonistic social interaction. Each agent's dominance rank value, **Dom**, is adjusted after any fight involving that agent. This variable determines both the agent's rank and its probability of winning a given fight. The first step of the interaction is a 'mental battle' in which the acting agent compares its own **Dom** value with the **Dom** of the other agent it has seen. If its own value is higher than or equal to the other's, the agent begins a full-scale dominance interaction. If not, the active agent will stay put. Because of the limits provided by the **field of view**, it is possible the dominant agent currently in its **personal space** will move off without ever having 'seen' the nearby subordinate agent.

The outcome of a dominance interaction is calculated with the following formula (from Hemelrijk, 2002, p. 734):

$$w_i = \begin{bmatrix} 1 & \frac{Dom_i}{Dom_i + Dom_j} > Random(0, 1) \\ 0 & otherwise \end{bmatrix} \tag{19.1}$$

where Random(0, 1) produces a random real value between 0 and 1.

In this calculation, w_i represents whether agent i has lost or won. Here, 1 means victory and 0 defeat. The relative dominance value between the two agents is compared with a randomly drawn number between 0 and 1. If the relative dominance is greater than the drawn number, the agent wins. This means that the higher an agent's rank is relative to its opponent, the more likely the agent is to win, while two similarly ranked agents each have an even chance of winning.

After a dominance interaction, the dominance values of both agents are adjusted according to the interaction's outcome, using roughly the same information:

$$Dom_i = Dom_i + \left[w_i - \frac{Dom_i}{Dom_i + Dom_j}\right] \ StepDom$$
$$Dom_j = Dom_j - \left[w_i - \frac{Dom_i}{Dom_i + Dom_j}\right] \ StepDom.$$

(19.2)

The only exception to the above equations is that the lowest possible **Dom** value is fixed at 0.01, keeping all **Dom** values positive.

Hemelrijk calls this mechanism of determining dominance values a *damped positive feedback system*, since if a higher-ranking individual wins its dominance value increases only slightly, but if the lower-ranked agent wins its dominance value undergoes a greater change. For both agents the **Dom** is not changed much by an expected outcome, but it changes greatly for an unexpected one.

The final step of a dominance interaction is a change in physical position. The winner moves slightly towards the loser, 'chasing' it, while the loser turns in a direction roughly opposite of the agent and 'runs' a more significant distance away. There is a small variation added to the angle the loser turns to reduce the probability that the two agents will meet again in the immediate future.

19.3.3 DomWorld results

The contributions of DomWorld can be summarised as follows.

19.3.3.1 Gradients of dominance hierarchy

The primary result is a hypothetical explanation of variation and the tolerance–conciliation social axis. Hemelrijk proposes that having a larger difference between **Dom** values among a troop is equivalent to the troop being more despotic, whereas more similar dominance values correspond to egalitarianism. This hypothesis implies that there is no qualitative difference in how primates in an egalitarian society treat their superiors versus how those in a despotic one do, but rather that every individual will show an equal amount of respect for a troop-mate with twice its absolute (real-valued) dominance. She uses a topographical metaphor to describe this, saying that despotic species have a steeper dominance profile. The main metric Hemelrijk uses for this is the *coefficient of variation of dominance values*. This coefficient indicates the average variation between dominance ranks of the individuals in the troop. A large coefficient indicates a steep gradient and therefore despotism, a small one egalitarianism.

In DomWorld, these differences in position along the tolerant–conciliatory axis are accounted for entirely by the intensity of aggression. Aggression is modelled using **StepDom** (Hemelrijk, 2002). The principle result then is that high levels of **StepDom** lead to greater variations in **Dom** within the troop (see Figure 19.3). Notice though that this aggression intensity value, **StepDom**, has no direct impact on whether a dominance interaction occurs or who wins it (see Equation (19.1)). Rather, its only direct impact is on the adjustment to **Dom** *after* the fight. Through this mechanism though, **StepDom** does have an indirect impact on future fight probabilities and outcomes.

19.3.3.2   Troop spatial structure

Another key result from DomWorld is a replication of the spatial organisation attributed to real troops (Hemelrijk, 2004). Hamilton (1971) suggests that one selective pressure for dominance might be protection of the highest-quality individuals by keeping them central to a group. There is almost no field evidence of primates adopting this strategy, though Hall and Fedigan (1997) report observing it in wild capuchins. The dynamics of DomWorld motion behaviour already described produce this phenomenon with no additional cognitive strategy required for the agents. *Centrality* is measured as the sum of the unit vectors (vectors with accurate direction but fixed length) from an agent towards every other agent in the troop. The shorter this summed vector, the more the directions of the other troop members cancel each other, and thus the more central the agent is. This is the same metric used in Hemelrijk's DomWorld papers. Independently, Christman and Lewis (2005) have shown it is the most reliable metric for centrality. In DomWorld, centrality correlates with **Dom**.

Centrality is not a main focus of our present analysis, but it *is* a primary result for DomWorld and we will return to it while discussing the extension of this model in Section 19.4.4.

19.3.3.3   Sexual attraction during tumescence

In most primate societies, most males are more dominant than most females. This is probably due to differences in body size and physical strength. Generally speaking, in a primate society dominant animals have priority access to any desirable resources. This changes, however, during females' receptive periods (i.e., when they are capable of reproduction). During these periods, females of most primate species develop genital swellings as an obvious physical signal. This is called *tumescence*. During tumescence, females are often the beneficiaries of special privileges, for example priority access to food, in apparent exchange for copulation opportunities (Yerkes, 1940). This is frequently seen as a cognitive strategy by males, with the assumption that apparently altruistic acts directed towards receptive females lead not only to satisfying the males' reproductive drive but also to an increase in their total number of offspring (Goodall, 1986; de Waal and Luttrell, 1989; Stanford, 1996).

Hemelrijk proposes a much simpler explanation (Hemelrijk, 2002; Hemelrijk *et al.*, 2003). She starts from a highly parsimonious theory that the only real difference in the animals' action selection is the apparent one – that at the time of tumescence males are more likely to approach females. Due to the dynamics of dominance interactions (as displayed in DomWorld) this leads to more fights between males and females, which in turn leads to a greater number of low-probability events such as a female winning a fight against a higher-ranking male. Because of the dynamics of Equation (19.2), this can in turn lead to a female who has won several unexpected victories to outrank at least some males. In this case, the apparent shift in behaviour, where males tolerate female access to resources, is in fact simply the normal respect a subordinate shows a dominant.

To model this theory, the only modification necessary to the standard DomWorld is the addition of one *run-dependent parameter*, **attraction**. The behaviour algorithm is modified such that when **attraction** is *on*, males move towards females when they are inside of **near view**. The increased fighting that results from this attraction can indeed in some conditions lead to an increased number of females with high rank, though on average no more than half of them would be (see full results below). When a tumescent female does come to outrank a male, the males are still attracted towards the females, but then sit still once they have entered the dominant female's **personal space**, since she now outranks them.

19.3.3.4   Female dominance over males

In most species of primates, dominant animals tend to be male, though some females may outrank some males. However, in a few species (particularly lemurs) females routinely and sometimes even entirely outrank males. Hemelrijk *et al*. (2008) claim that DomWorld can entirely account for these species – the model shows that the proportion of dominant females in a troop increases as the proportion of males in a population increases. This result required no change to the standard DomWorld model other than altering the proportion of males in a run.

19.4   Analysis of DomWorld

We now evaluate DomWorld as a general explanation of the despotic–egalitarian continuum in primate behaviour. As reviewed earlier, this continuum is best documented in the genus *Macaca*. We adopt the proposal of Thierry *et al*. (2004) that this genus should serve as a model (in the biological sense) for primate social organisation in general.

Following the approach described in Section 19.2, our analysis is in three phases. The first phase is a replication of the DomWorld experiments. This replication allows us not only to confirm their results but also to determine which aspects of the model are critical to its performance. The second phase of our analysis considers the correlations between these critical aspects of the model's agents and real primates, and makes a series of predictions based on the consequences of the model. The third phase tests these 'predictions' against the primate social behaviour literature. The third phase could involve gathering more data from the field, but in the present case the extant literature proves sufficient to answer the key questions derived in the second phase.

19.4.1   Replication

The original DomWorld was implemented in Object Pascal and Borland Pascal 7.0 Hemelrijk (2002) and has to date not been made publicly available. We implemented our version in NetLogo (Wilensky, 2005). As a purpose-built modelling tool, NetLogo provides a relatively easy high-level language for quickly constructing models and visualising results. The exact parameter settings of our model are matched to those in the previously published accounts of DomWorld. The details of our replication are described in Bryson *et al.* (2007); the code, including these parameter settings, is available as an electronic supplement to that article and from the authors' web pages.

In our experience, the model does not appear overly sensitive to most of the parameter values, although at the same time none of them can be eliminated and still maintain the action-selection model. However, the model *is* particularly sensitive to changes in the length of the waiting period. This may be because constant dominance interactions not only look unnatural but also make the troop so chaotic that spatial measurements of troop coherence and rank become less meaningful. The documentation of the waiting period is not as conspicuous in Hemelrijk's papers as other aspects of her model (e.g., it is not mentioned in her flow diagrams of her control system), so this sensitivity may account for why some modellers have reported difficulty in replicating her results.

19.4.1.1   Results

Our experiments were run under the four conditions specified by Hemelrijk (2002). For each of the despotic and egalitarian cases, ten runs were made under each of two conditions of *sexual attraction*, where either there was none (a replication of the basic DomWorld) or where all males were attracted to all females (the tumescent case). The total number of runs was therefore 40. Our results match Hemelrijk's wherever we used the same analysis, that is, most of the results reported here.

To match Hemelrijk's figures, we show typical individual exemplar results, rather than averaging over the ten runs. Figure 19.1 replicates the Hemelrijk (2002, p. 739) Figure 19.3*A*. It shows (over time in each of the four conditions) the sum over all females of the number of males which rank below that female. For example, if two females each outrank two males, one outranks one male and the other outranks no males, this value would be 5. We can see that, as reported in Hemelrijk, the female dominance in conditions with high **StepDom** increases over time, but stays constant in the egalitarian conditions with a low **StepDom**.

Figure 19.2 shows the classic DomWorld result concerning Hemelrijk's explanation of despotic and egalitarian species. In Hemelrijk (2002), it replicates Figure 4*A* (p. 741). The figure shows the distribution of the coefficient of variation of dominance values for both sexes (see discussion in Section 19.3.3). If **StepDom** is high, the difference between **Dom** values will be larger. By Hemelrijk's account, this models higher aggression leading to a despotic-style social structure. Sexual attraction amplifies this result, and females are more likely to outrank some males in this condition.

Figure 19.3 shows the change of dominance values for both the sexes in conditions with high and with low levels of aggression. Again, here we show typical instances from single runs. In each figure, all four males initially have a **Dom** value of 16, while the four females have an initial **Dom** value of 8. Figure 19.3a corresponds to Figure 4*B* in Hemelrijk (2002, p. 741). With high **StepDom** the dominance structure is enormously dynamic, with an increasing coefficient of variation for each sex. Figure 19.3b corresponds to Figure 4*C* in Hemelrijk (2002, p. 741). With a low **StepDom** there is very little change in the dominance values. This creates a relatively stable hierarchy, thus no females gain higher positions in the troop.

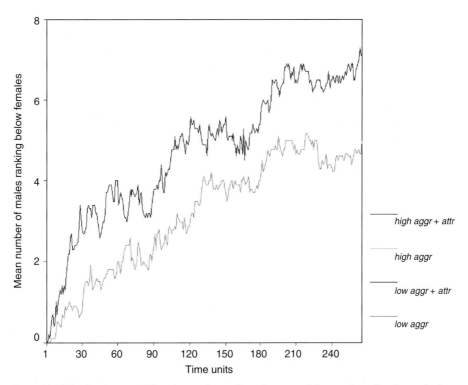

Figure 19.1 The dominance of females as shown from the sum of the number of males ranked below each female at different times in different conditions. The egalitarian (*low aggr*) conditions are not visible because they are equivalent to the *x*-axis, that is, they are constantly zero; *high aggr + attr*: despotic and tumescent; *high aggr*: despotic with no tumescence; *low aggr + attr*: egalitarian and tumescent; *low aggr*: egalitarian with no tumescence; *aggr*: aggression; *attr*: attraction.

Figure 19.4 has no equivalent in Hemelrijk (2002) but shows data derived from our replication which is significant to our analysis (Section 19.4.2). In this figure, the total number of aggressive interactions initiated by female agents is compared across the four different conditions used in the experiment, and averaged across all 10 runs in each condition. The number of female dominance interactions increases significantly in conditions with sexual attraction at both intensities of aggression (low: Mann-Whitney, $N = 10$, $U = 0$, $p < .001$, two-tailed; high: Mann-Whitney, $N = 10$, $U = 0$, $p < .001$, two-tailed). This means females are involved in considerably more interactions when they are attractive. Higher **StepDom** amplifies this result, though this effect is rather weak (Mann-Whitney U-Test, $N = 10$, $U = 24$ $p < .049$, two-tailed).

19.4.2   Analysis of model correlates

Having successfully replicated DomWorld and achieved a good understanding of its components and their dynamics, the next phase of our analysis is to consider what the natural analogues of those components and behaviours are, and what they imply, explain,

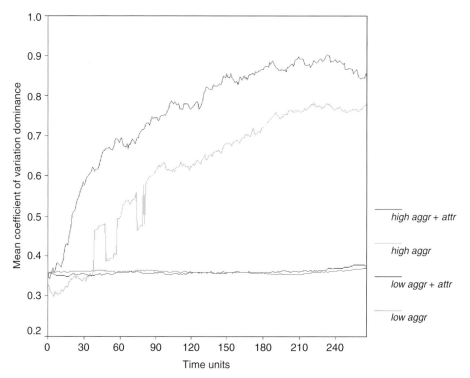

Figure 19.2 Distribution of the *coefficient of variation* of dominance values in different conditions for both sexes. The definitions are the same as those for Figure 19.1.

or predict about real primate behaviour. For example, the most basic model results show that only in groups with a high **StepDom** are females able to gain higher **Dom** values than males. Sexual attraction amplifies this effect, but plays a secondary role. Hemelrijk uses **StepDom** to model intensity of aggression, and **Dom** to model dominance rank. If we examine real animals substituting these terms into the results, will the results hold?

For this phase of our analysis, we compiled the following list of questions based on the model but rephrased in primatological terms:

1. If one agent defeats another that vastly outranks it in a dominance interaction, does this have more impact on its rank than if it defeats a near peer? In other words, is a more unexpected outcome from a fight likely to have a more significant effect? If this is true, it would validate the use of relative dominance values in Equation (19.2).
2. Within species, if a fight is more violent (e.g., if blood is drawn compared to mild beating, or if there is mild beating compared to a non-physical interaction) does the fight have more impact on the dominance hierarchy? If so, then it makes sense to refer to **StepDom** as 'intensity of aggression', since the level of aggression would determine the increment of **Dom**) and it would further validate its use in Equation (19.2).
3. Are females more likely to engage in fights when they are tumescent? If not, this model cannot account for their increased dominance (Figure 19.4).

(a)

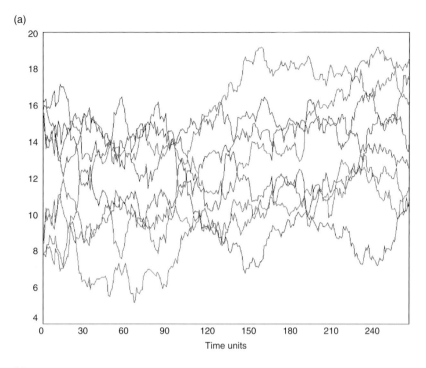

(b)

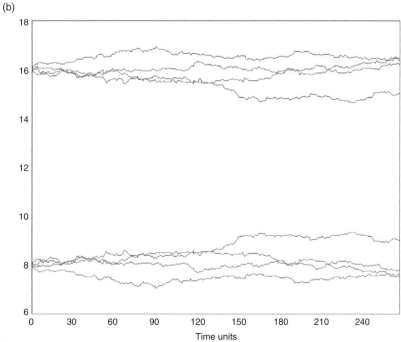

Figure 19.3 Distribution of Dom values at (a) a high level and at (b) a low level of StepDom. In both conditions, the males initially have twice the Dom value of the females.

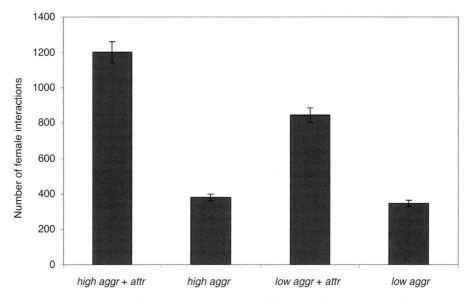

Figure 19.4 Total number of female interactions under different conditions. The definitions are the same as those for Figure 19.1.

4. Do females only become dominant during their tumescence in despotic species? Given that the prime indication in Hemelrijk's model of increased dominance for the females is the males' increased tolerance of them, discriminating an increase of rank in an egalitarian species may be difficult, since these species are definitionally more tolerant towards all group members. However, if there is any increase in favouritism towards egalitarian females, this model does not account for it.

5. When an animal in an egalitarian species is *clearly* outranked by another animal, are those two animals' interactions similar to two more nearly ranked animals in a more despotic species? Or is there a qualitative difference in how different species behave with respect to dominance hierarchies? The answer to this question will serve to validate whether the coefficient of variance is a good indicator of location along the tolerance–conciliation axis – is it sufficient to discriminate an egalitarian from a despotic species?

Each of these questions seeks to validate or invalidate some part of the DomWorld model. When we first framed these questions (Lehmann *et al.*, 2005), we could not be certain what data would be easy or hard to come by, therefore some of these questions test the same parts of the model but in different ways.

19.4.3   Evaluating the model

When answering questions of the sort just posed there are two obvious possible outcomes: either existing data may answer a question decisively, or, if there is not sufficient existing data, the question may motivate a new field study. However, at least three of the questions above fall into a third category. Existing data is not sufficient to answer the questions conclusively, but this is not because insufficient studies have been run. Rather, in order for data to give statistically significant indications, particular types of social events would have to occur at a frequency which is not observed in real animals. Thus a question that appears to be well-posed from the perspective of the model is not directly answerable. However, the discrepancy between the model and the target system that leads to the problematic question is itself information useful for evaluating the model.

Question 1 in Section 19.4.2 is an example of this third category of question. Particularly in despotic macaque species, unexpected outcomes in conflict are so rare that there can be no statistically significant results concerning them. Despotic conflicts are almost always unilateral, from a dominant to a subordinate. For there to be a statistically significant result either for or against the model, we would need to see a reasonable number of subordinate animals becoming superordinate (dominant) as a result of unlikely 'wins' in dominance interactions, then determine how the rate of their ascension correlates to their number of improbable outcomes. However, in macaques at least, changes in dominance ranking are very infrequent. Most variation comes as a consequence of aging (both juveniles becoming stronger and adults becoming weaker) or new arrivals in a troop. In both these rare cases, dominance rank change tends to be gradual, with the formerly subordinate animals challenging sequentially the troop members just above their own rank, working their way gradually up the hierarchy. Thus, the unlikely outcomes that drive the rank volatility in DomWorld are not a feature of the target system in nature.

If we consider the situation of DomWorld as shown in Figure 19.3b, there are four females with an average **Dom** of approximately 8, and four males with an average of approximately 16. A very average male and female might be expected to be separated by three or four individuals (the high ranking females and low ranking males), yet if they engage in a dominance interaction, the female would have a 1-in-3 ($8/(8 + 16)$) chance of defeating an agent very much her superior. This high number of 'improbable' outcomes is what creates the dynamicism of the ranking system in DomWorld. The difference between the two conditions, despotic and egalitarian, is a direct consequence of a larger multiplier (**StepDom**) exaggerating the effects of these improbable outcomes.

The fact that dominance order for adult macaques almost never changes makes question two above equally difficult to answer, at least from observations of captive troops. It further calls into doubt the plausibility of results such as are shown in Figure 19.3a, and therefore in turn the results shown in Figure 19.2a. The large and widening coefficient of variation comes not from an increasing and well-delineated order in the dominance ranking of the 'despotic' species, but rather from high-gain random fluctuations. These problems call into question the DomWorld account of **Dom** values and therefore its explanation of the difference between despotic and egalitarian social orders.

Standard DomWorld results like those shown in Figures 19.1 and 19.2 are simple consequences of the fact that DomWorld's damped positive feedback system (Section 19.3.2.3) ultimately produces a perfectly random dominance hierarchy. **StepDom** functions as a gain, determining how fast this process takes place. Thus the analysis performed by Hemelrijk (2002) – and subsequently in Hemelrijk et al. (2008) (replicated in Figure 19.1) is deceptive. While appearing to show a steady increase in female dominance, in fact, this increase will always asymptote when the females' ranks are randomly distributed with the males'. The rise is the consequence of having started from order, with the females all more lower ranked, then moving to disorder. The randomising process is accelerated in the female-attraction (tumescent) condition because there are more interactions involving the initially-lowest-ranked members of the troop (Figure 19.4).

Contrary to Hemelrijk *et al.* (2008), DomWorld could never account for complete female dominance, unless the starting condition had the females already in a dominant position, and **StepDom** was too low to randomise their position during the number of time units allocated for the experiment. The apparent rise in female dominance is only a trend towards complete randomness. Adding males to the system increases the rate at which random order is achieved because males have a higher **StepDom** than females and thus the average amount of 'violence' per interaction increases with the proportion of males. Since the experimental run times are truncated at an arbitrary but fixed period of time before the ordering of agents is perfectly random, the rate of change determines the proportion of dominant females.

One question that *can* be directly answered is question 3 in Section 19.4.2. Aujard *et al.* (1998) show that egalitarian macaque females in tumescence are involved in, if anything, *fewer* agonistic interactions, not more. Aujard *et al.* (1998) document a large range of behaviours with respect to the female reproductive cycle. Social grooming with males and 'affiliative interactions' with males all peak at or just before tumescence. For agonistic interactions, there is no significant change but a downward trend throughout this period, followed by a sharp increase several days *after* tumescence (Aujard *et al.*, 1998, particularly Figure 2, p. 293, and the following discussion). This work was done with semi-free-ranging Tonkeans, one of the species Thierry (2006) puts in the most egalitarian cluster.

As we showed in Figure 19.4, the Hemelrijk (2002) model of female preference predicts increased fighting for both egalitarian and despotic females. Further, DomWorld results indicate that there should be no increase in preferential treatment of females of egalitarian species. Thus the above results counter not only our question 3, but also the basic hypothesis that preferential behaviour towards females can be explained in this manner.

Eaton *et al.* (1980) document an increase of dyadic inter-sex and male-on-male violence in a similarly semi-free-ranging troop of Japanese macaques (*M. fuscata*) during their breeding season. Thierry (2006) assigns *M. fuscata* to the most highly despotic category. There is, however, a significant downturn of aggression either by females on females or by groups on females during this period, though there is an increase of violence in groups on males. Because this study does not include hormonal analysis, it is difficult to be certain whether this violence is occurring during the fertile period of individual animals or shortly after, as was reported by Aujard *et al.* (1998). Also, this species does not technically experience a period of tumescence – female fertility in Japanese macaques is not signalled by genital swelling. Nevertheless, if the level of violence *does* increase in periods of tumescence, but only in despotic species, then this would be evidence that DomWorld is not a sufficient model of the difference between egalitarian and despotic species. If, on the other hand, an increase in the despotic species' violence occurs *after* the females are no longer fertile as it does in the egalitarian Tonkeans, then the results for despotic agents shown in Figure 19.4 are also invalid.

The Aujard *et al.* (1998) data for the egalitarian Tonkeans also bear on question 4. While Aujard *et al.* do not specifically document tolerance of food access, the significant increases of affiliative behaviour *other* than (and as well as) grooming and sexual behaviour does seem an indication of the sort of favouritism the Hemelrijk (2002) extension of DomWorld is intended to explain. Thus egalitarian tumescent females *should* also be accounted for in DomWorld, but are not.

There is a further problem with DomWorld's model of female dominance rising in despotic species: other than the behaviours Hemelrijk calls 'tolerant', there is no indication that a tumescent female's dominance rank really changes. In many species, dominance can be recognised by a set of social signals (Preuschoft and van Schaik, 2000). With respect to these and other indicators, there is no change in a female's troop standing during her tumescence. In particular, other females treat a tumescent female no differently, and after tumescence males treat her just as they did before (Thierry, 2005, personal communication; Samuels *et al.*, 1987). DomWorld does not account for a female returning to her exact previous rank after tumescence, nor for her difference in rank in the eyes of male and female agents.

Our final question 5, about the difference between egalitarian and despotic species, is again difficult to answer with quantitative data. For one thing, dominance hierarchies in extremely egalitarian species are not well defined except at the very top ranks. But the answer again seems to be 'no'. There are many affiliative and conciliatory behaviours that all members of egalitarian species engage in and no members of despotic species do, for example, clasping (Thierry, 1985; de Waal and Luttrell, 1989; Thierry *et al.*, 2004). Thus absolute difference in **Dom** alone probably does not account for all the discrepancies between egalitarian and despotic species. However, this question is not really a fair evaluation of DomWorld, because it neglects the level of abstraction of the model. It is possible that a more complete model based on the same basic interactions could show the evolution of extra conciliatory behaviour. It is not really justified to ask a model to explain data outside its remit.

In summary then, while DomWorld does account for several primate social phenomena – including the propensity for dominant animals to be in the middle of the troop, the difference between egalitarian and despotic species, and the special treatment given females during their tumescence – we have found several failures of correspondence between this model and our target genus, macaques. In particular, despotic species are not well characterised by rapidly fluctuating dominance rankings, but these are the main mechanism DomWorld uses to explain both the tolerant/conciliatory access and female favouritism during tumescence. In nature, neither type of macaque species experiences significant numbers of victories by significantly subordinate animals in disputes, yet this is what drives the rank fluctuations in DomWorld. Finally, females in at least some species of macaques are not subject to significantly more agonistic interactions during their periods of tumescence, and again these are essential to the Hemelrijk (2002) account.

19.4.4   Partial recovery of the model

This chapter has two aims: to review the use of ABM as a methodological tool in science, and to present a case study for the analysis of existing models. Our analysis has shown some significant failures of correspondence between DomWorld and live macaque data. However, ABMs, like most scientific models, are not brittle – unlike analytic models or mathematical proofs. Even if a flaw is found in some aspect of a model, it does not necessarily invalidate the entire construction. While occasionally scientific theories are totally abandoned, more often scientific progress is gradual, and theories are refined and improved (Kuhn, 1970).

We continue our case study now by demonstrating that DomWorld has this property of robustness. We show that DomWorld's centrality result still holds even if our criticism is addressed with a slight modification to the model. The modification is simple – we assume that the motion dynamics aspects of dominance interactions are just as described earlier (Subsection 19.3.2.3). However, we change our *interpretation* of those dynamics with respect to their correlations to the target system. Also, we assume that dominance levels are entirely stable – we do not update any **Dom** values. While this new model no longer accounts for what changes *do* occur in dominance structures, it may be a better representation of average daily lives for most macaques.

In this modification of the DomWorld model, interactions are less likely to represent actual fights than *displacement* (sometimes called *supplantation*). Displacement is a common behaviour observed in macaques and other species where a dominant animal will come towards a subordinate, and the subordinate will get up and move out of the way (Rowell, 1966). The dominant will then sit in or near the location previously occupied by the subordinate. This behaviour may be seen simply as a power move, an assertion of dominance, but it is also possible that a dominant may take advantage of resources discovered by the subordinate. In the only study reporting centrality in primates we were able to find in the literature, Hall and Fedigan (1997) report that in capuchins the central position was held with no visible conflict, and conclude that subordinates simply avoid dominants.

In a further replication of DomWorld, Ando *et al.* (2007) show that centrality remains a characteristic of behaviour dynamics that are otherwise identical to DomWorld even if **Dom** values are held constant.

In this replication, we have tested what aspects of the behaviour dynamics of a dominance interaction are necessary to maintain this centrality result. We originally hypothesised that the 'fleeing' aspect of the motion might be sufficient to explain the effect, but as Figure 19.5 shows, this is not the case. These statistics were gathered for 20 individuals in time units 50–250 of a simulation otherwise as described above, except that the **Dom** values were set as run-dependent parameters with each agent given a unique **Dom** from 1–20. These results show that displacement is a sufficient explanation for

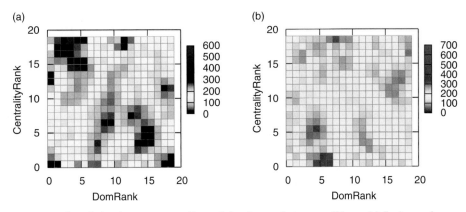

Figure 19.5 Correlation between centrality and dominance in two conditions: (a) fleeing and pursuing and (b) just fleeing. More dominant animals have a higher Dom rank, while agents closer to the centre have a lower centrality rank. The darker regions show the higher correlations.

centrality, but only if it involves the dominant animal coming closer to the subordinate's former position than it would have by chance wandering.

Taken in general, these results demonstrate the robustness of agent-based models, and their suitability for being not only replicated but also extended. This supports our position that ABM are a form of scientific hypothesis.

19.5 Conclusions and discussion

This chapter examines a leading paradigm for furthering the scientific understanding of actions selection: ABM. In addition to the extended case study in this chapter, four other chapters in this book demonstrate the diversity of action-selection research that is being explored using ABM (see chapters by Hill *et al.*, Laver *et al.*, Seth, and Rands *et al.*, this volume). The main theme of the present chapter has been to emphasise ABM as a *scientific* modelling technique. Models are a vector for communicating theory between scientists, as well as a mechanism to check ramifications of our theories that go beyond the computational ability of individual rational consideration (Kokko, 2007). The main argument, that ABMs can and should be treated like any other scientific hypothesis, can be extended from ABM to cover most, if not all, of the experiment-based techniques demonstrated in this volume.

To demonstrate and communicate our point, we have presented a thorough analysis of one of the most widely published ABMs in biology, Hemelrijk's DomWorld, a model of primate social dynamics. We have examined this model through a three-phase process: first, replicating the model, and in the process coming to understand its dynamics and important parameters; second, producing a list of testable predictions or assumptions by considering these important model attributes in terms of their target-system analogues; and, third, evaluating these predictions and assumptions in the light of the extant primate literature. We had originally expected to motivate novel research to test the predictions, but in fact the existing literature was sufficient to answer the questions once they were well-specified.

19.5.1   DomWorld as a model of primate social behaviour

We found several points where DomWorld did not correspond to the behaviour of the target system we chose for analysis, the genus *Macaca*. We chose this genus because it has previously been presented as a well-documented model for the sorts of primate social behaviour DomWorld models (Thierry *et al.*, 2004). The main problems we found were:

- The rate of change of the dominance rankings is quite exaggerated, and many of the effects claimed for the system were entirely based on this, e.g., increased female dominance (Hemelrijk, 2002; Hemelrijk *et al.*, 2008).
- The probability of success of subordinate animals in aggressive interactions is also exaggerated – this generates the first inconsistency, the size of the effect is determined by the StepDom, a proxy for the violence of the aggression in the interaction.
- The Hemelrijk (2002) account of special treatment for tumescent females (increased ordinary rank) is not predictive of actual observed behaviour (number of fights, return to previous rank after tumescence concludes).
- The Hemelrijk *et al.* (2008) account of female dominance is false because DomWorld cannot explain more than 50% of females, on average, being dominant in the long run.

Of course, the model was not originally built to model macaques. MIRROR was built to model social insects, and Hemelrijk originally applied it to her principle area of expertise, chimpanzee behaviour. However, DomWorld has been proposed as a general model of egalitarianism and despotism in primates (Hemelrijk, 2000; Hemelrijk *et al.*, 2008).

ABMs are not fragile analytic proofs which collapse in the face of an error in a premise. Like any conventional biological theory, an ABM can be augmented, extended, or restricted. We have demonstrated that if the part of the model we dispute (the mechanism for changing dominance rank) is excised, one of the other significant results (the emergent centrality of dominant animals to the troop) still holds. It would also be interesting to find whether in species that *do* have relatively dynamic dominance patterns the model holds better. In free-ranging baboons, for example, although the ranks of females are remarkably stable, the dominance ranks of males can change as often as once a month, because of the frequent migrations of males between troops (Kitchen *et al.*, 2005).

19.5.2   Agent-based models as hypotheses and vectors of scientific communication

Our perspective on AI models as an ordinary part of the scientific method is not universally held, although its acceptance seems to be spreading. However, some practitioners are less willing to take such an absolute stance. For example, although Axelrod (1997) describes ABM as 'a third way to do science' (induction and deduction being the other two), he also states that 'the purpose of agent-based modelling is to aid intuition. Agent-based modelling is a way of doing thought experiments.' (Axelrod, 1997, p. 4). Despite the fact that Hemelrijk validates her data statistically against real animal behaviour, she has also taken this perspective (Hemelrijk, 2006, personal communication).

We believe this perspective is not taking modelling seriously enough, or put another way, is taking the rest of science as something somehow more certain or special than it really is. No model describes all the known phenomena about a target species, but neither does any other form of scientific theory. Models and other theories are necessarily abstractions, constrained by the cognitive capacities of the scientists that hold and attempt to communicate them. In fact, some AI models might be criticised because they have become *too* precise and detailed to be comprehensible or communicated by individuals (related claims have been made about computer-generated mathematical proofs, cf. Bundy *et al.*, 2005). This leads us into an interesting position as a scientific community, analogous to what happens to story telling and history as cultures develop the innovation of literacy. AI models too large to be held in any one mind can still be communicated perfectly through digital copies without human comprehension. The process of validating and understanding them could thus become an evolutionary process similar to the scientific process itself. It is an open question whether such an approach would be *desirable*. It might, for example, increase our ability to make predictions, but reduce the probability of innovations based on insight.

Many modellers are in fact reluctant to make the digital versions of their models publicly available. This is primarily because models represent an enormous development effort. Some researchers are reluctant to fully share the outcomes of this effort, fearing perhaps that others might take better advantage of their work than they can themselves. King (1995, 2003) has addressed an equivalent concern in the social and political sciences, involving the datasets these scientists gather at great cost and effort. King (1995) argues that replication is a necessary part of the scientific process. Thus while data can sometimes be withheld either temporarily (to ensure the right of first publication) or permanently (due to confidentiality or national security issues), in general, withholding such work is a detriment both to the discipline *and* to the individual scientists. King's argument has now become a matter of policy for many political science journals (Gleditsch and Metelits, 2003). Further, Gleditsch *et al.* (2003) demonstrate empirically that there is an individual advantage of knowledge sharing, by performing extensive meta-analysis. Providing replication material actually improves the career of a scientist as their reputation and citation rate are both increased. Thus, researchers both benefit their own careers and accelerate scientific advance by sharing data sets, and presumably also ABMs. Hopefully, biology journals will follow suit with the social sciences and begin to require publication either in public repositories or as electronic supplements to an article any model on which a publication is based.

In conclusion, ABM is becoming a standard mechanism not only for conducting experiments into the consequences and validity of biological theories, but also for clearly communicating well-specified theories of action selection between scientists and laboratories. They provide a robust, algorithmic framework for expressing theories that can be described in terms of the consequences of an individual animal's behaviour in given contexts. We hope that sharing such models can further catalyse scientific progress in the study of social behaviour.

Acknowledgements

Bernard Thierry provided extensive assistance, comments, and references. Steve Butler also provided proofreading. JingJing Wang (2003) made the first version of the NetLogo model used in this replication. The NetLogo group at Northwestern University provided excellent and enthusiastic technical support. The modelling effort at Bath was funded by the British EPSRC grant number GR/S79299/01. Travel funding for collaboration between Bath and the Centre d'Ecologie, Physiologie and Ethologie was provided by the British Council Alliance: Franco-British Partnership Programme. All software used for the studies in this chapter is available on request from the authors or on demand from their websites.

References

Ando, Y., H. Lehmann, and J. J. Bryson (2007). The effects of centrality on the distribution of dominant animals in DomWorld. *Phil. Trans. Roy. Soc. B Biol. Sci.* **362**(1485): 1685–1698. Electronic supplement http://dx.doi.org/10.1098/rstb.2007.2061.

Aujard, F., M. Heistermann, B. Thierry, and J. K. Hodges (1998). Functional significance of behavioral, morphological, and endocrine correlates across the ovarian cycle in semifree ranging female Tonkean macaques. *Amer. J. Primatol.* **46**: 285–309.

Axelrod, R. (1985). *The Evolution of Cooperation*. New York: Basic Books.

Axelrod, R. (1997). *The Complexity of Cooperation: Agent-Based Models of Competition and Colloboration*. Princeton, NJ: Princeton University Press.

Axelrod, R. and W. D. Hamilton (1981). The evolution of cooperation. *Science* **211**: 1390–6.

Axelrod, R. and L. Tesfatsion (2006). A guide for newcomers to agent-based modeling in the social sciences. In *Handbook of Computational Economics*, ed. L. Tesfatsion, and K. L. Judd. Amsterdam: Elsevier, Appendix A.

Axtell, R. (2000). Why agents? On the varied motivations for agent computing in the social sciences. Technical Report 17, Brookings Institute: Center on Social and Economic Dynamics, Washington DC.

Axtell, R., R. Axelrod, J. M. Epstein, and M. D. Cohen (1996). Aligning simulation models: a case study and results. *Comput. Math. Org. Theor.* **1**(2): 123–41.

Balci, O. (1998). Verification, validation and testing. In *The Handbook of Simulation*, ed. J. Banks. New York: John Wiley and Sons, Chapter 10, pp. 335–93.

Box, G. E. P. (1979). Robustness in the strategy of scientific model building. In *Robustness in Statistics*, ed. R. L. Launer and G. N. Wilkinson. New York: Academic Press, pp. 201–236.

Bryson, J. J., Y. Ando, and H. Lehmann, (2007). Agent-based models as scientific methodology: a case study analysing primate social behaviour. *Phil. Trans. Roy. Soc. B Biol. Sci.* **362**(1485): 1685–98.

Bundy, A., M. Jamnik, and A. Fugard (2005). What is a proof? *Phil. Trans. Roy. Soc. A* **363**(1835): 2377–92.

Christman, M. C. and D. Lewis (2005). Spatial distribution of dominant animals within a group: comparison of four statistical tests of location. *Anim. Behav.* **70**(1): 73–82.

de Waal, F. B. M. (2000). Attitudinal reciprocity in food sharing among brown capuchin monkeys. *Anim. Behav.* **60**: 253–61.

de Waal, F. B. M. and D. L. Johanowicz (1993). Modification of reconciliation behavior through social experience: an experiment with two macaque species. *Child Dev.* **64**: 897–908.

de Waal, F. B. M. and L. Luttrell (1989). Toward a comparative socioecology of the genus *Macaca*: different dominance styles in rhesus and stumptailed macaques. *Amer. J. Primatol.* **19**: 83–109.

Delius, J. D. and M. Siemann (1998). Transitive responding in animals and humans: exaptation rather than adaptation? *Behav. Proc.* **42**(2–3): 107–137.

Eaton, G. G., K. B. Modahl, and D. F. Johnson (1980). Aggressive behavior in a confined troop of Japanese macaques: effects of density, season and gender. *Aggressive Behav.* **7**: 145–64.

Galef, B. G. J. (1988). Imitation in animals: history, definition, and interpretation of data from the psychological laboratory. In *Social Learning: Psychological and Biological Perspectives*, ed. T. Zentall, and B. G. J. Galef. Hillsdale, NY: Erlbaum, pp. 3–25.

Gleditsch, N. P. and C. Metelits (2003). The replication debate. *Int. Stud. Perspec.* **4**(1):72–79.

Gleditsch, N. P., Metelits, C., and Strand, H. (2003). Posting your data: will you be scooped or famous? *Int. Stud. Perspec.* **4**(1): 89–97.

Goodall, J. (1986). *The Chimpanzees of Gombe: Patterns of Behavior*. Cambridge, MA: Harvard University Press.

Hall, C. L. and Fedigan, L. M. (1997). Spatial benefits afforded by high rank in white-faced capuchins. *Anim. Behav.* **53**(5): 1069–82.

Hamilton, W. D. (1971). Geometry for the selfish herd. *J. Theor. Biol.* **31**: 295–311.

Hemelrijk, C. K. (1999). An individual-oriented model on the emergence of despotic and egalitarian societies. *Proc. Roy. Soc. B Biol. Sci.* **266**: 361–9.

Hemelrijk, C. K. (2000). Towards the integration of social dominance and spatial structure. *Anim. Behav.* **59**(5): 1035–48.

Hemelrijk, C. K. (2002). Despotic societies, sexual attraction and the emergence of male 'tolerance': an agent based model. *Behav.* **139**: 729–47.

Hemelrijk, C. K. (2004). The use of artificial-life models for the study of social organization. In *Macaque Societies: A Model for the Study of Social Organization*, ed. B. Thierry, M. Singh, and W. Kaumanns. Cambridge: Cambridge University Press, pp. 157–81.

Hemelrijk, C. K., G. J. van Laere, and J. A. R. A. M. van Hooff (1992). Sexual exchange relationships in captive chimpanzees. *Behav. Ecol. Sociobiol.* **30**: 269–75.

Hemelrijk, C. K., J. Wantia, and M. Dätwyler (2003). Female co-dominance in a virtual world: ecological, cognitive, social and sexual causes. *Behav.* **140**(10): 1247–73.

Hemelrijk, C. K., J. Wantia, and L. Gygax (2005). The construction of dominance order: comparing performance of five methods using an individual-based model. *Behav.* **142**(8): 1037–58.

Hemelrijk, C. K., J. Wantia, and K. Isler (2008). Female dominance over males in primates: self-organisation and sexual dimorphism. *PLoS One* **3**(7): e2678.

Hogeweg, P. (1988). MIRROR beyond MIRROR: Puddles of LIFE. In *Artificial Life: Santa Fe Institute Studies in the Sciences of Complexity*, ed. C. Langton. Reading, MA: Addison-Wesley, pp. 297–316.

Hogeweg, P. and B. Hesper (1979). Heterarchical selfstructuring simulation systems: concepts and applications in biology. In *Methodologies in Systems Modelling and Simulation*, ed. B. P. Zeigler, M. S. Ezas, G. J. Klir, and T. I. Ören. Amsterdam: North-Holland, pp. 221–31.

Hogeweg, P. and B. Hesper (1983). The ontogeny of the interaction structure in bumble bee colonies: a MIRROR model. *Behav. Ecol. Sociobiol.* **12**: 271–83.

Kennedy, R. C., X. Xiang, G. R. Madey, and T. F. Cosimano (2006). Verification and validation of scientific and economic models. In *Proceedings of Agent 2005: Generative Social Processes, Models, and Mechanisms*, ed. M. North, D. L. Sallach, and C. Macal. Chicago, IL: Argonne National Laboratory, pp. 177–192.

King, G. (1995). Replication, replication. *PS: Political Science and Politics*, **XXVIII**(3): 443–99, with comments from nineteen authors and a response, 'A Revised Proposal, Proposal'.

King, G. (2003). The future of replication. *Int. Stud. Perspec.* **4**(1): 100–105.

Kitchen, D. M., D. L. Cheney, and R. M. Seyfarth (2005). Male chacma baboons (*Papio hamadryas ursinus*) discriminate loud call contests between rivals of different relative ranks. *Anim. Cogn.* **8**: 1–6.

Kokko, H. (2007). *Modelling for Field Biologists and Other Interesting People*. Cambridge: Cambridge University Press.

Kuhn, T. S. (1970). *The Structure of Scientific Revolutions*. Chicago, IL: University of Chicago Press.

Kummer, H., G. Anzenberger, and C. K. Hemelrijk (1996). Hiding and perspective taking in long-tailed macaques (Macaca fascicularis). *J. Comp. Psychol.* **110**(1): 97–102.

Lehmann, H., J. Wang, and J. J. Bryson (2005). Tolerance and sexual attraction in despotic societies: a replication and analysis of Hemelrijk (2002). In *Modelling Natural Action Selecton: Proceedings of an International Workshop*, ed. J. J. Bryson, T. J. Prescott, and A. K. Seth. Edinburgh: The Society for the Study of Artificial Intelligence and the Simulation of Behaviour (AISB), pp. 135–42.

Preuschoft, S. and C. P. van Schaik (2000). Dominance and communication: conflict management in various social settings. In *Natural Conflict Resolution*, ed. F. Aureli, and F. B. M. de Waal. Berkeley, CA: University of California Press, Chapter 6, pp. 77–105.

Reynolds, C. W. (1987). Flocks, herds, and schools: a distributed behavioral model. *Comp. Graph.* **21**(4): 25–34.

Rowell, T. E. (1966). Hierarchy in the organization of a captive baboon group. *Anim. Behav.* **14**: 430–44.

Samuels, A., J. B. Silk, and J. Altmann (1987). Continuity and change in dominance relations among female baboons. *Anim. Behav.* **35**: 785–93.

Stanford, C. B. (1996). The hunting ecology of wild chimpanzees: implications for the evolutionary ecology of Pliocene hominids. *Amer. Anthropol.* **98**: 96–113.

te Boekhorst, I. J. A. and P. Hogeweg (1994). Self-structuring in artificial 'chimps' offers new hypotheses for male grouping in chimpanzees. *Behaviour* **130**(3–4): 229–52.

Thierry, B. (1985). Patterns of agonistic interactions in three species of macaque (*Macaca mulatta, M. fascicularis, M. tonkeana*). *Aggressive Behav.* **11**: 223–33.

Thierry, B. (2006). The macaques: a double-layered social organisation. In *Primates in Perspective*, ed. C. Campell, A. Fuentes, K. C. MacKinnon, M. Panger, and S. Bearder. Oxford: Oxford University Press, Chapter 13, pp. 224–39.

Thierry, B., Singh, M., and W. Kaumanns, eds. (2004). *Macaque Societies: A Model for the Study of Society Organization*. Cambridge: Cambridge University Press.

van Schaik, C. P. (1989). The ecology of social relationships amongst female primates. In *Comparative Sociecology of Mammals and Man*, ed. V. Standen and R. Foley. Oxford: Blackwell Scientific, pp. 195–218.

Wang, J. J. (2003). Sexual attraction and inter-sexual dominance among virtual agents: replication of Hemelrijk's DomWorld model with NetLogo. Master's thesis, Department of Computer Science, University of Bath.

Wilensky, U. (2005). *NetLogo ver. 2.1*. Evanston, IL, USA.

Wynne, C. D. L. (1998). A minimal model of transitive inference. In *Models of Action*, ed. C. D. L. Wynne, and J. E. R. Staddon. Mahwah, NJ: Lawrence Erlbaum Associates, pp. 269–307.

Yerkes, R. M. (1940). Social behavior of chimpanzees: dominance between mates in relation to sexual status. *J. Comp. Psychol.* **30**: 147–86.

20 An agent-based model of group decision making in baboons

Russell A. Hill, Brian S. Logan, William I. Sellers, and Julian Zappala

Summary

We present an agent-based model of the key activities of a troop of chacma baboons (*Papio hamadryas ursinus*) based on data collected at De Hoop Nature Reserve in South Africa. The construction of the model identified some key elements that were missing from the field data that would need to be collected in subsequent fieldwork. We analyse the predictions of the model in terms of how well it is able to duplicate the observed activity patterns of the animals and the relationship between the parameters that control the agent's decision procedure and the model's predictions. At the current stage of model development, we are able to show that, across a wide range of decision parameter values, the baboons are able to achieve their energetic and social time requirements. The simulation results show that decisions concerning movement (group action selection) have the greatest influence on the outcomes. Group decision making is a fertile field for future research, and agent-based modelling offers considerable scope for understanding group action selection.

20.1   Introduction

Group living is a common strategy among mammals and is key to understanding the success of the primate order in general and early humans in particular. For animals that forage or move in social groups, decisions about when and where to move often depend upon social interactions between group members (Krause and Ruxton, 2002; Couzin *et al.*, 2005). Little is actually known, however, about how groups of animals arrive at such collective decisions (Conradt and Roper, 2003). We focus on the problem of action selection in groups, i.e., where an individual's action choice is constrained by the choices of other members of the group.

We present an agent-based model of the key activities of a troop of chacma baboons (*Papio hamadryas ursinus*) based on data collected at De Hoop Nature Reserve in South Africa. Baboons (*Papio* sp.) are one of the most widely studied primate species and are ideal for studies of primate ecology since they often live in open, terrestrial habitats, and

Modelling Natural Action Selection, eds. Anil K. Seth, Tony J. Prescott and Joanna J. Bryson.
Published by Cambridge University Press. © Cambridge University Press 2012.

can be observed closely for long periods of time (Richard, 1985). This means that there are a wealth of data available documenting most aspects of their behaviour in great detail. Many of these studies have managed to quantify the activity patterns of individuals both in terms of durations and also the costs and benefits of the activity. *Papio* sp. are found across most of sub-Saharan Africa (Jolly, 2001), at a range of altitudes, with attendant large changes in average rainfall and temperature. Thus they can be said to inhabit a wide variety of habitats and ecotypes, and studies have shown that their diet and foraging varies in response to environmental determinants (Hill and Dunbar, 2002).

Our model extends that presented in Sellers *et al.* (2007). The model consists of two components: an environment model and a baboon model. The environment model is based on the 200 × 200 m map grid used for field data recording, and consists of 660 cells within an area 5.4 km by 8.4 km. Each cell contains a mixture of the six primary habitat types found at De Hoop, and each habitat type is characterised by a maximum food availability, food intake rate when foraging and travel-foraging, and replenishment rate for each month of the study period. The baboons are modelled as agents with physical parameters based on well-known baboon physiology. For ecological purposes, it has been shown that baboon activity can be well characterised by four behavioural categories: moving, foraging, socialising, and resting (Dunbar, 1992). At each timestep each agent selects, based on its physiological state, one of four possible actions (drinking, foraging, socialising, or resting) and whether it would prefer to move to a different habitat cell to allow it to perform its preferred action more effectively. As different agents may wish to move in different directions (or not to move at all), the agents utilise a voting-based mechanism to make consensus decisions whether to move and the direction of group travel. Such consensus decisions may result in a consensus cost for some agents, if they are not able to perform their preferred action as a result of a group decision to move in a particular direction.

While the agents in the Sellers *et al.* (2007) model were able to achieve their goals under a wide range of conditions, the model was less successful in predicting energy budgets and habitat utilisation. Sellers *et al.* speculated that the model's poor fit to the data may be due in part to the agents foraging too easily. Agents uniformly deplete 200 × 200 m cells without incurring additional search costs. In reality, local resource depletion occurs on a much finer scale with more rapidly diminishing foraging returns, and this is not captured in the model. In an attempt to address these issues, we have incorporated a simple model of diminishing foraging returns into the environment model. In our revised model, the rate of energetic return available to an agent in a given habitat cell declines at a rate which is proportional to the food remaining in the cell. This has the effect of making it progressively more difficult to obtain food at a given location, making it more likely that an agent will choose to forage in another cell at the next timestep. This new model allows us to test one of the hypotheses resulting from the original model, and to determine the sensitivity of the model of group decision making to changes in the agents' environment. We analyse the predictions of the revised model in terms of how well it is able to duplicate the observed activity patterns of the animals and the relationship between the parameters that control the agents' decision procedure and the model's predictions.

The remainder of the chapter is organised as follows. In Section 20.2 we review recent theoretical work on decision making in animal groups. In Section 20.3 we review the relevant agent-based modelling literature and motivate our modelling approach. In Section 20.4 we briefly summarise the field data on which our model is based and in Section 20.5 we outline our agent-based model and the decision procedure which the agents use to choose their activities, and explain how the model differs from that presented in Sellers *et al.* (2007). In Section 20.6 we present the results of a Monte-Carlo sensitivity analysis of the predictions of the model in terms of how well it is able to duplicate the observed activity patterns of the animals, and the relationship between the parameters that control the agent's decision procedure and the model's predictions. In Section 20.7 we discuss the results and outline directions for future work.

20.2   Decision making in animal groups

Animal groups must routinely arrive at collective decisions, such as when and where to feed and the location of nesting sites. Many group decisions will be crucial to the individual fitness of the group members, yet may also involve a conflict of interest between individuals since not all animals will have the same preference for an activity or travel destination. Consensus must nevertheless be reached or the group will split and members will forfeit many of the advantages of group living. The existence of collective decision making in animals that do not communicate verbally is a field of considerable current theoretical interest.

Conradt and Roper (2005) distinguish two conceptually different types of group decisions: *combined decisions* and *consensus decisions*. Combined decisions refer to situations where animals decide individually, but in a manner that is dependent on other group members. These decisions often affect the group as a whole, such as decisions to leave or join groups in fission–fusion species (Deneubourg *et al.*, 2002) or the allocation of tasks in eusocial insects (Beshers and Fewell, 2001). Consensus decisions, on the other hand, are made by spatially cohesive groups and concern issues such as movement direction (Couzin *et al.*, 2005), travel destination (Stewart and Harcourt, 1994), and activity timing (Conradt and Roper, 2003). Consensus decisions thus require mechanisms (such as voting) for groups to arrive at agreements. Although group decision making is an issue of fundamental importance in evolutionary biology, little is known about how animal groups arrive at such consensus decisions (Conradt and Roper, 2003).

Two mechanisms which represent the extremes of how groups can reach collective decisions are despotism and democracy (Conradt and Roper, 2003). Although democracy seems improbable for the majority of animal species given the perceived implicit cognitive requirements, empirical examples of 'voting' behaviours have been documented across a range of animal taxa (honey bees, *Apis mellifera*, Seeley and Buhrman, 1999; whooper swans, *Cygnus cygnus*, Black, 1988; African buffalo, *Syncerus caffer*, Prins, 1996; capuchins, *Cebus capucinus*, Leca *et al.*, 2003; gorilla, *Gorilla gorilla*, Stewart and Harcourt, 1994). Furthermore, models of group decision making have shown democratic decisions to be more beneficial than despotic decisions across a wide range of conditions (Conradt and Roper, 2003). Indeed, 'majority rules' appears to be a robust and highly adaptive form of decision making in groups (Hastie and Kameda, 2005). Nevertheless, there is also theoretical support for the emergence of effective leadership in certain contexts (Rands *et al.*, 2003; Couzin *et al.*, 2005). Group decision making is thus a field of considerable current theoretical interest (Simons, 2004; List, 2004; Conradt and Roper, 2005) that provides significant scope for further work. Agent-based modelling offers a valuable technique for exploring how animal groups arrive at consensus decisions.

20.3 Agent-based modelling

Individual-based ecological models have been growing in importance over the last 20 years and it has been predicted that this reductionist approach will provide valuable insight into system-wide properties (Lomnicki, 1992). Early work in Artificial Intelligence (AI) has shown that complex group behaviours such as flocking and following can be produced using simple rules applied to individuals (Reynolds, 1987). Agent-based modelling is an extension of this approach where each individual retains information about its current and past states, and its behaviour is controlled by an internal decision process. An agent in this context is a software system that perceives its environment and acts in that environment in pursuit of its goals. Agents integrate a range of (often relatively shallow) competences, such as goals and reactive behaviour, emotional state, memory, and inference. In agent-based modelling, the agents are situated in a simulated environment, and are equipped with sensors with differing ranges and directional properties (e.g., smell, hearing, vision) and the ability to perform a range of actions which change the state of the environment or the perceptible characteristics of the agent. The environment may contain passive objects (e.g., topography) and active objects and processes which change spontaneously during the course of the simulation (e.g., weather) and/or in response to the actions of the agents (e.g., food-bearing plants).

Agents are commonly described using anthropomorphic terms such as *beliefs* (what the agent believes the state of the environment and other agents to be), *desires* (those states of the environment it is designed to bring about), and *intentions* (the state(s) of the environment it is currently engaged in bringing about) – indeed the so-called *Belief–Desire–Intention*, or BDI, model of agency (Rao and Georgeff, 1991) is perhaps the dominant paradigm in agent theory, (see, e.g., Georgeff *et al.*, 1999). In some cases the agent's beliefs and desires are explicitly represented within the software state of the agent. However, not all agents represent beliefs and goals explicitly, even though they act in a goal-directed manner. For example, the behaviour of an agent may be controlled by a collection of decision rules or reactive behaviours which simply respond to the agent's current environment. In such cases it can still be useful to view the agent as an *intentional system*, that is we ascribe to it the beliefs and goals it *ought* to have, given what we know of its environment, sensors, and (putative) desires (Dennett, 1987, 1996). For example, an agent which has an 'avoid obstacles' behaviour, can be said to have a goal of 'avoiding collisions' even though this goal is not explicitly represented in the agent. This approach, which Dennett (1987) calls 'adopting the intentional stance', allows us to ascribe propositional attitudes to agents which do not explicitly represent beliefs and goals, and is licensed on the grounds that viewing an agent as an intentional system is more likely to yield useful insights than would a description couched in terms of the low level details of the agent's implementation.

The outcomes determined by an agent-based model depend on the set of desires and goals within each individual agent, its current internal state (which may include an internal world model), and the sensory information it receives. This reliance on individual choice makes agent-based modelling especially useful when dealing with animals which live in groups, since it is likely that the optimal strategy for an individual depends on the strategies adopted by others in the group (Milinski and Parker, 1991). Moreover, while the factors influencing the decisions made by an individual may vary as the environment changes, the decision process itself is likely to be conserved, and an agent with a robust decision procedure will demonstrate reasonable behaviour under a wide range of conditions. Such models can therefore be used to explore the potential effects of situational changes: climate, food distribution, and body size can all be altered and the effects on the agents' behaviour can be observed. If we are confident that the decision procedure is robust, then we can use the behaviour of the agents to predict the behaviour of real populations.

There are a number of different types of 'agent-based' model, and different terms are used in the literature for essentially the same kind of model. In some cases, for example, in population ecology models, the emphasis is on tracking the properties of individuals and/or of the population as a whole, with little or no interaction between the individual agents or between the agents and their environment. For example, Robbins and Robbins (2004) have developed a model to simulate the growth rate, age structure, and social system of mountain gorillas in the Virunga Volcanoes region. The model uses a one-year time step and is based on the probabilities of life history events (e.g., birth rates, mortality rates, dispersal patterns) as determined by census data from habituated research groups of gorillas. The gorillas do not interact with an environment model (or each other) and the only decisions the gorillas make as individuals is whether to move to a new group.

In other cases, the agents do interact with each other and/or their environment. In these models, individuals base their decisions on their beliefs about the state of the environment and/or the state of other agents, and their actions (e.g., changing position, eating food) change the environment perceived by other agents, which may in turn change their state and influence the decisions they make. This focus on interaction through the medium of the environment means that these models are often *spatially explicit*, i.e., the individuals are associated with a location in geometrical space. Such spatially explicit agent systems are sometimes called *situated* in the agent literature (e.g., Ferber, 1999).

Situated models allow consideration of social and spatial interactions between individuals. As a result, they have become a popular technique for modelling interactions in humans and non-human primates. Much of the work on agent-based modelling of non-human primates has been done by Charlotte Hemelrijk and her colleagues. They have developed an agent-based model which has been used to investigate dominance interactions in primates (Hemelrijk, 1999a, 1999b, 2000, 2002; Hemelrijk and Wantia, 2005; Hemelrijk *et al.*, 2003, 2005). For example, Hemelrijk (2002) presents a model of primate social behaviour in which agents have two tendencies, to group and to perform dominance interactions, and shows how increased levels of aggression can induce female dominance over males. (See Bryson and Lehmann in this issue for an analysis of the Hemelrijk, 2002, results.) Bryson and Flack (2002) have used an agent-based model to investigate primate social interactions. The agents are represented as 2D rectangles in a walled enclosure which alternate between two behaviours: grooming neighbours and wandering (feeding in relative isolation). The model investigated the effect of a 'tolerance behaviour' on the amount of time spent grooming. These models explicitly take into account the spatial position and orientation of individuals: in the Hemelrijk (2002) model, cohesiveness is determined by the 'SearchAngle', the angle by which an agent will rotate to locate other agents when there are none in sight; in the Bryson and Flack model, grooming requires being adjacent to and properly aligned with another agent.

Although agent-based models are increasingly finding acceptance, such computer simulations are not without their critics. John Maynard-Smith famously described these approaches as 'fact-free science' (Maynard-Smith, 1995). To overcome such objections and to enable us to use this technique as a tool for exploring primate behavioural ecology, the models produced must be tested by using them to predict behaviours in a given population and comparing the predictions with field observations. For example, the predictions of the model developed by Robbins and Robbins (2004) are directly comparable with future population data from this region, and Hemelrijk *et al.* (2003) have proposed model-guided studies of female dominance in real animals.

Existing agent-based models have tended to focus on interactions between the agents and their environment, or pairwise interactions (e.g., dominance interactions) between individuals and emergent properties arising from such interactions. There has been relatively little work to date on agent-based modelling of decision making in animal groups. However, work on social insects in particular allows good experimental testing of the role of individuals in group decisions such as the classic work on honeybees (Seeley *et al.*, 1991) as well as more recent agent-based modelling approaches using ants (Pratt *et al.*, 2005). While there is an extensive literature on agent-based models of human behaviour in a wide range of domains including resource exploitation, economics, and politics (e.g., Laver *et al.*, this volume), this work has not been applied (and in many cases would be difficult to apply) to group decision making in animals. In AI there is a substantial literature on joint actions (e.g., Grosz and Sidner, 1990; Cohen and Levesque, 1991; Tambe, 1997). However, this work has tended to view actions by individuals within a group as directed towards the achievement of a joint intention, with each agent committing to performing a (possibly different) action from a shared or team plan, rather than the selection of an action which is performed by all agents but which only serves the interests of a subset.

Table 20.1 Home range composition, vegetation food availability and predation risk
of the major habitat types at De Hoop.

Habitat Type	Proportion of range (%)	Food availability	Predation risk
Acacia woodland	15.8	High	High
Burnt acacia woodland	1.2	Low	Intermediate
Burnt fynbos	27.6	Low	Intermediate
Climax fynbos	25.7	Low	High
Grassland	11.0	Intermediate	Low
Vlei	18.7	High	Low

In the remainder of this chapter we present a model of group action selection in
baboons. Each baboon is modelled as an agent which chooses actions and interacts with
its environment (and indirectly with other agents) based on its individual state. A key
feature of the model is that an agent's choice of which action to perform is constrained
by a group-level decision whether the group as a whole will move at the next timestep,
which in turn is determined by the actions proposed by the other agents. To the best of
our knowledge this integration of individual-and group-level action selection (where all
the members of the group participate in the selection and execution of a common action)
has not been addressed in previous work.

20.4   Field data

The model is based on data from a study of chacma baboons (*Papio hamadryas ursinus*)
at De Hoop Nature Reserve, a coastal reserve in Western Cape Province, South Africa.
The baboons ranged in an area surrounding the De Hoop Vlei, a large landlocked body
of brackish water lined by cliffs along its eastern edge and fed by several freshwater
springs. Due to its southerly latitude, De Hoop is a highly seasonal environment with
significant annual variation in rainfall, temperature, and day length that has important
implications for the behavioural ecology of this population (Hill, 2005; Hill *et al.*,
2003, 2004). Vegetation is dominated by coastal fynbos, a unique and diverse vegetation
type comprising Proteacae, Ericaceae, Restionaceae, and geophyte species. Six distinct
habitat types were classified on the basis of vegetation structure within the home range
of the baboons (Hill, 2006a) (Table 20.1; see Hill (1999) for detailed descriptions and
further information on the ecology of the reserve).

The data presented here are for a seven-month period (June to December 1997) from
a single troop of chacma baboons that ranged in size from 40 to 44 individuals over
the course of the study. Data were collected by means of instantaneous scan samples
(Altmann, 1974) at 30-minute intervals, with 2–4 adult males and 12 adult females
sampled for a minimum of five full days each month. At each sample point, information
was recorded on the identity, habitat type, and activity state (feeding, moving, socialising,
or resting) of all visible individuals. Each scan lasted a maximum of five minutes. A

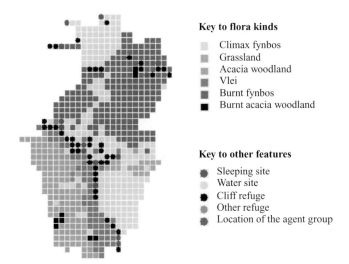

Key to flora kinds

Climax fynbos
Grassland
Acacia woodland
Vlei
Burnt fynbos
Burnt acacia woodland

Key to other features

Sleeping site
Water site
Cliff refuge
Other refuge
Location of the agent group

Figure 20.1 Graphical output from the simulator showing the habitat types and distributions. See plate section for colour version.

more detailed description of the data collection methods is given in Hill (1999), with further information on patterns of habitat use in Hill and Weingrill (2006).

20.5   The model

Based on the field data, we developed and implemented an agent-based model of baboon behaviour and used this to simulate a troop of 50 baboons over a seven-month period (June–December). The model determined the activity chosen by each baboon at each timestep and the resulting energy balance, time between drinking, time spent socialising, and time spent resting.

The simulation model consists of two components: the environment model and the baboon model. The environment model is based on the 200×200 m map grid used for field data recording, and consists of 660 cells within an area 5.4 km by 8.4 km. Each cell contains a mixture of the six primary habitat types found at De Hoop (acacia woodland, burnt acacia woodland, climax fynbos, burnt fynbos, grassland and vlei) and may also include one or more 'special features': water sources, sleeping sites, and refuges (primarily cliffs). When more than one habitat type occurs in a cell, it is assumed that they are present in equal proportions. Each habitat type is characterised by a maximum food availability, food intake rate when foraging and travel-foraging, and replenishment rate for each month of the study period. The energy value of the food available was estimated at 13.98 kJg^{-1} (Stacey, 1986) for all habitat types. The habitat types and distributions are illustrated in the graphical output of the simulator, shown in Figure 20.1.

The second component of the simulation is the baboon model. Each baboon is modelled as an agent with physical parameters based on well-known baboon physiology. In addition, each agent maintains an individual score for water, energy, and social time which function as 'drives' in biasing the agent's choice of preferred activity. At each timestep, an agent can perform one of four actions corresponding to the activities recorded for the baboons at De Hoop: foraging, moving (travel foraging), socialising, or resting. In addition, an agent can perform an instantaneous drinking action which can be combined with any of the other four actions (assuming the agent is in a cell which contains a water source). Foraging, moving, socialising, and resting actions have an associated energy cost which decreases the agent's energy score. Energy costs were calculated using the formulae given in Tucker (1970) for an average adult female baboon with a body mass of 16.1 kg (with the heavier males offset by the lighter infants and juveniles) and assuming that the baboons moved relatively slowly 0.5 ms^{-1} since they customarily foraged whilst moving. Thus foraging requires 36.71 W, moving (travel foraging) 50.59 W, socialising 64.04 W, and resting 34.63 W. These values are not directly based on the field data from De Hoop so must be viewed as approximate. The agents rest at night, and the energy this requires is also subtracted from their energy score. In addition to its energy cost, each action also updates the energy, water, and social time scores. Thus foraging increases the agent's energy score depending on the type of food consumed (i.e., the habitat type(s) of the current cell).

In Sellers *et al.* (2007) it is evident that the agents spend considerably less time foraging than their natural counterparts yet still achieve their energetic requirements. The authors speculated that this disparity was a consequence of the relatively coarse granularity of the environmental model, and specifically the constant rate at which resources are depleted by the agents. In an attempt to address these issues, we have extended the model presented in Sellers *et al.* (2007) to incorporate a model of diminishing foraging returns. The diminishing returns model assumes that the food in a cell is uniformly distributed and uniformly depleted by the agents. Under these assumptions the rate of energetic return in each cell at time t, r_t, is equal to the product of the maximum possible rate of return r_{max} and the ratio of the remaining energetic resource e_t to maximum available energetic resource e_{max} in the cell. That is:

$$r_t = r_{\max} \times \frac{e_t}{e_{\max}}. \tag{20.1}$$

The model, which relies solely on information present in the simulation, exhibits the intuitive behaviour that as resource within each cell becomes increasingly sparse the agents must spend proportionately more time foraging to obtain the same energetic return, i.e., once the resource available in a cell has halved, twice as much time must be spent foraging to obtain the same energetic return.

The agents also forage while moving, which increases the agent's energy score at a lower travel-foraging rate. Drinking adds one to the agent's water score. Socialising increases the agent's social time score by the length of the timestep. Not drinking causes the agent's water score to decrease by the reciprocal of the timestep, and any action other than socialising causes the social score to decrease by the length of the timestep.

The baboon model simulates the activities of each baboon during daylight hours at a five minute timestep. At the beginning of each timestep the agents execute a two stage decision procedure which determines the action performed by each agent at this timestep. In the first phase, each agent chooses a preferred action and whether it would prefer to move to allow it to perform the action more effectively. In the second phase, a group decision is taken to determine whether the agents actually move to another cell. This may force some agents to choose an alternative less-preferred action, as explained below.

In the first phase of the decision procedure, each agent's preferred action is determined by a combination of individual constraints and the agent's goals. The agents have a single individual constraint: they must return to a sleeping site to rest each night. In addition they have three goals: to maintain their energy balance (i.e., to eat sufficient food to make up for the energy expended each day), to drink (i.e., visit a grid cell constraining a water source) at least once every two days, and to spend two hours a day in social activity. The requirement that the agents must return to a sleeping site each night constrains the choice of the preferred action (and ultimately the preferred cell) so that the agent can always reach a sleeping site in the time remaining before nightfall. If the individual constraint does not force the agent to move at this timestep, the agent's preferred action is determined using a weighted random function with weights proportional to the current desire to forage, drink, and socialise. Desires are linear functions of the corresponding scores with gradients proportional to relative importance values for each action: W_F (the relative importance of foraging), W_D (the relative importance of drinking), and W_S (the relative importance of socialising). These desire functions fall to zero when the target amount has been reached and when they are all zero the agent will opt to rest. By aiming to keep all desires at zero, the agents will eat enough food to balance their energy expenditure, drink on average once per day, and socialise on average two hours per day.

The agent then determines whether it could perform its preferred action more effectively in another cell. The agent will *vote to move* if the best grid cell within a search radius, S, is more than an action-specific threshold better than the current cell for its preferred action. (If the search radius is greater than the maximum distance the baboon can travel and still reach the closest sleeping site by dusk, only cells within the maximum travel distance are considered.) In the case of foraging the threshold is denoted by T_F, and depends on the food availability, in the case of socialising and resting the thresholds (denoted by T_S, T_R) are a measure of predation risk. For example, if the agent would prefer to forage, it will vote to move if the best cell within the search radius has more than T_F times as much food as the current cell. It is assumed that the agent has perfect information about food availability and predation risk for all cells within the search radius of its current position, and that the agent knows where the nearest water source is, irrespective of search radius.

In the second phase, the votes for all the agents are counted, and a *group decision* is taken on whether *all* the agents will move. If the number of agents voting to move is higher than a user specified threshold, V, then the whole group moves in the most commonly preferred direction (i.e., each agent performs a move action in the specified direction at this timestep). If fewer than V agents opt to move, then the agents which voted to move choose their most preferred action for the current cell at this timestep. This is because the group decision not to move may invalidate an individual's initial

Table 20.2 Interaction between individual and group level decisions.

Group decides to move	Individual votes to move	
	yes	no
yes	travel-forage in the most preferred direction	
no	choose best available action for the current cell	perform preferred action in the current cell

choice of preferred action: for example, it is impossible to drink if there is no water in the current cell, or if the current cell's predation risk is greater than T_K then the agent will not want to socialise or rest.

The interaction between individual- and group-level decisions is summarised in Table 20.2. Note that the adoption of the group-level decision by all agents may involve an element of coercion for some agents. If the group decision is not to move, then all the agents that did not vote to move get to perform their preferred action and those that did vote to move are forced to choose another action to execute in the current cell. This could be the same action as their first choice (but in this case they are forced to perform it in the current cell which is at least T_X worse than their preferred cell for this action). In other cases it may be impossible or too risky to perform their preferred action in the current cell and they must choose another action. If, on the other hand, more than V agents voted to move, then those that preferred to stay in the current cell are coerced to move (travel-forage) in the most commonly preferred direction. Moreover, since the group decision is to move in the most preferred direction, it is possible that some of the agents that voted to move will ultimately not be able to perform their preferred action in their preferred cell. For example, an agent that wants to move west to a water source may be forced to move east towards a cell which is better for foraging or resting/socialising.

The agents then spend the next five minutes either moving in the chosen direction or performing their chosen action, and their scores in terms of energy, water, and social time are adjusted accordingly. If the agent's preferred action is to forage, socialise or rest, the agent will opportunistically drink if it finds itself in a grid cell containing a water source.

Critically, the actions of the agents also affect the environment, which in turn affects the action chosen by the agents at the next timestep. For example, foraging and travel-foraging causes the food available in the grid cell containing a baboon to be depleted at the appropriate food-intake rate for each habitat type occurring in the cell. While food consumed is replaced at the replenishment rate for the current simulation month for each of the habitat type(s) occurring in the grid cell, this is lower than the corresponding food intake rate. Foraging therefore reduces the availability of food at the next timestep (relative to other cells within the agents' perceptual range), making it more likely that an agent will choose to forage in another cell (or perform some other action) at the next timestep.

For the revised version of the model presented here, the original simulation was reimplemented using the MASON multiagent simulation toolkit (Luke *et al.*, 2005).

To verify that the reimplementation was identical to that in Sellers *et al.* (2007) we performed a replication and validation study. The original and reimplemented simulation (without diminishing returns) were run on the same input data and using an identical stream of random numbers (Will and Hegselmann, 2008). This approach accounts for the stochastic elements within the model, and allows direct comparison of the internal state of both simulations. The re-implementation was shown to exhibit numerical identity (Axtell *et al.*, 1996) when compared to the original simulation (Zappala, 2008).

The replication revealed a small number of minor defects in the original implementation relating to choice of direction and group action selection under extremely rare conditions. These defects were corrected and the revised and original models were statistically compared for distributional equivalence (Axtell *et al.*, 1996) using a two-tailed *t*-test for matched pairs ($n = 1001, p < 0.05$). A total of 1001 sets of parameter values were randomly chosen from the original Monte Carlo parameter ranges used in Sellers *et al.* (2007) and the corresponding outputs analysed for each simulation. While there are statistically significant differences between the results of the original and revised models, the changes in the mean time spent in each activity and in each habitat type were relatively small ($< 20\%$), and the change in the mean success rate with respect to V (a key finding of Sellers *et al.*, 2007) was less than 5% (Zappala, 2008). We take this as an indication that these defects did not materially affect the original findings of Sellers *et al.* The replication also gives us greater confidence that the results presented in Sellers *et al.* (2007) were not due to artefacts of the original implementation.

20.6   Sensitivity analysis

We do not currently have values for the parameters used in the agents' decision procedure. Some we may be able to estimate empirically with more detailed field observations, but others are essentially unknowable. To overcome this we chose plausible ranges for each decision parameter and performed a Monte-Carlo sensitivity analysis (Campolongo *et al.*, 2000) where the simulation was repeated a large number of times and the values of the parameters randomly sampled from the appropriate ranges for each run. This allows us both to estimate the importance of a particular parameter on the outcome and to calculate the range of possible outcomes. Sensitivity analysis was chosen as our primary interests in this initial study to see whether the range of possible outcomes predicted by the model were able to bracket those observed in the field and to highlight gaps in the field data, rather than trying to find the parameter values that produced the best fit to the field data (although this will be a goal of future work). The parameter ranges used in the analysis are shown in Table 20.3.

We analysed the predictions of the model in terms of how well it was able to duplicate the observed activity patterns in the baboon field data. The model was run 100 000 times sampling the parameters from Table 20.3 each time. Table 20.4 shows the success of the agents in achieving their goals for both the reimplemented (constant returns) model and the new diminishing returns model. We consider the agents successful if they achieve their energetic requirements (maintaining an energy intake of approximately 3500 kJ

Table 20.3 Key parameters in the decision procedures showing the ranges used in the Monte-Carlo sensitivity analysis.

Parameter	Min	Max
V vote to move threshold	0.1	0.9
S search radius	200	2200
W_F relative importance of foraging	1	10
W_S relative importance of social activity	1	10
W_D relative importance of drinking	1	10
T_F move to forage threshold	1	3
T_S move to socialise threshold	1	3
T_R move to rest threshold	1	3
T_K predation risk threshold	0	0.25

Table 20.4 Percentage of simulations in which the agents successfully achieved their goals for the reimplemented constant returns model and the new diminishing returns model.

	Constant returns		Diminishing returns	
	Success	Failure	Success	Failure
Water	69.6	30.4	66.0	34.0
Energy	79.4	20.6	77.3	22.7
Social	92.9	7.1	92.7	7.3
Total	69.4	30.6	65.9	34.1

depending on the activity pattern), water requirements (an interval between drinking of less than two days), and social requirements (a target of two hours of social activity). We consider a run successful if all these requirements are achieved simultaneously by all agents for the entire duration of the simulation.

It is clear from Table 20.4 that the correction of the original constant returns model (Sellers *et al.*, 2007) has resulted in an increase in the success of agents in achieving their goals. Nevertheless, the agents still fail to achieve their goals in over 30% of simulations and, as with the original simulation, this is primarily due to not meeting their water requirements. As with the original simulation, therefore, certain combinations of input criteria lead to significant levels of failure. Similar patterns are observed for the diminishing returns model, although the increased foraging costs in this model results in higher rates of failure on all criteria, with less than two thirds of simulations successful overall. It is clear, therefore, that the addition of a model of diminishing foraging returns has made it more challenging for the agents to achieve their goals. In the remainder of this section we examine parameters that account for the success and failure of each run and examine the degree to which the new diminishing returns model is able to predict observed time budgets and habitat utilisation for the De Hoop baboons.

Table 20.5 presents the results of a forward logistic regression analysis to determine which of the nine parameters in the model's decision procedure have significant effects on the success and failure of each run. Since the relationship between success or failure

Table 20.5 Results of a logistic regression analysis to determine which factors within the model have the greatest effect on whether the agents succeed or fail in achieving their goals.

Model	Nagelkerke r^2 0.585	−2 Log L 73337.7	X^2 55040.2	df 21	p <000001
Variables included	r^2 change	B	Wald	df	p
V	0.437		23884.3	15	<0.0001
W_D	0.083	0.049	8307.1	1	<0.0001
W_F	0.026	−0.269	3021.3	1	<0.0001
W_S	0.018	−0.224	2147.6	1	<0.0001
T_F	0.017	0.981	2041.8	1	<0.0001
T_K	0.004	3.757	448.4	1	<0.0001
T_S	0.001	0.046	4.7	1	<0.0001
Variables excluded			Score	df	P
S			2.05	1	0.152
T_R			0.89	1	0.346

of the model and the voting threshold was nonlinear (see Figure 20.2), the vote to move threshold was recoded as a categorical variable for analysis, with each category representing a proportional increase in threshold of 0.05. As in Sellers *et al.* (2007), despite seven parameters being significant determinants of the success or failure of the agents, it is clear that V, the proportion of agents required to vote in order to move, has the greatest effect. Furthermore, it is evident from Figure 20.2 that only intermediate vote to move threshold values produce successful outcomes, with thresholds between 0.40 and 0.70 consistently leading to successful runs of the model. In contrast, simulations with low or very high voting thresholds rarely result in the agents achieving their requirements, indicating that majority decision making is the key to a successful foraging strategy within the model.

By comparing the distribution of successful runs with respect to V for constant and diminishing returns we can investigate the response of the model to the introduction of diminishing returns. From Figure 20.2 we can see that for values of V between 0.10 and 0.50, the agents are consistently more successful with constant returns than with diminishing returns. However, as V tends towards 0.5 the number of successful runs reduces nonlinearly, until the number of successful runs converge. Perhaps surprisingly, for values of V between 0.70 and 0.85 the agents are more successful in the diminishing returns model than the model with constant returns.

Further differences with the logistic regression model of Sellers *et al.* (2007) are also evident, however, with the search radius no longer a significant predictor of the success of the model. Interestingly, T_F is now significant, suggesting that the increased foraging requirements of the diminishing returns model place far greater significance on the move to forage threshold in determining the agents' ability to achieve their energetic requirements.

Although the factors underpinning the success of the model are similar to those in Sellers *et al.* (2007) it is clear that the diminishing returns model is better able to predict the observed baboon activity budgets (Figure 20.3a). In particular, the diminishing

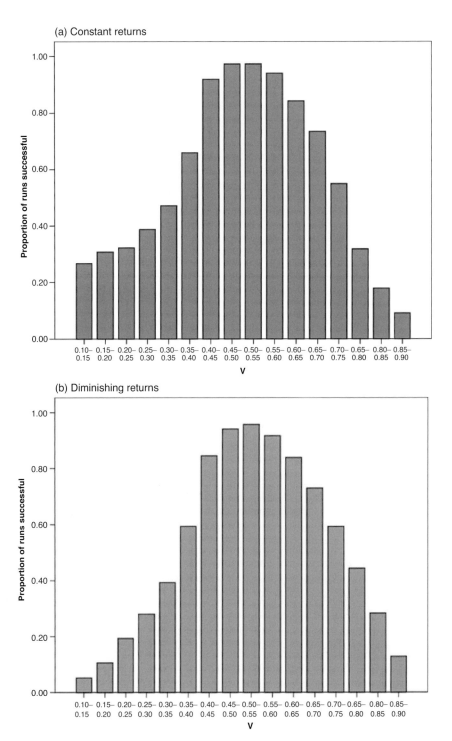

Figure 20.2 Proportion of runs resulting in the agents successfully achieving their goals against proportion of agents required in order to vote to move V.

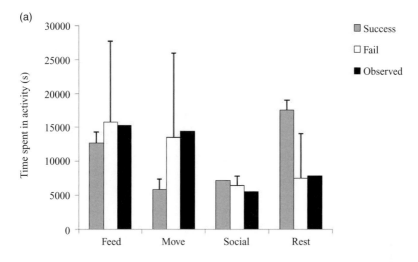

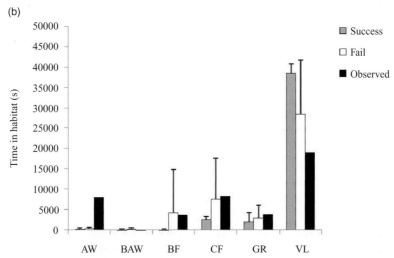

Figure 20.3 Mean (+SD) duration of time spent in (a) each of the four activities and (b) each habitat type in successful and failed runs of the model compared with the values from the field data. AW: acacia woodland; BAW: burnt acacia woodland; BF: burnt fynbos; CF: climax fynbos; GR: grassland; VL: vlei.

returns model results in a significant increase in time spent foraging (12 679 s compared to 6513 s in the constant returns model) although the observed value still lies over one standard deviation from the mean of the successful simulations. In turn this results in a reduction in resting time relative to the earlier model (17 544 s versus 23 391 s), although the simulated values still greatly exceed those observed. Similarly, as with Sellers *et al.* (2007), the successful simulations predict the agents to move far less than observed and social time is in line with that predicted.

The diminishing returns model does little to improve the fit with the observed habitat use relative to the model of Sellers *et al.* (2007). Figure 20.3b illustrates that in the successful simulations the agents use the vlei habitat significantly more than observed within the field data, with the acacia woodland habitat significantly underutilised. Since the vlei habitat is both high in food availability and low in predation risk these results suggest that, on average, the agents are able to satisfy their foraging requirements without needing to move to the more distant and risky acacia woodland. Overall, therefore, it is clear that while the diminishing returns model represents a significant improvement in terms of matching the foraging costs in the observed data, the model still does not adequately capture all of the parameters constraining patterns of baboon activity and habitat use.

20.7   Discussion

Although the diminishing returns model represents a significant improvement to the original model presented in Sellers *et al.* (2007), it is nevertheless clear that it is still relatively easy for the agents to satisfy their energetic requirements over a broad range of parameter values. It is important to remember though that we would never expect a model to precisely match the observed activity patterns at even a monthly level, let alone daily or hourly timescale, although the results presented here do suggest that this should be possible. Nevertheless, further developments are clearly required if this is to be achieved.

Despite the diminishing returns model providing far greater ecological realism in terms of foraging costs, we noted in Sellers *et al.* (2007) that the coarseness of our environmental model (where groups are foraging in 200×200 m patches) may prevent an accurate simulation of observed behaviour. Even with the diminishing returns model the agents are able to deplete the 200 m grids evenly without additional moving costs, whereas in reality baboons will of course cause local resource depletion on a much finer scale with more rapidly diminishing foraging returns. As a consequence, the animals are likely to make frequent movements over small distances between discrete food patches within a cell and these elements are currently not captured in our model. A significant improvement may therefore be achieved if we were to simulate baboon foraging at an appropriate temporal and spatial scale (such as 1 m^2 at sub-minute intervals). Although our current ecological data do not permit such an approach, a number of studies have recently started to incorporate landscape dynamics and geographic information systems (GIS) data into individual-oriented models (Gimblett, 2002; Topping *et al.*, 2003). In future, coupling multi-agent simulation tools with GIS mapping data will offer opportunities for the production of highly realistic multi-agent simulations of individual behaviour and population processes within precise spatial contexts (Schüle *et al.*, 2004).

While the need for more detailed environmental models is clear, there are a number of other areas where additional parameters could also be beneficially incorporated into the current model. First, the incorporation of a full diet model may be essential. While the agents' preference for foraging within the vlei habitat may be explained in terms of its proximity to sleeping sites and the nature of resource depletion ensuring that it always offers high energetic returns, it may be equally true that in nature the baboons move on in order to seek a more diverse diet (Hill, 2006b; Post, 1982). In reality, the vlei had only limited diversity in terms of food types (Hill, 1999), but since the model only examines energy intake this may explain why the more food species diverse habitats such as acacia woodland and burnt climax fynbos are underutilised in the simulations. A full diet model would be easy in modelling terms but difficult in terms of validation, since it would require much more detailed chemical and calorific analysis of what the baboons actually eat in different areas. While this is not possible with our existing ecological data, it does serve to highlight the value of agent-based modelling in identifying areas of empirical data that are important for future field studies.

Some improvements in relation to foraging costs should nevertheless be achievable within the framework of the current model. Over 56% of food items consumed within the vlei are subterranean, compared to less than 1% in acacia woodland, the other high food availability habitat. Although subterranean items are often of high quality in terms of energy they are generally considered to be fallback items due to their high costs of excavation (Hill and Dunbar, 2002). As a consequence, foraging within the vlei is likely to be more energetically expensive than in other habitats and this fact may account for why our simulations overestimate the time spent in this habitat. Although accurate estimates of the energetic costs of digging are not currently available for primates, it should still be possible to more accurately account for the different foraging costs for each habitat in a future iteration of the model. This alone should significantly improve the fit with the habitat usage observed for the De Hoop baboons.

Given the ease with which agents appear to be able to forage within our model, it is extremely interesting that the agents fail to achieve all of their goals simultaneously in over one-third of simulations. The results of the Monte-Carlo sensitivity analysis indicate that while the agents are able to achieve their minimum requirements across a range of decision parameter values, unsuccessful runs are most likely to arise from individuals gaining insufficient access to water. The primary determinant of the success of the model, however, is determined not by W_D, the relative importance of drinking, but instead by the proportion of individuals voting to move. Only in situations where a majority is required for movement (and thus changes in activity and location) does the model consistently result in the agents achieving their minimum requirements. In fact, the voting threshold is also the primary variable underlying variation in the time spent in various behaviours and in the different habitat types (Sellers *et al.*, 2005). This is almost certainly because democratic decision making tends to produce less extreme decisions (Conradt and Roper, 2003) and it is certainly true that the unsuccessful runs produce far more variable output (Figure 20.3). While all grid cells in the model contain at least some food, and many habitats are suitable for socialising and resting, water is restricted to just a few localities. As a consequence, while it is probably still possible for individuals to adequately forage, socialise, and rest under less democratic voting thresholds because suitable habitats are still likely to be encountered, low (and to a lesser degree very high) voting thresholds can lead to more extreme variation in drinking intervals resulting in the agents being unable to meet their drinking requirements in many cases. The introduction of diminishing returns creates a more challenging environment for the agents, in that more time is required to achieve a similar energetic intake. Intuitively, one might expect that this would reduce the success rate for all values of V; however, this is not the case. Although the introduction of diminishing returns does produce a noticeable (3.5%) reduction in overall success rates, this difference is almost entirely accounted for by runs in which V is less than 0.5. As it becomes more difficult for the agents to achieve their goals, super-majority ($V > 0.5$) decision strategies, which demand greater commitment from the group, are preferable to sub-majority ($V < 0.5$) decision strategies where lower group commitment is required.

Although the voting procedure employed in this chapter might be considered unrealistic, anecdotal observations of wild baboons have reported voting behaviours where a simple majority determines changes in group activity based on movement (Byrne 2000), or where the majority of adults decides on the direction of travel through body orientation (Norton 1986). Perhaps most importantly, a recent study on the De Hoop baboons has the shown the timing of departure and travel direction seemed to be a partially shared consensus decision with adult males contributing more to the decision outcome (Stueckle and Zinner 2008). While constraining a social group to remain together, the voting mechanism in our model may have greater similarities to natural systems than might be supposed. Nevertheless, while this study adds to the growing body of evidence that democracy and majority decision making should be widespread across a range of animal taxa, it is clear that the questions of how animal groups coordinate movement and reach decisions are a fertile field for future research.

It would also be interesting to extend the model to explore the relationship between individual and group-level action selection in more detail. For example, it would be straightforward to incorporate a weighted voting scheme in which the votes of some individuals have a greater effect on action choice (and in the limit some subset of individuals determines group actions). Such a modification would allow us to explore whether the empirical data reported by Stueckle and Zinner (2008), where males have greater voting weights, allow us to better predict the other elements of observed behaviour. It would be more interesting, however, to try to model the emergence of group-level action selection from the sum of interactions between individual agent's action choices (i.e., without an explicit voting scheme). This would require a much finer grained model of baboon sensing and behaviour, and a greater time resolution of the model. Nevertheless, agent-based modelling offers the potential to address these issues, and the current model should provide a valuable springboard for examining the relationship between individual-and group-level action selection.

Acknowledgements

RAH gratefully acknowledges the financial support of the Leverhulme Trust in contributing to this project.

References

Altmann, J. (1974). Observational study of behaviour: sampling methods. *Behaviour* **49**: 227–67.

Axtell, R., R. Axelrod, J. M. Epstein, and M. D. Cohen (1996). Aligning simulation models: a case study and results. *Computat. Math. Organiz. Theor.* **1**(2): 123–41.

Beshers, S. N. and J. H. Fewell (2001). Models of division of labor in social insects. *Ann. Rev. Entomol.* **46**: 413–40.

Black, J. M. (1988). Preflight signalling in swans: a mechanism for group cohesion and flock formation. *Ethology* **79**: 143–57.

Bryson, J. J. and J. C. Flack (2002). Action selection for an artificial life model of social behavior in non-human primates. In *Proceedings of the International Workshop on Self-organization and Evolution of Social Behaviour*, ed. C. Hemelrijk. Switzerland: Monte Verita, pp. 42–5.

Byrne, R. W. (2000). How monkeys find their way: leadership, coordination, and cognitive maps of African baboons. In *On the Move*, ed. S. Boinski and P. Garber. Chicago, IL: University of Chicago Press, pp. 491–518.

Campolongo, F., A. Saltelli, T. Sorensen, and S. Taratola (2000). Hitchhikers' guide to sensitivity analysis. In *Sensitivity Analysis*, ed. A. Saltelli, K. Chan, and E. M. Scott. Chichester, UK: Wiley, pp. 15–47.

Cohen, P. R. and H. J. Levesque (1991). Teamwork. *Nous* **25**(4): 487–512.

Conradt, L. and T. J. Roper (2003). Group decision-making in animals. *Nature* **421**: 155–8.

Conradt, L. and T. J. Roper (2005). Consensus decision making in animals. *Trends Ecol. Evol.* **20**: 449–56.

Couzin, I. D., J. Krause, N. R. Franks, and S. A. Levin (2005). Effective leadership and decision-making in animal groups on the move. *Nature* **433**: 513–16.

Deneubourg, J. L., A. Lioni, and C. Detrain (2002). Dynamics of aggregation and emergence of cooperation. *Biol. Bull.* **202**: 262–7.

Dennett, D. C. (1987). *The Intentional Stance*. Cambridge, MA: MIT Press.

Dennett, D. C. (1996). *Kinds of Minds: Towards an Understanding of Consciousness*. New York: Basic Books.

Dunbar, R. I. M. (1992). Time: a hidden constraint on the behavioural ecology of baboons. *Behav. Ecol. Sociobiol.* **31**: 35–49.

Ferber, J. (1999). *Multi-agent Systems*. Boston, MA: Addison Wesley Longman.

Georgeff, M. P., B. Pell, M. E. Pollack, M. Tambe, and M. Wooldridge (1999). The belief-desire-intention model of agency. In *Intelligent Agents V. Agent Theories, Architectures, and Languages, 5th International Workshop ATAL'98 Proceedings*, ed. J. P. Müller, M. P. Singh, and A. S. Rao. Berlin: Springer, Vol. 1555, pp. 1–10.

Gimblett, H. R. (2002). *Integrating Geographic Information Systems and Agent-based Modelling Techniques for Simulating Social and Ecological Processes*. New York: Oxford University Press.

Grosz, B. J. and Sidner, C. L. (1990). Plans for discourse. In *Intentions in communication*, ed. P. R. Cohen, J. Morgan, and M. Pollack. Cambridge MA: MIT Press, pp. 417–45.

Hastie, R. and T. Kameda (2005). The robust beauty of majority rules in group decisions. *Psychol. Rev.* **112**(2): 494–508.

Hemelrijk, C. J. (1999a). Effects of cohesiveness on intersexual dominance relationships and spatial structure among group-living virtual entities. In *Proceedings of the Fifth European*

Conference on Artificial Life (ECAL99), ed. D. Floreano, J.-D. Nicoud, and F. Mondada. Berlin: Springer, pp. 524–34.

Hemelrijk, C. J. (1999b). An individual-oriented model of the emergence of despotic and egalitarian societies. *Proc. Roy. Soc. B Biol. Sci.* **266**: 361–9.

Hemelrijk, C. J. (2000). Towards the integration of social dominance and spatial structure. *Anim. Behav.* **59**(5): 1035–48.

Hemelrijk, C. J. (2002, June). Self-organization and natural selection in the evolution of complex despotic societies. *Biol. Bull.* **202**(3): 283–8.

Hemelrijk, C. J. and J. Wantia (2005). Individual variation by selforganisation. *Neurosci. Biobehav. Rev.* **29**(1): 125–36.

Hemelrijk, C. J., J. Wantia, and M. Datwyler (2003). Female co-dominance in a virtual world: ecological, cognitive, social and sexual causes. *Behaviour* **140**: 1247–73.

Hemelrijk, C. J., J. Wantia, and L. Gygax (2005). The construction of dominance order: comparing performance of five methods using an individual-based model. *Behaviour* **142**: 1043–64.

Hill, R. A. (1999). Ecological and demographic determinants of time budgets in baboons: implications for cross-populational models of baboon socioecology. PhD dissertation, University of Liverpool.

Hill, R. A. (2005). Day length seasonality and the thermal environment. In *Primate Seasonality: Implications for Human Evolution*, ed. D. K. Brockman and C. P. van Schaik. Cambridge: Cambridge University Press, pp. 197–212.

Hill, R. A. (2006a). Thermal constraints on activity scheduling and habitat choice in baboons. *Amer. J. Phys. Anthropol.* **129**: 242–9.

Hill, R. A. (2006b). Why be diurnal? Or, why not be cathemeral? *Folia Primatol.* **77**: 72–86.

Hill, R. A., L. Barrett, D. Gaynor, *et al.* (2003). Day length, latitude and behavioural (in)flexibility in baboons. *Behav. Ecol. Sociobiol.* **53**: 278–86.

Hill, R. A., L. Barrett, D. Gaynor, *et al.* (2004). Day length variation and seasonal analyses of behaviour. *S. Afr. J. Wildl. Res.* **34**: 39–44.

Hill, R. A. and Dunbar, R. I. M. (2002). Climatic determinants of diet and foraging behaviour in baboons. *Evol. Ecol.* **16**: 579–93.

Hill, R. A. and Weingrill, T. (2006). Predation risk and habitat use in chacma baboons (Papio hamadryas ursinus). In *Primates and their Predators*, ed. S. Gursky and K. A. I. Nekaris. New York: Kluwer, pp. 339–54.

Jolly, C. J. (2001). A proper study for mankind: analogies from the papionin monkeys and their implications for human evolution. *Yearb. Phys. Anthropol.* **44**: 177–204.

Krause, J. and G. D. Ruxton (2002). *Living in Groups*. Oxford: Oxford University Press.

Leca, J.-B., N. Gunst, B. Thierry, and O. Petit (2003). Distributed leadership in semifree-ranging white-faced capuchin monkeys. *Anim. Behav.* **66**: 1045–52.

List, C. (2004). Democracy in animal groups: a political perspective. *Trends Ecol. Evol.* **19**: 168–9.

Lomnicki, A. (1992). Population ecology from the individual perspective. In *Individual-based Models and Approaches in Ecology*, ed. D. L. DeAngelis and L. J. Gross New York: Chapman and Hall, pp. 3–17.

Luke, S., C. Cioffi-Revilla, L. Panait, K. Sullivan, and G. Balan (2005). MASON: a multiagent simulation environment. *Simulation* **81**(7): 517–27.

Maynard-Smith, J. (1995). Life at the edge of chaos. *New York Rev. Books*, March **2**: 28–30.

Milinski, M. and Parker, G. A. (1991). Competition for resources. In *Behavioural Ecology*, J. R. Krebs and N. B. Davies. Oxford: Blackwell, pp. 137–168.

Norton, G. W. (1986). Leadership: decision processes of group movement in yellow baboons. In *Primate Ecology and Conservation*, ed. J. Else and P. Lee. Cambridge: Cambridge University Press, pp. 145–56.

Post, D. G. (1982). Feeding behaviour of yellow baboons in Amboseli National Park. *Int. J. Primatol.* **3**: 403–430.

Pratt, S. C., D. J. T. Sumpter, E. B. Mallon, and N. R. Franks (2005). An agent-based model of collective nest choice by the ant *Temnothorax albipennis. Anim. Behav.* **70**: 1023–36.

Prins, H. H. T. (1996). *Ecology and Behaviour of the African Buffalo*. London: Chapman and Hall.

Rands, S. A., G. Cowlishaw, R. A. Pettifor, J. M. Rowcliffe, and R. A. Johnstone (2003). The spontaneous emergence of leaders and followers in a foraging pair. *Nature* **423**: 432–34.

Rao, A. S. and M. P. Georgeff (1991). Modeling rational agents within a BDI architecture. In *Proceedings of the Second International Conference on Principles of Knowledge Representation and Reasoning*, pp. 473–84.

Reynolds, C. W. (1987). *Flocks, herds and schools: a distributed behavioral model.* In *Proceedings of the 14th Annual Conference on Computer Graphics and Interactive Techniques*. New York: ACM Press, pp. 25–34.

Richard, A. F. (1985). *Primates in Nature*. New York: W.H. Freeman and Company.

Robbins, M. M. and Robbins, A. M. (2004). Simulation of the population dynamics and social structure of the Virunga mountain gorillas. *Amer. J. Primatol.* **63**(4): 201–223.

Schüle, M., R. Herrler, and F. Klüg (2004). Coupling GIS and multi-agent simulation: towards infrastructure for realistic simulation. In *Multiagent System Technologies: Proceedings of the Second German Conference, (MATES 2004)*, Vol. 3187, ed. G. Lindemann, J. Denzinger, I. J. Timm, and R. Unland. Berlin: Springer, pp. 228–42.

Seeley, T. D. and Buhrman, S. C. (1999). Group decision making in swarms of honey bees. *Behav. Ecol. Sociobiol.* **45**: 19–31.

Seeley, T. D., S. Camazine, and J. Sneyd (1991). Collective decision-making in honey bees: how colonies choose among nectar sources. *Behav. Ecol. Sociobiol.* **28**: 277–290.

Sellers, W. I., R. A. Hill, and B. Logan (2005, July). Biorealistic modelling of baboon foraging using agent-based modelling. In *Modelling Natural Action Selection: Proceedings of an International Workshop*, ed. J. J. Bryson, T. J. Prescott, and A. K. Seth. Edinburgh, UK: AISB Press, pp. 127–134.

Sellers, W. I., R. A. Hill, and B. Logan (2007). An agent-based model of group decision making in baboons. *Phil. Trans. Roy. Soc. B Biol. Sci.* **362**(1485): 1699–710.

Simons, A. M. (2004). Many wrongs: the advantage of group navigation. *Trends Ecol. Evol.* **19**: 453–5.

Stacey, P. B. (1986). Group size and foraging efficiency in yellow baboons. *Behav. Ecol. Sociobiol.* **18**: 175–87.

Stewart, K. J. and Harcourt, A. H. (1994). Gorilla vocalisations during rest periods: signals of impending departure. *Behaviour* **130**: 29–40.

Stueckle, S. and D. Zinner (2008). To follow or not to follow: decision making and leadership during the morning departure of chacma baboons. *Anim. Behav.* **75**: 1995–2004.

Tambe, M. (1997). Towards flexible teamwork. *J. Artif. Intell. Res.* **7**: 83–124.

Topping, C. J., T. S. Hansen, T. S. Jensen, J. J. F. Nikolajsen, and P. Odderskaer (2003). Almass, an agent-based model for animals in temperate European landscapes. *Ecol. Model.* **167**: 65–82.

Tucker, V. (1970). The energetic cost of locomotion in animals. *Comp. Biochem. Physiol.* **34**: 841–6.

Will, O. and Hegselmann, R. (2008). A replication that failed: on the computational model in 'Michael W. Macy and Yoshimichi Sato: Trust, Cooperation and Market Formation in the US and Japan. Proceedings of the National Academy of Sciences, May 2002'. *J. Artif. Soc. Social Simul.* **11**(3): 3.

Zappala, J. (2008). Multi-agent simulation of group decision making in animals. Master's thesis, School of Computer Science, University of Nottingham, UK.

21 Endogenous birth and death of political parties in dynamic party competition[1]

Michael Laver, Ernest Sergenti, and Michel Schilperoord

21.1 'Spatial' models of political competition

People who talk about politics talk sooner or later about *positions* of political actors, be these citizens, voters, activists, or politicians. It is hard to have a serious discussion about the substance of real politics without referring to *where* key actors stand on important matters. Position implies distance (between two positions); distance implies movement; movement involves direction and can only be described relative to some benchmark. Indeed, it is difficult to analyse real political competition *without* using positional language and reasoning. This is why the spatial model is one of the 'workhorse' models of political science (Cox, 2001).

Spatial models of party competition typically involve two species of agent: voters and politicians. Voters have preferences about political outcomes. Politicians compete for voters' support by offering policy packages, in essence promised outcomes that appeal to these preferences. Voters' preferences are typically assumed to be *single-peaked* over the set of potential outcomes. This implies an *ideal point* for each voter, describing the most-preferred outcome. Less-preferred outcomes are described as points in some cognitive space that are increasingly far from this ideal. Although not a logical necessity, many models of party competition assume the set of voter ideal points to be both exogenously given and mapped into a common space. Basis vectors of real-world political spaces are typically interpreted as *policy dimensions*. Examples of such policy dimensions include economic left-right, social liberal-conservative, and foreign policy hawk-dove. In the 'proximity-voting' models that are common characterisations of voting in large electorates, each voter is assumed to support the politician offering the policy package closest to their ideal point. More complex assumptions may be made about strategic behaviour by voters. While these may be appropriate in small voting bodies where the voter has some realistic rational expectation that a single vote will affect the outcome, we do not consider these assumptions realistic in relation to voting in very large electorates,

---

[1] This is a radically revised version of a paper first published as Laver, M. and M. Schilperoord (2007). 'Spatial models of political competition with endogenous political parties.' Philosophical Transactions of the Royal Society B: Biology 362: 1711–1721. It also draws from work forthcoming in Laver, M. and E. Sergenti (2010). Party Competition: an Agent-Based Model. Princeton: Princeton University Press.

Modelling Natural Action Selection, eds. Anil K. Seth, Tony J. Prescott and Joanna J. Bryson.
Published by Cambridge University Press. © Cambridge University Press 2012.

which is the setting we concern ourselves with here. Hinich and Munger provide an accessible introduction to spatial models of party competition (Hinich and Munger, 1994, 1997). Austen-Smith and Banks provide a comprehensive technical overview (2000, 2005).

When more than one independent dimension of policy is important to voters, as seems plausible in any real setting, the game of spatial location played between politicians who compete for the support of voters is directly analogous to the 'Voronoi Game'. This is the generic geometric game of competitive spatial location, with widespread applications in many quite different fields, that is well-known to specialists in computational geometry. Assume a d-dimensional real space in which there are n voter ideal points and p party positions. The party positions generate a 'Voronoi tessellation' (tiling) of the policy space. This is an exclusive and exhaustive partition of the space into regions, each region associated with a generating point, such that any locus in the region is closer to the region's generating point than to any other generating point. Okabe *et al.* provide an exhaustive and authoritative review of the geometry of spatial tessellations (Okabe, *et al.* 2000), which Aurenhammer describes as a 'fundamental geometric data structure' (Aurenhammer, 1991). Any voter with an ideal point in a party's Voronoi region is closer to that party than to any other. If voters support their closest party, which is the assumption of proximity voting models, then each party's Voronoi region contains the ideal points of all its supporters. The Voronoi Game involves agents (party leaders in this case) competing to maximise the volumes of their Voronoi regions by manipulating the locations of their generating points. This game has been extensively analysed and proved formally intractable in spaces of more than one dimension (Teramoto *et al.*, 2006).

The formal intractability of the multidimensional Voronoi Game has two important consequences for spatial models of party competition. For *analysts*, it implies computational investigation of the voting model rather than formal analysis; no such formal analysis is possible. Much more importantly in our view, formal intractability has the *behavioural* implication that *agents playing the game*, absent formally provable best-response strategies, must rely on decision heuristics – rules of thumb that can in practice be very effective but can never be proven formally to be best responses to any conceivable state of the world. This shifts attention to the particular decision rules that real agents actually use, a fundamentally *empirical* question. What now interests us is how particular rules of thumb perform when pitted against each other in this analytically intractable setting. This is a classic argument for using agent-based models (ABMs) which, paradigmatically, involve computational investigation of interactions between agents deploying well-specified rules of thumb to make their decisions.

The complexity of this decision problem goes well beyond formal intractability of the underlying game of competitive spatial location, however. Mainstream spatial models of party competition are static: key model parameters and rules of interaction are fixed exogenously; the core intellectual mission is to specify a model and solve for equilibrium. Most informed observers of real politics, however, see party competition as a system in continual motion, and as a system with an endogenous dynamic. Thus, what agents do at tick t of the political process feeds back to affect the entire process at tick $t + 1$. This characterises political competition as an evolving complex system.

For the reasons we just outlined, there is a developing body of recent work in political science that analyses this evolving complex dynamic system using ABMs (De Marchi, 1999, 2003; Fowler and Smirnov 2005; Kollman *et al.* 1992, 2003; Laver 2005). A key feature of this work is that the number of political parties competing for votes is fixed exogenously. The innovation we present here is a dynamic spatial model of political competition in which the number and identity of competing parties is an endogenous *output* of the model, not an exogenous *input* to it. We achieve this by modelling the *birth* and *death* of political parties.

The rest of the chapter is organised as follows. We review current ABMs of party competition in Section 21.2. In Section 21.3, we specify an ABM of party competition that includes the birth of new parties and the death of existing ones. In Section 21.4 we report results from a systematic computational investigation of this model. In Section 21.5 we conclude and set out an agenda for future work.

21.2   Agent-based spatial models of party competition

The emerging literature on dynamic ABMs of party competition can be traced to an influential early paper by Kollman, Miller and Page (1992), who specified a dynamic model of two-party competition in a multidimensional policy space. Subsequent work in this tradition typically retains a US-oriented focus on two-party incumbent-challenger competition (De Marchi, 1999, 2003; Kollman *et al.*, 1998). The underlying spatial characterisation of policy preferences in these models is the same as in traditional spatial models, though computational implementations assume agents occupy one of a small number of discrete positions on a finite set of issue dimensions.

These ABMs follow traditional spatial models in assuming voters to be both policy-motivated and well-informed about published party policy positions, supporting the party position closest to their ideal point. However, they depart from traditional static models in assuming party leaders are not perfectly informed, either about the preferences of every single voter or about the uncertainties associated with these. Instead, party leaders are assumed to gather information, using private opinion poll and/or focus group feedback, on the impact of counterfactual policy moves on their electoral support levels, using this private information to select policy positions.

Laver (2005) built on this work with a multidimensional spatial model of multi-party competition that defined simple behavioural rules for setting party policy positions, rules that do not involve Kollman *et al.*'s complex counterfactual private polling. Each rule makes use of freely available public information about the history of the party system: published party policy positions and vote shares. As with the traditional static spatial model, Laver assumes voter ideal points are located in a real policy space, with voters supporting the party with the closest policy position to their ideal points. Following a random start of the system that is of course a model artefact and is burnt off before systematic interrogation of the model begins, party policy positions and citizens' party support patterns evolve continuously in the loop described in Figure 21.1. Voters support the party with the position closest to their ideal point; in light of observed patterns

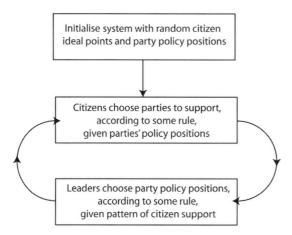

Figure 21.1 Complex dynamics of multi-dimensional, multiparty competition.

of support, party leaders use one of a number of simple decision rules to pick a new policy position; in light of these new party policy positions, voters support the party that is now closest; and so on. This process iterates forever.

The decision rules defined and investigated by Laver (2005) included:

- STICKER: never change position (an 'ideological' party leader).
- AGGREGATOR: set party policy on each dimension at the mean preference of all party supporters (a 'democratic' party leader).
- HUNTER: if the last policy move increased voter support, make the same move; else, reverse heading and make a unit move in a heading chosen randomly within the half-space now being faced (a Pavlovian vote-forager).

A significant limitation of both the Laver and Kollman *et al.* ABMs, together with most analytical spatial models, is that the set of political parties is fixed exogenously by nature. But the real world is full of examples of new political parties. Most of these parties are ephemeral and ultimately doomed to failure, but a small number succeed and all new parties, however unsuccessful, demonstrate the theoretically and substantively crucial *possibility* of new parties in any democratic system. Static models can ignore this by working with the set of parties that exist at any given time, setting aside the matter of how these parties came into existence. Dynamic models cannot do this, and must either assume the set of parties is fixed for all time, or model party 'birth' and 'death'. Self-evidently, by far the most plausible thing to do is to treat the set of competing parties as an endogenous *outcome* of political competition, not an exogenous *input* to this.

21.3   Birth and death of political parties

The endogenous 'entry' of new parties has by no means been ignored by scholars working with 'static' spatial models using traditional formal analysis. Key aspects of this work are reviewed by Shepsle; more recent writing, mostly by economists, is discussed by Dhillon and by Austen-Smith and Banks (Austen-Smith and Banks 2005; Dhillon 2005; Shepsle 1991). One prominent and widely cited approach focuses on incentives for individual policy-motivated citizens to run as 'citizen candidates' (Besley and Coate 1997; Osborne 2000). In what follows, we port this citizen candidate approach to the complex dynamic setting of the Laver ABM, extending this model so that the identity and number of parties is endogenous to the process of political competition. We model births of new parties in the spirit of the citizen candidate approach, as endogenous changes of agent type from voter to party leader, motivated by dissatisfaction of voters with the existing offer of party policies. If new parties are to be born into the system, some existing parties must 'die' if we are not to move inexorably towards an absurd situation with an infinite number of parties. In this sense modelling party birth implies modelling party death, which we do in terms of the inability of a party to maintain its updated fitness, defined precisely below, above some de facto survival threshold which is a feature of the party system as a whole.

Laver and Schilperoord (2007) implemented these ideas, endogenising the set of competing parties by endogenising party birth and death. This chapter consolidates and revises this work, taking account of recent theoretical and methodological progress. Thus Fowler and Laver designed a computer 'tournament' model for assessing relative effectiveness of different decision rules in long-running simulations; their model involved automatic party birth but endogenous party death (Fowler and Laver, 2008). Laver and Sergenti focus on the need for rigorous design, implementation, and analysis of computer simulations if inferences from these are to have the same order of robustness and reliability as those derived from formal analysis (Laver and Sergenti, 2007, 2011). These developments allow us, in what follows, to specify and investigate a more robust model of party birth and death.

21.3.1   The distribution of voter ideal points

The original Laver ABM, and subsequent work by Laver and Schilperoord (2007) and by Fowler and Laver (2008), model every voter as an independent agent. Reported simulations involve 1000 voters, with each voter in each simulation given an ideal point drawn randomly from the symmetric bivariate normal density distribution. However, *replications of model runs with the same parameter settings generate different outcomes*, not just because some decision rules have stochastic components but also because each replication uses a different draw of ideal points. We must thus replicate simulation runs many times for the same parameter settings if we want to ensure results are not a product of some random draw, adding immensely to our computational load. Since voters are in effect automata in our model, we tackle this problem by replacing a finite population of voting agents with ideal points drawn randomly from an underlying bivariate normal density function, with a 'landscape' of voters described by the underlying density function itself. The function describes vote density at any location in the space, and the same configuration of party policy positions always generates the same configuration of party support in a given landscape, since party support never depends upon details of some random draw. This approach is directly analogous to the 'electoral landscapes' used by Kollman *et al.* (1998) and by de Marchi (1999). In other work (Laver and Sergenti, 2011) we report results from modelling party competition with more generic asymmetric distributions of voter ideal points.

21.3.2   Voter dissatisfaction at tick *t*

Our citizen candidate model of party birth involves voters who are dissatisfied, in some well-specified sense we define below, having an increased probability of changing state from ordinary decent voter to political candidate. We thus need to model voter dissatisfaction and we do this by adapting the voter utility functions that underlie static spatial models of party competition. These almost invariably contain a term for 'policy loss'. This is the disutility for a voter with an ideal point at i, arising from outcome j, described as some increasing function of the Euclidean distance, d_{ij}, between i and j. There are differences between models in terms of whether voter disutility is modelled as a linear or quadratic function of d_{ij}. The most common assumption, typically justified by vague behavioural claims about risk-aversion in politics, is that policy loss should be modelled as a quadratic function, that is as $-d_{ij}^2$. We follow this assumption in order to align our work with that of conventional spatial modellers.

This begs a key question about the identity of the policy point j that, relative to the ideal point i, provides the generating point for citizen dissatisfaction. Which j we specify depends upon our behavioural model of politics. The seminal spatial model (Downs, 1957) and many of its direct intellectual descendents, assume 'proximity' voting by citizens. Each citizen supports their closest party and suffers more disutility, the more distant this closest party. This describes non-strategic behaviour by citizens who make no attempt to anticipate the consequences of their vote, which is after all most unlikely to have any observable consequence whatsoever in a large electorate, for long-term post-electoral policy outcomes. Voting is thus seen as an *expressive* action involving what amounts to consumption at the time of the election, rather than an *instrumental* action designed to influence downstream policy outcomes following: an election; government formation; government policy making; policy implementation; realised outcomes of implemented policies. Models of strategic instrumental voting certainly exist (Austen-Smith and Banks, 1988; Kedar, 2005). But these assume extraordinarily high levels of citizen rationality and instrumental behaviour in settings where a rational citizen will likely calculate that they are unlikely to make one iota of difference. Furthermore, results derived from such models are brittle and typically do not generalise beyond three parties and one policy dimension.

Our behavioural assumption is thus, quite simply, that a voter derives greater satisfaction from voting for a party with a position closer to her own ideal point. If j is the position at tick t of the party with the position closest to a voter with an ideal point at i, and if the Euclidean distance between i and j at tick t is d_{ijt}, we define the utility of voter i at tick t as $-d_{ijt}^2$.

21.3.3   Updating citizen dissatisfaction

It seems most implausible in a dynamic setting to assume agents respond only to the current *instantaneous* state of the system and ignore anything that happened even seconds before this. While this is never explicit in existing accounts of party competition, it seems more plausible to treat citizens as using new information they get at tick t to *update rather than completely determine* their evaluations of the party system. We thus define *updated* citizen dissatisfaction using a simple updating model. This defines D_{it}, the updated dissatisfaction at tick t of a citizen with an ideal point at i, in the following recursive manner:

$$D_{it} = a_m \times D_{i(t-1)} + (1 - a_m) \times d_{ijt}^2. \tag{21.1}$$

In this equation, α_m is a memory parameter describing *how much* voters update their dissatisfaction on the basis of new information about party positions at tick t. Thus, if $\alpha_m = 0$, voters have a 'goldfish memory'; their updated dissatisfaction is the quadratic Euclidean distance between their voter ideal point and the *current* instantaneous position of their closest party. If $\alpha_m = 1$, voters *never* update their dissatisfaction with the configuration of party positions, no matter what (crazy) positions any party adopts. When $0 < \alpha_m < 1$, the memory parameter α_m determines the extent to which voters update their (previously updated) dissatisfaction with the party system at tick t-1, using information about the configuration of party positions at tick t. This type of update is analogous to updates modelled in the extensive literature on reinforcement learning, to which Sutton and Barto (1998) provide an excellent introduction.

We added α_m to our parameter space in exploratory runs, investigating effects on model outputs of sweeping different values of this parameter. However, we found no statistically significant difference in model outputs for different values of α_m. In what follows, therefore, and budgeting our finite computational resources, we take a cue from some recent work in neuro-economics and set $\alpha_m = 0.50$ (Glimcher *et al.*, 2005). This implies, for example, that a voter's updated dissatisfaction eight elections previously contributes about 1% of their updated dissatisfaction in the current election.

21.3.4   Mean citizen dissatisfaction as a welfare output of party competition

Having defined D_{it}, the updated dissatisfaction of a citizen with ideal point i at tick t, we can easily compute the aggregate dissatisfaction of all voters. We can think of aggregate voter dissatisfaction, thus measured, as a welfare index for the party system as a whole. It describes how well the evolved configuration of party positions 'represents' the ideal points of the population of voters. This is one of the main output metrics we investigate in the analyses that follow.

21.3.5   The birth of political parties

The driving motivation behind our model of updated voter dissatisfaction was a desire to specify a citizen candidate model of party birth. We assume every voter always has the implicit option of forming a new party by changing state from rank-and-file voter to party leader. Specifically, we assume that the probability, p_{it}, that a voter with an ideal point at i changes state to a party leader at tick t, increases in direct proportion to this voter's updated dissatisfaction with the configuration of party positions. Thus $p_{it} = \beta \cdot D_{it}$, where β is a 'birth' parameter, measuring how sensitive is the voter's probability of changing state to her updated dissatisfaction with the evolving configuration of party positions. The birth parameter β is scaled to the units in which policy distances, and thus D_{it}, are measured. Substantively realistic values of β are a function of how we calibrate the model to real time. This is because they are associated, for a given point in the model's parameter space, with an expected number of new party births per election. Absent real time calibration, different values of β have the effect of controlling for how *fast* the system evolves, rather than *how* it evolves in a substantive sense. For this reason, we do not investigate different values of β in the simulations that follow.

When a voter changes state to party leader, the new party enters the system at the location of the ideal point of the founding voter. In the 'tournament' model we report here, the new party leader selects a decision rule at random from the available set (Sticker, Aggregator, Hunter). In other work, we report results both using a much larger rule set, and using an evolutionary model in which the probability of each rule being selected is proportional to the rule's updated fitness. But our purpose here is the same as that of the Fowler–Laver tournament. We want to observe the evolution of the party system, and in particular party birth and death, in settings where there is a diverse rule set. And we impose this diversity by specifying equi-probable random rule selection each time a new party is born. This avoids the admittedly very interesting situation that often arises with the evolutionary model, whereby one successful rule drives out all others.

21.3.6   The fitness and death of political parties

Just as new parties may be born, existing parties may 'die'. A natural way to think about this is to model the *fitness* of political parties, and then model party death as occurring when party fitness falls below some de facto *survival threshold* that is a feature of the general environment for party competition.

In modelling party fitness, we extend an approach used by Fowler and Laver (2008) who specified a recursive algorithm for updating information about the relative fitness of different *decision rules*. The updating algorithm is directly analogous to the algorithm we specified for updating voter dissatisfaction. Let f_{pt} be party p's fitness at time t. This is p's fitness at t-1, updated by new information observed at time t. It seems plausible to assume that the new information used to update p's fitness at time t is p's vote share at time t, labelled v_{pt}. This gives the following recursive algorithm:

$$f_{pt} = a_f \times f_{p(t-1)} + (1 - a_f) \times d_{pt}. \tag{21.2}$$

The extent of this update is determined by a memory parameter, α_f. When $\alpha_f = 0$, we have the situation implicitly assumed by most current models, a goldfish memory regime in which a party's fitness is simply its fitness this second, with no weight attached to a history of past fitness. When $\alpha_f = 1$, party fitness never updates from its initial starting value, whatever new information is observed. When $0 \le \alpha_f \le 1$, α_f reflects the relative weight agents give to the history of a party's past success at winning votes, and new information about the party's current success. Thus α_f is an interesting model parameter and we analyse its effects on model outputs in the computational work reported below.

Having modelled party fitness, we now consider the de facto survival threshold that is such an important feature of the general environment for party competition. This is a trickier matter than it might seem at first sight. It is well-known that both explicit and implicit thresholds for party representation in the legislature are embedded in all *electoral systems*. These arise from the interaction of electoral formulae, constituency size, and constituency-level concentrations of party support (Cox, 1997). It is less commonly appreciated that, considering the system of elections more generally, de facto thresholds for party representation are generated by all sorts of matters such as candidate nomination procedures, campaign finance laws, public funding of political parties, and so on.

The tricky question arises because it is clear that many political parties continue to survive, in some sense at least, even when they fall far below formal representational thresholds. Indeed principles of free speech typically indicate that nearly any eligible voter can set up what they might choose to call a 'political party' and run for election. For this reason, all models of party competition of which we are aware implicitly exclude political parties deemed in some sense to be 'below the radar' of mainstream party competition. For example, models of British party politics invariably exclude the Official Monster Raving Loony Party (OMRLP; www.omrlp.com), led for a long time by former rock musician Screaming Lord Sutch, who ran for election 42 times between 1966 and 1997 and only once (in the Rotherham by-election of 1994) won more than 1000 votes. In effect the OMRLP is informally deemed 'below the radar' in the sense that it is held to have no measurable effect on the behaviour of any other party and nearly all voters.

In our terms, therefore, the de facto survival threshold, τ, is a feature of the general environment for party competition that rolls together a lot of different things, from formal representational thresholds in the electoral system to informal perceptions by voters of which parties are 'serious' political contenders. A party with an updated fitness that is below the survival threshold is not necessarily non-existent, but is invisible below the political radar to all other agents.

21.3.7   'Campaign' ticks and 'election' ticks

The Laver ABM treated party competition as a continuous process with, no particular feature, such as an election, distinguishing one model tick from another. Since elections do happen in the real world, this is substantively unrealistic. Following Fowler and Laver (2008), we make a distinction between:

campaign ticks, in which politicians select actions in response to published information about levels of party support;

election ticks in which, in addition to the above: voters select which party to vote for; rewards and punishments are administered; existing parties may die; new parties may be born; a range of measures are updated.

Assuming a fixed electoral schedule with election campaigns running continuously between elections, we define an election scheduling parameter, Ψ, which specifies the frequency of election ticks relative to campaign ticks. At the end of each of the $\Psi - 1$ campaign ticks that happen between elections, party leaders select policy positions and their estimated support levels are made public, in effect in a public opinion poll. But politicians are not subject to realised rewards and punishments at the end of a campaign tick. In line with question wording in real opinion polls, published party support at the end of campaign ticks reflects how people *would have voted if there had been an election that day*, offering crucial feedback to candidates. There is an election every Ψ ticks, with voters actually voting rather than answering opinion polls and outcomes have binding consequences for success and failure of political parties. This means that *updates* to voter dissatisfaction and party fitness take place at the end of *election* ticks, not at the end of campaign ticks. Parties may thus adapt continuously during the campaign, but births and deaths take place only following an election. What parties may do *between* elections is to explore implications of alternative actions; it is what happens *at* elections that generates rewards and punishments.

21.3.8   Analysing the birth and death of political parties

21.3.8.1   Specifying the model

Our main interest is in characterising endogenous party birth and death in the competitive environment we describe with our model. We do this by observing birth and death locations of parties, measured in terms of the *eccentricity* of the party position, which is defined as the Euclidean distance of this position from the centroid of voter ideal points. We also measure: party *longevity*, in terms of elections survived between birth and death; mean *fitness* of the set of parties using each decision rule; mean *dissatisfaction* of the population of voters. Our model has three party system parameters of interest. We investigate the effects of these using an experimental design that involves 1000 very long runs of the model, each run with a 'Monte Carlo parameterisation'. That is, we draw random values for each model parameter from a uniform distribution on intervals that we take to be substantively plausible. Specifically, these intervals were:

- α_f: memory parameter for party fitness; floating point numbers on the [0.00, 0.99] interval;
- τ: de facto survival threshold; floating point numbers on the [0.05, 0.30] interval;
- Ψ: number of campaign ticks/election; integers on the [5, 25] interval.

As we noted above, outputs from the dynamic model we described above are ergodic time series, distributed around long-run stationary means. This means that independent very long runs with the same parameterisation converge on the same estimated mean. These long runs are Markov chains and our diagnostic tests for convergence thus use the R-Hat statistic developed for Markov-Chain Monte Carlo (MCMC) methods (Brooks and Gelman 1998). Diagnostic tests described by Laver and Sergenti (2007, 2011) allow us to conclude that the random start has burnt off and outputs of interest have converged on long-run means, despite their clearly periodic structure, in runs with 20 000 elections. In a nutshell, longer runs, or additional 20 000-election runs with the same parameterisation, would yield effectively identical estimates. Since model outputs of interests are highly autocorrelated time series, means and standard errors of interest must be estimated using standard time series methods, once each output series has been checked for stationarity. In what follows, we report means and standard errors of quantities of interest estimated using AR(1) regressions on the burnt-in portion of each of the 1000 output chains, each chain with 20 000 elections.

This is a fairly heavy computational load, but one that we are confident statistically gives us very robust and reliable results. Indeed, readers may take comfort in the fact that the simulation experiment we report below has been rerun several times in the course of our exploratory work and has always yielded identical results. The model set out above was programmed in NetLogo and interrogated using the Harvard–MIT high-performance cluster of about 180 machines. Code was written to control the NetLogo program so as to run the program 1000 times for 20 000 elections, each run with a Monte Carlo parameterisation. The 1000 large output files were then automatically formatted and analysed, using code programmed in R, to estimate burn-in. They were then automatically analysed, using Stata, to derive the AR(1) estimates. These estimates were then automatically harvested from Stata output and placed in a single summary file. Of the 1000 runs in the simulation experiment reported below, 19 runs failed our diagnostic tests for convergence and were dropped from the analysis, which was confined to the 981 converged runs.

It is worth emphasising in this context that 'heavy-duty' computational work of this type is not really feasible without automated running of the model, chained to automated analysis of model outputs and compilation of results. Rerunning this entire experiment would involve just a few minutes work followed by a long but tranquil wait for the computing cluster to spit out the results. The need to rerun this experiment by hand would trigger a nervous breakdown and involve person-months of error-prone work.

21.3.8.2   Party system sizes

Figure 21.2 summarises a lot of information about the long-run mean party system sizes that typically arise from various parameterisations of our model of dynamic multiparty competition. Rather than plot 981 individual estimates for each of four quantities in each of these figures, we summarise each cloud of 981 points using a median spline. Note before looking at Figure 21.2 that there is an *axiomatic upper bound on the number of parties in any party system*. This is $1/\tau$, the reciprocal of the survival threshold. Self-evidently, if the survival threshold is 0.10, for example, no more than ten parties can get 0.10 of the vote or more, and then only if all parties are of perfectly equal size. The solid line in Figure 21.2a plots the typical number of surviving parties for a given survival threshold and shows a similar reciprocal relationship. (If the x-axis is $1/\tau$ rather than τ the plots in Figure 21.2a are straight lines.)

Figure 21.2 gives substantively interesting insight into dynamic party systems with endogenous parties. It shows, for example: that a survival threshold of 0.10 of the vote tends to be associated over the long run with a six-party system; that a threshold of

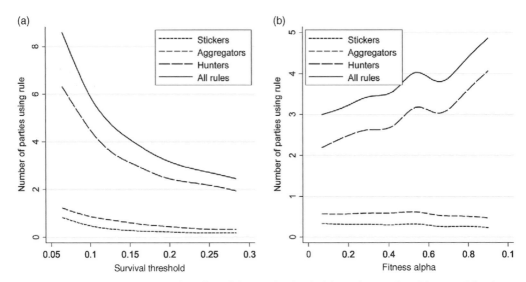

Figure 21.2 Mean number of surviving parties, by decision rule, τ and α_f. Lines are 8-band median splines summarizing AR(1) estimates from the burnt-in era of 1000 runs, each run with 20 000 elections. Settings of τ and α_f for each run were randomly selected from uniform distributions on the intervals shown on the horizontal axes of each figure. Cases are dropped if the R-hat measure for any quantity of interest was less than 1.1 or of the ratio of the AR(1) standard error to the standard deviation for any quantity of interest was greater than 0.10. A total of 19 cases were dropped for this reason. Our very long converged runs for each estimate have the effect that the AR(1) standard errors on any one of these 981 estimates of the number of parties using each rule are very low – on average 0.03 for Hunters and Aggregators, 0.02 for Stickers.

0.25 tends to be associated with a three party system; and so on. If we believe in the model, then this allows us to 'back out' the de facto party survival threshold, for a real party system of interest, from the number of surviving parties observed over the long run. Thus, if we tend to observe six surviving parties in a system of interest, this implies a de facto threshold of about 0.10; a two-party system implies a threshold of about 0.30 and so on.

Figure 21.2a also shows that *Hunter comfortably outperforms the other decision rules* in this setting, measuring performance in terms of the number of surviving parties using each rule. Since new parties choose rules at random in this environment, this implies parties using the adaptive Hunter rule are less likely to fall below the survival threshold and die than parties using other rules. We also see that the number of Hunters increases disproportionally as the survival threshold gets lower. With lower survival thresholds there are not only more parties, there are in particular more Hunter parties.

The solid line in Figure 21.2b shows that the other party system parameter with an effect on the number of parties is α_f, the memory parameter for fitness updating. The lower α_f, the smaller the number of surviving parties and in particular the fewer surviving Hunter parties. When α_f is very low, updated fitness is almost the same as the update on current party support; a party dies as soon as its current support falls below the survival threshold. High-alpha systems are more 'forgiving' in this sense, updating more slowly,

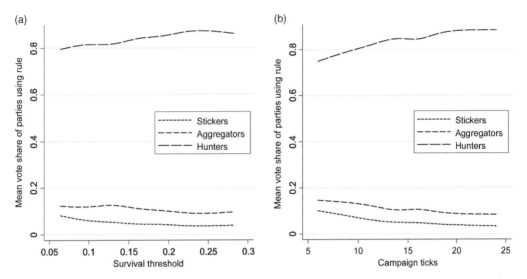

Figure 21.3 Mean vote share of sets of surviving parties, by decision rule, τ and ψ. See caption to Figure 21.2.

'remembering' past successes and allowing parties to survive if their current support falls below the threshold for an election or two but then moves back over the threshold. For this reason, fewer parties tend to die in high-alpha systems and there tend to be more surviving parties. This discussion of 'memories of past success' is novel in the context of modelling party competition. It is very important to note that we cannot even frame such a discussion in terms of a static model but that, once we move to a fully dynamic model, *such a model will axiomatically have an updating regime, however implicit this might be, and that the parameterisation of this updating regime is likely to have an impact on the evolution of party competition.*

21.4 Performance of sets of parties using different decision rules

We have just seen that Hunter was the most successful rule in our dynamic system of party competition with endogenous parties, measuring success in terms of the number of surviving parties using each rule. Figure 21.3 plots another measure of success, the aggregate vote share of sets of surviving parties using each rule. This shows the relative success of the Hunter rule very clearly. The i.i.d. mean (standard deviation) of the AR(1) estimated vote shares won by the set of Hunter parties over the burnt-in era of each of the 20 000 elections, for each of the 981 converged Monte Carlo parameterisations of the model, was 0.83 (0.07). Equivalent figures for the sets Sticker and Aggregator parties were 0.06 (0.04) and 0.11 (0.03) respectively.[2]

---

[2] AR(1) standard errors on any one of these 981 estimated vote shares for each rule set are on average 0.006 for Hunters, 0.005 for Aggregators and Stickers.

Figure 21.3 shows that the relative success of Hunter is somewhat, though not dramatically, affected by parameters of party competition. In particular, Figure 21.3b shows that Hunter tends to do worse when ψ, the number of campaign ticks per election, is low. This is because, of the three rules we investigate here, Sticker never adapts its position, while Aggregator instantly adapts to the centroid of its supporters' ideal points. Hunter, in contrast, adapts in a sequence of unit moves. The lower is ψ, the shorter the sequence of moves enabling Hunters to adapt their policy positions between elections, and the less well they perform. As we will see below, this is to a large extent a product of the fact that endogenous party births tend to be at peripheral policy locations, so that short election campaigns do not give Hunters 'enough' time to adapt away from these before the first visit, scheduled by ψ, of the electoral grim reaper.

21.4.1   Policy locations of party births, deaths, and survivors

Figure 21.4 plots policy positions of endogenous party births and deaths, and of surviving parties, in our simulated environment for dynamic multiparty competition. Figure 21.4a shows that our citizen candidate model of party birth tends to generate new parties at the ideal points of dissatisfied voters who are, on average, 1.8 standard deviations from the voter centroid. The mean (standard deviation) over all runs of AR(1) estimated birth eccentricities was 1.79 (0.03). Substantively, this means that endogenously generated *new parties tend strongly to come into existence at quite peripheral policy positions.*

Since Stickers never move and thus die precisely where they are born, *loci* of Sticker deaths are identical to those of all party births, which Figure 21.3 shows are only very slightly affected by the party survival threshold. Where Aggregators and Hunters tend to die, however, depends on parameters of the party system. This is most easily understood in relation to typical policy locations of *surviving* parties using each decision rule, shown in f Figure 21.4b.

This shows another piece of headline news. *Surviving Aggregators and Hunters tend to be found in very different positions in the policy space.* Means (standard deviations) over all runs of AR(1) estimated surviving Aggregator and Hunter party eccentricities were 1.39 (0.17) and 0.61 (0.15), respectively. Indeed, over the entire suite of 981 converged runs, *the full ranges of mean surviving Hunter and Aggregator locations never overlapped*, at [0.37, 0.96] and [1.10, 1.90], respectively.[3] Substantively this implies that, if we believe the model, *we can confidently back out the decision rule being used by each party by observing its typical policy locations.* Considering the three rules we investigate here, *parties typically locating less than one standard deviation away from the voter centroid are almost certainly Hunters.*

Figure 21.4b also shows, however, that typical policy locations are quite strongly influenced by the survival threshold. Lower thresholds imply more parties, as we have seen, which implies more diverse and on average more eccentric party policy positions.

---

[3] AR(1) standard errors on any one of these 981 estimates of party eccentricities are on average 0.002 for Hunters and 0.003 for Aggregators.

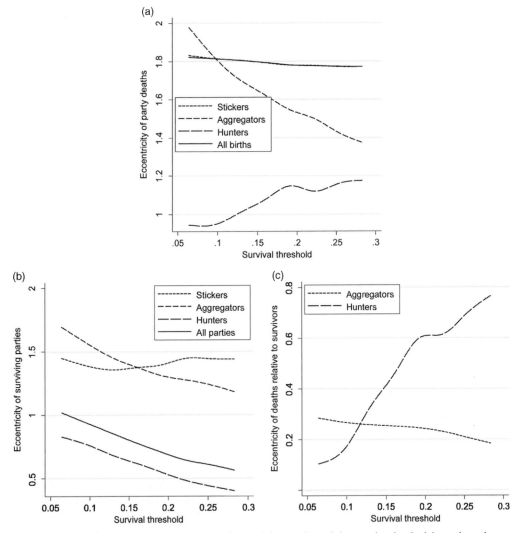

Figure 21.4 Policy eccentricities of new, dying, and surviving parties, by decision rule and survival threshold. See caption to Figure 21.2.

Returning to consider where parties tend to die, Figure 21.4c plots the difference between the death location of parties using each rule and the typical location of surviving parties using the same rule. *This measure is always positive, showing that parties tend strongly to die at more eccentric policy positions than those of surviving parties using the same rule.* The mean extra eccentricity of dying parties over all runs is 0.23 for Aggregators and 0.48 for Hunters though Figure 21.4c shows this is *strongly* affected by the survival threshold for Hunters. When survival thresholds are high and the number of parties consequently low, the Hunters that tend to die are those that stray far from typical Hunter policy locales.

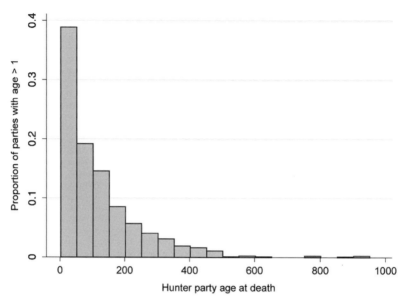

Figure 21.5 Distribution of Hunter party longevities in a sample model run ($\tau = 0.10$; $\alpha_f = 0.50$; $\Psi = 20$. Mean party age at death $= 107.5$; median age $= 65$).

21.4.2   Life expectancy of political parties

The life expectancy of political parties in an endogenously evolving dynamic party system, their typical 'age' at death measured in terms of elections survived, is the result of a survival process – ability to stay above a de facto survival threshold. Figure 21.5 shows a frequency distribution of ages at death of Hunter parties for a particular simulation run. It plots precisely the type of exponential age distribution we expect to observe when parties are subject to a constant hazard rate of dying at each successive election. Given this skewed age distribution, we use *median* age at party death as the most informative summary of the life expectancy of a 'typical' party in a given setting.

Figure 21.6 shows typical party longevities are strongly affected by the survival threshold, increasing exponentially as the survival threshold goes down. Lower survival thresholds imply that all parties, and particular Hunter parties, tend to live very much longer. A large part of the relative success of the Hunter rule arises because Hunter parties tend to live longer, especially when survival thresholds are low.

21.4.3   Representativeness of the party system

Before reporting computational results on representativeness of the evolving set of party positions, we consider findings from computational geometry that should be of great interest to social scientists more generally. 'Centroidal Voronoi tessellations' (CVTs) are a special class of Voronoi tessellation, in which each generating point is at the centroid of its Voronoi region. Du *et al.* (1999) show that a set of generating points that is a CVT

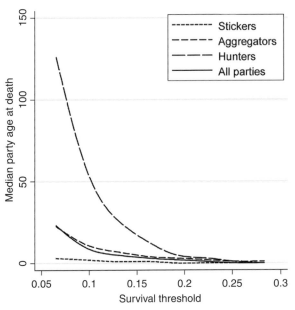

Figure 21.6 Median party ages at death, by decision rule, τ, ψ, and α_f. See caption to Figure 21.2.

is an 'optimal representation' of the space, defining optimal representation in the *precise* sense we use above, as minimising aggregate quadratic (or linear) distances between all points in the space and their closest generating point (Du *et al.*, 1999: 644–646). This result is used in computational work on a huge variety of applications, for example data compression in image processing as well as the reverse problem, image intensification. A set of *n* generating points in a CVT is the most efficient representation of a larger set of points, at a level of precision given by *n*. This tells us that *representativeness of any n-party system is maximised when the n party positions are in a CVT*, a very useful result indeed.

A widely used computational procedure for *finding* a CVT from an arbitrary starting configuration of generating points is Lloyd's Algorithm (Lloyd, 1982). This recursive algorithm is simple: (1) generate a Voronoi tessellation of the space; (2) move each generating point to the centroid of its Voronoi region; (3) go to (1). There are formal proofs in the computer science literature that a CVT can be found using Lloyds Algorithm for any arbitrary *one-dimensional* space and starting configuration of generating points (Du *et al.*, 1999). More generally, there is a strong and widely accepted *conjecture* in information science that Lloyds Algorithm converges on a CVT, in finite time, for any finite level of precision. This conjecture has been deployed in a wide variety of heavy-duty computational applications (such as image compression and intensification). It has never been reported to have failed but has never been proved formally. This work is crucially important in the context of dynamic models of party competition because *a party system in which all party leaders use the Aggregator rule is, precisely, deploying Lloyds Algorithm*. Thus we know from the work in computational geometry that party

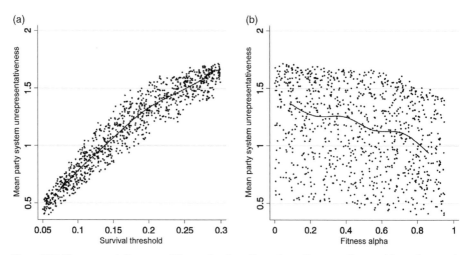

Figure 21.7 Unrepresentativeness of the evolved configuration of party policy positions, *by* τ and αf. See caption to Figure 21.2.

positions in an all-Aggregator system will (1) converge on a CVT of the policy space that will maximise the representativeness of the configuration of party policy positions and (2) for an arbitrary level of precision determined by the floating point precision of the computation, reach steady state in finite time. Laver (2005) did indeed find, and we have subsequently confirmed in of all of our own extensive computational work, that all-Aggregator party systems do always converge on a steady state, at the level of floating point precision used by the computing environment in which algorithms were programmed.

These results tell us something of great normative interest. *A steady state policy configuration of an n-Aggregator party system maximises representativeness of the party system* as we measure this; no other configuration of *n* party positions is more representative. This emergent phenomenon arises despite the fact that leaders of individual Aggregator parties never try to maximise *overall* representativeness of the party system, but simply to represent the ideal points of their own current supporters.

Figure 21.7 plots the relationship between representativeness party system and party system parameters. It shows both the cloud of AR(1) estimates from the 981 converged runs of 20 000 elections each, as well as the median splines summarising these. Figure 21.7a shows the big though not unexpected news; *party system representativeness is very strongly affected by the survival threshold*. Lower thresholds imply more parties, which in turn leads to a more representative configuration of party positions.

Tight clustering of points around the summary line in Figure 21.7a suggests that other party system parameters have much smaller effects, and the left panel shows the more attenuated effect of the memory parameter for fitness updating, α_f, on party system representativeness. Higher values of this are associated with more representative party systems. We saw in Figure 21.2 that high-alpha systems are more 'forgiving' of short-term dips in support, tending to be associated with more parties and thus, other things equal, with more representative party systems.

Table 21.1 OLS regressions of mean party system unrepresentativeness on party system parameters.[4]

	Model 1	Model 2	Model 3
Survival threshold (τ)	4.71***	3.29***	3.40***
	(0.031)	(0.037)	(0.037)
Fitness alpha (α_f)	−0.32***	−0.33***	0.35***
	(0.008)	(0.006)	(0.007)
Number of parties		−0.16***	
		(0.004)	
Number of Hunters		0.13***	
		(0.005)	
Aggregators/Hunters			−0.67***
			(0.024)
Constant	0.48***	0.97***	1.07***
	(0.007)	(0.012)	(0.014)
Adj. R²	0.96	0.99	0.99
n	981	981	981

$N = 981$. Significance levels: *** ≤ 0.001; ** ≤ 0.01; * ≤ 0.05

An important pattern is hidden in these bivariate plots, however, and arises directly from the fact that all-Aggregator party systems generate CVTs and thereby optimise representation. We know from Figure 21.2 that most surviving parties in these endogenously evolving party systems are *not* Aggregators. We know from Figure 21.4 that surviving Hunters tend to have positions *much* closer to the voter centroid than do surviving Aggregators. This suggests that party system representativeness is likely to be enhanced, the more Aggregators there are, and reduced the more Hunters there are.

Table 21.1 tests this conjecture. Model 1 is a multiple OLS regression of the effects of τ and α_f on representativeness of the configuration of party positions, estimated in 981 converged runs, and characterises the effects plotted in Figure 21.7. Higher survival thresholds, and lower alphas, are associated with more unrepresentative systems. Model 2 adds two variables, the number of surviving parties, and the number of surviving *Hunters*. We now see clearly that it is indeed the case that, while having more parties increases representativeness, it is also the case that, holding the number of parties constant, *having more Hunters reduces representativeness*. Model 3 expresses this in another way, using the ratio of Aggregator to Hunter parties as the independent variable of interest. *The more Aggregators there are, relative to the number of Hunters, the more representative the evolved configuration of party positions.*

We see this as an interesting and normatively important 'paradox', in the context of what we take to be a naïve view about party competition: that having parties compete with each other for votes by trying to find popular policy positions will result in an evolved configuration of party positions that is a good representation of voter ideal points. This is self-evidently true when there is only a single party, but we now see it

---

[4] See Figure 21.2. Estimates for each of the 981 retained runs are also plotted as points.

is not at all true when multiple *endogenous* parties are engaged in competitive spatial location. Parties using Hunter are *much* more successful than parties using other rules at winning votes, and will be rewarded for this in an evolutionary system with endogenous parties. But such vote-seeking parties tend to search for support much 'too close' to the centre of the distribution of voter ideal points; the more successful these parties are, the less well represented are voters. The paradox is that representativeness of the evolved configuration of party policy positions is *not* enhanced by endogenous parties who compete with each other by seeking popular policy positions. The results from the computational geometry of competitive spatial location tell us this, and our model illustrates a realisation of this phenomenon in endogenous party systems with three possible decision rules, Aggregator, Hunter, and Sticker. These results tell us, in effect, that the best way to optimise representation in an *n*-party system is to let loose a herd of *n* Aggregator parties.

21.5   Discussion and further work

We moved on quite far in this chapter from a dynamic model of party competition in which Nature exogenously specifies a set of parties that never changes. Modelling endogenous birth and death of political parties involves developing the original Laver model in a number of ways. We define and measure 'fitness' of parties and specify how this is updated each election by new information about current party performance. This allows us to model death of political parties in terms of a de facto survival threshold, with parties 'dying' as their updated fitness falls below this. We adapt a citizen candidate model of new party birth; new parties form at ideal points of dissatisfied voters, with a probability proportional to some measure of voter dissatisfaction. We measure voter dissatisfaction as the quadratic distance between the voter ideal point and the closest party position. Aggregating this measure for the entire voting population gives us a 'welfare' measure of the extent to which an evolved configuration of party position 'represents' the distribution of voter ideal points. Having specified the theoretical model, we then specify a rigorous computational method that ensures our key estimates, derived from dynamic and periodic model output, have converged to stationary means that are ergodic in the long run. This allows us to design and run simulation experiments that involve 1000 long (20 000 election) burnt-in runs of the model, each run with a Monte Carlo parameterisation, that is with parameter values drawn randomly from uniform distributions of within substantively plausible ranges.

The main results can be succinctly summarised. Our endogenous party system evolves to an ergodic state with the number of competing parties largely determined by the survival threshold, and to a lesser extent the rate of fitness updating. This is significant since, to the extent we believe the model, we can 'back out' a party system's de facto survival threshold from empirical observations of the long run mean of the number of competing parties. Observing that we typically have six competing parties, for example, implies a de facto survival threshold of 0.10 of the total vote. We also see that the Hunter rule, which is after all the only rule explicitly programmed to search for increased vote share, evolves to have a far greater updated fitness, denominated in backwards discounted ability to win votes. This implies there will typically be more parties using the Hunter rule, in an endogenous party system, than using either of the other rules. We saw that Hunter parties seek support *much* closer to the voter centroid than Aggregators. Since we know that a system with only Aggregators will optimise representation by party positions of voter ideal points, it was not surprising to confirm that party systems with more Hunters tend to be less representative. Hunters compete very effectively, having a good algorithm for finding popular policy positions, but paradoxically this competition *reduces rather than increases* the extent to which the evolved configuration of party positions represents the distribution of voter ideal points. Crudely speaking, our results on this matter tell us that, if we were social planners setting out to increase representativeness of a party system, we would (1) lower party survival thresholds, perhaps by reforming electoral law and/or (2) force parties to set policy positions that reflect the wishes of *current* supporters, rather than changing positions to attract *new* supporters, perhaps by mandating more internal party democracy.

The next steps involve generalising the distribution of voter ideal points and implementing a major expansion of the set of available decision rules (Laver and Sergenti, 2011). The latter is achieved both by specifying new decision algorithms, such as predation and generalised hill-climbing, and by characterising a space of 'rule features' that in effect parameterise many different decision rules. Such features include: satisficing, by implementing a given rule only when some output metric falls below some comfort threshold; the 'speed' with which the decision rule can change party policy positions in any one model tick; parameterised shocks to both the current policy position (jittering) and to the specified direction of forward movement (wobbling). Laver and Sergenti (2011) then implement a more evolutionary regime driven by a replicator–mutator system according to which, when a new party selects a decision rule, the probability any given rule is selected is a function of that rule's updated fitness, subject to some small probability of random replication errors whereby some given rule is indicated by the replicator system but some other rule is selected. They then move on to discuss effects of parties having non-policy 'valence' characteristics, such as leadership charisma or scandals, that also attract or repel voter support. They finally move on to endogenise the distribution of voter ideal points by implementing a standard social-psychological model of the effects on preferences of both random and structured interactions between voters.

References

Aurenhammer, F. (1991). Voronoi diagrams: a survey of a fundamental geometric data structure. *ACM Comput. Surv.* **23**(3): 345–405.

Austen-Smith, D. and J. S. Banks (1988). Elections, coalitions and legislative outcomes. *Amer. Pol. Sci. Rev.* **82**: 405–22.

Austen-Smith, D. and J. S. Banks (2000). *Positive Political Theory I: Collective Preference.* Ann Arbor, MI: University of Michigan Press.

Austen-Smith, D. and J. S. Banks (2005). *Positive Political Theory II: Strategy and Structure*. Ann Arbor, MI: University of Michigan Press.

Besley, T. and S. Coate (1997). An economic model of representative democracy. *Quart. J. Econ.* **112** (1): 85–106.

Brooks, S. P. and A. Gelman (1998). General methods for monitoring convergence of iterative simulations. *J. Comput. Graph. Stat.* **7**: 434–55.

Cox, G. (1997). *Making Votes Count: Strategic Coordination in the World's Electoral Systems*. Cambridge: Cambridge University Press.

Cox, G. (2001). Introduction to the Special Issue. *Polit. Anal.* **9**(3): 189–91.

De Marchi, S. (1999). Adaptive models and electoral instability. *J. Theor. Polit.* **11**: 393–419.

De Marchi, S. (2003). A computational model of voter sophistication, ideology and candidate position-taking. In *Computational Models in Political Economy*, ed. K. Kollman, J. H. Miller and S. E. Page. Cambridge, MA: MIT Press, pp. 143–58.

Dhillon, A. (2005). *Political parties and coalition formation. In Group Formation in Economics: Networks, Clubs, and Coalitions*, ed. G. Demange and M. Wooders. Cambridge: Cambridge University Press, pp. 289–311.

Downs, A. (1957). *An Economic Theory of Democracy*. New York: Harper & Row.

Du, Q., V. Faber, and M. Gunzburger (1999). Centroidal Voronoi tessellations: applications and algorithms. *Soc. Indust. Appl. Math. Rev.* **41** (4): 637–76.

Fowler, J. H. and M. Laver (2008). A tournament of party decision rules. *J. Confl. Res.* **52**(1): 68–92.

Fowler, J. H. and O. Smirnov (2005). Dynamic parties and social turnout: an agent-based model. *Amer. J. Sociol.* **110** (4): 1070–94.

Glimcher, P. W., M. C. Dorris, and H. M. Bayer (2005). Physiological utility theory and the neuroeconomics of choice. *Game. Econ. Behav.* **52**(2): 213–16.

Hinich, M. J. and M. C. Munger (1994). *Ideology and the Theory of Political Choice*. Ann Arbor, MI: University of Michigan Press.

Hinich, M. J. and M. C. Munger (1997). *Analytical Politics*. Cambridge: Cambridge University Press.

Kedar, O. (2005). When moderate voters prefer extreme parties: policy balancing in parliamentary elections. *Amer. Pol. Sci. Rev.* **99**(2): 185–199.

Kollman, K., J. Miller, and S. Page (1992). Adaptive parties in spatial elections. *Amer. Polit. Sci. Rev.* **86**: 929–37.

Kollman, K., J. Miller, and S. Page (1998). Political parties and electoral landscapes. *Brit. J. Polit. Sci.* **28**: 139–58.

Kollman, K., J. Miller, and S. Page (2003). *Computational Models in Political Economy*. Cambridge, MA: MIT Press.

Laver, M. (2005). Policy and the dynamics of political competition. *Amer. Polit. Sci. Rev.* **99**(2): 263–81.

Laver M. and M. Schilperoord (2007). Spatial models of political competition with endogenous political parties. *Phil. Trans. R. Soc. B* **362**(1485): 1711–21.

Laver, M. and E. Sergenti (2007). Rigorous characterization of the output of agent-based models of party competition. American Political Science Association Annual Meetings, Chicago.

Laver, M. and E. Sergenti (2011). *Party Competition: An Agent-Based Model*. Princeton, Princeton University Press.

Lloyd, S. P. (1982). Least squares quantization in PCM. *IEEE T. Inform. Theory* **28**(2): 129–37.

Okabe, A., B. Boots, K. Sugihara, and S. N. Chiu (2000). *Spatial Tessellations: Concepts and Applications of Voronoi Diagrams*, 2nd edn. New York: John Wiley.

Osborne, M. (2000). Entry-deterring policy differentiation by electoral candidates. *Math. Soc. Sci.* **40**: 41–62.

Shepsle, K. A. (1991). *Models of Multiparty Electoral Competition*. New York: Harwood Academic Publishers.

Sutton, R. S. and A. G. Barto (1998). *Reinforcement Learning: An Introduction*. Cambridge, MA, MIT Press.

Teramoto, S., E. Demaine, and R. Uehara (2006). Voronoi game on graphs and its complexity. 2nd IEEE Symposium on Computational Intelligence and Games, Reno, Nevada, pp. 265–71.

22 On optimal decision making in brains and social insect colonies[1]

James A. R. Marshall, Rafal Bogacz, Anna Dornhaus, Robert Planqué, Tim Kovacs, and Nigel R. Franks

Summary

The problem of how to compromise between speed and accuracy in decision making faces organisms at many levels of biological complexity. Striking parallels are evident between decision making in primate brains and collective decision making in social insect colonies: in both systems separate populations accumulate evidence for alternative choices, when one population reaches a threshold a decision is made for the corresponding alternative, and this threshold may be varied to compromise between the speed and accuracy of decision making. In primate decision making simple models of these processes have been shown, under certain parameterisations, to implement the statistically optimal procedure that minimises decision time for any given error rate. In this chapter, we adapt these same analysis techniques and apply them to new models of collective decision making in social insect colonies. We show that social insect colonies may also be able to achieve statistically optimal collective decision making in a very similar way to primate brains, via direct competition between evidence-accumulating populations. This optimality result makes testable predictions for how collective decision making in social insects should be organised. Our approach also represents the first attempt to identify a common theoretical framework for the study of decision making in diverse biological systems.

22.1   Introduction

Animals constantly make decisions. Habitat selection, mate selection, and foraging require investigation of, and choice between, alternatives that may determine an animal's reproductive success. For example, many animals invest considerable time and energy in finding a safe home (Franks *et al.*, 2002; Hansell, 1984; Hazlett, 1981; Seeley, 1982).

[1] This chapter previously appeared in the *Journal of the Royal Society: Interface* (volume 6, pages 1065–1074): Marshall, J. A. R., Bogacz, R., Dornhaus, A., Planqué, R., Kovacs, T., and Franks, N. R. (2009) On optimal decision making in brains and social insect colonies (doi: 10.1098/rsif.2008.0511).

Similarly an animal may frequently have to deal with ambiguous sensory information in deciding whether a predator is present or not (Trimmer *et al.*, 2008).

There has been ongoing speculation as to whether decision-making mechanisms in brains and in colonies of social insects might be closely related to each other, beginning at least with Douglas Hofstadter (Hofstadter, 1979) and generating continued interest (Passino *et al.*, 2008; Seeley and Buhrman, 2001; Visscher, 2007). In this chapter, we examine a model of decision making in the primate brain (Usher and McClelland, 2001), and compare it to three new models of collective decision making during house-hunting by social insect colonies. These models are based on a proposed model for emigration in the rock ant *Temnothorax albipennis* (Pratt *et al.*, 2002), and two models proposed for nest-site selection in the honeybee *Apis mellifera* (Britton *et al.*, 2002). The similarities are striking: both systems are modelled with mutually interacting populations, in both systems a decision is made when one population exceeds some threshold, and in both systems this threshold can be varied to mediate between the speed and accuracy of the decision-making process. As well as examining the structural similarities and differences between the neuron model and social insect models, we examine optimality criteria for decision making in the social insect models. Bogacz *et al.* (2006) showed how the model of decision making in the brain proposed by Usher and McClelland (Usher and McClelland, 2001) can be parameterised to implement the statistically optimal strategy for choosing between two alternatives. Here we analyse to what extent each of the social insect models can implement or approximate this statistically optimal strategy. This gives testable predictions for how social insects should behave when house-hunting in order to optimise their decision making. The analysis we present represents the first step in establishing a common theoretical framework for the study of decision making in biological systems, that is based on the interactions between their components rather than the details of the components themselves. Hence this framework should prove applicable to diverse biological systems at many levels of biological complexity.

22.2   Optimal decision making

Decision making is a process in which uncertain information must be processed in order to make a choice between two or more alternatives. We can illustrate decision making with a simple perceptual choice task, in which a primate subject is presented with a display filled with moving dots. The subject is required to decide if the majority of dots move to the left or right and to make an eye movement in the same direction. The proportion of the displayed dots that move in a coherent direction can be varied to make the decision task easier or harder, and the rewards for correct choices can be modified to vary the optimal compromise between the speed and the accuracy of the decision.

The above description is just one example of a decision-making problem, but diverse organisms face a wide variety of decision problems exhibiting the key features of variable difficulty and a dynamic tension between the speed and the accuracy of the decision-making process (Chittka *et al.*, 2003; Edwards, 1965). Based on the analysis

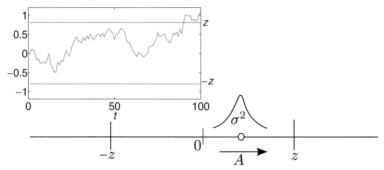

Figure 22.1 The diffusion model of decision making can be thought of as a random walk with normally distributed step size (Wiener process or Brownian motion) along a line where the positive direction corresponds to increasing evidence for one of the available alternatives, and the negative direction to increasing evidence for the other alternative. The random walk is subject to a constant drift A, a tendency to move along the line towards the better alternative, whose strength is the difference between the expectations of the incoming data on the available alternatives. The variance in the random walk (proportional to σ^2) represents the uncertainty in these incoming data. The diffusion model of decision-making implements the statistically optimal Sequential Probability Ratio Test, and by varying the decision threshold z can compromise between speed and accuracy of decision making. Inset: a sample trace of the diffusion model: at time $t = 0$, when decision making starts, there is no evidence in favour of either alternative. As time passes evidence accumulated so far varies stochastically, but consistently tends to increase in favour of one of the two alternatives. At approximately time $t = 90$, the positive decision threshold is reached and the corresponding alternative is chosen.

of human reaction-time distributions in decision tasks, psychologists proposed the 'diffusion model' of decision making (Ratcliff, 1978; Stone, 1960), which represents the process abstractly as Brownian motion on a line representing relative evidence for the two alternatives, with constant drift towards the correct hypothesis (Figure 22.1).

The diffusion model of decision making is, in fact, a special case of the more general Sequential Probability Ratio Test (SPRT).[2] The SPRT provably achieves optimal decision making over two alternatives (Wald and Wolfowitz, 1948), as it makes use of the Neyman–Pearson lemma familiar to statisticians and scientists (Neyman and Pearson, 1993). The SPRT works by continuing to gather evidence for the two alternative hypotheses until the log of their likelihood ratio exceeds a positive or negative threshold; this is the test that, among all possible tests, minimises decision time for any desired decision error rate. Through adjustment of this threshold the test can achieve the optimal trade-off between decision accuracy and decision speed.

The diffusion model of decision making has recently been shown to fit reaction-time data better than models that do not implement statistically optimal decision making (Ratcliff and Smith, 2004). Moreover, neural recordings from cortical regions in monkeys undertaking the moving-dots decision task are better described by the diffusion model

---

[2] This special case is obtained when information gain over time becomes continuous: the standard SPRT works with discrete evidence samples.

than by other, non-optimal models (Ratcliff *et al.*, 2003). This suggests that neural decision networks can be parameterised in a way that allows optimal decision making, as we shall discuss in the next sections.

22.3   Decision making in the cortex

The neural bases of decision making are typically studied in the context of the moving-dots experiment described in the preceding section. Neuronal activity recordings from single cells in the monkey cortex suggest that decision making during this task involves two main brain areas.

First, the neurons in the medial temporal area (MT) process the motion present in the visual field. Each of the MT neurons responds proportionally to the magnitude of motion in a particular direction (Britten *et al.*, 1993). Hence the neurons in the MT area that are selective for motion in different directions provide sensory evidence supporting the corresponding alternatives. However, this sensory evidence is uncertain due to the noise present in the stimulus and the neural representation itself.

Second, the neurons in the lateral intra-parietal area (LIP) and the frontal eye field are concerned with controlling eye movement. These neurons are selective for the direction of eye movement. During the motion discrimination task, it has been observed that the neurons corresponding to the correct alternative gradually increase their firing rate (Roitman and Shadlen, 2002; Schall, 2001; Shadlen and Newsome, 2001). Detailed studies of their activity provide strong evidence that the LIP neurons integrate input from the corresponding MT neurons over time (Hanks *et al.*, 2006; Huk and Shadlen, 2005). Hence, as time progresses in the task, the sensory evidence accumulated in the LIP neurons becomes more and more accurate.

It has been observed that when the activity of the LIP neurons exceeds a certain threshold, the decision is made and an eye movement in the corresponding direction is initiated (Roitman and Shadlen, 2002; Schall, 2001; Shadlen and Newsome, 2001). This arrangement of neural populations with decision thresholds lends itself to representation by a simple model, as described in the next section.

22.4   The Usher–McClelland model

The Usher–McClelland model represents decision making using neural populations that act as mutually inhibitory, leaky integrators of incoming evidence (Figure 22.2). In the moving-dots decision task described above, these integrator populations would represent the LIP neural populations corresponding to the different possible eye movement decisions. Each population of integrator neurons receives a noisy input signal which it integrates, subject to some constant loss. Each population also inhibits the activation of the other to a degree proportional to its own activation. So, as one population becomes highly activated, the suppression it exerts on the activation of the other grows stronger.

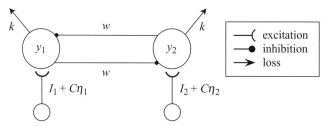

Figure 22.2 In the Usher–McClelland model of decision making in the primate visual cortex, neural populations represent accumulated evidence for each of the alternatives. These populations y_1 and y_2 integrate noisy inputs I_1 and I_2, but leak accumulated evidence at rate k. Each population also inhibits the other in proportion to its own activation level, at rate w. When $w = k$ and both are large the Usher–McClelland model reduces to the diffusion model of decision making (Figure 22.3).

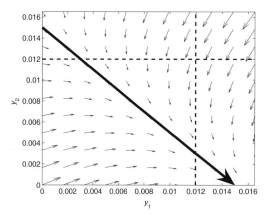

Figure 22.3 The expected dynamics of the Usher–McClelland model, plotted as activation of population y_1 against activation of population y_2. When decay equals inhibition ($w = k$) the system converges to a line (bold arrow) and diffuses along it, until a moveable decision threshold is reached (dashed lines). Along the attracting line the Usher–McClelland model is equivalent to the optimal diffusion model of decision making (Figure 22.1).

For a binary choice the linear version of the system is formally described as a pair of coupled stochastic ordinary differential equations:

$$\begin{cases} \dot{y}_1 = I_1 + c\eta_1 - y_1 k - y_2 w, \\ \dot{y}_2 = I_2 + c\eta_2 - y_2 k - y_1 w, \end{cases} \tag{22.1}$$

where y_i is the activity of population i, $\dot{y}_1$ is the change in that activity over time, I_i is the strength of the input signal for alternative i, $c\eta_i$ is the noise in that input signal described as a Wiener process with mean zero and standard deviation proportional to c, w is the rate at which one population inhibits the activation of the other, and k is the rate at which a population's activation level decays. The decision is made by the model if the activity of either of the populations reaches a threshold value.

Choosing different coordinates, $x_1 = (y_1 - y_2)/\sqrt{2}$ and $x_2 = (y_1 + y_2)/\sqrt{2}$, the model can be decoupled into two independent random processes (see Appendix A):

$$
\begin{cases}
\dot{x}_1 = (w - k)x_1 + \dfrac{I_1 - I_2}{\sqrt{2}} + c\eta_{1'}, \\[3mm]
\dot{x}_2 = (-k - w)x_2 + \dfrac{I_1 - I_2}{\sqrt{2}} + c\eta_{2'},
\end{cases}
\tag{22.2}
$$

where $c\eta_1' = (c\eta_1 - c\eta_2)/\sqrt{2}$, and similarly for $c\eta_2'$. If $w = k$, then x_1 simply undergoes a biased random walk. Moreover, taking both these parameters to be large, x_2 quickly converges to a limiting value (Figure 22.3).

Since x_2 quickly converges, the decision is made when the difference between integrated evidence, x_1, exceeds a positive or negative threshold (Bogacz et al., 2006). This corresponds to the statistically optimal diffusion model of decision making (Figure 22.1). Thus when $w = k$ and both of these parameters are relatively high, the Usher–McClelland model approximates optimal decision making.

22.5   Decision making in social insect colonies

The rock ant *Temnothorax albipennis* lives in colonies of up to a few hundred individuals, inhabiting small enclosed cavities such as rock crevices, which break down over time. Colonies of the honeybee *Apis mellifera* are substantially larger, often comprising more than 50 000 workers nesting in large cavities in hollow trees. For both species the need to hunt for a new nest site arises when the nest degrades or is destroyed, or when the colony grows or propagates. To minimise exposure, colonies must minimise the duration of the emigration, while still gathering substantial information about potential nest sites. 'Scout' individuals leave the old nest (or the bee swarm) to search for new suitable sites. When an individual has located a new site, this is thoroughly inspected according to multiple criteria (Franks et al., 2005, 2003b, 2006b, 2007a, Mallon and Franks, 2000).

A unanimous decision among the discovered nest sites is required, and the highest quality site should be identified to maximise future success. To achieve all of this, both rock ants and honeybees use a process of quality-dependent recruitment to nest sites, causing positive feedback, coupled with quorum sensing, ultimately leading to a collective decision (Visscher, 2007).

In *T. albipennis*, scouts recruit nestmates to a site they have discovered by tandem-running, teaching others the route (Franks and Richardson, 2006; Möglich, 1978; Möglich and Hölldobler, 1974; Richardson et al., 2007). The recruiters take longer to recruit to poor nests than they do for good nests (Mallon et al., 2001; Robinson et al., 2007, 2011). Recruits inspect the new nest and also start recruiting, leading to a positive feedback, with more ants arriving faster at higher-quality nest sites. When a certain number of ants, a quorum, have accumulated in the new site, all ants that are committed to it switch from tandem-running to carrying nest mates. This represents a switch to decision implementation, as brood items and passive ants are carried to the chosen nest site. The colony's collective decision for a new nest is thus usually for the site that first attracts the quorum number of ants. By adjusting this number, the ants opt for a quick but error-prone, or a slower but more accurate decision, depending on their group size and external conditions (Dornhaus *et al.*, 2004; Dornhaus and Franks, 2006; Franks *et al.*, 2003a).

In *A. mellifera*, scouts similarly start recruiting to discovered nest sites, here using the honeybee waggle dance (Lindauer, 1955; Seeley, 1982; von Frisch, 1967). The probability of performing waggle dances, as well as their duration, depends on the quality of the discovered site. Positive feedback thus arises only if recruits become recruiters, which happens only for superior sites (Seeley and Buhrman, 1999, 2001). Eventually all recruitment is for a single site, which is then chosen by the honeybee swarm (Seeley, 2003). Honeybees may also use a quorum at the new site to determine whether this decision has been made (Seeley and Visscher, 2004b).

Both of these decision-making mechanisms operate without central control, and individuals use only local information (Mallon *et al.*, 2001). Both species can select the best nest site even if news of it arrives late in the decision-making process (Britton *et al.*, 2002; Franks *et al.*, 2007b). However, there are some differences between the two collective decision-making systems. In the bees, the decision-making process is separated from the execution of the decision: the flight of the swarm to the new site occurs after the decision has been made, and is guided by a small number of informed individuals (Beekman *et al.*, 2006, see also Couzin *et al.*, 2005). In the ants, these processes are integrated, introducing a logistics problem into the decision problem (Planqué *et al.*, 2007). Note that the decision problem solved by colonies during emigration is one of optimal consensus decision making, and thus differs from the problem of distributed resource intake maximisation that colonies tackle during foraging (e.g., Seeley, 1995).

22.6   Models of house-hunting by social insect colonies

In the following sections we will examine how social insect colonies might implement optimal decision making, through formal analysis and numerical simulations of mathematical models. We propose three new models based on one published model of house-hunting by *T. albipennis* (Pratt *et al.*, 2002) and two published models of house-hunting by *A. mellifera* (Britton *et al.*, 2002). Our aim is to examine which model or models can implement optimal decision making, and use this to generate testable hypotheses about how social insects should behave if they are to decide optimally.

To understand how collective decision making may be optimised in situations characterised by uncertainty, our models are stochastic differential equations, as in the neural case. This departs from previous modelling efforts using deterministic differential equations (Britton *et al.*, 2002; Pratt *et al.*, 2002), population matrix models (Myerscough, 2003), or individual-based models (Marshall *et al.*, 2006; Pratt *et al.*, 2005). All the models represent flows between populations of individuals having different behavioural states. The structure of all of these models is very similar, and one such model is presented by way of illustration in Figure 22.4; the models differ, however, in the details of the rates at which individuals flow between these populations.

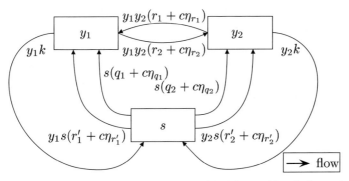

Figure 22.4 In the direct-switching model of decision making during emigration by the honeybee *A. mellifera*, populations of scouts y_1 and y_2 discover two alternative potential sites and compete with each other to recruit uncommitted scouts s and scouts committed to the other alternative. If there is no decay from commitment ($k = 0$) then once all scouts are committed to one alternative or the other subsequent decision making is exactly equivalent to the statistically optimal diffusion model of decision making (based on a model by Britton *et al.*, 2002)

22.6.1   House-hunting in *Temnothorax albipennis*

We begin with the model of emigration by *T. albipennis* (Pratt *et al.*, 2002). The full model considers the complete emigration process both before and after the quorum threshold is satisfied at a potential site: thus the model includes both tandem-running behaviour and carrying. In accordance with current biological understanding, we model only the decision-making process up to quorum satisfaction, considering that after this point a collective decision has been made and all that remains is its implementation (Pratt *et al.*, 2002). This view is not without its problems (Franks *et al.*, 2007b; Planqué *et al.*, 2007), but is an acceptable simplification for our purposes. We further simplify the original model by removing the intermediate class of assessor ants; ants thus switch directly from uncommitted to committed.

   Our simplified version of the Pratt *et al.* model (Pratt *et al.*, 2002) thus considers only ants discovering nest sites and recruiting to them through tandem-running. Ants leave the class of uncommitted scouting ants s, discover and become recruiters y_i for nest site i at rate q_i; this rate is proportional to the nest site's quality and ease of discovery, and is subject to noise $c\eta_{q_i}$. Recruiters for a site recruit uncommitted scouts in class s at noisy, quality-dependent rate $r_i'(s)$ where

$$r_i'(s) = \begin{cases} r_i' + c\eta_{r_i'} & \text{if } s > 0, \\ 0 & \text{otherwise.} \end{cases} \tag{22.3}$$

Finally, recruiters for a site spontaneously switch to recruiting for the other site at rate r_i, or switch to being uncommitted to any site at rate k_i. These rates are subject to noise $c\eta_{r_i}$ and $c\eta_{k_i}$ respectively. In this model, as in the other stochastic models below, we only consider stochasticity in any process related to quality assessment of the available alternatives. This enables our analysis to concentrate on how this relevant noise is processed by the system. This strategy has already been used implicitly in the Usher–McClelland model: there decay and inhibition are modelled deterministically, yet corresponding neural processes in the real world will of course be noisy.

Thus the ants' decision-making process is described by the following equations:

$$\begin{cases} \dot{y}_1 = (n - y_1 - y_2)(q_1 + c\eta_{q1}) + y_1 r_1'(s) + y_2(r_2 + c\eta_{r2}) \\ \quad - y_1(r_1 + c\eta_{r1}) - y_1(k_1 + c\eta_{k1}), \\ \dot{y}_2 = (n - y_1 - y_2)(q_2 + c\eta_{q2}) + y_2 r_2'(s) + y_1(r_1 + c\eta_{r1}) \\ \quad - y_2(r_2 + c\eta_{r2}) - y_2(k_2 + c\eta_{k2}), \end{cases} \tag{22.4}$$

where population size is constant $s = n - y_1 - y_2$, and hence the equation for $\dot{s}$ is redundant.

In the (x_1, x_2) variables, we seek to parameterise the model so that the random process $\dot{x}_1$ is independent of the random process $\dot{x}_2$, and is identical to the diffusion model of decision making. It can easily be shown that this parameterisation requires the decay parameters and switching rate parameters to be set according to the qualities of both the alternative nest sites under consideration (see Appendix B). In other words, optimal decision making can only be achieved under this model if individuals have global knowledge about the alternatives available. Given our understanding of social insects' house-hunting mechanisms, we do not expect all committed individuals to have quantitative knowledge of the qualities of both alternatives. Hence optimal parameterisation of our model of house-hunting in *T. albipennis* seems biologically unrealistic.

22.6.2   House-hunting with indirect switching in *Apis mellifera*

In this section and the next, we consider two models of house-hunting in *A. mellifera* due to Britton *et al.* (2002). These models differ only in whether or not they allow scouts committed to one site to switch directly to commitment to the alternative site. First we consider the case in which scouts cannot directly switch: that is, they can only change their commitment by first becoming completely uncommitted.

We adapt the model of (Britton *et al.*, 2002) so that, as in the Pratt *et al.* (2002) model, we have one population of uncommitted scouts, s, and two populations of recruiters, y_1 and y_2 for the two alternative sites under consideration. This is a simplification of the full Britton *et al.* model, in that we dispense with their populations of committed but inactive recruiters. We make a further small modification to the Britton *et al.* model by adding spontaneous discovery of alternative sites by uncommitted scouts at rates q_1 and q_2. We make these rates independent of site quality, to agree with the modelling approach of Britton *et al.* and with current biological understanding of *A. mellifera* (Seeley, 2003), however they may vary according to how distant, or how hard to discover, a potential nest site is.

Using the same notation as in Equations (22.4), our indirect-switching model of house-hunting by *A. mellifera* is described by the following equations:

$$
\begin{cases}
\dot{y}_1 = (n - y_1 - y_2)(q_1 + c\eta_{q1}) - y_1(k_1 + c\eta_{k_1}) \\
\quad + y_1(n - y_1 - y_2)(r_1' + c\eta_{r_1'}), \\
\dot{y}_2 = (n - y_1 - y_2)(q_2 + c\eta_{q2}) - y_2(k_2 + c\eta_{k_2}) \\
\quad + y_2(n - y_1 - y_2)(r_2' + c\eta_{r_2'}).
\end{cases}
\tag{22.5}
$$

It is easy to show that the indirect-switching model can neither be reduced to two independent random processes, nor does it asymptotically converge to the diffusion model of decision making (see Appendix C). Thus the indirect-switching model of decision making in *A. mellifera* cannot be (asymptotically) reduced to one dimension and therefore cannot be made exactly or approximately equivalent to the diffusion model of decision making. This does not rule out the possibility that indirect switching may be an effective decision-making strategy, but it does rule out it being a statistically optimal decision-making strategy.

22.6.3 House-hunting with direct switching in *Apis mellifera*

We now consider the Britton *et al.* (2002) model in which scouts can directly switch their commitment between alternative sites (Figure 22.4). The equations for this decision-making system are:

$$
\begin{cases}
\dot{y}_1 = (n - y_1 - y_2)(q_1 + c\eta_{q1}) + y_1(n - y_1 - y_2)(r_1' + c\eta_{r_1'}) \\
\quad - y_1 k + y_1 y_2 (r_1 - r_2 + c\eta_{r1} - c\eta_{r2}), \\
\dot{y}_2 = (n - y_1 - y_2)(q_2 + c\eta_{q2}) + y_2(n - y_1 - y_2)(r_2' + c\eta_{r_2'}) \\
\quad - y_2 k - y_1 y_2 (r_1 - r_2 + c\eta_{r1} - c\eta_{r2}).
\end{cases}
\tag{22.6}
$$

The key differences between the model described above for *A. mellifera*, and the *T. albipennis* model of Equations (22.4), are in the nature of the recruitment mechanism. In the *T. albipennis* model of the preceding section, the number of ants recruited per unit time is a linear function of the number of recruiters (as long as recruits are still available). In the honeybee recruitment occurs through waggle dancing, which is a process in which both parties meet (von Frisch, 1967), thus in the *A. mellifera* model number of bees recruited per unit time depends both on numbers of recruiters and on numbers of potential uninformed recruits. If either is small, the growth of new recruiter numbers is limited.

Unlike the *T. albipennis* model, it is not possible to make the random process $\dot{x}_1$ independent of the random process $\dot{x}_2$. However, we can analyse how $\dot{x}_1$ behaves in the limit when x_2 converges. By setting the decay rate $k = 0$, all scouts will become recruiters over time so x_2 approaches $n/\sqrt{2}$. In this limit, the dynamics of $\dot{x}_1$ are described as

$$
\dot{x}_1 = \left(\frac{n^2}{2} - x_1^2 \right) \left(\frac{r_1 - r_2}{\sqrt{2}} + c\eta_r \right).
\tag{22.7}
$$

In this random process both noise and strength of drift vary quadratically with x_1. Choosing an appropriate nonlinear coordinate transformation to x (see Appendix D) we find by the chain rule that the random process can be expressed as

$$\dot{x} = \frac{dx}{dx_1} \frac{dx_1}{dt} = A + c\eta, \tag{22.8}$$

where $A = (r_1 - r_2)/\sqrt{2}$.

Thus when $k = 0$ decision making asymptotically converges to the diffusion model (Figure 22.1), a decision-making process that is exactly equivalent to the statistically optimal strategy. We therefore describe the direct-switching model without decay as *asymptotically optimal*.

Optimal decision making in the model occurs when no uncommitted scouts remain in the colony. For honeybees, we presume that this usually occurs, as swarms typically take hours or days to reach a decision. As the emigration progresses more and more honeybees enter the decision-making process, and the number of sites considered by the colony reduces as known alternatives are eliminated and new alternatives are discovered less and less frequently (Seeley and Buhrman, 1999; Visscher and Camazine, 1999b). Before this full-commitment stage is reached, decision making will be governed by differences in discovery (q_i) and recruitment rates (r_i') for the available alternatives, and by availability of information on the alternatives. These rates can depend not only on the quality of the available sites, but on their distance, or the difficulty of their discovery. Thus an easy to discover, close but inferior site may attract more recruitment effort early on due to positive feedback than a more distant, hard to discover, but superior site. Once all scouts are committed, however, no new information on other alternatives can arrive (as there are no scouts searching), and decision making between the available alternatives is made optimally, solely on the basis of their relative quality. The only deviation from purely optimal diffusion decision making will be bias in the starting point of the decision-making process on the line $x_2 = n/\sqrt{2}$, resulting as just described. This will either tend to favour or disfavour selection of the best available alternative, depending on the relative ease of discovery, and distance, of the available alternatives. Nevertheless, we expect that setting decay $k = 0$ will lead robustly to faster, more accurate decision making, regardless of how easy or hard nest sites are to find and recruit to. In the following section we undertake numerical simulation of the model to test this optimality hypothesis.

22.7   Numerical simulation

To test whether decision making in the *A. mellifera* direct-switching model is optimised by setting decay $k = 0$, we conducted a numerical sensitivity test of the model (see Supporting Information in Marshall *et al.*, 2009): we simultaneously varied the differences in the initial discovery and recruitment rates, $q_1 - q_2$ and $r_1' - r_2'$ respectively, so that they either favoured or disfavoured selection of the superior nest site (site 1). The difference in the recruitment rates between the two populations of committed scouts,

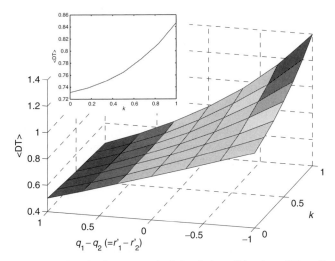

Figure 22.5 Results from numerical simulation of the *A. mellifera* direct-switching model. When decay $k > 0$, decision making is more strongly affected by the difference in discovery rates and recruitment rates from the home nest ($q_1 - q_2$ and $r'_1 - r'_2$); if these differences are in favour of the superior alternative site (site 1), then decision time can be reduced by increasing k, however if the differences favour the inferior alternative then increasing k increases decision time. Inset: if all differences are equally likely then mean decision time (y-axis) is minimised when k (x-axis) equals zero. See plate section for colour version.

$r_1 - r_2 = 2$, reflects the true relative qualities of the two alternatives. We then simulated the model with decay k varying between 0 and 1. The results (Figure 22.5) show that, although the benefit or cost of increasing k for decision time varies according to whether the superior site is easier or harder to find than its inferior alternative, setting $k = 0$ is robustly optimal as it minimises expected decision time across all scenarios considered.

22.8   Discussion

We have presented the first optimality hypothesis for collective decision making during emigration for social insect colonies. We have also presented the first formal investigation of similarities between certain neural decision-making processes, and collective decision making in social insect colonies, similarities which others have previously discussed (Hofstadter, 1979; Passino *et al.*, 2008; Seeley and Buhrman, 2001; Visscher, 2007). In both brains and social insect colonies, mutually interacting populations must reach an activation threshold to precipitate a decision. We argue that the interaction patterns between populations are the crucial part of the decision-making process at both these levels of biological complexity, organismal and super-organismal. Notwithstanding their impressive individual abilities (Koch, 1999), neurons are simple in comparison to individually sophisticated social insects (Chittka *et al.*, 2003; Franks and Richardson, 2006; Franks *et al.*, 2003b; Giurfa *et al.*, 2001; Richardson *et al.*, 2007). Simple interaction patterns in both these systems, however, may implement robust, efficient decision making regardless of how sophisticated their individual components are. Thus one could really think of social insect colonies as performing 'colony-level cognition' (Marshall and Franks, 2009), and we feel that the understanding of collective and individual decision-making systems can benefit from developing a common theoretical framework.

Why should we expect diverse natural systems, at such different levels of biological complexity as social insect colonies and the vertebrate brain, to solve similar decision problems using similar mechanisms? In this, we are using optimality theory as a guiding principle. For decision making, Bayes-optimal decision rules, of which the sequential probability ratio test is an example, provide a theoretically ideal solution to the problem at hand (see, for example, Berniker *et al.* in this volume, and Trimmer *et al.* (2011). Of the models presented here only one approximates statistically optimal (Bayesian) decision making in a biologically plausible manner. This is the direct-switching model of house-hunting by the honeybee *A. mellifera*, based on a model proposed by Britton *et al.* (2002) in which scouts switch their commitment between alternatives due to direct recruitment by others. Thus our optimality hypothesis is that such direct switching through recruitment should occur in social insect colonies if they are to implement optimal decision making. Lack of direct switching does not imply ineffective decision making, but does imply departure from statistical optimality, and also weakens the analogy between cross-inhibition in neural decision-making circuits and in social insect colonies. We do not expect natural selection necessarily to result in optimal behaviour (see, for example, Houston *et al.*, this volume), but we do expect natural selection to achieve the optimal compromise between benefits of optimal behaviour, and costs of overcoming developmental or other constraints on that behaviour. Of course, our optimality hypothesis remains useful in this case, by providing a gold-standard of optimal behaviour that we can use to theoretically quantify the cost a real biological system incurs by deviating from optimality, and set against this the cost of overcoming any constraints on that system (Parker and Maynard Smith, 1990).

Considerable discussion has focussed on whether direct recruited switching, or indirect switching via decay to being uncommitted, is more biologically plausible, both for *A. mellifera* and *T. albipennis*. In both species, significant numbers of scouts have been observed to visit more than one alternative site (Mallon *et al.*, 2001; Seeley and Buhrman, 1999), yet experimentation and argument have suggested that direct comparison is not necessary (Britton *et al.*, 2002; Pratt *et al.*, 2002; Visscher and Camazine, 1999a). More recently, further evidence on the ability of *T. albipennis* scouts to directly switch commitment has been presented (Franks *et al.*, 2007b). While the optimal direct-switching model of Equations (22.6) was proposed by Britton *et al.* (2002) as a model of honeybee decision-making, experimental evidence now suggests that honeybees may not be influenced in their switching by the activities of recruiters for other alternatives (Seeley, 2003), but may simply decay from their commitment to a site over time as in the indirect-switching models of Britton *et al.* (2002) and this chapter. However, researchers have recently observed production of the 'stop-signal' during decision making by honeybee swarms (Seeley and Visscher, 2004a). This signal inhibits the production of waggle dances (Nieh, 1993), and it has been suggested that this could serve the same purpose as the inhibitory connections postulated by the Usher–McClelland neuronal model (Visscher, 2007). Inhibition followed by recruitment is functionally similar to direct recruited switching. This hypothesis may be tested empirically by observing whether the targets of stop signals subsequently might follow dances for, and become committed to, alternative sites. The direct-switching nonlinear model also seems to be a plausible description of pre-quorum decision making in *T. albipennis*. We reanalysed the experimental data of Pratt *et al.* (2002) from a binary emigration experiment with *T. albipennis*, and found that 14% of commitment switches from poor to good nests occurred through recruitment, compared to 3.8% of switches from good to poor nests.[3] Such relative levels of switching are consistent with the optimal parameterisation of our direct-switching model presented here, in that, while switching occurs in both directions, more individuals switch from poor to good sites, as they would if the colony were implementing a diffusion process in reaching its decision. In general, for both species the data available on direct switching are sparse yet very interesting, and deserve closer examination supplemented by additional experiments investigating mechanisms such as the honeybee's stop signal. If such examination conclusively shows that direct switching does occur in honeybees, then our optimality hypothesis will be supported. If, however, direct switching is shown definitely not to occur, then our optimality hypothesis will enable us to quantify theoretically the cost of deviation from optimality, in terms of speed and accuracy of decision making.

In this chapter, we have considered only the binary decision case, for which the Sequential Probability Ratio Test (SPRT) is provably optimal. Much experimental work undertaken with social insect colonies involves binary choice experiments. However, in the real world it seems unlikely that a colony will only ever be faced with a choice between two alternatives. Optimal decision making becomes more difficult in the presence of more than two alternatives, and a provably optimal strategy is not known. However a decision-making strategy that is asymptotically optimal (as required error rate goes to zero) is known in the form of the Multihypothesis Sequential Probability Ratio Test (MSPRT) (Veeravalli and Baum, 1995), and it has recently been proposed that the vertebrate basal ganglia could implement this test (Bogacz *et al.*, this volume; Bogacz and Gurney, 2007). Other work has shown that the simple SPRT applied to multiple alternatives can be very effective when some of the alternatives are much better than the others (Bogacz *et al.*, 2007), a scenario that may be common in nature, and that both *T. albipennis* (Franks *et al.*, 2003b; Franks *et al.*, 2006a) and *A. mellifera* (Seeley and Buhrman, 2001) colonies have been experimentally demonstrated to perform well under.

One complicating factor for our analysis is that in social insect colonies, decision making is conflated with decision implementation. In *T. albipennis* colonies, once the quorum is satisfied only those scouts that know the location of the new site will be able to undertake the transportation of the remainder of the colony: ants transported by carrying are carried in a pose unsuitable for learning the route. Hence, the quorum threshold must be optimised not just for optimality of decision making, but for efficiency of decision implementation (Planqué *et al.*, 2007). This may account for other

---

[3] These rates were despite the physical proximity of the nests (10 cm apart), which reduces the need for recruitment processes to augment independent discovery and switching (Pratt, 2008).

authors' observations of a reduced effect of quorum threshold on emigration time during computer simulations of *Temnothorax* emigrations (Pratt and Sumpter, 2006). A similar, but arguably less acute, situation occurs in *A. mellifera* colonies, where a sufficiently large minority of informed scouts must guide the entire swarm to the new nest site (Beekman *et al.*, 2006; Couzin *et al.*, 2005). To increase confidence in the theoretical predictions from our models, which are necessarily simplified for analytical tractability, it could be interesting to attempt to validate these predictions using more biologically plausible individual-based models, such as those of Marshall *et al.* (2006), Passino and Seeley (2006), and Pratt *et al.* (2005).

An additional complication arises because, in real emigrations, news about all the alternatives is not available to the colony from the beginning: discovery of potential nest sites by scouts is a stochastic process, and the best available alternative may not be discovered until quite late in the decision-making process. Experimental (Franks *et al.*, 2007b) and theoretical (Britton *et al.*, 2002) work has examined the robustness of social insects' collective decision making to this kind of late information. Our analysis shows how such robustness might be understood because under the direct-switching model, once all scouts are committed and no further information on new alternatives can arrive, decision making proceeds optimally between the available alternatives based on their quality: the only departure from optimality is the bias in the starting point of the decision process based on the relative discovery times of the alternatives.

The previous point brings us to one final observation, that social insect colonies may face a subtly different decision problem to neural circuits in the vertebrate brain. A social insect colony must actively acquire information from its environment, whereas in the visual decision-making task considered in this chapter information on both alternatives arrives at an equal and unvarying rate. Scouts stochastically discover alternative sites, but once some potential sites are known the colony is faced with the traditional explore/exploit dilemma: should the colony send more scouts to assess the known alternatives and gain a better estimate of their quality, or should it allocate scouts to attempt the discovery of unknown, potentially better, alternatives? As previously noted (Marshall *et al.*, 2006), the colony is thus faced with a decision problem that is a hybrid of the bandit problem, in which trials must be allocated across noisy alternatives of unknown quality in order to maximise long-term gain, and the minimal decision time problem that the SPRT addresses. To our knowledge, no attempt has previously been made to formalise or analyse such a problem. We believe that analysis of the social insects' behaviour, and models thereof, could provide a fruitful avenue for tackling this new decision problem. We expect this problem will also reveal further similarities between collective and neural decision-making processes, leading to further extension of the general decision-making framework outlined here.

Acknowledgements

Thanks to P. Holmes, A. I. Houston, and P. Trimmer for comment and discussion. This work was partially supported by EPSRC Grant No. GR/S78674/01, and by an Emmy Noether Fellowship awarded to A.D. by the Deutsche Forschungsgemeinschaft.

Appendix A   Reduction of the Usher–McClelland model to one dimension

Transformation of the Usher–McClelland model into the new coordinate system $x_1 \times x_2$ is given by

$$x_1 = \frac{y_1 - y_2}{\sqrt{2}} \tag{A.1}$$

and

$$x_2 = \frac{y_1 + y_2}{\sqrt{2}}. \tag{A.2}$$

Then

$$\dot{x}_1 = \frac{\dot{y}_1 - \dot{y}_2}{\sqrt{2}} \tag{A.3}$$

and

$$\dot{x}_2 = \frac{\dot{y}_1 + \dot{y}_2}{\sqrt{2}}, \tag{A.4}$$

hence the transformation between Equations (22.1) and Equations (22.2) is achieved (Bogacz *et al.*, 2006).

Appendix B   Reduction of the *Temnothorax albipennis* model to one dimension

Applying Equations (A.1) through (A.4) to the model described by Equations (22.5) gives

$$\dot{x}_1 = \frac{n}{\sqrt{2}}(q_1 - q_2 + \sqrt{2}c\eta_q)$$
$$+ x_1 \left(\frac{r_1'(n - \sqrt{2}x_2) + r_2'(n - \sqrt{2}x_2) + \sqrt{2}c\eta_{r'} - k_1 - k_2 + \sqrt{2}c\eta_k}{2} \right.$$
$$\left. -r_1 - r_2 + \sqrt{2}c\eta_r \right)$$
$$+ x_2 \left(\frac{r_1'(n - \sqrt{2}x_2) - r_2'(n - \sqrt{2}x_2) + \sqrt{2}c\eta_{r'} - k_1 + k_2 + \sqrt{2}c\eta_k}{2} \right.$$
$$\left. -r_1 - r_2 + \sqrt{2}c\eta_r + q_1 - q_2 + \sqrt{2}c\eta_q \right) \tag{A.5}$$

and

$$\dot{x}_2 = \frac{n}{\sqrt{2}}(q_1 + q_2 + \sqrt{2}c\eta_q)$$
$$+ x_1 \left(\frac{r_1'(n - \sqrt{2}x_2) - r_2'(n - \sqrt{2}x_2) + \sqrt{2}c\eta_{r'} - k_1 + k_2 + \sqrt{2}c\eta_k}{2} \right)$$
$$+ x_2 \left(\frac{r_1'(n - \sqrt{2}x_2) + r_2'(n - \sqrt{2}x_2) + \sqrt{2}c\eta_{r'} - k_1 - k_2 + \sqrt{2}c\eta_k}{2} \right.$$
$$\left. - q_1 - q_2 + \sqrt{2}c\eta_q \right), \tag{A.6}$$

where all noise terms are derived as described in the main text from their constituent noise terms; as the mean of the distribution for each noise source is 0 we can write all noise terms as being added to their associated rate even if, algebraically, they should be subtracted.

Examining Equation (A.5) we see that to have the random process $\dot{x}_1$ independent of its state and of the random process $\dot{x}_2$, disregarding noise, we must have

$$
\begin{aligned}
0 &= \frac{r_1'(n - \sqrt{2}x_2) + r_2'(n - \sqrt{2}x_2) - k_1 - k_2}{2} - r_1 - r_2 \\
&= \pm\left(\frac{r_1'(n - \sqrt{2}x_2) - r_2'(n - \sqrt{2}x_2) - k_1 + k_2}{2}\right).
\end{aligned}
\tag{A.7}
$$

Simplifying Equation (A.7) gives us the condition

$$
r_1'(n - \sqrt{2}x_2) - k_1 - 2r_1 = q_1 - q_2
\tag{A.8}
$$

or

$$
r_2'(n - \sqrt{2}x_2) - k_2 - 2r_2 = q_2 - q_1
\tag{A.9}
$$

demonstrating that optimal parameterisation of recruitment and decay rates for one nest site (the left hand side of Equations (A.8) and (A.9)) requires knowledge of the qualities of *both* alternative sites (the right hand side of those equations).

Appendix C   Reduction of the *Apis mellifera* indirect-switching model to one dimension

Applying Equations (A.1) through (A.4) to the model described by Equations (22.5) gives

$$
\begin{aligned}
\dot{x}_1 = {}&\frac{n}{\sqrt{2}}(q_1 - q_2 + \sqrt{2}c\eta_q) \\
&- \frac{x_1 x_2}{\sqrt{2}}(r_1' + r_2' + \sqrt{2}c\eta_{r'}) - \frac{x_2^2}{\sqrt{2}}(r_1' - r_2' + \sqrt{2}c\eta_{r'}) \\
&+ x_1\left(\frac{n(r_1' + r_2' + \sqrt{2}c\eta_{r'}) - (k_1 + k_2 + \sqrt{2}c\eta_k)}{2}\right) \\
&+ x_2\left(\frac{n(r_1' - r_2' + \sqrt{2}c\eta_{r'}) - (k_1 - k_2 + \sqrt{2}c\eta_k)}{2} - (q_1 - q_2 + \sqrt{2}c\eta_q)\right)
\end{aligned}
\tag{A.10}
$$

and

$$\dot{x}_2 = \frac{n}{\sqrt{2}}(q_1 + q_2 + \sqrt{2}c\eta_q)$$

$$-\frac{x_1 x_2}{\sqrt{2}}(r_1' - r_2' + \sqrt{2}c\eta_{r'}) - \frac{x_2^2}{\sqrt{2}}(r_1' + r_2' + \sqrt{2}c\eta_{r'})$$

$$+x_1 \left(\frac{n(r_1' - r_2' + \sqrt{2}c\eta_{r'}) - (k_1 - k_2 + \sqrt{2}c\eta_k)}{2} \right)$$

$$+x_2 \left(\frac{n(r_1' + r_2' + \sqrt{2}c\eta_{r'}) - (k_1 + k_2 + \sqrt{2}c\eta_k)}{2} - (q_1 + q_2 + \sqrt{2}c\eta_q) \right).$$

$$(A.11)$$

Once again all noise terms are derived as described in the main text and are written as being positive terms regardless of their algebraic sign (see Appendix B).

In attempting to reduce the above decision-making system to one dimension, we quickly see that $\dot{x}_1$ (Equation (A.10)) cannot be made independent of both x_1 and x_2 through simple parameterisation, as to do so would require all relevant rates (q_i, r_i' and k_i) to be 0.

We next consider whether Equation (A.10) can asymptotically approximate the constant drift diffusion model of decision making, as we show for the direct-switching *Apis mellifera* model (Appendix D). To do this we must find a limiting value of x_2 that is independent of x_1, then analyse how $\dot{x}_1$ behaves with this fixed x_2. The condition for $\dot{x}_2$ to be independent of x_1 is

$$0 = x_1 \left(\frac{n(r_1' - r_2') - (k_1 - k_2)}{2} - \frac{x_2}{\sqrt{2}}(r_1' - r_2') \right). \tag{A.12}$$

Solving for x_2 the condition becomes

$$x_2 = \frac{n}{\sqrt{2}} - \frac{k_1 - k_2}{\sqrt{2}(r_1' - r_2')}. \tag{A.13}$$

Assuming that k_i and r_i' are negatively correlated as would be required for effective switching behaviour, the second term of Equation (A.13) is always negative, hence we find that the required value of x_2 can never be attained as it is greater than the maximum value $n/\sqrt{2}$ that x_2 can take.

Thus the indirect-switching model of decision making in *A. mellifera* cannot be (asymptotically) reduced to one dimension and therefore cannot be made exactly or approximately equivalent to the diffusion model of decision making.

Appendix D   Reduction of the *Apis mellifera* direct-switching model to one dimension

Applying Equations (A.1) through (A.4) to the model described by Equations (22.6) gives

$$\dot{x}_1 = \frac{n}{\sqrt{2}}(q_1 - q_2 + \sqrt{2}c\eta_q) - \frac{x_1^2}{\sqrt{2}}(r_1 - r_2 + \sqrt{2}c\eta_r)$$

$$+ \frac{x_2^2}{\sqrt{2}}(r_2' - r_1' + r_1 - r_2 + \sqrt{2}c\eta_{r'} + \sqrt{2}c\eta_r) - \frac{x_1 x_2}{\sqrt{2}}(r_1' + r_2' + \sqrt{2}c\eta_{r'})$$

$$+ x_1 \left(\frac{n(r_1' + r_2' + \sqrt{2}c\eta_{r'}) - k}{2} \right)$$

$$+ x_2 \left(\frac{n(r_1' - r_2' + \sqrt{2}c\eta_{r'})}{2} - (q_1 - q_2 + \sqrt{2}c\eta_q) \right) \tag{A.14}$$

and

$$\dot{x}_2 = \frac{n}{\sqrt{2}}(q_1 + q_2 + \sqrt{2}c\eta_q) - \frac{x_1 x_2}{\sqrt{2}}(r_1' - r_2' + \sqrt{2}c\eta_{r'}) - \frac{x_2^2}{\sqrt{2}}(r_1' + r_2' + \sqrt{2}c\eta_{r'})$$

$$+ x_1 \left(\frac{n(r_1' - r_2' + \sqrt{2}c\eta_{r'})}{2} \right)$$

$$+ x_2 \left(\frac{n(r_1' + r_2' + \sqrt{2}c\eta_{r'}) - k}{2} - (q_1 + q_2 + \sqrt{2}c\eta_q) \right). \tag{A.15}$$

Again all noise terms are derived as described in the main text and written as being positive terms regardless of their algebraic sign (see Appendix B).

If we assume that there is no decay from commitment to an alternative, then $k = 0$ and according to Equation (A.15) the value of x_2 asymptotically approaches $n/\sqrt{2}$. When $x_2 = n/\sqrt{2}$, Equation (A.14) simplifies to give Equation (22.7).

Although the noise and drift in the limit of the direct-switching model (when $k = 0$) vary quadratically, they both vary with the same quadratic coefficient. This nonlinear decision-making system is thus equivalent to the diffusion model of decision making, which has constant drift and noise, under a nonlinear coordinate transform. We now derive that transform.

Let us define the diffusion model of decision making as per Equation (22.8)

$$\dot{x} = A + c\eta, \tag{A.16}$$

where A is the strength of the drift and c is the standard deviation of the normally distributed noise.

Changing notation, we wish to make use of the chain rule to find the derivative dx/dx_1 that will yield the equality $dx/dt = dx_1/dt$. Assuming dx_1/dt as given by

Equation (22.7), and assuming dx/dt as given by Equation (A.16) with $A = (r_1 - r_2)/\sqrt{2}$, we find

$$\frac{dx}{dx_1} = \frac{1}{\left(\frac{n^2}{2} - x_1^2\right)}.$$ (A.17)

We next integrate Equation (A.17) to find the nonlinear transform of x_1 to x that we require is

$$x(x_1) = \frac{\sqrt{2}}{n} \operatorname{arctan} h \left(x_1 \frac{\sqrt{2}}{n}\right).$$ (A.18)

References

Beekman, M., R. Fathke, and T. Seeley (2006). How does an informed minority of scouts guide a honeybee swarm as it flies to its new home? *Anim. Behav.* **71**(1): 161–71.

Bogacz, R., E. Brown, J. Moehlis, P. Holmes, and J. D. Cohen (2006). The physics of optimal decision making: a formal analysis of models of performance in two-alternative forced choice tasks. *Psychol. Rev.* **113**: 700–765.

Bogacz, R. and K. Gurney (2007). The basal ganglia and cortex implement optimal decision making between alternative actions. *Neural Comput.* **19**:442.

Bogacz, R., M. Usher, J. Zhang, and J. L. McClelland (2007). Extending a biologically inspired model of choice: multi-alternatives, nonlinearity and value-based multidimensional choice. *Phil. Trans. Roy. Soc. B Biol. Sci.* **362**:1655–70.

Britten, K. H., M. N. Shadlen, W. T. Newsome, and J. A. Movshon (1993). Responses of neurons in macaque mt to stochastic motion signals. *Vis. Neurosci.* **10**: 1157–69.

Britton, N. F., N. R. Franks, S. C. Pratt, and T. D. Seeley (2002). Deciding on a new home: how do honeybees agree? *Proc. Soc. Roy. Soc. B Biol. Sci.* **269**:1383–8.

Chittka, L., A. G. Dyer, F. Bock, and A. Dornhaus (2003). Bees trade off foraging speed for accuracy. *Nature* **424**: 388.

Couzin, I. D., J. Krause, N. R. Franks, and S. A. Levin (2005). Effective leadership and decision-making in animal groups on the move. *Nature* **433**: 513–6.

Dornhaus, A. and N. Franks, (2006). Colony size affects collective decision-making in the ant *Temnothorax albipennis*. *Insectes Sociaux* **53**: 420–7.

Dornhaus, A., N. R. Franks, R. M. Hawkins, and H. N. S. Shere (2004). Ants move to improve: colonies of *Leptothorax albipennis* emigrate whenever they find a superior nest site. *Anim. Behav.* **67**: 959–63.

Edwards, W. (1965). Optimal strategies for seeking information: models for statistics, choice reaction times, and human information processing. *J. Math. Psychol.* **2**: 312–29.

Franks, N. R. and T. Richardson (2006). Teaching in tandem-running ants. *Nature* **439**: 153.

Franks, N., A. Dornhaus, C. Best, and E. Jones (2006a). Decision making by small and large house-hunting ant colonies: one size fits all. *Anim. Behav.* **72**: 611–16.

Franks, N. R., A. Dornhaus, J. P. Fitzsimmons, and M. Stevens (2003a). Speed versus accuracy in collective decision making. *Proc. Soc. Roy. Soc. B Biol. Sci.* **270**: 2457–63.

Franks, N. R., A. Dornhaus, G. Hitchcock, *et al.* (2007a). Avoidance of conspecific colonies during nest choice by ants. *Anim. Behav.* **73**: 525–34.

Franks, N. R., A. Dornhaus, B. G. Metherell, *et al.* (2006b). Not everything that counts can be counted: ants use multiple metrics for a single nests. *Proc. Soc. Roy. Soc. B Biol. Sci.* **273**: 165–9.

Franks, N. R., J. Hooper, C. Webb, and A. Dornhaus (2005). Tomb evaders: house-hunting hygiene in ants. *Biol. Lett.* **1**:190–2.

Franks, N. R., J. W. Hooper, M. Gumn, *et al.* (2007b). Moving targets: collective decisions and flexible choices in house-hunting ants. *Swarm Intell.* 181–94.

Franks, N. R., E. B. Mallon, H. E. Bray, M. J. Hamilton, and T. C. Mischler (2003b). Strategies for choosing between alternatives with different attributes: exemplified by house-hunting ants. *Anim. Behav.* **65**: 215–23.

Franks, N. R., S. C. Pratt, E. B. Mallon, N. F. Britton, and D. J. T. Sumpter (2002). Information flow, opinion polling and collective intelligence in house-hunting social insects. *Proc. Soc. Roy. Soc. B Biol. Sci.* **357**: 1567–83.

Giurfa, M., S. Zhang, A. Jenett, R. Menzel, and M. V. Srinivasan (2001). The concepts of 'sameness' and 'difference' in an insect. *Nature* **410**: 930–33.

Hanks, T. D., J. Ditterich, and M. N. Shadlen (2006). Microstimulation of macaque area lip affects decision-making in a motion discrimination task. *Nature Neurosci.* **9**: 682–9.

Hansell, M. H. (1984). *Animal Architecture and Building Behaviour*. London: Longman.

Hazlett, B. A. (1981). The behavioral ecology of hermit crabs. *Ann. Rev. Ecol. Syst.* **12**: 1–22.

Hofstadter, D. R. (1979). *Gödel Escher Bach: An Eternal Golden Braid*. New York: Basic Books.

Huk, A. C. and M. N. Shadlen (2005). Neural activity in macaque parietal cortex reflects temporal integration of visual motion signals during perceptual decision making. *J. Neurosci.* **25**:10420–36.

Koch, C. (1999). *Biophysics of Computation: Information Processing in Single Neurons*. New York: Oxford University Press.

Lindauer, M. (1955). Schwarmbienen auf wohnungssuche. *J. Comp. Physiol. A: Sens. Neural Behav. Physiol.* **37**: 263–324.

Mallon, E. B. and N. R. Franks (2000). Ants estimate area using Buffon's needle. *Proc. Soc. Roy. Soc. B. Biol. Sci.* **267**: 765–70.

Mallon, E. B., S. C. Pratt, and N. R. Franks (2001). Individual and collective decision-making during nest site selection by the ant *Leptothorax albipennis. Behav. Ecol. Sociobiol.* **50**: 352–9.

Marshall, J. A. R., R. Bogacz, A. Dornhaus, *et al.* (2009). On optimal decision making in brains and social insect colonies. *J. Roy. Soc. Interface*, doi: 10.1098/rsif.2008.0511.

Marshall, J. A. R., A. Dornhaus, N. R. Franks, and T. Kovacs (2006). Noise, cost and speed-accuracy trade-offs: decision-making in a decentralized system. *J. Roy. Soc. Interface* **3**: 243–54.

Marshall, J. A. R. and N. R. Franks (2009). Colony-level cognition. *Curr. Biol.* **19**: R395–R396.

Möglich, M. (1978). Social organization of nest emigration in *Leptothorax* (Hym., Form.). *Insectes Sociaux* **25**: 205–225.

Möglich, M. and B. Hölldobler (1974). Social carrying behavior and division of labor during nest moving in ants. *Psyche* **81**: 219–36.

Myerscough, M. R. (2003). Dancing for a decision: a matrix model for nestsite choice by honeybees. *Proc. Soc. Roy. Soc. B Biol. Sci.* **270**: 577–582.

Neyman, J. and E. Pearson (1993). On the problem of the most efficient tests of statistical hypotheses. *Phil. Trans. Roy. Soc. A* **231**: 289–337.

Nieh, J. C. (1993). The stop signal of honey bees: reconsidering its message. *Behav. Ecol. Sociobiol.* **33**: 51–6.

Parker, G. A. and J. Maynard Smith (1990). Optimality theory in evolutionary biology. *Nature* **348**(6296): 27–33.

Passino, K. and T. Seeley (2006). Modeling and analysis of nest-site selection by honeybee swarms: the speed and accuracy trade-off. *Behav. Ecol. Sociobiol.* **59**(3): 427–42.

Passino, K. M., T. D. Seeley, and P. K. Visscher (2008). Swarm cognition in honeybees. *Behav. Ecol. Sociobiol.* **62**: 401–414.

Planqué, R., F. X. Dechaume-Moncharmont, N. R. Franks, T. Kovacs, and J. A. R. Marshall (2007). Why do house-hunting ants recruit in both directions? *Naturwissenschaffen* **94**: 911–18.

Pratt, S. C. (2008). Efficiency and regulation of recruitment during colony emigration by the ant *Temnothorax curvispinosus*. *Behav. Ecol. Sociobiol.* **62**: 1369–76.

Pratt, S. C., E. B. Mallon, D. J. T. Sumpter, and N. R. Franks (2002). Quorum sensing, recruitment, and collective decision-making during colony emigration by the ant *Leptothorax albipennis*. *Behav. Ecol. Sociobiol.* **52**: 117–27.

Pratt, S. C. and D. J. T. Sumpter, (2006). A tunable algorithm for collective decision-making. *Proc. Nat. Acad. Sci. USA* **103**: 15906–10.

Pratt, S. C., D. J. T. Sumpter, E. B. Mallon, and N. R. Franks (2005). An agent-based model of collective nest choice by the ant *Temnothorax albipennis*. *Anim. Behav.* **70**:1023–36.

Ratcliff, R. (1978). A theory of memory retrieval. *Psychol. Rev.* **85**: 59–108.

Ratcliff, R., A. Cherian, and M. A. Segraves (2003). A comparison of macaque behavior and superior colliculus neuronal activity to predictions from models of two choice decisions. *J. Neurophysiol.* **90**: 1392–407.

Ratcliff, R. and P. L. Smith (2004). A comparison of sequential sampling models for two-choice reaction time. *Psychol. Rev.* **111**: 333–67.

Richardson, T., P. Sleeman, J. McNamara, A. I. Houston, and N. R. Franks (2007). Teaching with evaluation in ants. *Curr. Biol.* **17**: 1520–6.

Robinson, E. J. H., N. R. Franks, S. Ellis, S. Okuda, and J. A. R. Marshall (2011). A simple threshold rule is sufficient to explain sophisticated collective decision making. *PloS One* **6**(5): e19981.doi:10.1371/journal.pone.0019981.

Robinson, E. J. H., F. D. Smith, K. M. E. Sullivan, and N. R. Franks (2009). Do ants make direct comparisons? Proc. R. Soc. B **276**: 2635–41.

Roitman, J. D. and M. N. Shadlen (2002). Response of neurons in the lateral intraparietal area during a combined visual discrimination reaction time task. *J. Neurosci.* **22**: 9475–89.

Schall, J. D. (2001). Neural basis of deciding choosing and acting. *Nat. Rev. Neurosci.* **2**: 33–42.

Seeley, T. (1995). *The Wisdom of the Hive: The Social Physiology of Honey Bee Colonies*. Cambridge, MA: Harvard University Press.

Seeley, T. D. (1982). How honeybees find a home. *Sci. Amer.* **247**: 158–69.

Seeley, T. D. (2003). Consensus building during nest-site selection in honey bee swarms: the expiration of dissent. *Behav. Ecol. Sociobiol.* **53**: 417–24.

Seeley, T. D. and S. C. Buhrman (1999). Group decision making in swarms of honey bees. *Behav. Ecol. Sociobiol.* **45**: 19–31.

Seeley, T. D. and S. C. Buhrman (2001). Nest-site selection in honey bees: how well do swarms implement the 'best-of-N' decision rule? *Behav. Ecol. Sociobiol.* **49**: 416–27.

Seeley, T. D. and P. K. Visscher (2004a). Group decision making in nest-site selection by honey bees. *Apidologie* **35**: 101–16.

Seeley, T. D. and P. K. Visscher (2004b). Quorum sensing during nest-site selection by honeybee swarms. *Behav. Ecol. Sociobiol.* **56**: 594–601.

Shadlen, M. N. and W. T. Newsome (2001). Neural basis of a perceptual decision in the parietal cortex (area lip) of the rhesus monkey. *J. Neurophysiol.* **86**: 1916–36.

Stone, M. (1960). Models for choice reaction time. *Psychometrika* **25**: 251–60.

Trimmer, P. C., R. Bogacz, A. I. Houston, *et al.* (2008). Mammalian choices: combining fast-but-inaccurate and slow-but-accurate decision-making systems. *Proc. Soc. Roy. Soc. B Biol. Sci.* **275**: 2353–61.

Trimmer, P. C., A. I. Houston, J. A. R. Marshall, *et al.* (2011) Decision-making under uncertainty: biases and Bayesians. *Anim. Cogn.* doi: 10.1007/s10071-011-0387-4.

Usher, M. and J. L. McClelland (2001). The time course of perceptual choice: the leaky, competing accumulator model. *Psychol. Rev.* **108**: 550–92.

Veeravalli, V. V. and C. W. Baum (1995). Asymptotic efficiency of a sequential multihypothesis test. *IEEE Trans. Inf. Theor.* **41**: 1994–7.

Visscher, P. K. (2007). Group decision making in nest-site selection among social insects. *Ann. Rev. Entomol.* **52**: 255–75.

Visscher, P. K. and S. Camazine (1999a). Collective decisions and cognition in honeybees. *Nature*, **397**: 400.

Visscher, P. K. and S. Camazine (1999b). The mystery of swarming honeybees: from individual behaviours to collective decisions. In *Information Processing in Social Insects*, ed. C. Detrain, J. L. Deneubourg and J. M. Pasteels. Basel, Switzerland: Birkhäuser, pp. 355–78.

von Frisch, K. (1967). *The Dance Language and Orientation of Bees*. Cambridge, MA: Belknap Press.

Wald, A. and J. Wolfowitz (1948). Optimum character of the sequential probability ratio test. *Ann. Math. Stat.* **19**: 326–39.

23 State-dependent foraging rules for social animals in selfish herds

Sean A. Rands, Richard A. Pettifor, J. Marcus Rowcliffe, and Guy Cowlishaw

Summary

Many animals gain benefits from living in groups, such as a dilution in predation risk when they are closely aggregated (referred to as the 'selfish herd'). Game theory has been used to predict many properties of groups (such as the expected group size), but little is known about the proximate mechanisms by which animals achieve these predicted properties. We explore a possible proximate mechanism using a spatially explicit, individual-based model, where individuals can choose to rest or forage on the basis of a rule of thumb that is dependent upon both their energetic reserves and the presence and actions of neighbours. The resulting behaviour and energetic reserves of individuals, and the resulting group sizes, are shown to be affected both by the ability of the forager to detect conspecifics and areas of the environment suitable for foraging, and by the distribution of energy in the environment. The model also demonstrates that if animals are able to choose (based upon their energetic reserves) between selecting the best foraging sites available, or moving towards their neighbours for safety, then this also has significant effects upon individuals and group sizes. The implications of the proposed rule of thumb are discussed.

23.1   Introduction

When animals form groups, it is often assumed that each individual faces various costs and benefits of group membership (Giraldeau and Caraco, 2000; Krause and Ruxton, 2002; Pulliam and Caraco, 1984). For example, within a foraging group, benefits could come through an increased likelihood of finding food or detecting predators, while costs could come through increased competition for resources, or increased visibility to predators. Much theoretical work has been conducted examining how the trade-off between these costs and benefits can determine the stable size of a group (Clark and Mangel, 1984; Ekman and Rosander, 1987; Giraldeau and Caraco, 2000; Higashi and Yamamura 1993; Sibly, 1983), and how these predictions match with empirical observations (Krause and Ruxton, 2002). However, although these studies have considered which

Modelling Natural Action Selection, eds. Anil K. Seth, Tony J. Prescott and Joanna J. Bryson.
Published by Cambridge University Press. © Cambridge University Press 2012.

group sizes should be stable from a functional perspective, little work has been conducted examining the proximate mechanisms resulting in the formation of these groups: recent models (e.g., Flierl *et al.*, 1999; Juanico *et al.*, 2003) have considered the actions of individuals following extremely simple rules of thumb. However, as noted by Krause and Ruxton (2002), little consideration has been given to making these rules realistic. State-dependent models of behaviour (Clark and Mangel, 2000; Houston and McNamara, 1999) offer us a means of predicting realistic rules, by considering which behaviours at a particular moment in time an animal with a given state set (such as its energy reserves, or the environment it currently occupies) should conduct in order to maximise some measure of its fitness. Therefore, unlike previous spatially-explicit models considering group formation behaviour, the model presented in this chapter bases its rules upon the results of state-dependent models (Rands and Johnstone, 2006; Rands *et al.*, 2003, 2008).

The moment-to-moment decisions about movement made by an animal will depend upon a number of factors. For example, if it is foraging, it may move in order to visit patches which yield the highest nutrient content. However, if the environment is dangerous, it may choose its movements in order to minimise its risk of predation, which could be done by altering its behaviour (Houston and McNamara, 1999) or by choosing its environment according to its relative level of risk (Cowlishaw, 1997). Within groups, other predation-reducing behaviours are available: in joining a group, the risk to an individual is diluted, and its spatial position within the group may be important (Krause 1994; Stankowich, 2003). Hamilton (1971) explored this 'selfish herd' concept, and demonstrated that in order to reduce predation risk (where it is assumed that a randomly appearing predator will attack the nearest prey item) an individual should minimise the amount of unoccupied space around itself from which a predator would selectively target it as a victim. Furthermore, choosing when to forage in relation to what neighbours are doing may bring benefits through increased predator detection or energetic gain (Rands *et al.*, 2003, 2008), where theory suggests that the activities of the foragers should become highly synchronised if there is a fitness-increasing advantage to foraging or resting together. However, in conducting 'selfish herding' behaviour, the forager faces a trade-off; although its predation risk is reduced, it is likely that its energy intake will be reduced as well (Krause and Ruxton, 2002).

In this chapter, we describe a spatially explicit model where foraging animals follow a rule-of-thumb behaviour that reflects the emphasis that an individual puts on protective herding versus individual foraging behaviour, with the individual basing its decisions upon both its energy reserves and the location and actions of its neighbours (see also Rands *et al.*, 2006, for an extension of these models, considering what happens when there are rule differences between individuals). We consider how this rule of thumb affects both the behaviour and foraging success of both individuals within groups, and the groups themselves, in response to changes in the foraging/predation trade-off, the distribution of foraging resources in the environment, and the perceptual range over which individuals are able to detect colleagues and resources.

23.2   Methods

23.2.1   Outline of the model

An individual-based model was created using NetLogo 1.3 for Mac OS X (Wilensky, 1999). A number of simulations were conducted, using the parameter sets described in Section 23.2.2. At the beginning of each simulation, a two-dimensional (51×51) grid of square cells was created, with sides joined to form a torus. The arena was seeded by randomly choosing a set number (*SEED*) of cells. Having chosen these, all the cells within a randomly chosen radius (using an integer-discretised normal distribution with a mean of 2.5 ± 1.2 cell length units ($\pm$ SD)) of each seeded cell were filled with a randomly allocated integer amount of energy (using a discretised normal distribution with a mean of 10 ± 1.2 energy units). Twenty individuals were randomly placed at unoccupied points. Each of these individuals was randomly allocated an initial level of energy reserves (using a discretised normal distribution with a mean of 225 ± 37.5 energy units) and a randomly chosen initial direction of movement (in one of the four directions described below). Once initialised, a simulation was run for 1500 timesteps, where every individual conducted one behavioural action at each timestep.

At any given timestep, the action of an individual (to either rest or forage) was determined by its energy reserves, as summarised in Figure 23.1. Rules are based upon those suggested by Rands *et al.* (2003, 2008), where individuals can choose between resting and foraging (both of which incur an energetic cost, with foraging incurring the greater cost). If reserves were above an upper satiation threshold t_{upper} of 300 units, the individual rested. If reserves fell to zero units, the individual was assumed to have starved to death, and was removed from the current simulation. For other reserve levels, the animal could choose to either rest or forage, according to the rules described below. If the individual rested, it did not move, and its energy reserves were reduced by $c_{rest} = 0.7$ units. If it foraged, reserves were reduced by c_{rest} plus an extra cost of foraging, $c_{forage} = 0.3$ units.

At a given period of time (assuming that the animal makes consecutive decisions about which action it should conduct until it makes its next decision), if the reserves of an animal fell at or below a lower threshold t_{lower} (set at 150 units), the animal foraged, regardless of the actions of any neighbours, using the behaviour described below for selecting the best available cell. Above this threshold, the actions of an individual depended upon whether there was another animal within detection radius (defined as the area within a circle with a radius of *DET*, centred on the focal individual): if there were detectable neighbours, the focal individual copied the action (rest or forage) of the closest (if there was more than one nearest neighbour, the focal individual randomly chose which of these to copy); whereas, if there was no detectable neighbour, the focal individual rested.

However, the form of foraging taken by the focal individual was dependent upon its energetic reserves. If it was foraging due to copying the actions of a neighbour, its movement pattern was determined according to either the location of the best available

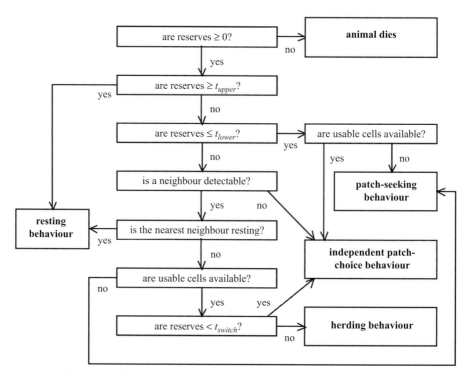

Figure 23.1 Summary of how an individual chooses its behaviour during a timestep of the model.

food patch, or the position of its neighbours (essentially, a trade-off between foraging and predation risk). If the forager was moving to the best available food, it foraged as described above, maximising its energetic intake; if instead it conducted a selfish-herding behaviour, it moved one cell towards a safer position (defined as the point between its two closest neighbours if two are detectable, or towards a single neighbour), harvesting a potentially suboptimal amount of energy from the cell it moved to. The choice between these independent best-patch behaviour and risk-minimising herding behaviours was governed by an intermediate switching threshold t_{switch} (where $t_{lower} \leq t_{switch} \leq t_{upper}$ and $t_{lower} < t_{upper}$), determined using the independence parameter IND, defining the proportional value between t_{lower} and t_{upper} at which t_{switch} should occur:

$$t_{switch} = IND \times (t_{upper} - t_{lower}) + t_{lower}. \tag{23.1}$$

With $IND = 0$, all individuals with reserves above t_{lower} conduct herding behaviour, whilst $IND = 1$ means all individuals between t_{lower} and t_{upper} conduct independent foraging. If reserves fell below t_{switch}, the forager conducted independent foraging; otherwise, it conducted herding behaviour. The value of t_{switch} could therefore be used to explore differences in the perception of predation risk by foragers; for example, when animals are in high-risk habitats or belong to a vulnerable age-sex class (low IND), or when animals are in low-risk habitats or belong to an age-sex class that is rarely predated (high IND). We assume that herding behaviour occurs when the animal has higher energy reserves, and therefore does not need to forage to avoid starvation.

If the forager chose to move to the best available cell, the energy contents of its current cell and those of the four neighbouring cells that were unoccupied were compared to ascertain which had the highest energy content: if its current cell had the highest value the forager remained in the cell; otherwise, it moved to the best neighbour, or randomly selected between best neighbours if there were more than one. If instead the forager chose to reduce its predation risk by herding, it moved to the usable neighbouring cell (where a usable cell is defined as one which contains at least a threshold minimum level of energy, set at 2 units) that took it closest to the point midway between the two nearest neighbours within detection range (or towards its neighbour if only one is detectable).

If at all possible, a forager should move to an unoccupied usable cell: this behaviour was also followed when herding, even if this forced the forager to move in the direction away from its colleagues (this behaviour was necessary to avoid excessive numbers of individuals starving during the simulation). If the individual could not move to a usable cell (due to either no neighbouring cells containing sufficient energy, or being occupied by a colleague), it moved to the neighbouring unoccupied cell (or randomly chose between them if several were available) that took it closest to the cell within its radius of detection that had the highest amount of energy. If no suitable cells were detectable, the animal moved according to a sinuous random walk, with a 50% chance of moving one cell forwards in the same direction it moved in the previous round, and 25% chances each of moving one cell forwards at 90° or 270° to this previous direction.

Once a forager had moved (or decided to stay in its current cell), it harvested 2 units of energy from the target patch (and the cell's energy content is reduced by the same amount), which were added to its current energy reserves. Once all the live foragers within the simulation had conducted their movement for the timestep, any cells within the arena that had energy levels below their initially determined level at the start of the simulation had their energy levels increased by the minimum value of either 0.05 units or the amount needed to achieve the initial level.

23.2.2 Model exploration

An experimental data set was generated using a crossed design. The detection radius of each forager, *DET*, was either 5 or 10 cells. The independence parameter *IND* took a value in the set {0.0, 0.25, 0.5, 0.75, 1.0}. The number of initial cell seeds in the environment, *SEED*, was a value from in the set {25, 50, 75, 100}. (This meant that the following proportions of the arena ($\pm$ SD) contained energy when *SEED* = 25: 0.208 $\pm$ 0.036; 50: 0.358 $\pm$ 0.045; 75: 0.499 $\pm$ 0.046; 100: 0.614 $\pm$ 0.041. The mean numbers of discrete patches when *SEED* = 25: 14.55 $\pm$ 2.14; 50: 17.00 $\pm$ 3.26; 75: 12.80 $\pm$ 4.76; 100: 6.95 $\pm$ 3.56.) Twenty randomly generated environments (including the initial positioning of the 20 individuals within the simulation), denoted *ENV*, were simulated for each value of *SEED*. The parameter set chosen for the models presented were chosen arbitrarily: qualitatively similar results to those presented were obtained for a number of other simulations conducted with different initial parameter sets.

Table 23.1 Results of general linear models for group size (the mean cluster size within a simulation, where e, the estimated error degrees of freedom of ENV(SEED), is 52.65); proportion foraging ($e = 78.67$); mean reserves ($e = 93.12$); mean number of moves ($e = 124.03$); and mean moves variation ($e = 117.94$). See text for details of transformations used.

	d.f.	group size		proportion foraging		mean reserves		mean number of moves		mean moves variation	
		F	p	F	p	F	p	F	p	F	p
DET	1,76	1693.83	<0.001	0.67	0.417	682.90	<0.001	541.83	<0.001	8.50	0.005
SEED	3,76	8.72	<0.001	20.67	<0.001	1.46	0.232	123.18	<0.001	128.05	<0.001
IND	4,304	18.11	<0.001	17.64	<0.001	33.76	<0.001	1131.83	<0.001	429.96	<0.001
ENV(SEED)	76,e	1.32	0.146	1.22	0.188	1.48	0.036	4.82	<0.001	1.53	0.018
DET×SEED	3,76	4.82	0.004	2.25	0.089	7.89	<0.001	12.74	<0.001	29.20	<0.001
DET×IND	4,304	30.79	<0.001	2.14	0.075	31.41	<0.001	17.69	<0.001	8.48	<0.001
DET×ENV(SEED)	76,304	1.08	0.331	1.44	0.017	1.60	0.003	1.69	0.001	1.78	<0.001
SEED×IND	12,304	1.59	0.093	5.62	<0.001	10.07	<0.001	23.19	<0.001	12.01	<0.001
IND×ENV(SEED)	304,304	1.00	0.517	1.23	0.034	1.41	<0.001	1.85	<0.001	1.78	<0.001
DET×SEED×IND	12,304	1.22	0.266	1.23	0.256	1.02	0.434	1.82	0.044	0.99	0.454

Statistics were determined based upon the positions and attributes of all survivors at period 1500 of each simulation. For each simulation, we determined: the mean cluster size (measured here as the number of individuals in a nearest-neighbour cluster, as described by Hamilton (1971), where a self-contained cluster is composed of all individuals that have at least one of the other members of the cluster as their nearest detectable neighbour); the mean energetic reserves of all the individuals within a simulation set; the mean number of moves made during the simulation by an individual and its variation within a simulation set (measured as the standard error of the mean); and the proportion of individuals foraging during the period. We also calculated the mean value for each simulation of a summary statistic ψ describing the degree of synchronisation within a detection nearest-neighbour cluster of at least two individuals, where $\psi = 2 \times$ [max(proportion foraging within cluster, proportion resting within cluster) – 0.5]. $\psi = 0$ shows complete asynchrony with half a cluster engaged in each activity, whilst $\psi = 1$ shows complete synchrony, regardless of the activity all the members of the group are conducting.

23.2.3 Statistical analysis

The data were analysed using Minitab, V. 12.1 (Minitab Inc., 1998). General linear models were constructed, using the model DET | IND | SEED | ENV(SEED) – DET × IND × ENV(SEED), where ENV was a random factor. Where necessary, data were transformed to conform to model assumptions: the proportions foraging were arcsine transformed, mean reserves were exponentiated, the standard errors of the mean number of moves were log-transformed, and the mean numbers of moves were calculated to the power -3.5. Mean cluster sizes did not need adjusting. The mean value of ψ could not be adjusted suitably, and so a summary value of this term was calculated by averaging over the 20 ENV datapoints, and fitted with the general linear model DET | IND | SEED – DET × IND × SEED. In discussing the results, significant interaction terms are only discussed where the effects seen gave further insights into the patterns observed.

23.3 Results

Mean size of nearest-neighbour clusters was extremely dependent upon detection distance (Figure 23.2a; Table 23.1), where longer detection distances increased the likelihood that two animals would be within a suitable range for formation of nearest-neighbour clusters. Number of seeds had a significant effect upon cluster size, where the largest clusters were found in the environments with the lowest seed number (Figure 23.2a); foragers tend to stay within a region of connected usable cells until all the resources within the region are depleted below a critical threshold; a lower initial seed count means that it is likely that within a region of usable connected cells there are fewer cells, and so foragers aggregated within these regions are more likely to be within detection range, leading to a higher number of animals sharing nearest neighbours. The value at which independent foraging switched to herding also had a significant

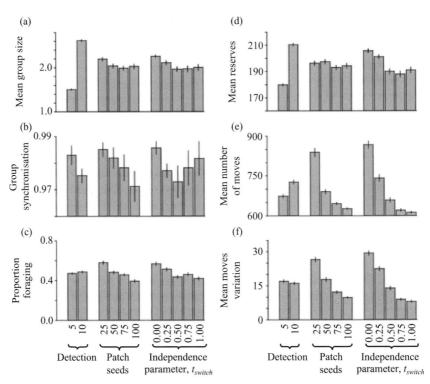

Figure 23.2 Effects of detection distance, number of initial cell seeds and the switch-point t_{switch} upon mean values ($\pm$ SD) of: (a) nearest-neighbour cluster size; (b) degree of synchronisation ψ within a multi-player nearest-neighbour cluster; (c) proportion of a simulation set foraging during period 1500; (d) energetic reserves of individuals; (e) number of moves made by an individual; (f) variation in move numbers shown within a simulation set.

effect (Figure 23.2a; Table 23.1), and larger clusters occurred when the switch-point was low (meaning individuals would be more likely to keep within detection range of each other).

Synchrony levels within nearest-neighbour clusters with two or more members were very close to unity (Figure 23.2b), meaning that all the members of a cluster were likely to be conducting the same behaviour. As would be expected, neither detection distance, initial number of seeds, or the herding switch-point had a significant effect upon synchronisation (Table 23.2).

The proportion of a simulation set foraging was not significantly related to detection distance (Figure 23.2c; Table 23.1). The foraging proportion was highly related to the initial seeding of the environment (Figure 23.2c; Table 23.1), where proportion foraging decreased with an increase in available cells (with more usable environment, individuals should spend less time in empty cells, and so should replenish energy reserves more rapidly, ultimately spending less time foraging). Similarly, the proportion foraging was greater where the independent foraging switch-point was low (Figure 23.2c). In this case, individuals would be affected by both a reduction in intake caused by the shift from intake maximisation to herding behaviour, as well as an increased likelihood of copying foraging behaviour (because a herding animal is more likely to be within

Table 23.2 Results of general linear models, for the summarised proportion of individuals surviving and the summarised mean proportion of individuals synchronised in their behaviour within a multi-individual nearest-neighbour clusters, as summarised by the ψ statistic.

	d.f.	proportion synchronised	
		F	p
DET	1,12	2.38	0.149
SEED	3,12	1.41	0.287
IND	4,12	0.74	0.583
DET × SEED	3,12	1.13	0.375
DET × IND	4,12	0.78	0.558
SEED × IND	12,12	0.36	0.956

detection range of a neighbour, meaning that it will copy the neighbour's behaviour if its own reserves are above t_{lower}, rather than just rest, as would occur if there were no neighbour available to copy).

The mean energetic reserves of an individual within a simulation group were significantly lower when detection distance was low (Figure 23.2d; Table 23.1), which may be related to foragers travelling through regions of empty cells being less likely to detect and move to the cells with the highest energy content. Mean reserves were not significantly affected by the number of seeds in the environment (Figure 23.2d). The switch-point between independent and herding behaviour had significant effects upon reserves and variation in reserves (Figure 23.2d), where individuals with higher values of t_{switch} (and therefore more likely to be following independent foraging behaviour) had lower mean reserves, with reserves varying less within an environment.

The mean number of movements made by an individual increased with detection distance (Figure 23.2e; Table 23.1), and the variation within a simulation fell (Figure 23.2f; Table 23.1), presumably because the actions of individuals were more likely to be dictated by the actions of neighbours. Both mean number and variation in the number of moves fell with an increase in the initial number of seeds (Figure 23.2e and f; Table 23.1), where individuals were less likely to travel long distances over bad environments to find energy supplies. Mean number and variation in number of moves also fell with an increase in the switch-point between independent foraging and herding (Figure 23.2e and f; Table 23.1), with individuals becoming more likely to move to high-energy regions and remain within them until they were depleted, rather than being forced to move to low energy regions closer to neighbours, and so work harder to maintain reserves at a suitable level.

23.4   Discussion

This model has demonstrated that we can use state-dependent social foraging rules taken from optimality models to explore their effects upon group behaviour. Some of the results we present are intuitively obvious (such as many of the patterns seen in response to increasing the amount of energy available in the environment), but these results confirm that our model is following realistic patterns, and thus give us confidence that those model results that are less intuitively obvious are likely to be robust. Moreover, the model does present a number of predictions (discussed below) that are novel, relating to effects upon group size, and how individuals should behave, given differing levels of environmental predation risk.

In our model, group size is quantified using the surrogate measure of nearest-neighbour cluster size: the number of individuals connected by a nearest-neighbour network, as considered by Hamilton (1971). Although the size of clusters may appear small, it is a useful means of quantifying the size of the social groups formed. Social behaviour within the model framework depends upon the actions of nearest neighbours, and therefore it is more meaningful to consider a group as consisting of the set of individuals that can affect each other's actions, rather than using some arbitrary definition such as an aggregation of individuals within a specific radius of each other. The statistic allows us to quantify the degree of association seen between individuals, showing us that group size should increase with an increase in perceptual range, and should tend to fall with an increase in energy available in the environment, or an increase in the degree of independent patch choice behaviour shown by an individual. Therefore, modulation of group size is an emergent feature of the simple rules followed by individuals (Camazine et al., 2001; Couzin and Krause, 2003).

Theoretical investigations of stable group sizes have suggested that the optimal size (at which some fitness-related currency is maximised) is unlikely to be seen (Clark and Mangel, 1984; Giraldeau and Caraco, 2000; Giraldeau and Gillis, 1985; Hamilton, 2000; Kramer, 1985; Pulliam and Caraco, 1984; Sibly, 1983). The model presented here does not make predictions about stable size because it is not an optimality model: it depends upon a mechanistic, rule-based procedure, rather than considering how the actions of the foragers could maximise some measure of their fitness (McNamara and Houston, 1986). Individual-based models of behaviour rely upon defining the rule set of individuals, and, if they are based on any biologically or socially relevant information, they are usually based upon straight assumptions about some proximate measure of the agent's physiology and its current environment (e.g., Bryson et al., 2007; de Vries, 2009; Duriez et al., 2009; Hemelrijk, 1999, 2000; Stillman et al., 1997, 2000, 2002). To interpret how the proximate mechanisms for group formation (modelled as the behaviours used within spatially explicit individual-based models) could have evolved, we must therefore consider how the responses of the foragers to external and internal stimuli are related to their fitness. This is indirectly addressed in the model described here, where the mechanisms leading to group formation are based upon a number of state-based rules that have been predicted by theory where it is assumed that the animal is maximising some measure of its fitness (Hamilton, 1971; Houston and McNamara, 1999; Rands et al., 2003, 2008). It would be desirable to base these rules upon the results of a single fitness-optimising model that incorporated all the elements considered, rather than piecing together a rule based upon several models, but this is computationally complex, and arguably it is equally desirable to gain a thorough understanding of the effects of each of these separate elements before attempting to address them together within a single framework. This is one of the inherent problems with modelling decision-making processes (Prescott *et al.*, 2007). Using predictions resulting from optimality modelling, as demonstrated here and in Rands *et al.* (2006), is arguably a sensible approach to generating rules for models, but we must always be mindful of whether we have correctly identified the process which is being optimised (Houston *et al.*, 2007), and whether the output we deliver aligns with any biological systems (Bryson *et al.*, 2007).

The model demonstrates that all the individuals of a given nearest-neighbour group will usually be conducting the same activity. This is perhaps predictable from the rule of thumb used, but it does demonstrate that synchronisation within groups can occur. Synchronisation of foraging behaviour is a phenomenon seen in many species (e.g., Rands *et al.*, 2008; Rook and Huckle, 1995; Ruckstuhl and Neuhaus, 2002), but little work has been done on the synchronisation of activity within local clusters of individuals; what our model suggests is that activities of nearest-neighbour groups may be highly synchronised, even if the behaviour of a local population is not.

Although the model described here did not include explicitly modelled predation events, we were nonetheless able to consider the indirect effects of differing environmental predation risks upon an individual's behaviour, such as the effects seen upon the number of movements made by individuals, and the likelihood an individual foraged. The rule of thumb we used did not allow an individual to alter its behaviour in response to a predation event (and hence including explicit predation in the model would not have been enlightening, especially if predation events were rare), but it did reflect a range of feasible behavioural responses to differing risks of predation (reflected by the changing value of the independence threshold, at which a forager switched from independent foraging to selfish herding behaviour). Furthermore, differences in predation risk could also be reflected in an altered value of t_{lower} (as demonstrated by Rands *et al.*, 2008), which could also affect the group behaviours seen. The action an animal takes in the model we present is based primarily upon its energy reserves. Our model suggests that the reserve levels of a forager are inversely related to the threshold at which it should swap between maximising its intake rate and seeking safety by approaching group members. If we interpret this to mean that the forager will have higher reserves when predation risk is high, this is contrary to predictions from theory (Houston and McNamara, 1993, 1999; McNamara *et al.*, 1994), where the optimal level of reserves falls as predation risk increases (although it should be noted that these models considered energetic expenditure as a mass-dependent cost; it is possible that including mass-dependence in the current model will have an effect upon results, although it is unclear whether mass-dependence would have a large qualitative effect within the dynamic game proposed by Rands *et al.*, 2003, 2008). Experiments testing these predictions by manipulating the perceived predation risk of individuals have shown that in some cases animals decrease their energetic reserves in response to an increase in risk. However, other experiments have yielded an increase in reserves (reviewed in Rands and Cuthill, 2001). This has been suggested to be because the animals are responding to the predator interrupting their foraging routine, which can be countered by an increase in stored reserves (a result also predicted by theory). Although these experiments have not considered how social behaviour should affect reserves, the model presented here suggests that, with the added complexities of group-related behaviours, we should be careful how we apply the results of models optimising the fitness of an individual acting alone to individuals interacting in groups.

In the model presented here, an individual bases its herding rule solely on its nearest neighbour or pair of neighbours. Other theoretical explorations of selfish herding behaviour have considered how simple movement rules can lead to realistic aggregations of animals (Morrell and James, 2008; Morton *et al.*, 1994; Schreiber and Vejdani, 2006; Viscido *et al.*, 2001, 2002), and demonstrate that the greatest reductions in predation risk occur when an animal is able to base its movements relative to a larger number of close neighbours. It should be noted however that the assumptions made in these models have been criticised as being biologically unrealistic (James *et al.*, 2004). Other models have also considered the rules about how attraction and repulsion between individuals work (Hancock and Milner-Gulland, 2006; Hancock *et al.*, 2006), whilst other work has considered the effects of rule differences between individuals based upon dominance (de Vries, 2009; Hemelrijk, 1999, 2000; Rands *et al.*, 2006). In the model we present here, paying attention to one or two nearest neighbours proved sufficient to affect the group sizes seen, but further realism in the rules used could be added in future models by allowing an individual to consider the locations and actions of other group members within its detection range. Furthermore, decisions may be made collectively by aggregating individual decisions at the group level, such as through consensus processes (King and Cowlishaw, 2007, 2009; Sellers *et al.*, 2007); much realism could therefore be added to these individual-based models by allowing groups of individuals to aggregate (and then act on) the information that is possessed by all the members of the group.

Through considering detection distance, the model showed that the perceptual range of the forager could be important in determining both the behaviour and decisions of an individual, and the size of the group. Perceptual ranges may be very important in determining the movement behaviours shown by an animal (Zollner, 2000; Zollner and Lima, 1999), especially where resources are clumped in a patchy environment. Perceptual ranges will also have effects upon group structure: if detection range is small but group benefits are high, groups will have to remain closely packed to allow cohesion, with repercussions on competition and visibility to predators. The limits of perceptual ranges, and therefore group structure, could also be exacerbated by a spatially complex environment (such as thick vegetation). These findings also highlight the potential importance of contact calls and food calls in extending the perceptual range of social foragers, thus influencing group structure. For example, recent research has shown that such calls are given more frequently when group dispersion is high and when visibility conditions are poor (Uster and Zuberbühler, 2001).

As urged by Krause and Ruxton (2002), it is important that individual-based models examining social behaviour attempt to use realistic rules. This allows us to make accurate predictions about group sizes and behaviours, which could be crucial for our understanding and management of natural populations (Conroy *et al.*, 1995; Ruckelshaus *et al.*, 1997). Models based upon rules derived from state-dependent optimality theory, such as the one presented here, are an effective way of incorporating this necessary element of realism.

Acknowledgements

The work described in the original version of this paper (Rands *et al.*, 2004) was supported by a Natural Environment Research Council research grant awarded to G.C., R.A.P., J.M.R., and Rufus Johnstone (University of Cambridge). S.A.R. created the model in discussion with G.C. S.A.R. coded the simulations, conducted the statistical analysis, and was responsible for the initial draft of the manuscript. Many thanks to Sasha Dall, Andy Fenton, Rufus Johnstone, Jens Krause, and two anonymous referees for comments.

References

Bryson, J. J., Y. Ando, and H. Lehmann (2007). Agent-based modelling as scientific method: a case study analysing primate social behaviour. *Phil. Trans. R. Soc. B* **362**: 1685–1699.

Camazine, S., J.-L. Deneubourg, N. R. Franks, *et al.* (2001). *Self-organization in Biological Systems*. Princeton, NJ: Princeton University Press.

Clark, C. W. and M. Mangel (1984). Foraging and flocking strategies: information in an uncertain environment. *Am. Nat.* **123**: 626–41.

Clark, C. W. and M. Mangel (2000). *Dynamic State Variable Models in Ecology: Methods and Applications*. New York: Oxford University Press.

Conroy, M. J., Y. Cohen, F. C. James, Y. G. Matsinos, and B. A. Maurer (1995). Parameter estimation, reliability, and model improvement for spatially explicit models of animal populations. *Ecol. Appl.* **5**: 17–19.

Couzin, I. D. and J. Krause (2003). Self-organization and collective behavior in vertebrates. *Advances in the Study of Behaviour* **32**: 1–75.

Cowlishaw, G. (1997). Trade-offs between foraging and predation risk determine habitat use in a desert baboon population. *Anim. Behav.* **53**: 667–86.

de Vries, H. (2009). On using the DomWorld model to evaluate dominance ranking methods. *Behaviour* **146**: 843–869.

Duriez, O., S. Bauer, A. Destin, *et al.* (2009). What decision rules might pink-footed geese use to depart on migration? An individual-based model. *Behav. Ecol.* **20**, 560–9.

Ekman, J. and B. Rosander (1987). Starvation risk and flock size of the social forager: when there is a flocking cost. *Theor. Popul. Biol.* **31**: 167–77.

Flierl, G., D. Grünbaum, S. Levin, and D. Olson (1999). From individuals to aggregations: the interplay between behavior and physics. *J. Theor. Biol.* **196**: 397–454.

Giraldeau, L.-A. and T. Caraco (2000). *Social Foraging Theory*. Princeton, NJ: Princeton University Press.

Giraldeau, L.-A. and D. Gillis (1985). Optimal group size can be subtle: a reply to Sibly. *Anim. Behav.* **33**: 666–7.

Hamilton, I. M. (2000). Recruiters and joiners: using optimal skew theory to predict group size and the division of resources within groups of social foragers. *Am. Nat.* **155**: 684–95.

Hamilton, W. D. (1971). Geometry for the selfish herd. *J. Theor. Biol.* **31**: 295–311.

Hancock, P. A. and E. J. Milner-Gulland (2006). Optimal movement strategies for social foragers in unpredictable environments. *Ecology* **87**: 2094–2102.

Hancock, P. A., E. J. Milner-Gulland, and M. J. Keeling (2006). Modelling the many-wrongs principle: the navigational advantages of aggregation in nomadic foragers. *J. Theor. Biol.* **240**: 302–310.

Hemelrijk, C. K. (1999). An individual-orientated model of the emergence of despotic and egalitarian societies. *Proc. Roy. Soc. B* **266**: 361–9.

Hemelrijk, C. K. (2000). Towards the integration of social dominance and spatial structure. *Anim. Behav.* **59**: 1035–1048.

Higashi, M. and N. Yamamura (1993). What determines group size? Insider-outsider conflict and its resolution. *Am. Nat.* **142**: 553–63.

Houston, A. I. and J. M. McNamara (1993). A theoretical investigation of the fat reserves and mortality levels of small birds in winter. *Ornis Scand.* **24**: 205–219.

Houston, A. I. and J. M. McNamara (1999). *Models of Adaptive Behaviour: An Approach Based on State*. Cambridge: Cambridge University Press.

Houston, A. I., J. M. McNamara, and M. D. Steer (2007). Do we expect natural selection to produce rational behaviour? *Phil. Trans. R. Soc. B* **362**: 1531–43.

James, R., P. G. Bennett, and J. Krause (2004). Geometry for mutualistic and selfish herds: the limited domain of danger. *J. Theor. Biol.* **228**: 107–113.

Juanico, D. E., C. Monterola, and C. Saloma, (2003). Allelomimesis as a generic clustering mechanism for interaction agents. *Physica A* **320**: 590–600.

King, A. J. and G. Cowlishaw (2007). When to use social information: the advantage of large group size in individual decision making. *Biol. Lett.* **3**: 137–9.

King, A. J. and G. Cowlishaw (2009). Leaders, followers, and group decision-making. *Commun. Integr. Biol.* **2**: 147–50.

Kramer, D. L. (1985). Are colonies supraoptimal groups? *Anim. Behav.* **33**: 1031–2.

Krause, J. (1994). Differential fitness returns in relation to spatial position in groups. *Biol. Rev.* **69**: 187–206.

Krause, J. and Ruxton, G. D. (2002). *Living in Groups*. Oxford: Oxford University Press.

McNamara, J. M. and A. I. Houston (1986). The common currency for behavioral decisions. *Am. Nat.* **127**: 358–78.

McNamara, J. M., A. I. Houston, and Lima, S. L. (1994). Foraging routines of small birds in winter: a theoretical investigation. *J. Avian Biol.* **25**: 287–302.

Minitab Inc. (1998). Minitab 12.1 for Windows 95/NT. State College, Philadelphia.

Morrell, L. J. and R. James (2008). Mechanisms for aggregation in animals: rule success depends on ecological variables. *Behav. Ecol.* **19**: 193–201.

Morton, T. L., J. W. Haefner, V. Nugala, R. D. Decimo, and L. Mendes (1994). The selfish herd revisited: do simple movement rules reduce relative predation risk? *J. Theor. Biol.* **167**: 73–9.

Prescott, T. J., J. J. Bryson, and A. K. Seth (2007). Modelling natural action selection. *Phil. Trans. R. Soc. B* **362**: 1521–9.

Pulliam, H. R. and T. Caraco (1984). Living in groups: is there an optimal group size? In *Behavioural ecology: an evolutionary approach*, ed. J. R. Krebs and N. B. Davies. Oxford: Blackwell Science, pp. 122–47.

Rands, S. A., G. Cowlishaw, R. A. Pettifor, J. M. Rowcliffe, and R. A. Johnstone (2003). The spontaneous emergence of leaders and followers in a foraging pair. *Nature* **423**: 432–34.

Rands, S. A., G. Cowlishaw, R. A. Pettifor, J. M. Rowcliffe, and R. A. Johnstone (2008). The emergence of leaders and followers in foraging pairs when the qualities of individuals differ. *BMC Evol. Biol.* **8**: 51.

Rands, S. A. and I. C. Cuthill (2001). Separating the effects of predation risk and interrupted foraging upon mass changes in the blue tit *Parus caeruleus. Proc. R. Soc. B* **268**: 1783–90.

Rands, S. A. and R. A. Johnstone (2006). Statistical measures for defining an individual's degree of independence within state-dependent dynamic games. *BMC Evol. Biol.* **6**: 81.

Rands, S. A., R. A. Pettifor, J. M. Rowcliffe, and G. Cowlishaw (2004). State-dependent foraging rules for social animals in selfish herds. *Proc. Roy. Soc. B* **271**: 2613–20.

Rands, S. A., R. A. Pettifor, J. M. Rowcliffe, and G. Cowlishaw (2006). Social foraging and dominance relationships: the effects of socially mediated interference. *Behav. Ecol. Sociobiol.* **60**: 572–581.

Rook, A. J. and C. A. Huckle (1995). Synchronization of ingestive behaviour by grazing dairy cows. *Anim. Sci.* **60**: 25–30.

Ruckelshaus, M., C. Hartway, and P. Kareiva (1997). Assessing the data requirements of spatially explicit dispersal models. *Conserv. Biol.* **11**: 1298–306.

Ruckstuhl, K. E. and P. Neuhaus (2002). Sexual segregation in ungulates: a comparative test of three hypotheses. *Biol. Rev.* **77**: 77–96.

Schreiber, S. J. and M. Vejdani (2006). Handling time promotes the coevolution of aggregation in predator-prey systems *Proc. Roy. Soc. B* **273**: 185–91.

Sellers, W. I., R. A. Hill, and B. S. Logan (2007). An agent-based model of group decision making in baboons. *Phil. Trans. Roy. Soc. B* **362**: 1699–710.

Sibly, R. M. (1983). Optimal group size is unstable. *Anim. Behav.* **31**: 946–51.

Stankowich, T. (2003). Marginal predation methodologies and the importance of predator preferences. *Anim. Behav.* **66**: 589–99.

Stillman, R. A., L. M. Bautista, J. C. Alonso, and J. A. Alonso (2002). Modelling state-dependent interference in common cranes. *J. Anim. Ecol.* **71**: 874–82.

Stillman, R. A., J. D. Goss-Custard, and R. W. G. Caldow (1997). Modelling interference from basic foraging behaviour. *J. Anim. Ecol.* **66**: 692–703.

Stillman, R. A., J. D. Goss-Custard, A. D. West, *et al.* (2000). Predicting mortality in novel environments: tests and sensitivity of a behaviour-based model. *J. Appl. Ecol.* **37**: 564–88.

Uster, D. and K. Zuberbühler (2001). The functional significance of Diana monkey 'clear' calls. *Behaviour* **138**: 741–56.

Viscido, S. V., M. Miller, and D. S. Wethey (2001). The response of a selfish herd to an attack from outside the group perimeter. *J. Theor. Biol.* **208**: 315–28.

Viscido, S. V., M. Miller, and D. S. Wethey (2002). The dilemma of the selfish herd: the search for a realistic movement rule. *J. Theor. Biol.* **217**: 183–94.

Wilensky, U. (1999). *NetLogo.* Evanston: Center for Connected Learning and Computer-based Modeling, Northwestern University. Available online: http://ccl.northwestern.edu/netlogo/.

Zollner, P. A. (2000). Comparing the landscape level perceptual abilities of forest sciurids in fragmented agricultural landscapes. *Landscape Ecol.* **15**: 523–33.

Zollner, P. A. and S. L. Lima (1999). Search strategies for landscape-level interpatch movements. *Ecology* **80**: 1019–30.

Index